Table of Contents

Chapter 1 – Optics (Geometrical)

REFRACTION AT SINGLE SPHERICAL OR PLANE SURFACES

Curvature
R=1/r

1. Curvature and Sagitta

- **Curvature** (R) = 1/r, where r = radius
- **Sagitta** (s) is the distance from a surface to a chord (AB)

The formulas for Sag (s):

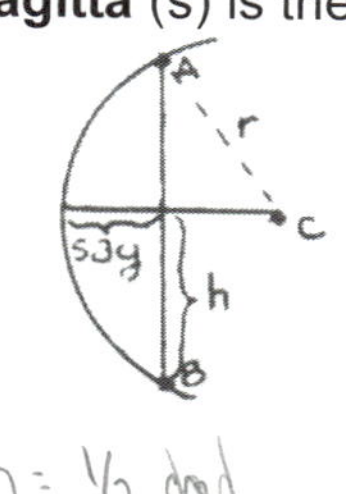

Exact Sag Formula:
$s = r - \sqrt{(r^2 - h^2)}$
$r = h^2/2s + s/2$
(use exact formula for contact lenses)

Approximate Sag Formula:
$s = h^2/2r$
$r = h^2/2s$
(use approximate formula for $h^2 << r^2$)

Example: *The distance between the moveable (center) pin and stationary pin of a lens clock is 2mm. The sag of a contact lens is measured to be 0.252mm. What is the contact lens' radius of curvature?*

h = 2mm
s = 0.252 mm
$r = \frac{h^2}{2s}$

Step 1) $r = h^2/2s + s/2$
Step 2) $r= [(2mm)^2/2(0.252mm)] + [(0.252mm)/2]$
Step 3) r = 8.06 mm

2. Refractive Index and Rectilinear Propagation

- Light travels at different speeds in different media, traveling fastest in a vacuum.
- A medium's **refractive index** (n) is proportional to the speed of light in a vacuum (v_c) to the speed of light through a material (v_m).
- The refractive index is always equal to or greater than 1.0, and indicates how much light has slowed down when entering a refractive media

$n = v_c/v_m$
$v_c = 3 \times 10^8$ m/sec

Common Refractive Indices	
Air	1.00
Water	1.33
Cornea	1.376
Plastic	1.44-1.49
Crown Glass	1.523
Polycarbonate	1.586

- **Rectilinear propagation** – light travels in a straight line (for our convention: light from left to right)

3. Vergence and Dioptric Power

- The **vergence** (in diopters) at a certain point (in a pencil of rays) is the reciprocal of the distance from a reference point (in meters).
- A **diopter** is a unit of accommodative amplitude. It describes the vergence of a waveworm at a specific distance from a source, and is also defined as the power of the lens. It is the reciprocal of distance (m).
- **Dioptric power** is the ability of a lens to alter incident light.

U=vergence of object at the lens
u= distance from the object to the lens
V= vergence of image rays
v= distance from the image to the lens
n= refractive index before refraction (object space)
– the medium in which the object resides
n'= refractive index after refraction (image space)
– the medium in which the image resides
P= lens or surface power (diopters)
r= radius of refracting surface in meters
f=primary focal length
f' = secondary focal length

<u>Incident vergence (U):</u>
U = n/u
<u>Emergent vergence (V):</u>
V = n'/v
<u>Simple Lens Formula:</u>
V = U + P
Thus, n'/v = P + n/u
<u>Dioptric power:</u>
P = (n' – n) / r
P = Δn/r
P= -n/f = n'/f'
r=f +f'

Note: Distances measured from the point of interest to the source or focus in the same direction that light travels are <u>positive.</u> If measured in the opposite direction that light travels, they are <u>negative.</u> Therefore, in a system where light travels from left to right, if the object on the left side of a lens, then its distance is measured as a negative value. If the object is on the right side of a lens, then its distance is measured as a positive value.
Note: If n' > n, P is positive, If n'< n, P is negative (This rule applies if C is to the right of the interface)

Example (Vergence):

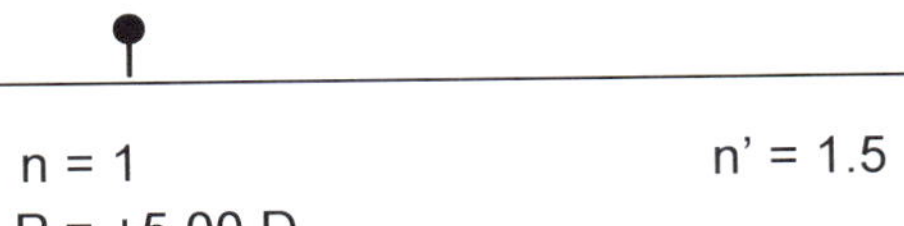

n = 1 n' = 1.5
P = +5.00 D
Object= 50cm to the left of the lens
Where would the image be located?

> ***Answer:***
> U= n/u = 1/-0.50m = -2.00D
> V = U + P = (-2.00) + (+5.00) = +3.00D
> v = n'/V = 1.5 / +3.00 = 0.50m
> (Image is located 50cm to the right of the surface.)

Example (Dioptric Power):
n = 1.0
n' = 1.5
r = 20 cm
What is the Dioptric Power of the lens?

> ***Answer:***
> P=Δn/r = (1.5 – 1.0) / 0.20m = +2.50D

Example:
What are f and f' in a +5.00D surface with n' = 1.5?
n = 1.0
P = +5.00
n' = 1.5

F←----f----→ | ←-----f'---→ F'

> ***Answer:***
> P = -n / f ⇒ f = -n / P = -1 / +5.00 = -0.20m
> (f is to the left)
> f' = n' / P = 1.5 / +5.00 = 0.30m
> (f' is to the right)

Note: For minus refractive surfaces, the focal points and focal length will switch sides compared to positive surfaces (as shown below.)

Example:

F'←---f'----→ | ←-----f---→F
Where is f'?

n=1.0
P=-5.00
n'=1.5

> ***Answer:***
> P = -n / f ⇒ f = -n / P = -1 / -5.00 = +0.20m
> (f is to the right)
> f' = n' / P = 1.5 / -5.00 = -0.30m
> (f' is to the left)

For plus and minus lenses:

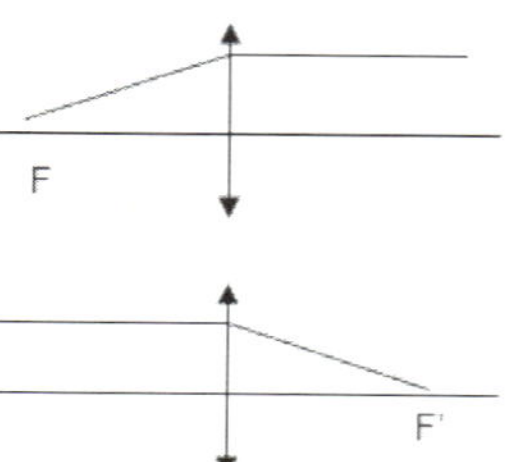

- An object at the primary focal point (F) will give parallel light leaving the system.
- Parallel light entering the system will focus at the secondary focal point (F')

4. Object-Image Relationships, including Apparent Depth

- The object-image relationships can be found by calculation with the above formulas or by ray tracing.
- **Real objects** give diverging light and are to the left of the lens optical system.
- **Real images** are formed by converging light and are to the right of the lens optical system.
- **Virtual objects** give converging light and are to the right of the lens optical system.
- **Virtual images** are formed by diverging light and are to the left of the lens optical system.

	Object	Image
Real	Diverging (left)	Converging (right)
Virtual	Converging (right)	Diverging (left)

Apparent Depth:

- When light enters a medium it can be:
  1) Reflected off the surface
  2) refracted (bent due to change in velocity when it hits the medium) or
  3) absorbed (changed into a different type of energy)

Looking at object X at the bottom of a tank of water, the oblique ray is refracted away from the surface normal (n' < n) and so object X appears at position Y.

only applies if n > n'

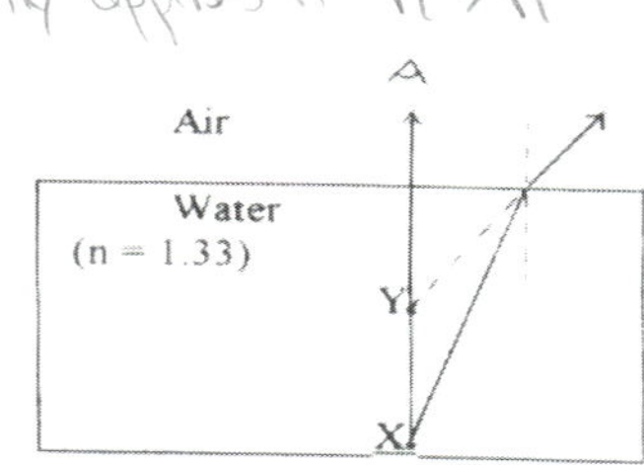

u = object's actual distance from interface
n = refractive index of object's media
v = apparent position of object from interface
n' = refractive index of viewing media

Apparent Depth:
n / u = n' / v

Example: *If object X is embedded 12cm deep under water, 12cm from the interface, how deep does the object appear to be when viewed by a person looking from above?*

n=1.33
n'=1.00
u=0.12 m

Answer:
n/u = n'/v ⇒ 1.33 / 0.12 = 1.00 / v ⇒ v = 0.09m
X appears to be 9 cm deep instead of 12 cm deep

5. Ray Tracing, Nodal Point, and Nodal Ray

- Ray tracing is used to find the image/object after refraction by the lens. There are three rays with predictable paths used.

Ray Tracing Rule	Ray Tracing Action
1. Rays parallel to the axis (from infinity) go through the secondary focal point (F').	1. Draw a line from the object to the lens, parallel to the axis. At the lens, draw a line to through F'
2. Rays through the center of curvature are undeviated	2. Draw a line from the object through the center of the lens, extending into image space
3. Rays through the primary focal point (F) leave parallel to the axis.	3. Draw a line from the object through F to the lens. At the lens draw a line parallel to the axis in image space

- The image is located at the intersection of these 3 rays.

Note: For minus surfaces, the rays must be dotted in order for them to intersect.

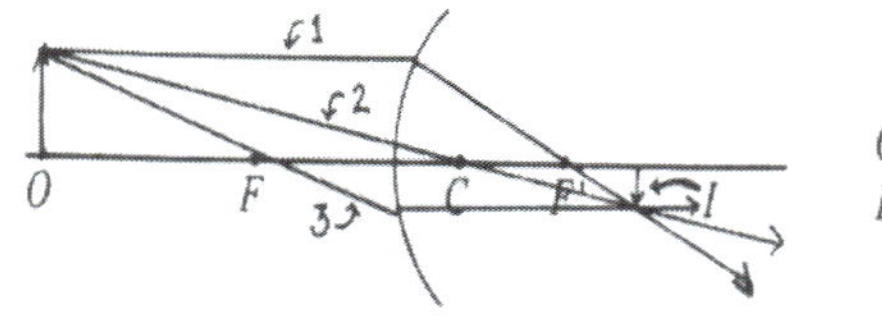

- Images on the same side as the object are erect. If the image is on opposite side of object, the image is inverted.

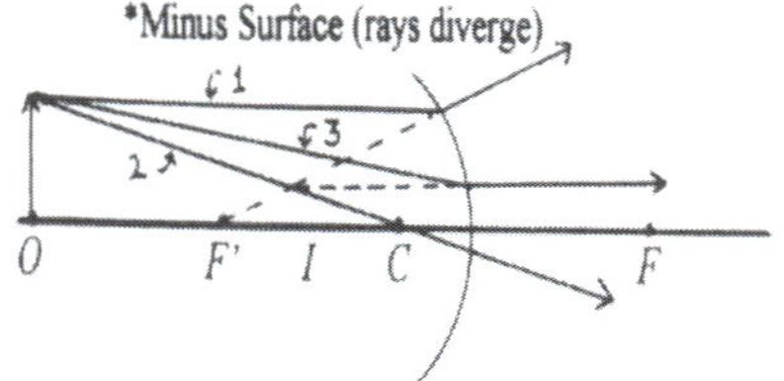

The following objects produce the following images:

Object	Positive Surface Image	Negative Surface Image
Real, outside F	Real Inverted Magnified	Virtual Erect Minified
Real, inside F	Virtual Erect Magnified	Virtual Erect Minified
Virtual, outside F	Real Erect Minified	Virtual Inverted Magnified
Virtual, inside F	Real Erect Minified	Real Erect Magnified

Remember: For positive lenses, the primary focal point (F) is to the left of the lens. For negatives lenses, the primary focal point (F) is to the right of the lens

Nodal Point: the center of curvature of the interface for Single Spherical Refractive Interfaces (SSRI)

Nodal Ray: Any ray that passes through the nodal point and passes straight through the interface.

6. Lateral (Translinear) and Angular Magnification

- **Lateral Magnification (M_T)** is the ratio of the image size to the object size, or the ratio of the image vergence to the object vergence
  - If LM is positive, the image is erect
  - If LM is negative, the image is inverted

    I=height of the image

    O=height of the object

Lateral Magnification:

M_T = I/O = U/V

M_T = (v - r) / (u - r) = nv / n'u

M_T = -f / x = -x' / f'

Example: *A 5cm tall object is 1 m away from a +2.50D lens, what is the LM?*

r = 20 cm

u=-1 m, then U = -1.00D

Answer:

V = U + P = +1.50D

⇒ v = n' / V = 1.5 / +1.50 = 1 m

r = Δn / P = (1.5 - 1) / 2.5 = 0.20 m

LM = (v - r) / (u - r)

= (1 m - 0.2 m) / (-1 m - 0.2 m)

= -0.667 X

The image is inverted (negative) and minified (less than 1)

Other ways of calculating LM

LM = nv / n'u = (1) (1) / (1.5) (-1) = -0.667 X

or **LM = U / V** = -1.00 D / +1.50D = -0.667 X or **LM = - f / x = -x' / f'**

x = distance from primary focal point to object (measured from f)

Above, LM = -f / x = -(-0.4 m) / -0.6 m = -0.667 X

(f = -n / P = -1 / +2.50 = -0.40 m)

(x = u - f = -1.0 m - (-.04 m) = - 0.6 m)

x' = distance from secondary focal point to image (measured from f')

Above, LM = -x' / f' = -(0.4m) / 0.6m = -0.667 X

(f' = n' / P = 1.5 / +2.50 = 0.6m)

(x' = v – f' = (1.5 / +1.50) – 0.6 m = 0.4m)

- **Angular Magnification (M_A)** -magnification of an object due to an optical system interposed between the object and the eye. The optical system produces a virtual image smaller than the original object but closer to the eye, giving it a larger angular subtense than the original object, and thus the appearance of being larger.
  - M_A is the angle subtended at the eye by the lens image, divided by the angle subtended at the unaided eye by the object at LDDV (Least Distance of Distinct Vision: covered more in the thin lens section).

7. Snell's Law of Refraction

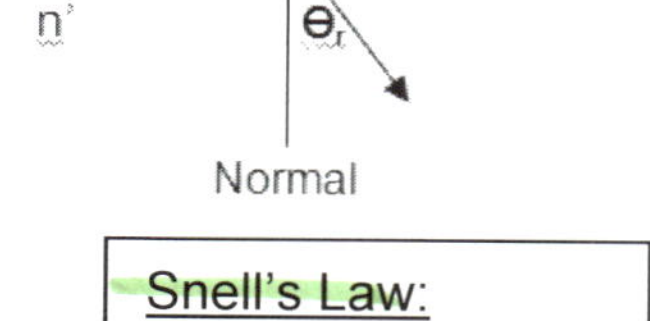

- **Refraction** is the bending of light when it travels between two media. It is a function of the incident angle and independent of the speed of light.
- **Normal** – an imaginary line perpendicular to the surface
- **Incident angle (Θ_i)** - the angle formed between the incident ray of light and the normal, when light it's the surface at less than a 90° angle.
- **Refracted angle (Θ_r)** - the angle formed between the emerging ray of light (on the other side of the interface) and the normal.
- **Snell's Law** the relationship between the incident and refracted angles of light.
  - If light enters a denser medium (n'>n), light is bent towards the normal
  - If light enters a less dense medium (n'<n), light is bent away from the normal
- If a beam of light perpendicular to the interface, enters a more dense medium, it emerges transmitted at a higher speed (Θ_i=0)

> Snell's Law:
> **$n \sin \Theta_i = n' \sin \Theta_r$**

Example: *If $\Theta_i = 30°$, Θ_r = ?*

air (n = 1) n' = 1.5

Answer:
n=1
n' = 1.5
(1) $\sin 30° = 1.5 \sin \Theta_r$
$\sin \Theta_r = 0.5 / 1.5$
$\Theta_r = 19.47°$

Note: If n'>n $\Rightarrow \Theta_r < \Theta_i \Rightarrow$ ray is bent toward the normal
If n'<n $\Rightarrow \Theta_r > \Theta_i \Rightarrow$ ray is bent away from the normal

> Critical Angle:
> **$\sin \Theta_c = n'/n$**
> **$\Theta_i \geq \Theta_c$** = total internal reflection

- **Critical Angle** (Θ_c) is the incident angle (Θ_i) at which the angle of refraction (Θ_r) is equal to 90°. This only occurs when light is going from a denser medium to a less dense (rarer) medium (n>n') and causes all light to be internally reflected.
  - Incident angles greater than the critical angle result in total internal reflection.

Example: *If n' = 1 and n = 1.5, then $\sin \Theta_c = 1/1.5$ and $\Theta_c = 41.81°$.*

THIN LENSES

1. Vergence: Dioptric and Effective Power

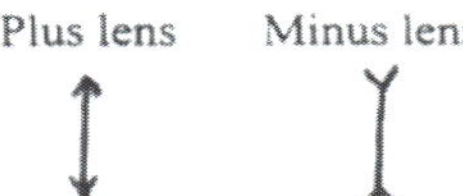

- A **thin lens** is a lens with a thickness that is negligible compared to the focal length of the lens
- Plus lenses add vergence, causing image light rays to converge
- Minus lenses reduce vergence, causing image light rays to diverge
- The surface power of a lens, $P=\Delta n/r$, is also called the refractive power, or power of a spherical refracting surface

Note: All formulas for thin lenses apply to single spherical refracting interfaces (SSRIs) except $f' = -f$.

- Draw thin lenses as straight lines

- The power of a thin lens (IOL) immersed in fluid:
  $\mathbf{P_{air}/P_{fluid} = (n_{IOL} - n_{air})/(n_{IOL} - n_{fluid})}$
- To determine the power of a lens, either use the **Lensmaker's Formula**, or break the lens into two surfaces, the front and the back and add.
- For a thin lens, the object and image distances are related by the boxed equation to the right, where i=image distance, and o=object distance

> Lensmaker's Formula
> $\mathbf{P = (n' - n)(1/r_1 - 1/r_2)}$
> or
> $\mathbf{P_T = P_1 + P_2}$
>
> $\mathbf{1/o + 1/i = 1/f}$

Example:

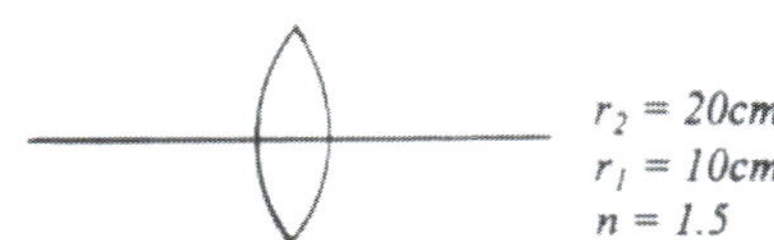

What is the dioptric power of this lens?

1. *Front surface*

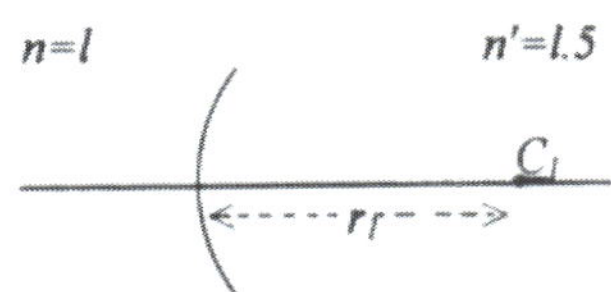

2. *Back surface*

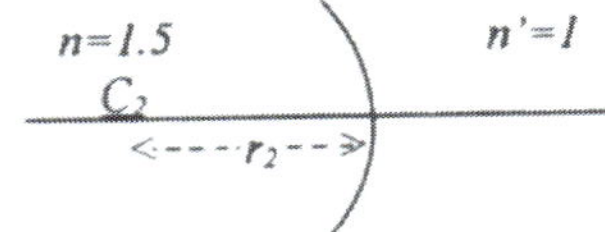

> ***Answer:***
> *Front Surface:*
> $P_1 = (n' - n)/r_1 = (1.5 - 1)/{+0.10\ m} = +5.00\ D.$
> Here, r_1 is positive because it is to the right of the surface.
>
> *Back Surface:*
>
> $P_2 = (n' - n)/r_2 = (1 - 1.5)/{-0.20\ m} = +2.50\ D.$
> Here, r_2 is negative because it is to the left of the surface.
>
> $P_t = P_1 + P_2 = +5.00\ D + 2.50\ D = +7.50\ D.$
>
> *Using lensmaker's formula,*
> $P = (1.5 - 1)(1/0.10\ m - 1/{-0.20}\ m)$
> $P = 0.5(10.00\ D + 5.00\ D) = +7.50\ D.$

- **Effective Power (P_{eff}):** the relative power of a lens as it is moved to a new location. Lens power depends upon its location in front of the eye (vertex distance)
  d- distance the lens has moved from original location
  - d is positive if lens is moved in the direction of light travel
  - d is negative if lens moved opposite the direction of light

> Effective Power
> $\mathbf{P_{eff} = P/(1 + dP)}$ for n=1.00

Note: As you move any lens away from your eye (increase vertex distance), you effectively increase the lens' plus power (decrease its minus power). This is why presbyopic patients find it useful to push their glasses down their nose (increase the plus power).

- **Correcting Lens Power (P_c):** when a new location of the lens (vertex distance) makes a lens effectively stronger/weaker, the correcting lens for

> Correcting Lens Power
> $\mathbf{P_c = P/(1 - dP)}$
> $\mathbf{P_c = P/1-(t/n)\ P}$

that patient at that vertex distance will need to be made weaker/stronger to compensate. This is why myopes need less minus and hyperopes need more plus when going from spectacles to contact lenses.

t=thickness, n=refractive index of lens, **d = t/n =reduced distance**

- Remember ***CAP- Closer Add Plus***
  - For spectacles, pushing a minus lens closer to the eye increases the P_{eff} of the lens(more minus)
  - Moving a plus lens away from the eyes increases the P_{eff} of the lens (more plus)

Example: *What is the new effective power of a +10.00 D lens just after you move the lens 5cm to the left? What correcting power of a lens would the patient need for this vertex distance?*

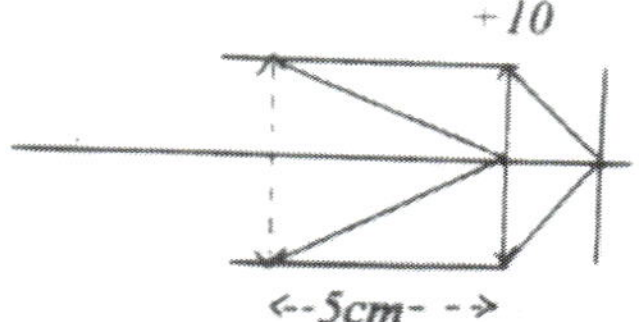

Answer:

d < 0 (because the lens is moved in the opposite direction of light travel).

$$P_{eff} = \frac{+10.00\text{ D}}{1+(-0.05\text{ m})(+10.00\text{ D})} = +20.00\text{ D}$$

- The new lens position makes the lens effectively too strong; hence, it focuses light in front of the screen.

$$P_c = \frac{+10.00\ D}{1-(-0.05\ m)(+10.00\ D)} = +6.67\ D$$

- To correct a patient at this new lens location, you would need a weaker plus lens.

2. Object-Image Relationships

- **Real Objects** have diverging rays and are on the same side as the incoming object rays
- **Virtual Objects** are not naturally occurring and have converging rays
- **Real Images** have a focal point that can be focused on a screen and on the same side as the outgoing rays
- **Virtual Images** cannot be focused on a screen and are always on the left side of the lens system
- A virtual object can have a virtual image
- Converging lenses (plus) have real, inverted images on the opposite side of the lens from the object
- Diverging lenses (minus) create virtual, erect images on the same side of the lens as the object

Summary of Image Formation for Plus(Converging) Lenses w/ Real Objects		
Object Position	**Image Position**	**Nature of Image**
At ∞ (infinity)	At F	Real, inverted, zero size
Between ∞ and 2F	Between F and 2F'	Real, inverted, minified
At 2F	At 2F'	Real, inverted, same size
Between 2F and F	Between 2F' and -∞	Real, inverted, magnified
At F	At - ∞	
Between F and 0	From +∞ to 0	Virtual, erect, magnified
At 0 (the lens)	At 0	Virtual, erect, same size

Summary of Image Formation for Minus (Diverging) Lenses w/ Real Objects		
Object Position	**Image Position**	**Nature of Image**
At ∞	At F'	Virtual, zero size
Between ∞ and 0	Between F' and 0	Virtual, erect, minified
At 0	At 0	Virtual, erect, same size

3. Lateral (Translinear) and Angular Magnification

- **Lateral Magnification (M_T):** same formulas as for SSRIs→ M_T**=I/O**
  Note that for thin lenses (vs. SSRIs), n = n' and f' = -f.
- **Angular Magnification (M_A): M_A = qU/(1 - dV)**
  d = distance of magnifier from eye
  q = least distance of distinct vision (use -25 cm if not specified) aka working distance

Lateral Magnification
M_L=image size/object size
Correcting Lens Power
M_A = qU/(1 - dV)

***Example**: A +8.00 D lens is held 5 cm from the eye, what is the AM for an object 8 cm in front of the lens?*

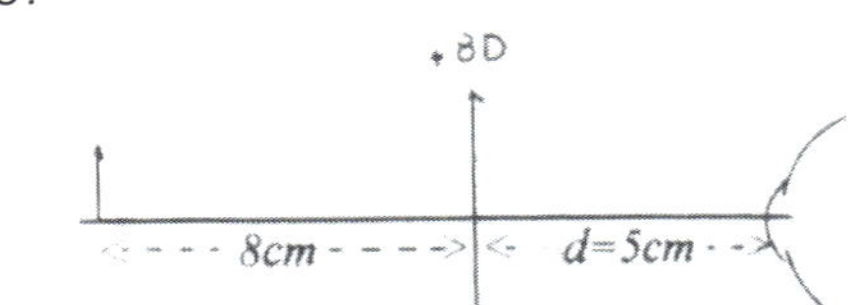

Answer:
U = 1/-0.08 m = -12.50 D
V = U + P = -12.50 D + 8.00 D = -4.50 D
M_A = qU/(1 - dV)
=(-0.25 m)(-12.50 D)/[1 - (-0.05 m)(-4.50 D)]
= 2.55X

4. Thin Lens Systems

- One can think of two thin lenses separated by some distance as a thick lens and vice versa.
- For several thin lenses together, use the image from the first lens as the object for the next lens and so on. This is called "successive imaging."

5. Prismatic Effect (Prentice's Rule and Prism Effectivity)

- Prisms are a transparent medium bound by two plane sides inclined at an angle used to deviate light but not change the vergence. Prisms do NOT focus light, they only bend light towards the base
- Image of an object formed by a prism is virtual and appears displaced towards the apex of the prism
- A **Prism Diopter** is a deviation of 1 cm at 1 meter.
- **Prentice's Rule** determines how much prismatic deviation you get when you look off center of a lens.
  - There is no prismatic power at the optical center of the lens
  - A plus lens can be thought of as 2 prisms joined at the base
  - A minus lens can be thought of as 2 prisms joined at the apex

  Z = prism power (in prism diopters)
  h = distance from optical center (in cm)
  P = lens power (in diopters)

Prentice's Rule
Z = hP

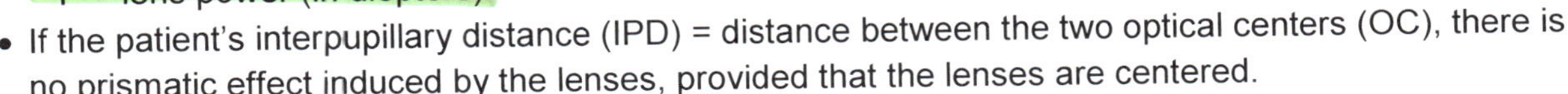

- If the patient's interpupillary distance (IPD) = distance between the two optical centers (OC), there is no prismatic effect induced by the lenses, provided that the lenses are centered.

***Example**: What is the prismatic power 5 mm from the optical center of a +3.00 D lens?*
Z = hP = (0.5 cm)(+3.00 D) = 1.5Δ

Net prismatic effect of 2 prisms:

- Horizontal prisms:
  - If the bases are in the same direction over both eyes (i.e. base out (BO) over both eyes or base in (BI) over both eyes), add the amounts of prism.
    ***Example**: 2Δ BI OD + 2Δ BI OS = 4Δ BI total*
  - If the directions are opposite (i.e. BI + BO) then subtract them and express the total prism as being in the direction of the larger amount of prism and over the eye with the larger amount of prism.
    ***Example**: 4Δ BI OD + 1Δ BO OS = 3Δ BI OD*

- Vertical prisms:
    - If both eyes have the same direction of prism (i.e. base up (BU) over both eyes or base down (BD) over both eyes), subtract the two amounts and express the total in the direction of the larger amount of prism and over the eye with the larger amount of prism.

      ***Example**: 3Δ BU OD + 2Δ BU OS = 1Δ BU OD*

    - If the prism base direction is opposite in the two eyes, then add the two amounts. Keep in mind that BD over one eye is the same as BU over the other eye. However, this thought does not apply to horizontal prisms (BI over one eye is NOT the same as BO over the other).

      ***Example**: 3Δ BD OD + 3Δ BU OS = 6Δ BD OD or 6Δ BU OS*

***Example**: A 5 D myope with a 58 mm PD (papillary distance) views through a pair of spectacles with the optical centers 64 mm apart. What is the total prism power the myope looks through?*

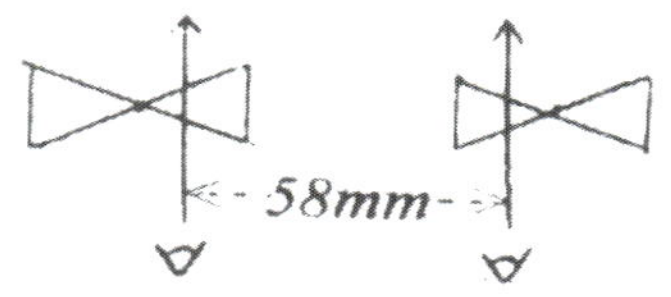

> ***Answer**:*
> h = 64 - 58 = 6 mm
> Z = hP = (0.6 cm)(-5 D)
> = 3Δ BI total (1.5Δ BI per lens)

In this example, the myopic lens acts as two prisms (one BO and one BI) connected at the apex. Here, the apex is the optical center (OC). Since the myope's pupils are closer together than the OC, the myope is looking through the BI part of the lens (as illustrated above).

- **Prism effectivity:** the effectivity of a prism changes as the object location changes. The effectivity increases as the object distance increases.

6. Ray Tracing, Optical Center, and Optical Axis

- **Optical Center:** the point on the lens axis through which the undeviated ray (or its projection) passes.
- **Optical Axis:** the line joining the centers of curvature of two lens surfaces or the line joining the vertex and center of curvature of a surface.

THICK LENSES

- Thick lenses are like 2 thin lenses except that now the medium between the lenses is lens material; consider each surface separately.

1. Cardinal Points

- The **cardinal** points are three pairs of points (6 points) located *on the optical axis* of an *ideal*, symmetric, focal optical system that are used to define the system itself: 2 principal points, 2 nodal points, and 2 focal points. The position of the cardinal points in an eye depend upon its structure and level of accommodation. *For an ideal system, assume sinΘ=Θ and cosΘ=1
- The location, orientation, and size of an image in an ideal system (plane mirror) are determined by the locations of cardinal points using 4 points (focal points and either principal or nodal points). The cardinal points can be used to approximate behavior of real, symmetric, focal systems.
- **Focal planes**
    - An object placed at the (light leaving the) **primary focal point (F)** will be imaged at infinity
    - An object placed at infinity (parallel light) will image at the **secondary focal point (F')**

- **Back focal length (f'_v):** distance from back of lens to secondary focal point of system.
- **Front focal length (f_n):** distance from front lens surface to primary focal point.
- **Back vertex power (P_v):** the effective power of a lens as measured from the surface toward the eye. BVP is often the "power" of a spectacle lens

  n_3' = refractive index of the medium that is on the right side of the lens

- **Front vertex power or neutralizing power (P_n):** reciprocal of the front vertex focal length.

  n_1 = refractive index of the medium on the left side of the lens

- **Equivalent Power (P_e):** Measure of the ability of an optical system to bend rays of light. The higher the power, the greater the ability to bend rays.

  P_e = equivalent power of the system
  P_1= Front surface power
  P_2 = Back surface power
  t = distance between surfaces (always positive)
  n_2 = refractive index between surfaces

- Two ways to find the focal points:
  1. Use Successive Imaging to find focal points.
  2. Use Equivalent Power

Back Vertex Power
$P_v = n_3'/f_v'$
BVP in air:
$P_v = 1/f_v'$
Front Vertex Power
$P_n = -n_1/f_n$
FVP in air:
$P_n = -1/f_n$
Equivalent Power
(Gullstrand's equation)
$P_e = P_1 + P_2 - (t/n_2)P_1P_2$

Example (Successive Imaging):

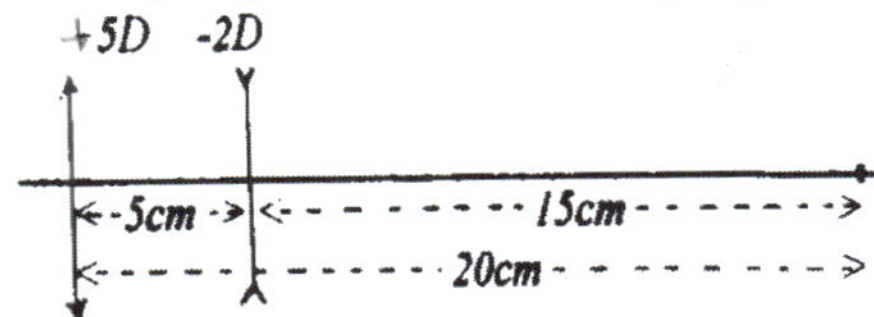

What are the secondary and primary focal points?

To find the **secondary focal point (F')**:
Parallel light in → $U_1 = 0$ →
$V_1 = U_1 + P_1 = 0 + 5\ D = +5\ D$ →
$v_1 = 1/V_1 = 1/+5\ D = +20$ cm
(Use 20 cm as object location for second lens)

$u_2 = +20$ cm - 5 cm = +15 cm →
$U_2 = 1/u_2 = 1/+0.15$ m = +6.67 D →
$V_2 = U_2 + P_2 = +6.67\ D + (-2.00\ D) = +4.67\ D$
[Back vertex power = +4.67 D.]

$v_2 = 1/V_2 = 1/+4.67\ D = +0.214$ m = +21.4 cm
[Thus, F' is 21.4 cm behind the -2.00 D lens, and the back focal length = +21.4 cm.]

To find the **primary focal point (F)**, turn the system around:

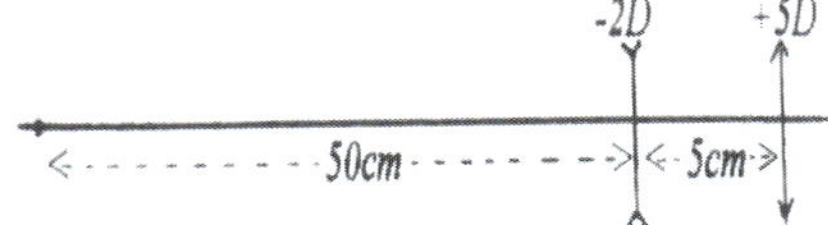

Parallel light in → $U_1 = 0$ →
$V_1 = U_1 + P_1 = 0 + (-2\ D) = -2\ D$ →
$v_1 = 1/V_1 = 1/-2\ D = -50$ cm
(Use -50 cm as object location for 2nd lens)

$u_2 = -50$ cm - 5 cm = -55 cm →
$U_2 = 1/u_2 = 1/-0.55$ m = -1.82 D→
$V_2 = U_2 + P_2 = -1.82\ D + 5.00\ D = +3.18\ D$
[Front vertex power = +3.18 D.]
$v_2 = 1/V_2 = 1/+3.18\ D = +0.314$ m = +31.4 cm
[Thus, F is 31.4 cm in front of the +5.00 D lens in the original system, and the front focal length = -31.4 cm.]

Example (Equivalent Power):

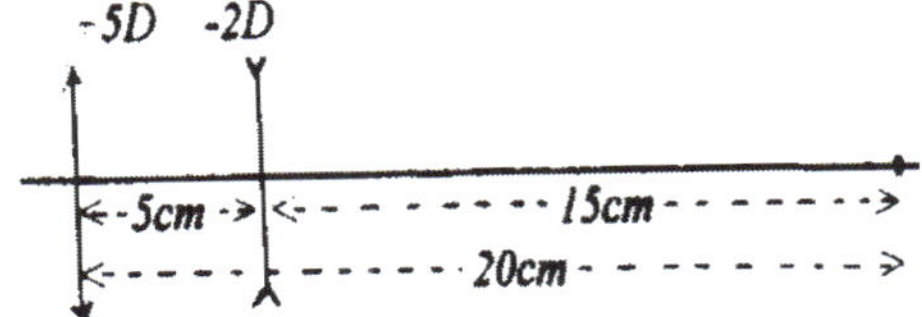

What are the secondary and primary focal points?

$P_e = +5\ D + (-2\ D) - (0.05\ m/1)(+5\ D)(-2\ D)$
$= +3.00\ D + 0.50\ D = +3.50\ D$

Now find focal lengths from equivalent power:
$f = -n_1/Pe = -1/+3.50\ D = -28.6$ cm
$f' = n_3'/P_e = 1/+3.50\ D = +28.6$ cm

- **Principal planes** – there are two principal planes in a system where a ray emerging from the lens *appears* to have crossed the **real (emergent) principal plane (H')** at the same distance from the axis that the ray *appears* to cross the **front (incident) principal plane (H).** The distance from the object and image from the incident and emergent principal planes determines the magnification of the system.
  - For a thin lens, the principle planes both lie at the location of the edge
  - The focal lengths are with respect to the principal planes.
- When **Ray Tracing Thick Lenses** you measure the focal length, object distance and image distance NOT from the center of the lens (thin lens) but rather the principal planes (where refraction is assumed to occur.
- **Principal points:** where principal planes intersect optic axis (assuming $n_1 = n_3'$, e.g. thick lens in air). The images are conjugate to each other so that transverse magnification is+1. If an object were placed at one of these points, an erect image of the same size would be formed at the other point.

- To find principal planes H and H':
  - Determine A_1H: the distance from the front surface to H
  - Determine A_2H: the distance from the back surface to H

To find principal planes H and H'
$A_1H = n_1(t/n_2)(P_2/P_e)$
$A_2H' = -n_3'(t/n_2)(P_1/P_e)$

Example (Equivalent Power):

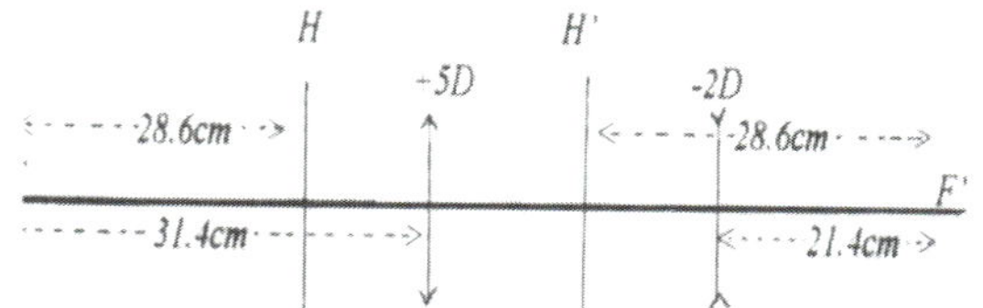

$A_1H = (1)(0.05 \text{ m}/1)(-2 \text{ D}/+3.5 \text{ D}) = -2.86$ cm
[H is 2.86 cm in front of first lens.]
$A_2H' = -(1)(0.05 \text{ m}/1)(+5 \text{ D}/+3.5 \text{ D}) = -7.1$ cm
[H' is 7.1 cm in front of second lens.]

Once you find H and H', you can use all thin lens formulas but with respect to H and H'. It is a simple system with an equivalent power of P_e and the principle planes H and H'.

***Example**: Object at 50 cm in front of system.*

$u = -0.471$ m since H is 2.86 cm in front of first lens → $U = 1/u = 1/-0.471 \text{ m} = -2.12$ D
$V = U + P_e = -2.12 \text{ D} + 3.50 \text{ D} = +1.38$ D (V is vergence leaving H') →
$v = 1/V = 1/+1.38 \text{ D} = +0.725$ m
Image is located 72.5 cm to right of H' or 65.4 cm to right of second lens.

- A **nodal ray** is a unique ray that enters a thick lens system from an off axis point and then leaves the lens system without being bent (i.e. the outgoing nodal ray is parallel to the incident nodal ray). When the off-axis is the point of fixation, the ray is called the **visual axis**.
- **Nodal points:** where the nodal rays intersect the optic axis. These two nodal points (**N** and **N'**) are conjugate to each other, so that the nodal ray from an off-axis point passing through **N** appears to pass through **N'** on the image side of the optical system.

2. Vertex Power and Equivalent Power

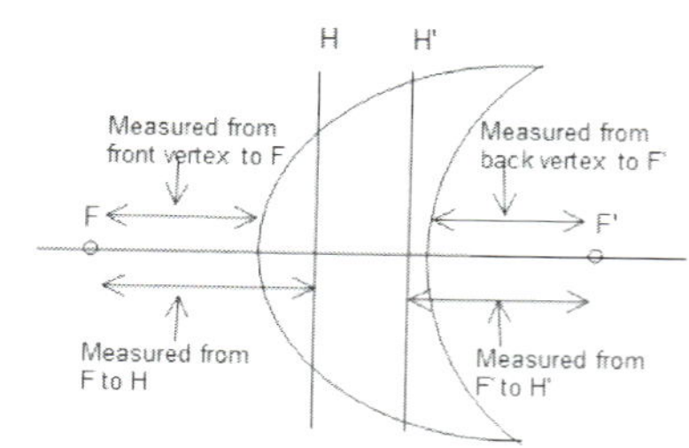

- The **Equivalent Power** is assigning one power to a two lens system (the position of the principal planes with respect to the first and second focal points.
- The **Lensmaker's equation [$P = (n' - n)(1/r_1 - 1/r_2)$]** for thin lenses does not take into account lens thickness and cannot be used with thick lenses. For thick lenses the Back Vertex Power

(P_v) and Front Vertex Power **(P_n)** must be calculated using the Front Surface Power **(P_1)** and the Back Surface Power **(P_2)** of the lens to determine the Equivalent Power of the system

Example (Continuing from above)

P1= +5D

P2= -2D

t=0.05m

n=1.00

Back vertex power:

$$P_v = \frac{+5\ D}{1 - (0.05\ m/1)(+5\ D)} + -2\ D = +4.67\ D$$

Front vertex power:

$$P_n = \frac{-2\ D}{1 - (0.05\ m/1)(-2\ D)} + 5\ D = +3.18\ D$$

Note: t is always positive

Back Vertex Power

$$\mathbf{P_v = n_3'/f_v'}$$

$$\mathbf{P_v = \frac{P_1}{1 - (t/n)P_1} + P_2}$$

$$\mathbf{P_v = \frac{P_e}{1 - (t/n_2)P_1}}$$

Equivalent Power

(Gullstrand's equation)

$$\mathbf{P_e = P_1 + P_2 - (t/n_2)P_1P_2}$$

Front Vertex Power

$$\mathbf{P_n = -n_1/f_n}$$

$$\mathbf{P_n = \frac{P_2}{1 - (t/n)P_2} + P_1}$$

$$\mathbf{P_n = \frac{P_e}{1 - (t/n_2)P_2}}$$

3. Lateral (Translinear) and Angular Magnification

- The **Linear Magnification** formula is the same, but all distances are measured from principal planes except: x is measured from F to object; x' is measured from F' to image

  O - object distance

  I – image distance

  Example (Continuing from above)

  LM = v/u = +72.5 cm/-47.1 cm = -1.54

- **Angular Magnification**:

  u_e= object distance with the unaided eye

  u_m= object distance with a magnifier

Linear Magnification

$$\mathbf{M_L = U/V = I/O = v/u = -f/x = -x'/f'}$$

Angular Magnification

$$\mathbf{M_A = \text{longitudinal mag} \times LM = |u_e|/|u_m| \times I/O}$$

4. Reduced Systems

- Used to equivalent distances in medium to distances in air. The thickness (d) of glass of index (n) is equivalent to an air thickness (d') of d/n. Whenever the refractive index (n) is greater than 1, the equivalent air distance (d') is less than the actual distance (d) and thus d' is often called the reduced distance. The system can be treated as if it is in air. Thus, the equations U=1/u and V=1/v can be applied.

Equivalent Air Thickness

d'=d/n

Example

A butterfly is imbedded 7cm deep in a plastic (n=1.44) slab. The plastic is covered by 16cm of water (n=1.33) and a 5cm layer of oil (n=1.72) is floating on the water. A camera is held in the air so that its lens is 10cm avobe the top surface of the oil. What distance must the camera be focused for?

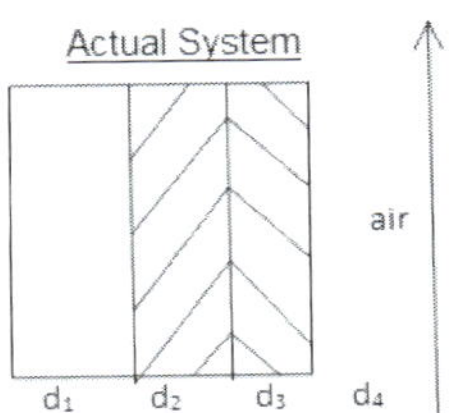

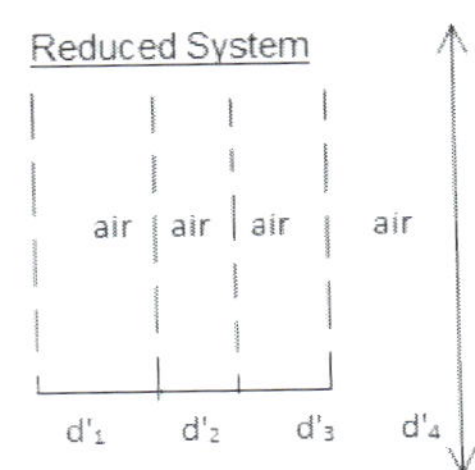

Answer

d'_1=7/1.44 = 4.86

d'2=16/1.33 = 12.03

d'3=5/1.72 = 2.91

d'4=10/1=10

u_{lens}=-(4.86+12.03+2.91+10)cm=-29.80cm

ABERRATIONS

Note: Throughout the preceding pages, we used the **paraxial approximation**. That is, we assumed that incident rays were all very close to the optic axis and close to being parallel to the optic axis. With this approximation, a point object has a point image. In reality, this is not true.

- **Monochromatic (Seidel) Aberrations**: spherical aberration, coma, oblique astigmatism, curvature of field, and distortion

1. Spherical

- **Spherical aberration** is an optical effect where there is increased refraction of light rays when they strike the periphery of a lens, causing an imperfect image to be formed.
  - **Positive SA**: Peripheral rays bent too much (See picture)
  - **Negative SA:** Peripheral rays not bent enough
- Shape dependent aberration that increases as you move towards the periphery of a lens (because the deviating power of the lens increases towards the periphery of the lens – **Prentice's Rule**).
- Spherical aberration is minimized with **biconvex** lenses and/or **aspheric** lenses (radius of curvature gets flatter in the periphery – less power at edge of lens)
  - The cornea is an aspheric surface that flattens in the periphery.
  - Incident rays further away from the optic axis (i.e., marginal rays) come to a focus closer to the lens than do paraxial rays. Marginal rays focus in front of the paraxial rays. The axial distance between the marginal ray focus (P') and paraxial ray focus (P") is the **longitudinal spherical aberration (LSA).**
  - **LSA** depends on the *square* of the aperture
  - **TSA (Transverse spherical aberration**) depends on the *cube* of the aperture
- SA is dependent on aperture size, controlled by lens form, and independent of aperture stop location

2. Coma

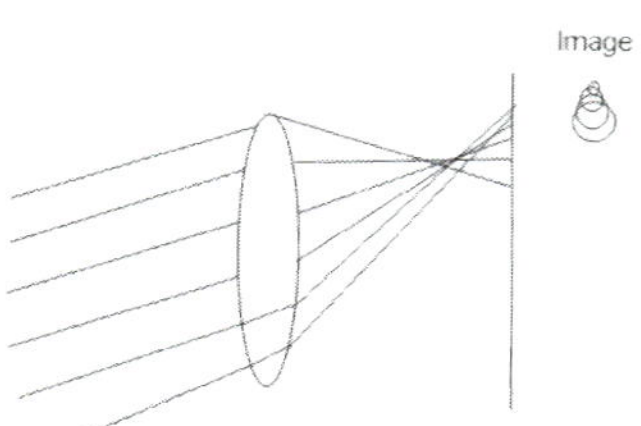

- **Coma** is a type of spherical aberration for off-axis objects produced by peripheral rays. The aberration produced is an asymmetric cusp or chromatic flare (comet shape). The pencil of rays from point P in the center of the lens is imaged at point P'. Rays passing through more peripheral parts of the lens produce an image of a circle below point P'. Intermediate zones are imaged as smaller circles in between. The net image formed is that of a coma.
- This is a problem for large aperture optical systems, but is negligent in spectacles which is limited by the size of the human pupil.
  - As you increase the aperture size, there is more coma.
  - Shorter objects have less coma.
  - Objects off axis have more coma
- Lens shape will minimize spherical aberration, but not eliminate coma
  - The closer the aperture to the lens, the greater the coma

3. Oblique (Marginal) Astigmatism

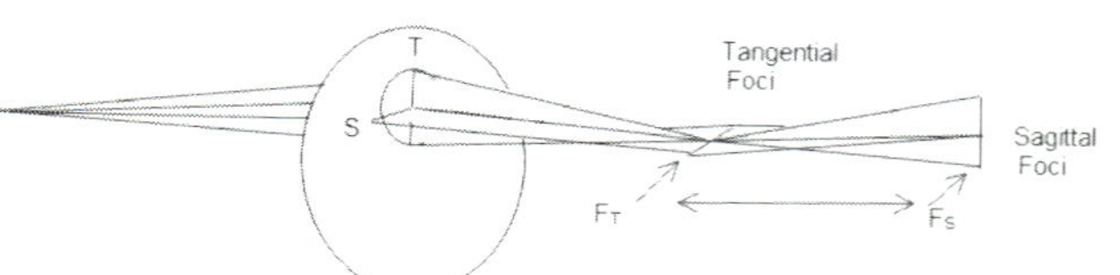

- **Oblique astigmatism** is a monochromatic aberration that occurs when a bundle of rays meet a lens surface obliquely (e.g., from below/above), and the beam forms an ellipse with a shorter tangential axis and a longer sagittal axis. Hitting a lens obliquely is like tilting the lens, similar to astigmatism in the human eye.

- **Tangential plane** – plane that includes the object point and the axis of symmetry. A meridional plane- vertical.
- **Sagittal plane** – plane perpendicular to the tangential plane that includes the object point and chief ray (not the optic axis)- horizontal. A skew plane (non-meridional)
- Sagittal and transverse rays form foci at different distances along the optic axis (Tangengial and Sagittal foci). The **Tangential Foci** is focused closer to the lens than the **Sagittal Foci**.
- The separation between F_T and Fs represents the magnitude of the marginal astigmatism

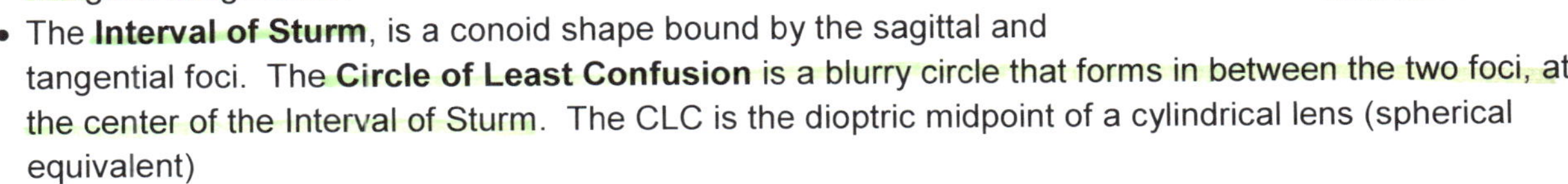

"Teacup and Saucer" Aberration

- The **Interval of Sturm**, is a conoid shape bound by the sagittal and tangential foci. The **Circle of Least Confusion** is a blurry circle that forms in between the two foci, at the center of the Interval of Sturm. The CLC is the dioptric midpoint of a cylindrical lens (spherical equivalent)
- Tilting a spherical lens induces astigmatism (cylinder power) with axis equal to the axis around which the lens was tilted. A plus lens induces plus cyl and a minus lens induces minus cyl with axis in the axis of tilt
    - If tilted along its horizontal axis, the increased astigmatism (plus/minus) will occur along axis 180.
    - To solve for new effective power when lens is tilted:
      P_s = new sphere power
      P_{so} = original sphere power
      P_c = new cylinder power
      θ = angle of lens tilt

Astigmatism of Oblique Incidence

$$\mathbf{P_s = P_{so}\,[1 + (\sin^2\theta/2n)]}$$
$$\mathbf{P_c = P_s \tan^2\theta}$$

- Oblique astigmatism varies with the angle of the incoming rays, so the separation of the foci for the tangential and sagittal axes varies. The foci are also sensitive to the location of the aperture stop.
- If the aperture is at the center of curvature, oblique astigmatism is eliminated because the rays are perpendicular to the lens surface. The image surface created by a lens with no radial astigmatism is the

4. Curvature of Field

- **Curvature of Field** is the aberration where a lens is unable to form a plane image of a plane object (produces a curved image). This is corrected by imaging the object on a curved plane (e.g. the retina).
- The **Petzval Surface** is a theoretical perfect surface where marginal astigmatism is absent. It is a function of the lens. The radius of this locus of focal points
- The **Far Point Sphere (FPS)** is a function of the eye, it represents the locus of points conjugate to the fovea as the eye rotates, assuming a COR at 27mm.
- Curvature of field is also called the **Power (Image Shell) Error.** It is the dioptric difference between the Petzval surface and the FPS.
- **Mean Oblique Power** is the position of the "CLC", which is the best position of least marginal astigmatism. It is the midpoint of T and S focus
- **Mean Oblique Error** describes where the MOP falls in relationship to the FPS. If MOP falls on FPS, than MOE=0

Curvature of Field

$\mathbf{r_{petz} = -nf'}$

$\mathbf{r_{FPS} = 0.027 - f'}$

Power Error = $\mathbf{P_{FPS} - P_{PS}}$

MOP = $\mathbf{(P_T + P_S/2)}$

MOE = $\mathbf{MOP - P_v}$

5. Distortion

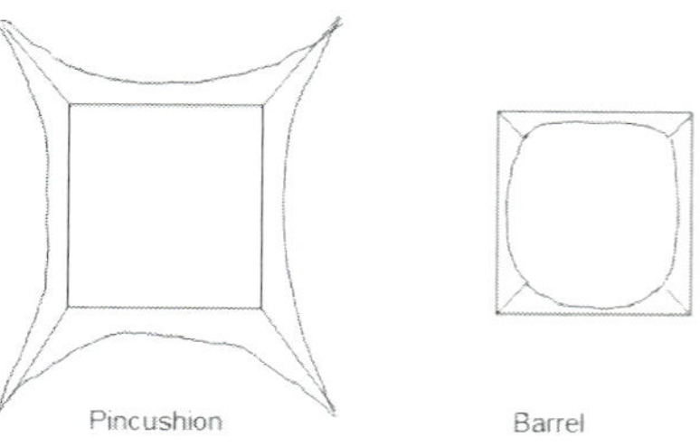

- **Distortion** is an aberration (of thick lenses) arising from a variation of lateral magnification with axial distance.
- **Pincushion:** rays in the center are less magnified than the rays off axis (magnification of the corners of a square object). The magnification increases with increasing axial distance, as with plus lenses.
- **Barrel:** rays in the center are more magnified than rays further off axis (minification of the corners of a square object more than the sides). The magnification decreases with axial distance, as with minus lenses.

6. Chromatic (Longitudinal and Lateral)

- **Chromatic (color) aberration** is the change in light refraction in materials with different refractive indices due to different wavelengths of light. Since the focal length of a lens is a function of the index of refraction and since the index varies with wavelength, a lens does not form a single image of light, but several images from each wavelength.
  - Blue light tends to bend more than red light, leading to chromatic aberration.
  - Chromatic aberration occurs strongly in the eye (3.00D difference in focus).
    - This is the basis of the red-green test for refinement of sphere power in refractions
- Chromatic aberration can be modified by changing 1) Lens shape 2) Lens refractive index 3) Aperture size 4) Position of the aperture.
- Since magnification depends on focal length, these images are also of different sizes. The nu value or Abbe value (v) of a material is a measure of chromatic aberration. Higher Abbe values correspond with less chromatic aberration.

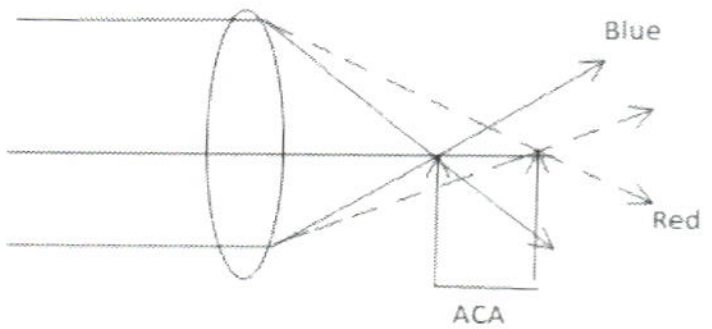

- **Axial (Longitudinal) Chromatic Aberration (ACA)** – variation of image distance with wavelength. Spreading of light is a function of how far you are away from the optical axis (peripheral rays). LCA is the dioptric separation between red and blue defocus.
- ACA of the eye has more axial aberration ~+2.25D than the spectacle lens

  P_D = dioptric power at the sodium D line
  n_F=blue line
  n_C= red line
  n_D= sodium

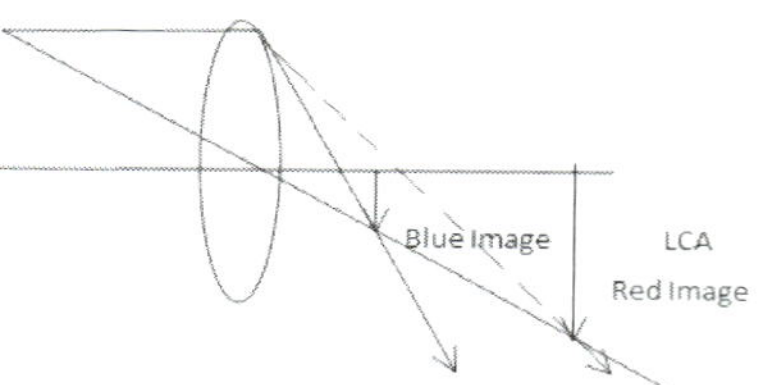

- **Lateral (Transverse) Chromatic Aberration (LCA)** – variation of image size. The further you look from the optical center of a lens, the more prismatic effect is induced. LCA is dependent upon the Abbe value. LCA can be applied to prisms using Prentice's Rule. Blue (short wavelength) light forms smaller images than red (longer wavelength) light.
- Significant amounts of LCA can lead to magnification differences.
- LCA of the eye has less lateral aberration than spectacle lenses Because it is limited by the aperture stop
- **Achromatic Doublet:** A system designed to reduce chromatic aberration by combining two lenses of different abbe values (different materials). The achromatic doublet can be created by using the

Chromatic Aberration

Abbe value (v) = $(n_D-1)/(n_F-n_C)$

$$ACA = (P_D)\frac{n_F-n_C}{n_D-1}$$

$$ACA = P_D/v$$

$$LCA_{Lens} = yP/v$$

$$LCA_{Prism} = \Delta/v$$

Achromatic Doublet - Lens

$$P_t = P_1+P_2$$

$$P_1/v_1 + P_2/v_2 = 0$$

Achromatic Doublet - Prism

$$Z_t = Z_1+Z_2$$

$$Z_1/v_1 = Z_2/v_2$$

following 2 equations, where

P_t = total power of two lenses

P_1=power of one lens

P_2=power of other lens

$\boldsymbol{v_1}$ and $\boldsymbol{v_2}$ are the respective abbe values

Z_T= total power of two prisms

Z_1= power of one prism

Z_2= power of other prism

Example

Design a +4.00D achromatic lens system using Crown Glass (nu=58) and polycarbonate (nu=30)

Answer:	
P1/58+P1/30=0; P1=-P2(58/30)=-1.93P2	-A +4.00D achromatic lens=
P1+P2=+4.00D; -1.93P2 +P2=+4.00D; P2=-4.30D	a +8.30D crown glass lens
P1=+4.00-(-4.30)=+8.30D	+ -4.30D polycarbonate lens

STOPS, PUPILS, PORTS

1. Entrance and Exit Pupils (Size and Location)

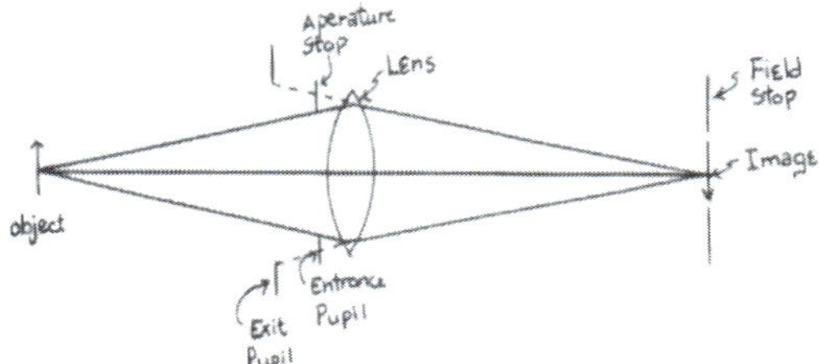

- **Aperture stop (AS)**: The element limiting the size of the light ray bundle (amount of light) from object space into image space. AS limits axial rays
  - **Chief Ray** – ray from a point on the object that goes through the center of the AS. It is the center of the blur circle, used for calculating magnification
- **Field stop (FS)**: Element limiting the size of the object which can be imaged by the system. It restricts the field of view as seen from the AS. FS limits chief rays
- **Entrance pupil**: The image of the aperture stop as seen from an axial object point on the object, imaged through those optical elements preceding the stop (from object space).
- **Exit pupil**: The image of the aperture stop as seen from an axial point on the image plane, through those optical elements behind the aperture stop (through image space).
- **Entrance port**: The image of the field stop as seen from an axial object point on the object, imaged through those optical elements preceding the stop (i.e., the field stop as seen in object space). It is the entrance pupil candidate that subtends the smallest angle at the entrance pupil.
- **Exit port**: The image of the field stop as seen from an axial point on the image plane, imaged through those optical elements behind the aperture stop (i.e., the field stop as seen in image space)..
- **Size and location**: To locate the positions of pupils and ports, use **V = U + P**. For size, use **m = v/u**.
- To find a field stop in a system:
  1) Image all elements into object space. AS is the real element conjugate to the pupil
  2) Entrance pupil is the candidate that subtends the smallest angle at the axial object point. AS is the physical element conjugate to the entrance pupil.
  3) Once the entrance pupil is found, the remaining candidate that subtends the smallest angle at the center of the entrance pupil is the entrance port
  4) The physical element conjugate to the entrance port is the field stop

***Example**: A +5.00D lens is located 6 cm in front of a -2.00D lens. Each lens has a 3.0 cm diameter. Find the aperture stop and entrance pupil for a real object 50 cm in front of the +5.00D lens.*

> ***Answer**:*
> To find the entrance pupil: Image of -2D through +5D
> V = U + P = 1/-0.06 + (+5) = -11.67
> v = -8.57cm
> m = v/u = I/O => I = Ov/u = [(3cm)(-8.57cm)]/6cm = 4.29cm
> - For +5D lens, q = Arctan 3cm/50cm = 3.43 °
> - For image of -2D lens, q = Arctan 4.29cm/58.57cm = 4.19 °
>
> * Since +5D lens subtends the smaller angle from the object plane it is the aperture stop. Also, since there are no lenses in front of it the +5D lens is also the entrance pupil
> ˉ The -2D lens being the only other candidate, is the field stop.

2. Depth of Focus, Depth of Field, Hyperfocal Distance

- **Depth of Focus**: The interval between the plane in front of the retina and the plane in back of the retina, in which an eye perceives an object to be in focus.
- **Depth of Field:** The interval between the plane in front of the fixation plane and the plane in back of the fixation plane, in which an object can be moved and still be perceived to be in focus (without accommodation).
- **Hyperfocal Distance:** The shortest distance for which a lens may be focused to permit satisfactory image definition of any object at infinity. This takes into account the small range of focus provided by depth of focus.

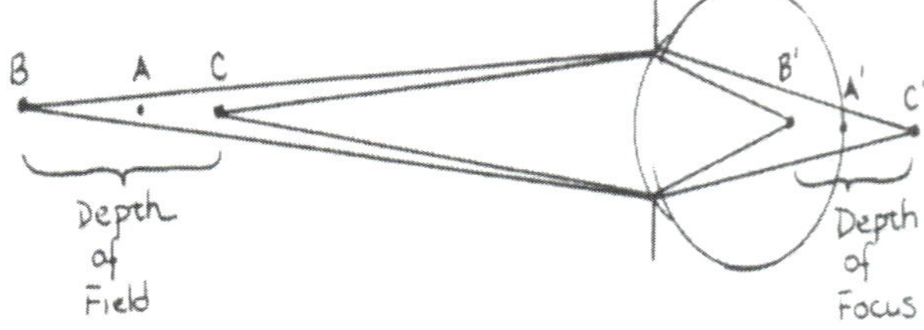

3. Field of View and Half Illumination

- **Field of view**: The angular subtense of the entrance port measured from the center of the entrance pupil. If a correcting lens is in front of the eye, the angular subtense must be measured from the image of the entrance pupil. Minus lenses will increase the field of view, and plus lenses will decrease the field of view. Remember that the field of view describes all that can be seen while fixating straight ahead. We conventionally use 17mm as the distance from the center of the entrance port to the center of the entrance pupil.

***Example:** Find entrance pupil image:*

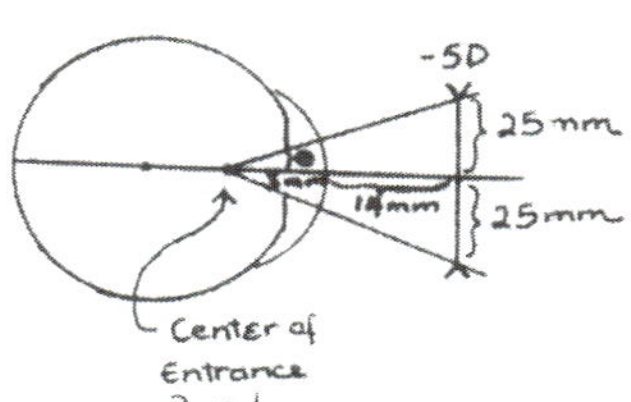

> ***Answer:***
> V = U + P = (1/-0.017m)+ -5.00 = -63.8D
> v = 1/V = 1/-63.8D = -0.0157M (behind lens)
> tan ϴ = 25/15.7 => ϴ = 57.9 °
> Field of view = 2 ϴ = 115.8 °

- **Field of Fixation**: The angular subtense measured from the center of rotation of the eye. Again, with a correcting lens, it must be measured from the image of the center of rotation. Minus lenses will increase the field of fixation and create a circle of diplopia around the lenses. Plus lenses will decrease the field of fixation and create a scotoma ring around the lenses. The field of fixation is smaller than the field of view. Remember that the field of fixation describes all that can be fixated on. (Usually 27mm)

Example: *Find center of rotation image:*

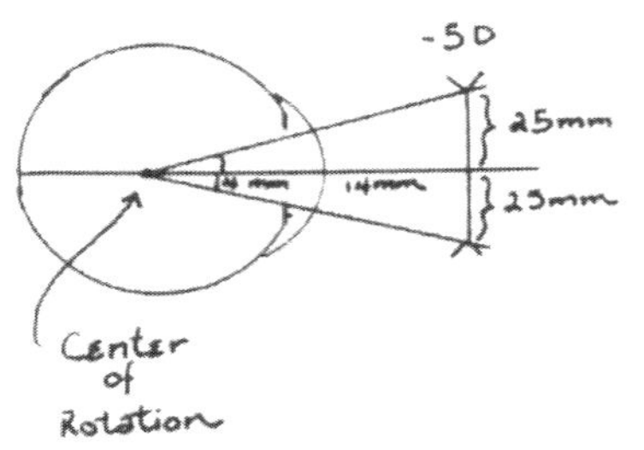

> ***Answer:***
> V = U + P = 1/-0.028m + (-5.00D) = -40.7D
> v = 1/V = -0.0246 (behind lens)
> tan ϴ = 25/24.6 => ϴ = 45.5 °
> Field of fixation = 2 ϴ = 91.0 °

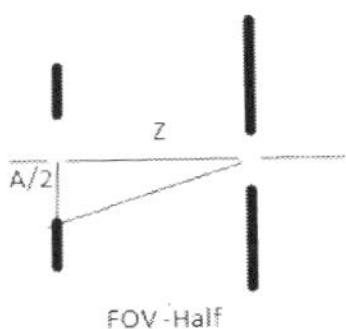

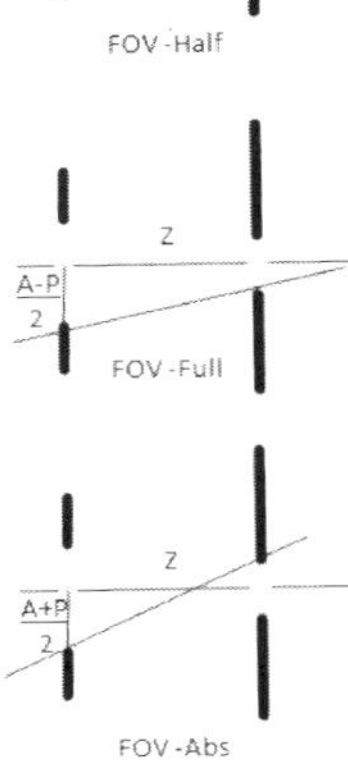

- There are 3 kinds of fields of view in entrance space, depending on the quantity of light getting through at different angles.
- **Field of Half Illumination** – area in the object plane from which light from a point source could completely fill half of the aperture stop
- **Field of Full Illumination** – area in the object plane from which light from a point source could completely fill the aperture stop.
- **Absolute Field of View** – area in the object plane from which light from a point source could send any light into image space. Vignetting is complete (intensity of viewed object is zero) **Vignetting** – limiting of one aperture by another

SPHEROCYLINDRICAL LENSES

1. Location of Foci, Image Planes, Principal Meridians, and Circle of Least Confusion

- A **spherocylindrical lens** has both a spherical component and a cylindrical component. It has two principal meridians, one that has greater power and the other that has less power. These two principal meridians are usually perpendicular to each other. The focus of a meridian is located at its focal distance from the lens (the reciprocal of the meridian's dioptric power). The image plane of each meridian can be found using V = U + P where P = power of the meridian of interest.
- The **circle of least confusion**, also known as the blur circle, is the point of best focus for the entire lens. To find it, take the reciprocal of the average power of the two principal meridians. It is this distance from the lens.
- The **interval of Sturm** is the distance between the two foci of the two principal meridians.

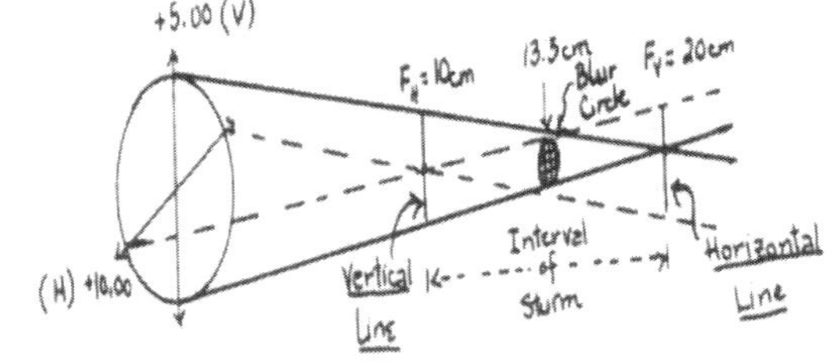

2. Obliquely Crossed Spherocylindrical Lenses

- Adding spherocylindrical lenses will give you a resultant spherocylindrical lens with the resultant axis between the 2 component axes.

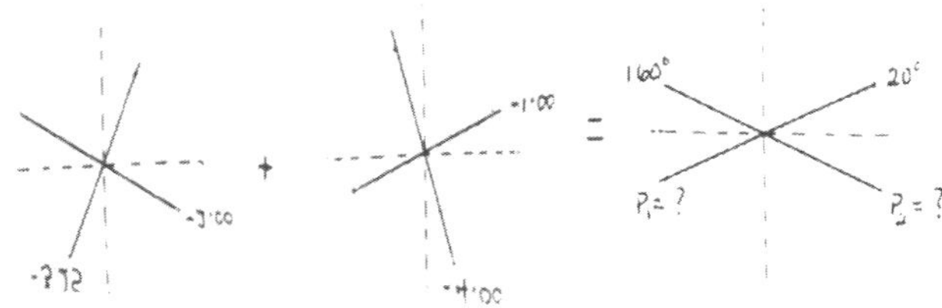

3. Transposition

- Going from (+) to (-) cylinder form and vice versa:
  - a) Algebraically add the sphere and cylinder value and put the new value as the new sphere.
  - b) Change the sign of the cylinder.
  - c) Change the axis by 90 degrees.

Example:

(-)cyl: -3.00 - 2.00 x 180 <----> (+)cyl: -5.00 +2.00 x 090

4. Prismatic Effect

- A spherical lens is a stack of prism with no deviation at the optical center of the lens. The farther one moves away from the optical center, the more prism that's in that part of the lens. If you move to the right of the optical center of a plus lens, you get base-left prism. If you move to the right of the optical center of a minus lens, you get base-right prism.
- To quantify, use Prentice's rule:
  - Z = prism diopters
  - h = cm away from optical center
  - P = lens power

Prentice's Rule
Z=hP

THIN PRISMS

- **Prisms**: a transparent medium bound by two plane sides that are inclined at an angle to each other

1. Unit of Measuerment (prism diopter)

- **One prism diopter** (1^{Δ}) is the amount of prism required to deviate a light 1cm at a distance of 1m .

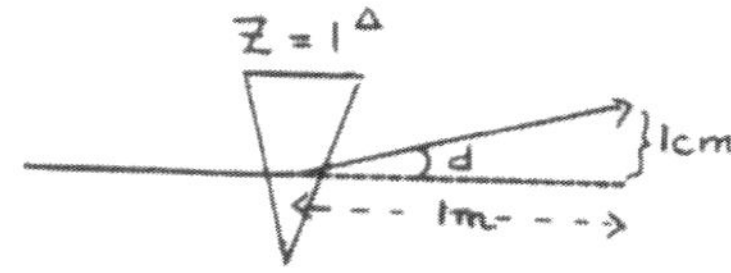

Z = deviation in Δ
d = deviation angle (in degrees)

Prism
Z = 100 tan(d)

2. Prism Deviation

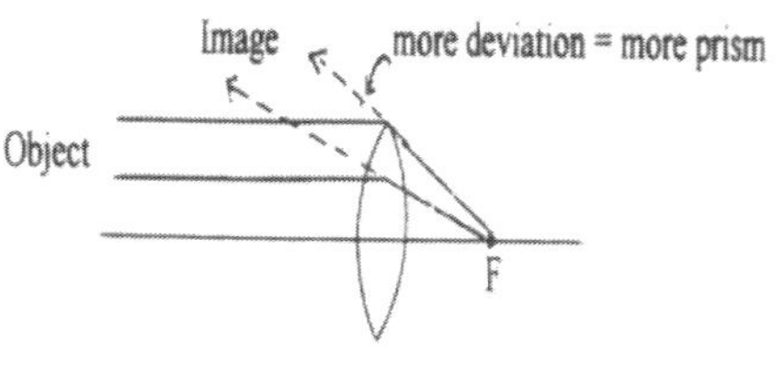

- Prism deviates light towards its base. Prism in glasses causes the image to deviate towards the apex of the prism. In spherical lenses, there is more deviation of light towards the edge of the lens; so there is more prism towards the edge of the lens. For a thin prism in air, the deviation only depends on the prism's refractive index (n) and the apex angle (A) -(for incident angles <20°)

Prism Deviation
d = (n-1)A

Example: *What is the deviation for a glass prism (n = 1.5) with a 5° apex angle?*

Answer:
d = (n-1)A = (1.5 -1)5° = 2.5°
To convert to prism diopters:
tan 2.5° = x cm/100cm
x = 4.4cm => 4.4 Δ

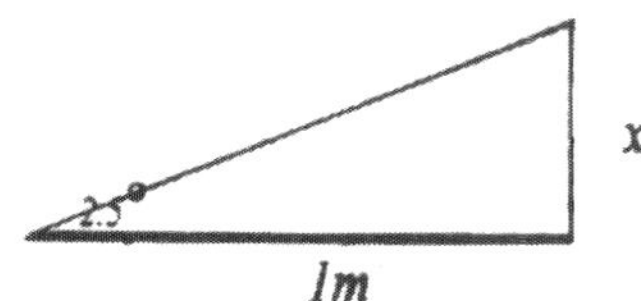

3. Combination of Thin Prisms

- When combining two prisms, they can be treated like vectors pointing in the direction of the base. The resultant vector is the resultant prism in magnitude and base direction.

$2^{\Delta}BU + 3^{\Delta}BR = $ Resultant 3.61^{Δ} (2^{Δ}, 3^{Δ}, $\theta = 33.7°$)

In the example, the Pythagorean theorem is used to determine the magnitude of the resultant vector ($c^{2=}a^2+b^2$, where c is the length of the hypotenuse).

4. Resolution of Oblique Prisms into Horizontal and Vertical Components

- Use the following trigonometric equations for the vertical component (Z_v) and the horizontal component (Z_H), where Θ is measured from the horizontal axis

Prism Components
Z_v = Zsin Θ
Z_h = Zcos Θ

Example: *Resolve 3.61^{Δ} @ 33.7° into horizontal and vertical components:*

$Zv = 3.61^{\Delta} (\sin 33.7°) = 2^{\Delta} BU$
$Zh = 3.61^{\Delta} (\cos 33.7°) = 3^{\Delta} BR$

$2^{\Delta}BU$
$3^{\Delta}BR$

Answer:
3.61^{Δ} @ 33.7°
$Z_v = 3.61^{\Delta} (\sin 33.7°) = 2^{\Delta}$ BU
$Z_h = 3.61^{\Delta} (\cos 33.7°) = 3^{\Delta}$ BR

5. Total Internal Reflection

- 100% of the incident light is reflected when: a ray of light approaches a boundary with a medium of smaller refractive index, and the angle of incidence of the ray is greater than the critical angle (Θ_c).

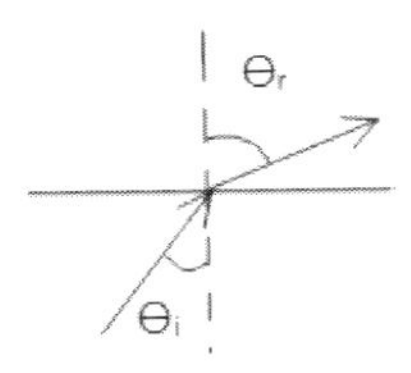

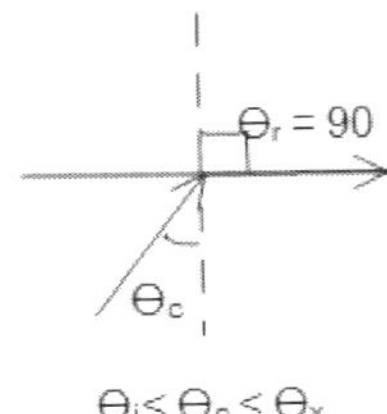

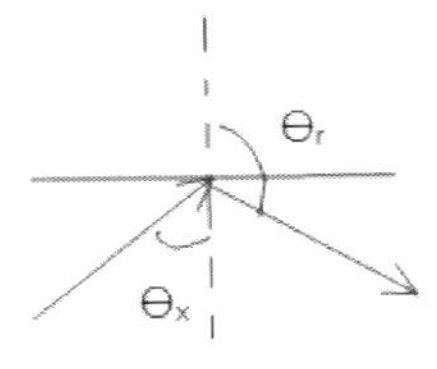

$\Theta_i < \Theta_c < \Theta_x$

Total Internal Reflection
$\sin \Theta_c = n'/n$ → When n > n'

OPHTHALMIC AND OPTICAL INSTRUMENTS

1. Ophthalmoscopes

- Direct and indirect ophthalmoscopes: An ophthalmoscope allows us to objectively examine the integrity of the interior eye. It can also be used to objectively approximate the spherical

Property:	**Direct**	**Indirect**
Field of View:	10 degrees	40 degrees
Magnification:	15x	3x
Position of image:	erect/virtual	inverted/real
Depth of focus:	small	large
Distance from patient:	close	farther

refractive error of the eye. There are two basic types of ophthalmoscopes - direct and indirect:

Direct Ophthalmoscope

- Magnification is based on the total refractive power of the eye. Using basic magnification formula M=P/4, an emmetropic eye of +60D would provide 60/4=15X. An aphakic eye of +40.00D would provide 40/4=10X.

-Illumination system:

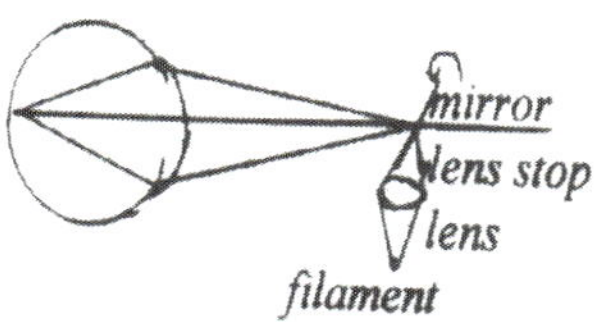

Observation system:

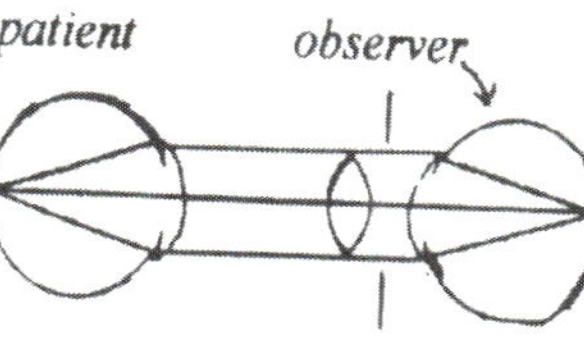

- The patient's and observer's retinas are conjugate.

Indirect Ophthalmoscope:

-Illumination system:

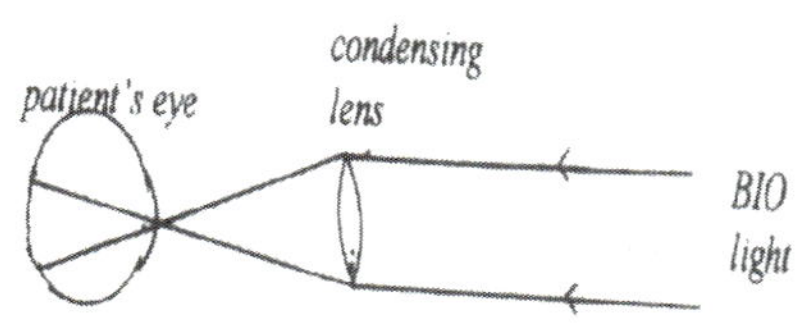

Observation system:

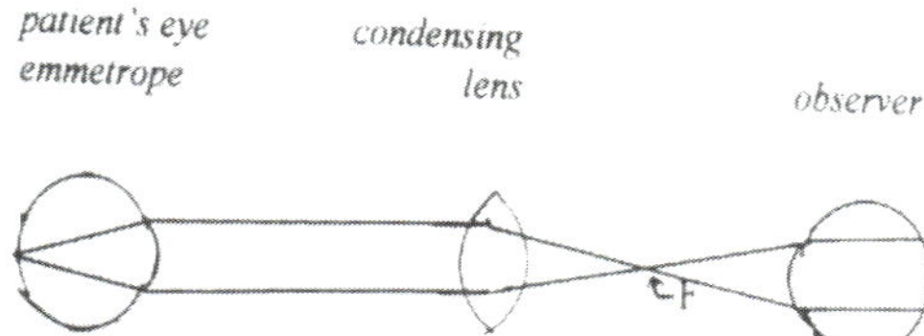

- Light is shone through a +13 to +30D biconvex condensing lens to illuminate the patient retina.
- Light reflected from the retina leaves as parallel rays. The condensing lens focuses light at its focal point, forming a real, inverted, reversed image. The observer's and patient's pupils are conjugate.
- As the power of the condensing lens decreases, the magnification increases.

2. Retinoscopy

- A **retinoscope** allows us to objectively determine a patient's spherocylindrical refractive error, irregular astigmatism, and evaluate opacities and irregularities of the cornea and lens. The basic principle of retinoscopy is Foucalt's method of determining the focal power of a lens by locating its conjugate foci in space. A neutral reflex is seen when the retinoscope is conjugate to the patient's retina. A retinoscope consists of two systems: illumination and observation.

emmetrope — light — -neutral reflex

myope — light shadow — - "against" motion

hyperope — shadow light — - "with" motion

- Retinoscopes use a **streak projection system**: A streak of light is reflected from a mirror or moved in relation to a convex lens (sleeve up), allowing light to leave the device as if it were from a point behind the retinoscope (plane mirror) or from between the examiner and patient (concave mirror).

> Retinoscope
> **Patient's Rx=NL-WD**
> NL=lens needed to neutralize the retinal reflex
> WD=distance between the patient and the observer

- Examiner is attempting to put the far point of the patient's eye at the plane of the examiner's pupil.
    - "Against" motion – far point plane lies between the patient's eye and examiner's eye (myopia)

- "With" motion- far point lies behind the examiner's eye (hyperopia, emmetropia, mild myopia)

3. Lensometry

- The standard **lensometer** measures the effective power (back **vertex power**) of lens, axis of cylindrical components, and power and directions of prisms.

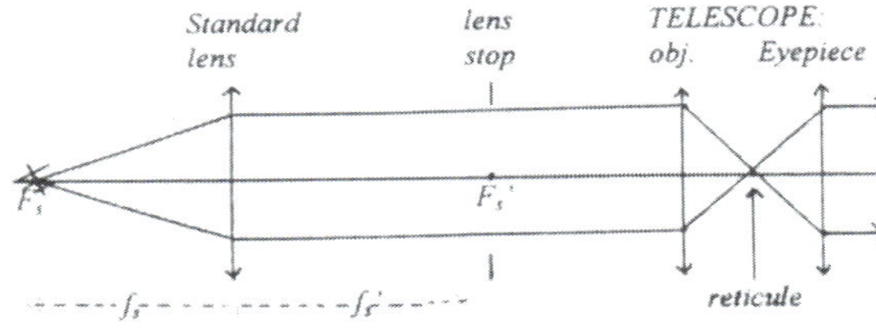

- The standard lensometer consists of a movable target, a standard lens (usually +20.00 or +25.00D) and a telescopic system. The maximum power of the test lens must be less than the power of the standard lens. The lensometer is based on the Badel Principle (Knapp's Law applied to lensometers) with the addition of an astronomical telescope for precise detection of parallel rays at neutralization
- The target is at the primary focal point of the standard lens. The test lens is at the secondary focal point of the standard lens (**the lens stop**).
- In order for the target to be focused, parallel light must enter the observer's eye. This means that parallel light must enter the telescope system and parallel light must leave the test lens. For parallel light to leave the test lens, light must approach the primary focal point of the test lens.
- For a **concave test lens**, converging light must exit the standard lens, and thus the target must be moved **away** from the standard lens.
- For a **convex test lens**, diverging light must exit the standard lens, and thus the target must be moved **toward** the standard lens.

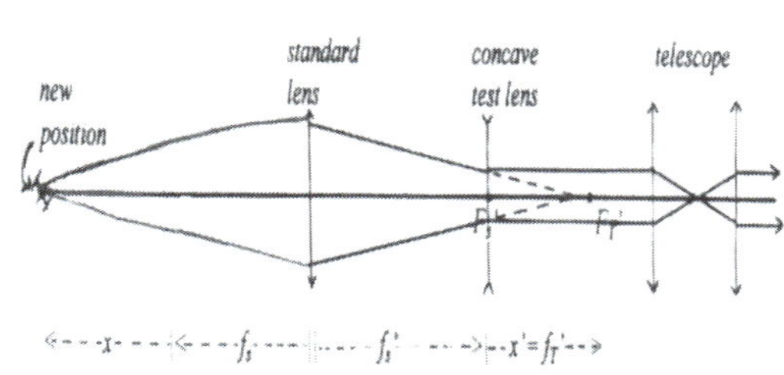

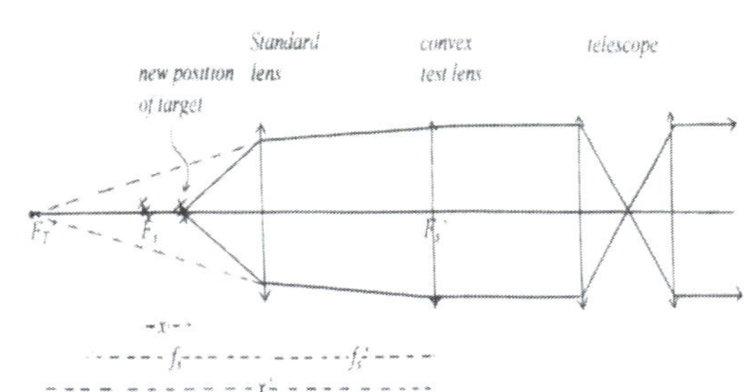

- There is a linear relationship between the distance the target is moved (x) and the back vertex power of the test lens (P_v). This relationship is demonstrated by **Newton's formula,** where x and x' are measured from F_s and F_s' respectively.
  - Since $f_s = - f_s'$, $xx' = - f_s^2$
  - Solving for x, $x = - f_s^2/x'$ (Eq.1)
  - Since the test lens is at F_s', $x' = - f_T'$
  - Substituting into Eq. 1,
    $x = - f_s^2/ - f_T' = f_s^2/ f_T'$
  - Since $1/ f_T' = P_v$, $x = f_s^2 P_v$ and $P_v = x/ f_s^2$

Newton's Formula
$\mathbf{xx' = f_s f_s'}$

4. Slit Lamp Biomicroscopy

- A Slit lamp biomicroscope functions in
  1) Examination of the anterior segment of the eye, specifically: tear film, cornea, eyelids, conjuctiva, anterior chamber, iris, and lens.

2) Grading the anterior chamber angle
3) Applanation tonometry (with the Goldmann tonometer).
4) Fundus and vitreous examination (with addition of the Hruby lens or other condensing lens).
5)Tear break-up time determination.

- The biomicroscope consists of an illumination system and observation system (a microscope). The two can be coupled (thus focused at the same time) or dissociated to obtain different types of illumination.
- Size of light beam can change from parallelepiped to an optic section.
- Direction of beam and microscope can vary, creating different types of illuminations.

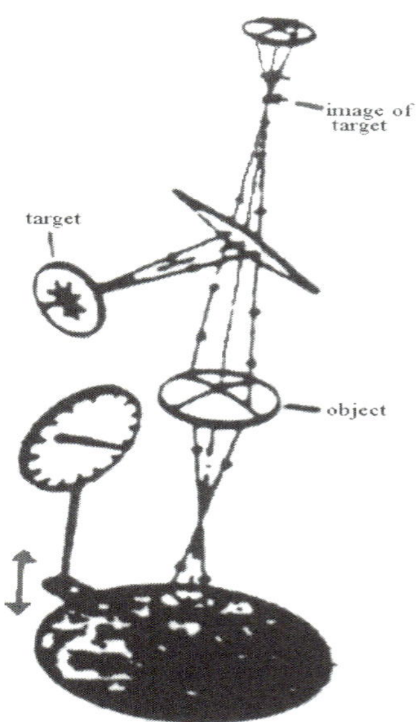

5. Radiuscopy

- A **Radiuscope** functions to measure the radii of curvature of contact lenses.
- The instrument consists of a compound microscope in which a target is projected along its axis. An image of this target will be seen through the microscope when it is focused upon a reflecting surface, such as a contact lens. The image will also be seen when the microscope is focused at the center of curvature of the concave or convex surface due to light being reflected back along its path. The distance between the two positions, where an in-focus target image is seen, equals the radius of curvature.

6. Keratometery

- A **Keratometer** functions to objectively measures the refractive power of the cornea (central 3mm) along the principle meridians and the axes of these meridians (thus measuring astigmatism). Also used to detect irregularities (eg. Keratoconus) and tear film stability after each blink.
- This instrument consists of a mire (the object), a telescope system to magnify The image reflected off the cornea, and a doubling system (which consists of two prisms, one for each meridian) to measure the image size.
- The cornea acts here as a convex mirror. Given the size of the mire, the size of the reflected image (which is measured) and the distance between the object and image, the radius of curvature can be determined from the mirror equation:

Mirror Equation
$1/v - 1/u = 2/r$
Refractive Power of Cornea
$P=(n_2-n_1)/r$

Note: The distance between object and image is a constant (fixed by mfg): this is assured by allowing the mire to be in focus only when the objective lens is brought to a fixed distance from the image. The keratometer is calibrated to give the refractive power of the cornea from using (r) (n_2 =1.3375).

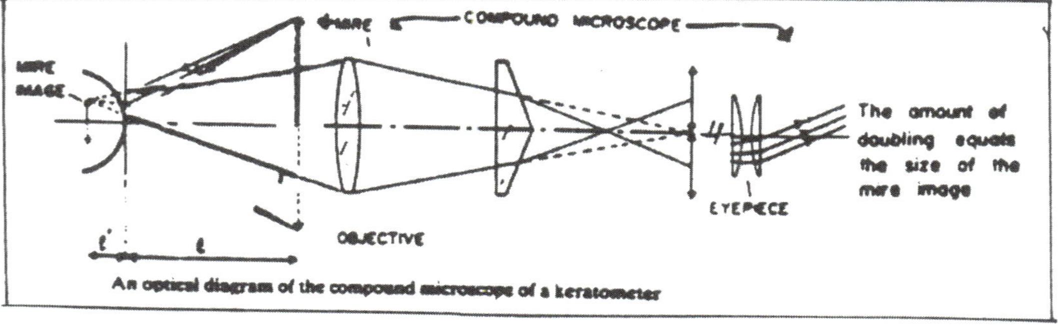

An optical diagram of the compound microscope of a keratometer

7. Gonioscopy

- A **Gonioscopic lens** allows us to visualize and assess the anterior chamber angle as we, as well as the peripheral fundus of dilated patients in greater magnification and detail
  - Its use is indicated for glaucoma suspects, narrow angles through Van Herrick estimation (determine if truly a narrow angle prior to dilation), history of trauma (angle recession via overexposure of the ciliary body suggests a damaged trabecular meshwork), and lesions or abnormalities of the angle.
- Indentation gonioscopy allows one to determine if a closed angle results from synechiae or mere apposition (which can be treated with Laser Peripheral Iridotomy).
- Due to **total internal reflection** (light trapped in the incident medium), it is normally not possible to view the anterior chamber angle because light from the angle undergoes total internal reflection at the air-tear film interface. Thus the light from the angle cannot leave the eye, making the angle impossible to visualize without the aid of a gonio lens.
- The gonio lens is a cone shaped device that is placed on the eye using a cushioning solution as an interface. The higher index of refraction of the lens compared to air allows viewing of the angle structures as light from the angle leaves the eye, enters the gonioscopic mirror and gets reflected by the gonioscopic mirrors
- Gonioscopic tilt angle should be 7.5° to the visual axis to minimize reflection and image distortion

8. Fundoscopy

- A **fundus lens** functions to view the posterior fundus through increased magnification and field of view.
- Used in conjunction with a slit lamp the fundus lens is placed near but not in contact with the eye. The slit lamp light source is shown through the lens and enables viewing of posterior structures of the eye such as the optic disc, retinal blood vessels, macula, foveal reflex, and posterior pole. The mid-peripheral or peripheral retina can be view by directing the patient's gaze.

Chapter 2 – Optics (Physical)

WAVE OPTICS

- The ray model for light cannot explain phenomena like interference, diffraction, and polarization
- Thus we must adopt a model to describe how light travels. Excited electrically charged particles radiate energy, which travels in waves.

1. Characteristics of Wave Motion

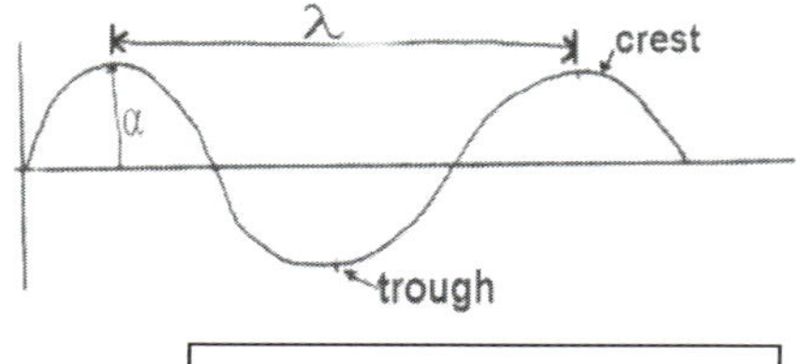

- **Transverse Wave:** energy propagates forward, but the oscillation of the wave is perpendicular to the direction of travel. You can move energy without transporting themedia
- Definitions of Wave Variables:
  - **-Amplitude (A)**: Maximum value of displacement
  - **-Crest**: Maxima
  - **-Trough**: Minima
  - **-Wavelength (λ)**: Distance between 2 adjacent crests on consecutive wave fronts. This is the linear distance of a cycle
  - **-Frequency (f)**: Number of waves passing a given point per unit time
    - **-Unit of Frequency**: Hertz: number of cycles/second
  - **-Period (T)**: Time for 1 cycle to pass a given point; T=1/f
  - **-Velocity (v)**: Speed of wave (measured in m/s)
  - **-Intensity (I)**: Amount of energy that flows per second across a unit area in direction of travel

Variable Relationships:

$\mathbf{I \propto A^2}$

$\mathbf{f=1/T}$

$\mathbf{\lambda=VT}$

$\mathbf{V=\lambda f=c/n}$

$\mathbf{\lambda=2\pi f=2\pi/T}$

$\mathbf{c=3x10^8 m/s}$

$\mathbf{\lambda_m=\lambda/n}$

- **Frequency Invariance**
  - -Speed of light changes as it goes through different media
  - -Frequency remains constant, so wavelength must change

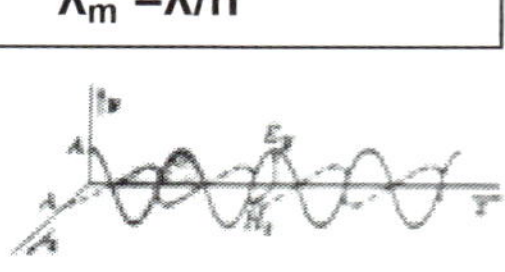

- Diagram of Electric and Magnetic Vectors in a Plane Polarized Wave: Each electric field is associated with its own magnetic field which makes up **electromagnetic radiation**

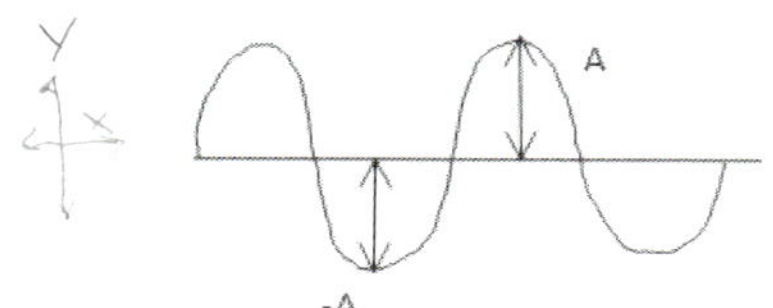

- **Simple Harmonic Motion (SHM)**: simple to and from motion in a continuous sine wave
  - Phase (p)- describes what part of the cycle the transverse wave is in
    - When phase is 0, y=0
    - When phase is 90, y=A.

Simple Harmonic Motion:

$\mathbf{y=A \sin (\lambda T)}$

$\mathbf{y=A \sin (p)}$

- **Superposition Principle:** When two or more low energy waves are superimposed in the same space, the waves travel independently and the resultant displacement of 2 or more waves is the sum of the displacement of their amplitude

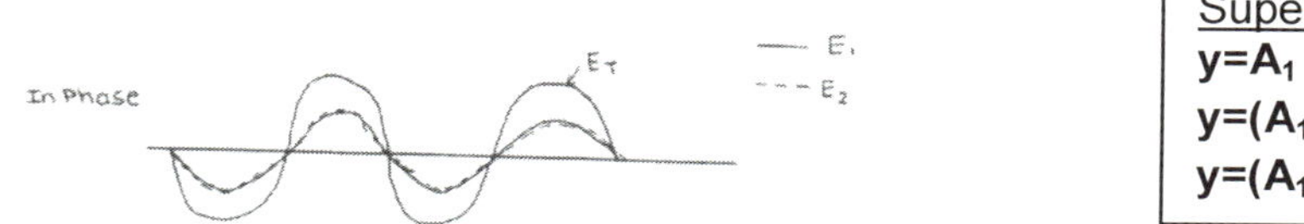

Superposition:

$\mathbf{y=A_1 \sin p_1 + A_2 \sin p_2}$

$\mathbf{y=(A_1+A_2)\sin p_1}$ (phase is the same)

$\mathbf{y=(A_1-A_2) \sin p_1}$ (phase is out by 180 deg)

- The **wave equation** represents the moving wave, and is represented by the propagation number (κ), angular frequency (ω) and the initial phase (ε). When ω is positive, the wave is traveling to the right, when ω is negative, the wave is traveling to the left.

Wave Equation:

$\mathbf{E=A\sin(\kappa x-\omega t+\varepsilon)}$

$\mathbf{\kappa=2\pi/\lambda}$ (propagation number)

$\mathbf{\omega=2\pi f}$ (angular frequency)

$\mathbf{\varepsilon=}$ initial phase (in radians)

2. Classification of the Electromagnetic Spectrum

- The **electromagnetic spectrum** is the range of all possible frequencies of electromagnetic radiation and is classified by wavelength or frequency. It ranges from 0.1A to 1000m (wavelength) or 10^{19}-10^{6} Hz (frequency) There are no sharp dividing lines between various portions of the spectrum, and there are no gaps in the EM spectrum. Adjacent portions overlap and the visible spectrum lies between 380-760nm

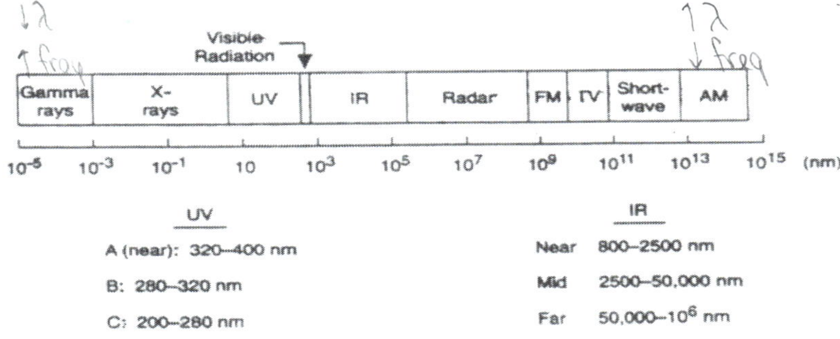

3. Total and Partial Coherence

- **Coherence** is a property of EM radiation from a source. The phase difference between waves is constant with time and the waves can be in or out of phase, as long as the relationship does not change. An example includes laser beams resulting from the stimulated emission that gives total coherence.
- **Mutually Coherent**: when the crest of the first wave is a fixed distance from the crest of the second wave. Resultant of two mutually coherent waves is a new amplitude and phase (same frequency and wavelength). Coherent light sources generally originate from the same light source
- **Incoherence** is where there is no fixed phase relationship, phase changes are completely random
- **Partial coherence** is between the two extremes of total coherence and incoherence. Either path or phase difference changes with time

> Coherence
> $\mathbf{E_1 + E_2 = A_r sin(p_r)}$
> $\mathbf{I_{coherent} = (E_1+E_2)^2}$
> $\mathbf{I_{incoherent} = E_1^2 + E_2^2 = A_1^2 + A_2^2}$

4. Diffraction

- **Diffraction** is the bending of light around an obstacle. It is an interference phenomenon because it takes into account the phase difference between rays passing through various parts of a slit (sub-slits).
- **Fraunhofer diffraction (far field)** is when the screen is far enough away from the slit or the slit is small enough so that all rays from the slit to a point on the screen are parallel.
- **Fresnel diffraction (near field)** occurs when a screen is relatively close to a slit or the slit is relatively wide. Fresnel diffraction becomes Fraunhofer as the screen is moved away

Single Slit Diffraction:

- When a single slit is very small, only one wavelet can come through and the resulting cross-sectional shape of the envelope is circular in shape (indicated a large amount of diffraction and lateral spreading). These secondary wavelets superpose and give a rippled irradiance distribution → the **single slit diffraction pattern**: central maximum area bordered by alternating dark and light bands. Intensity decreases as you move away from the central maxima on a diffraction pattern

  d = slit width
  D = distance from slit to screen
  D >> d

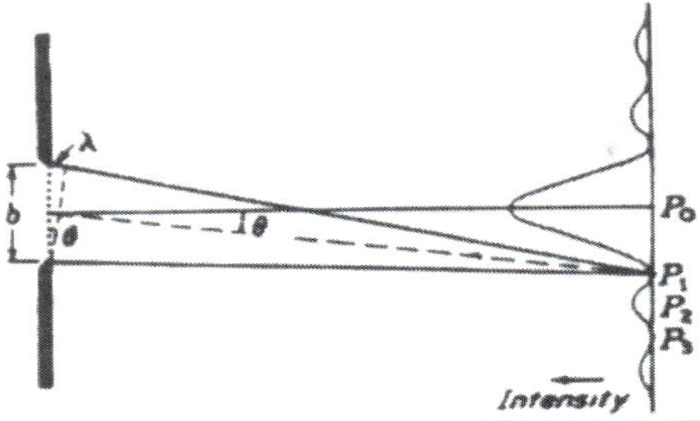

> Single Slit Diffraction
> **Path difference=dsinΘ**
> **Phase difference/2π= Path difference/λ**
> **ϕ/2π=Asin (Θ/λ)**
> Intensity Zeros
> **dsinΘ = mλ;** m = 1, 2, 3, (m= order or maxima)

- For m =0, (As $\Theta \rightarrow 0$ there is no path difference leading to central maximum where Θ is the angular subtense from slit center to first minima (as slit width increases the central maxima narrows).

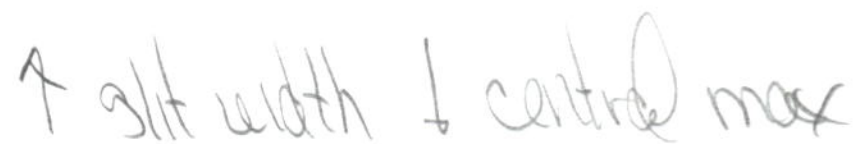

- **Electric Field Amplitude (E_Θ)** – the instantaneous amplitude of a light wave
- **Intensity Profile**: Can be determined by the following equations: given d and λ, for any Θ, intensity can be compared to I_{max} (when Θ=0).

> Electric Field Amplitude
>
> $$E_\Theta = E_{max} \frac{\sin(\phi/2)}{(\phi/2)}$$
>
> Intensity Profile
>
> $$\frac{I_0}{I_{max}} = \frac{\sin(\Theta/2)}{(\Theta/2)}^2 = \frac{\sin(\pi d \sin(\Theta/\lambda))}{\pi d \sin(\Theta/\lambda)}^2$$

Example: *For a 10 λ slit width, what is the angular subtense of the first minima?*

-Slit width =d=10λ m=1 (1st minima)

> **Answer:**
> -Since $d\sin\Theta = m\lambda$
> $10\lambda \sin\Theta = 1\lambda$, $\Theta = 5.73$ degrees

- **Circular Apertures:** When illuminated by a monochromatic plane wave of light, the waves are defracted equally in all directions, resulting a in a diffraction pattern with a central maximum bright disk surrounded by a first minimum (less bright ring) and a series of progressively less intense rings that are separated by rings of zero intensity. The smaller the aperture, the larger the diffraction. When the center maximum is surrounded by the first minimum, it is called **Airy's Disk.** The boundary for Airy's disk is given by the first minimum which has angular location given by the following equation.

  d = diameter of aperture

  Θ= measured from straight-ahead maximum to first zero ring

  - Airy's disk is larger with a larger Θ.
  - The longer the wavelength, the larger the diffraction pattern

> 1st Minimum Angular Location
> $$d \sin \Theta = 1.22 \lambda$$

***Example**: λ=600 nm. What is the diameter of the central maximum for a pinhole of 0.05 mm radius if the screen is 6m away?*

x

Θ

6m

d=0.10 mm

> **Answer:**
> $d\sin\Theta = 1.22\lambda$
> $(0.0001\text{m}) \sin\Theta = 1.22(600\text{x}10^{-9}\ \text{m})$
> $\Theta = 0.419$
> $\tan\Theta = x/6$
> x=0.044m; radius = 4.4cm or diameter = 8.8cm

- **Limits of Resolution**: Diffraction places a limit on the ability of a system to transmit perfect information about the object. For the human eye, the pupil forms a circular aperture. The smaller the aperture size, the greater the diffraction, and the larger Airy's disk. Two separate point sources will have their own Airy's disk. As the aperture size decreases the Airy's disks increase and overlap, until eventually the two point sources cannot be resolved from each other.

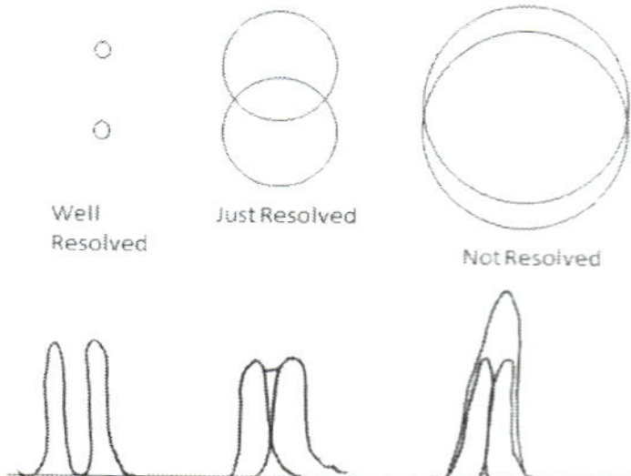

  - **Rayleigh Criterion** – 2 point sources can be resolved if diffraction patterns are small or sufficiently separated to be distinguished. This occurs when the first minimum of one coincides with the center maximum of the other.
  - It is this criterion that allows the human eye to see two stars in the sky as being separate entities (d=diameter of aperture)

> Rayleigh Criterion
> $$\Theta_{min} = 1.22\ \lambda/d$$

Example: Using a pinhole camera, how close can 2 dots 20 ft away be and still be resolved?

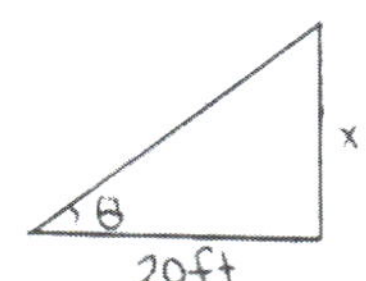

d=0.5mm, λ=555nm

Answer:

$\sin\Theta = 1.22\ \lambda/d$

$\sin\Theta = 1.22(555\text{x}10^{-9}\ \text{m})/(0.5\text{x}10^{-3}\ \text{m})$

$\Theta = 7.76\text{x}10^{-2}$

$\tan\Theta = x/20\ \text{ft}$

$x = 0.027\ \text{ft}$

- **Zone Plates**: Monochromatic plane waves are incident on a diffraction grating made of circular "slits." Due to the circular symmetry, the diffracted waves also have a circular symmetry and are diffracted inward or outward. This set of radially symmetric rings (Fresnel Zones) alternate between opaque and transparent. Light hitting the zone plate will diffract around the opaque zones. These zones can be spaced to make light contructively/destructively interfere to form a "point image."

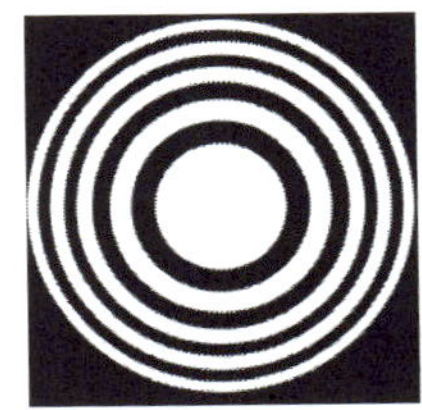
Binary Zone Plate

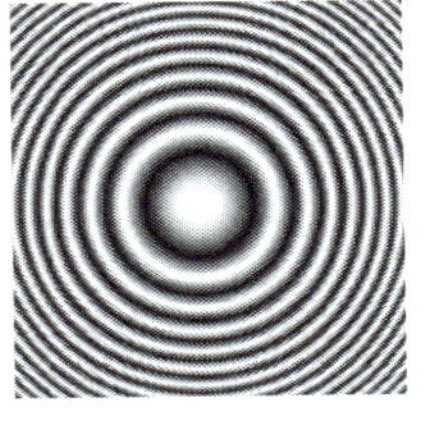
Sinusoidal Zone Plate

- By forming an extended image by diffraction, a zone plate can function like a lens. Zone plates have been used to block light waves so that the resulting zone plate acts like a lens with a focal length and dioptric power. Zone plates are able to focus light using diffraction instead of refraction like typical lenses.

5. Interference

Constructive interference:

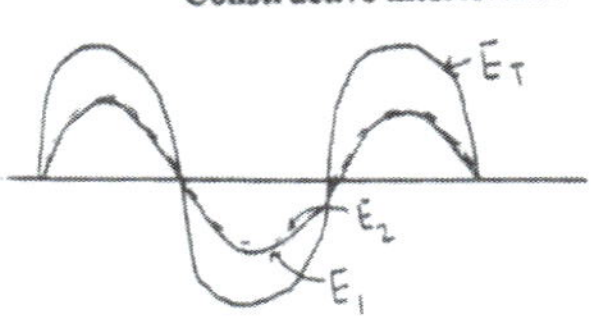

Destructive interference:

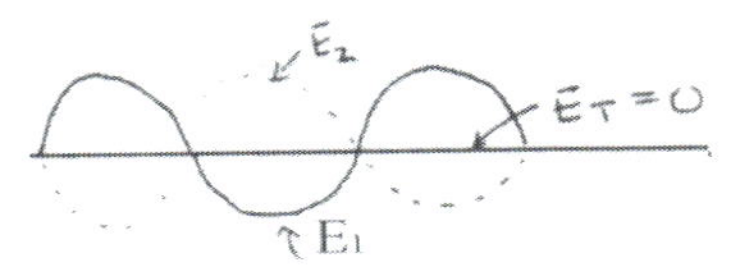

- Interference is the modification of intensity by superposition of 2 or more waves. It is based on the superposition principle so that the net effect is the sum of the separate effects.
- **Constructive Interference:** 2 waves are in phase; the resultant intensity is greater than the separate intensities (i.e., the waves are additive).
- **Destructive Interference:** 2 waves are out of phase; resultant intensity is zero or less than the intensities of each wave (i.e., the waves subtract one another)
- Resultant Intensity is 4 times that of 1 wave.

$$\frac{I_\alpha\ A^2}{I_\alpha\ A_o} = \frac{(2A_o)^2}{A_o^2} = \frac{4A_o^2}{A_o^2} = 4\text{x initial intensity}$$

Intensity
$I = (\text{Constant})\ A^2$
Resultant Intensity
$I_R = C\ (2A)^2 = 4I$

Young's Double Slit Interference:

- When passing a light source through 2 slits, one can generate an interference pattern by interfering the light with itself. The interference arises from the difference in path lengths between 2 mutually coherent sources of light

  d = distance between slits

  D = distance from screen to slits

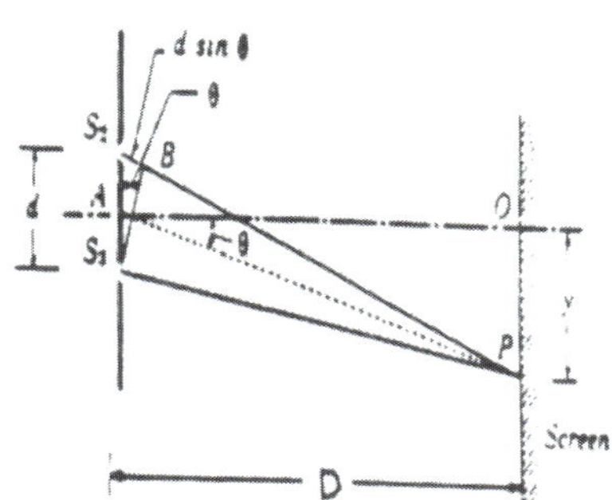

$\lambda << d$ there are several closely spaced fringes near 0, and Θ is small.

- Using small angle approximation:
  $\Theta = \sin\Theta = \tan\Theta$ so then $d\sin\Theta = d\tan\Theta = \Theta$
  $\tan\Theta = y/D$, By substitution: $d\Theta = dy/D = m\lambda$
  $Y_m = m\lambda D/d$ used to calculate λ,
  if you measure D, d, and Y_m
  Y_m is the distance to the "m"th fringe.

Intensity Maxima:
$d\sin\Theta = m\lambda_1$ $m = 0, 1, 2, 3....$
Intensity Minima:
$d\sin\Theta = (m+1/2)\lambda$
Double Slit
$Y = D\lambda/d$

***Example**: For 0.3mm slit separation, illuminated with 589nm light, to get a 2mm separation between light fringes, how far should the slits be from the screen?*

> ***Answer:***
> $X = D\lambda/d$
> $0.002m = D(5.89\times10^{-7}m)/0.0003m$
> $D = 1m$

Multiple Slit Interference:

- Diffraction gratings with multiple slits. You get diffraction and interference patterns superimposed. When a diffraction minimum equals an interference maximum, the interference maximum is not seen. Diffraction gratings are usually specified by # lines/inch.
  $d\sin\Theta = m\lambda$
  $m = 0,1,2,3...$ principal maxima
  1st order maxima: $m=1$
  2nd order maxima: $m=2...$
- The number of orders is limited by $\sin\Theta$ (remember $\sin\Theta$ cannot be >1). With increasing numbers of slits (n), you get n-z smaller, less intense maxima between major maxima. With a grating (large number of slits) – the intensity is more directed, there is a thinner principal maximum (narrow fringe), and the 2nd maximum gets smaller in intensity. When using phase diagrams: $\Delta\phi$ is the change in phase difference between adjacent slits or between the principle max and nearest zero.
  P = order of diffraction minima
  b = slit width
  m = order of interference maxima
  d = slit separation

Multiple Slit Interference
$P/b = m/d$

***Example**: If b= 10 and d= 30, what order interference maxima will be covered by the first order diffraction minima?*

> ***Answer:***
> p=1
> 1/10 = m/30
> m = 3, the third interference max

Thin Film Interference:

- When light hits a surface, it can be absorbed, transmitted, or reflected. Light can reflect off any interface where there is a change in refractive index.
- **Rule for Reflection**: when the index of refraction after the interface (n_2) is higher than the index of refraction before the interface (n_1), then the light upon reflection undergoes a 180° phase shift. When n_2 is lower than n_1 there is no phase shift.
- When light hits multiple layers, each layer can reflect light from the top surface and refract light through the medium. Of the refracted light, some is reflected off the bottom surface.

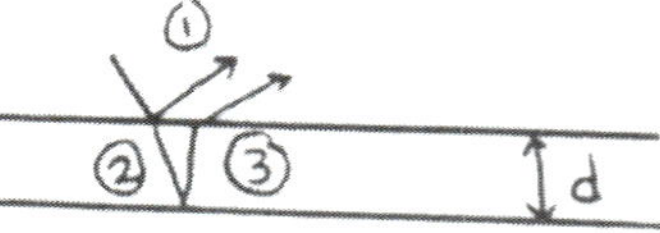

- The two reflected waves can interfere constructively or destructively. This depends on the round trip path difference (2d or 2t/n) and the phase shift of 180° if $n_2 > n_1$. This property is employed when manufacturers design anti-reflective coatings for lenses (see below).

n' > n 180° phase shift
n > n' no phase shift

- The **path difference** must be within the **coherence length** (length in space over which the light has a predictable phase)

  n = refractive index

  d = thickness

  Θ is found by Snell's Law

  If light travels from low n to high n = 180° phase shift.

  (nt is defined as the **optical thickness of the film**)
- Constructive interference occurs when the difference in waves is some integer multiple of the wavelength.

Path Difference
$2nd\cos\Theta$
Thin Film
$2t = \frac{1}{2}(\lambda_o/n)$
$nt = \lambda_o/4$ OT = λ/4
Constructive interference occurs at:
$2t = (m + \frac{1}{2})\lambda_o/n$
Destructive interference occurs at:
$2t = (m)\lambda_o/n$

Example: A glass slab of thickness λ/4 surrounded by air.

AIR	n=1.00
GLASS	n=1.53 ↕d
AIR	n=1.00

Wave 1 is reflected at the glass interface and is 180° out of phase from its original phase. Wave 2 travels λ/2 further then Wave 1 (2 x λ/4). It does not change phase when it reflects at the air-glass interface, so it is also 180° out of phase. Therefore Waves 1 and 2 are in phase with each other and the amplitudes add.

Anti-Reflective Coatings (ARCs):

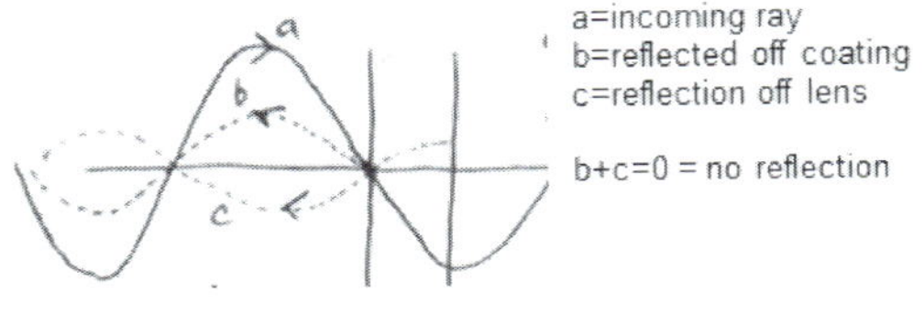

- By putting a coating on the surface of glasses, the amount of reflection is minimized through destructive interference, which automatically increases the amount of transmission. Destructive interference now occurs at $2t = (m + \frac{1}{2})\lambda_o/nf$ where m = 0, 1, 2, 3, etc.
- For complete destructive interference, the amplitudes of ray 1 and 2 must be the same ($r_1 - r_2 = 0$) → the reflectivity of the air-coating interface and the coating-glass interface must be the same:

  $r_1 = (n_c - n_{air})/(n_c + n_{air})$

  $r_2 = (n_g - n_c)/(n_g + n_c)$

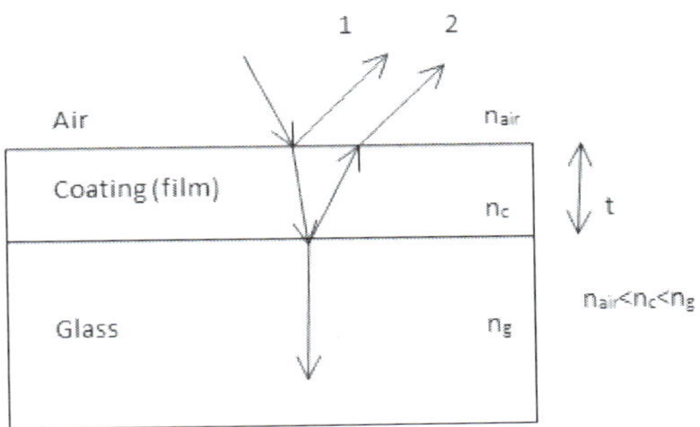

- Two conditions must be met for ARC:

  1. Amplitude condition: Resultant amplitude is the difference between the two amplitudes so total destructive interference occurs→$n_c = \sqrt{(n_g)(n)}$

  n_c = index of ARC

  n_g = index of underlying material (material coated by the ARC)

  2. Path condition: To achieve destructive interference of the light incident on the surface and the light emerging from the surface. →$t = \lambda/(4n_c)$

  t=thickness of the coating

  n_c=index of ARC
- ARC thickness of a single layer (t) is the same as the path condition

Reflectance Equation for Amplitude
$r = (n'-n)/(n'+n)$
Amplitude Condition
$n_c = \sqrt{(n_g)}$
Path Condition
$t_{dest} = \lambda/(4n_c)$
ARC Thickness
$t = \lambda/(4n_c)$

***Example**: What coating would be used for a crown glass lens in air?*

> ***Answer:***
>
> $n_c = \sqrt{(1.0)(1.523)}$
>
> $n_c = 1.23$ (closest coating is MgF_2 with an n=1.38)

Holography:

- A technique that utilizes a very complicated diffraction grating or zone plate that when properly illuminated, results in diffracted waves (maximums) that can be reconstructed to form images of an object when an imaging system (eye) is placed in the reconstructed light, even when the object is no longer there. The diffracted waves are actually reconstructions of the waves that would come from real objects. The observer viewing them sees the objects in three dimensions because the image changes as the position and orientation of the viewing system changes. The holographic recording itself it not an image, but consists of a random structure of varying intensity, density, and/or profile. How it works:

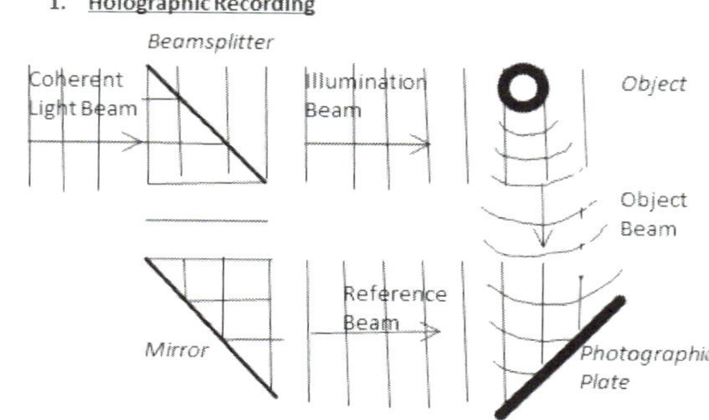

1. **Holographic Recording**
   - Light scattered from an object falls on a recording medium
   - A second "reference' light beam illuminates the recording medium to create interference between the two beams, which results in a light field generating a random pattern of varying light intensity (hologram).
2. Holographic Reconstruction
   - The original reference beam illuminates the hologram, the light gets **diffracted** to produce a light field identical to the previous light scattered by the original object. This is a **virtual image** (divergent rays)

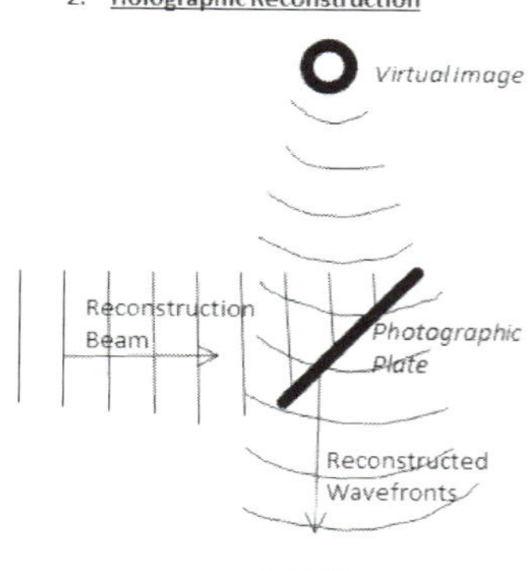

6. Scattering

- Scattering depends on the size of the particles, distance between particles, and the strength of the interaction between particles and light, which depends on refractive index and absorption strength of the particles
- **Rayleigh Scattering**: Describes scattering of light by particles whose size is must smaller than the wavelength of light (λ). It is *wavelength dependent*. Theoretically, the scattering dependence of the intensity of light depends directly on the 4th power of the wavelength. Blue (short wavelength) light is scattered 3.3 times more than red (long wavelength) light which is more transmitted, and thus scattering of sunlight off of the small transparent air molecules in the atmosphere causes the sky to appear blue.

Rayleigh Scattering
$\mathbf{I_{scat} = k\ (I/\lambda^4)}$

- **Tyndall Scattering:** Describes scattering of light by small particles which are somewhat similar in size to the wavelength of light (λ) and are suspended in liquid or gas. It is *wavelength independent*. The scattering of light by larger water molecules or ice crystals in clouds give them the appearance of being white, this is Tyndall Scattering. Tyndall effect can be demonstrated by the slit lamp biomicroscope and in blue irises. Due to the absence of melanin (which absorbs light), light can randomly pass and diffusely scatter through the translucent iris. Since scattering occurs more by shorter wavelengths, an iris without pigment that is translucent will appear blue due to reflection and scattering.

7. Dispersion

- **Dispersion** describes the property that different frequencies of EM radiation travel through a material at different speeds. Dispersion is responsible for **chromatic aberration** and as a consequence separates white light into its individual color wavelengths (prismatic effect).
- The phase velocity of light (v) depends upon the refractive index of the medium (n) in relation to the speed of light in a vacuum (c).
  - The higher the refractive index, the slower the wave travels through the medium.
- The velocity is also a function of the wavelength(λ) and frequency (f) of the incoming light, and thus refractive index is some function of frequency and wavelength of light.
  - The refractive index depends on density (δ) of the medium as well.
  - The wavelength dependency of the refractive index is related to the material absorption (k).
- According to Snell's law, the angle of refraction of light in a prism is dependent on the prism refractive index. Thus, the angle that light is refracted also depends on wavelength, which causes an angular separation of colors (**angular dispersion**) where blue light (higher refractive index) bends more than red light.
  - A path difference occurs due to small changes in λ.
  - Dispersion (D) = $\delta\Theta=\delta\lambda=m/d\cos\Theta_m$ at a given maximum m.

Dispersion
v=c/n=λf
(D) = $\delta\Theta=\delta\lambda=m/d\cos\Theta_m$

$n=\frac{c}{V_n}=\lambda(f)$ $n=\frac{\lambda_o}{\lambda_n}$

INTERACTION OF LIGHT AND MATTER

---

1. Atomic Energy Levels, Absorption, and Emission Line Spectra

- Light can be described as both a wave and a particle. The **quantum theory** of light describes electromagnetic radiation to be noncontinuous, and to come in packets of light called **photons**. Photons exhibit both wave and particle-like behavior.

  h = Planck's constant (**$6.63\text{x}10^{-34}$Js**)
  f = frequency
  E applies to both absorption & emission of energy.
  c= speed of light in a vacuum (**$3\text{x}10^{8}$m/s**)
  λ= wavelength (nm)

Energy of a Photon
E=hf=hc/λ

- The **Bohr Model** of the atom describes negatively charged electrons orbiting a positive atomic nucleus in discrete **atomic energy levels**. Each atom has certain allowable energy states. Normal state or "ground state" is the lowest energy level of an atom, and is the stable state of the atom. Excited states encompass all higher levels, and are not stable. Each atom has allowable electron energy levels. Bohr described the hydrogen atom where E_m represents the energy level, and m=0,1,2,3...
- An electron can jump to a lower energy level by emitting a photon and an electron can jump to a higher level by absorbing a photon.

Energy Levels of Hydrogen Atom
$E_m=\frac{-13.6eV}{(m+1)^2}$
E_0=-13/6eV –Ground state

***Example**: What is the energy and wavelength of a photon emitted when an electron in hydrogen jumps from E_3 to E_1?*

Answer:
E_3=-13.6eV/$(4)^2$= -0.85eV
E_1=-13.6eV/$(2)^2$= -3.4eV
ΔE= -0.85eV- (-3.4eV)=2.55eV
λ=1239eVnm/2.55eV=486nm

- **Line Spectra:** Are spectrum from a monatomic gas light source. Wavelengths emitted are characteristic of the element emitting the light. Absorption line spectrum is a dark series of lines corresponding to λ absorbed. **Absorption** occurs as the atom's internal energy increases and there is a decrease in the intensity of light.
- **Emission Line Spectra**: Occurs when an atom goes from an excited state to a lower state.
- **Continuous Spectra**: Incandescent solid or liquid light source. All λ are present. Energy is determined by temperature not by material.

2. Continuous Spectra

- **Black Body Radiator:** A blackbody is a material that absorbs most of the incident light. According to **Kirchoff's law**, the amount of electromagnetic radiation emitted (E) is proportional to the amount absorbed (A). An ideal blackbody (A=1) is the strongest emitter of radiant energy. Since the surface absorbs all incident radiant energy, it appears as black. According to **Wein's Displacement Law**, the peak wavelength (λ_{max}) is inversely related to the Temperature(Kelvin) of the blackbody radiator. The total irradiance (I_t) is directly proportional to the 4th power of the Temperature(K) according to the **Stefan-Boltzman Law**.
- A **Gray Body Radiator** is not a perfect absorber (A<1).

Kirchoff's Law

$$\mathbf{E_1=A_1I}$$

$$\mathbf{E_1/A_1=E_2/A_2}$$

Wien's Displacement Law

$$\boldsymbol{\lambda_{max} = \frac{2.9 \times 10^6\ (nm \cdot k)}{T(k)}}$$

Stefan-Boltzman Law

$$\mathbf{I_t = \frac{constant}{T^4}}$$

3. Fluorescence (Photons, Energy Levels

- Fluorescent materials absorb high frequency (short wavelength) radiation and transitioning them to a higher energy level ($E_0 \rightarrow E_2$). The electron then emits a photon of lower frequency (longer-wavelength) than what was absorbed. The re-emitted quantum is at a lower energy; loss of energy results in visible light. Thus, a fluorescent material can absorb UV light, and emit visible spectrum light
  - For fluorescence, the incident radiation must have the energy needed for the electron to jump from the ground state → $\Delta E=E_2-E_0$ must be a positive number.

Example: *Can a material with energy levels of E_0=-10.0eV, E_1=-8.0eV, and E_2=-5.5eV fluoresce? What incident wavelength is needed to excite the material? What wavelengths are emitted?*

Answer:

ΔE= -5.5eV – (-10.0eV)= +4.5eV

ΔE>1 so material is fluorescent.

Incident wavelength needed:

λ=1239nm-eV/4.5eV= 275nm (UV)

Emitted wavelengths:

$E_2 \rightarrow E_1$:

$$\lambda = \frac{1239\ \text{nm-eV}}{-5.5\text{eV} - (-8.0\text{eV})} = 496\text{nm}$$

$E_1 \rightarrow E_0$:

$$\lambda = \frac{1239\ \text{nm-eV}}{-8.0\text{eV} - (-10.0\text{eV})} = 620\text{nm}$$

4. Lasers

- Lasers (Light Amplification of Stimulated Emission of Radiation)
- LASERS produce an intense beam of coherent light (in phase).
- **Theory of Operation**: A photon is used to trigger a stimulated emission resulting in 2 coherent photons (same wavelength) traveling in the same direction, which stimulate another emission of 4 coherent photons. The mechanism of **light amplification** requires that atoms be in a higher energy state with electrons lingering longer than usual. More electrons are in an excited meta-stable state (E_1) than normal and emitted photons reflect back and forth (in a closed chamber) through excited

atoms and perpetuate the process. This creates an **inverted population** (more atoms in higher state than lower state) so that there is a net emission instead of absorption, resulting in amplification.

- **The Speckle Pattern**: Speckles are the granular appearance of diverged laser beam; they always appear sharp. They are created at the retina and are interference patterns of diffusely reflected coherent light. Light reflected from a surface enters the eye producing speckles that cause constructive interference on the retina. Motion parallax occurs when the ametropic observer moves his head sideways. This can be used for laser refraction. With increased viewing distance the granules increase in size.
    - **Emmetrope**: sees no motion
    - **Hyperope**: sees with motion
    - **Myope**: sees against motion

5. Spectral Transmission

- Light incident on an object is transmitted after it is reflected or absorbed. The amount of light transmitted depends upon the thickness of the material, and the material's transmittance factor. The color of a lens will tent to transmit color of its own wavelength and absorb the color farthest from it in the spectrum.

    I_x=amount of transmitted light

    I_o=amount of light passing front surface

    x=number of units of equal thickness having a transmittance factor q

    q=transmittance factor- represents the transmission characteristics of the lens

- Transmission is given in %, Transmittance is given in decimal point
- **Total transmission** takes into account the reflection of light off the front of the lens.

    I_f=light incident on the front

    R_f=reflection of light at the front

- **Opacity (O)** – reciprocal of transmittance
- **Optical Density (OD)**- Absorbance

Transmission

$I_x = I_o(q^x)$

Total Transmission

$T = [(I_f - R_f)q^x]\ [1 - R_f]$

$T = (1 - R_f)^2 q^x$ if $I_f = 1$

Optical Density

$OD = \log_{10} O$

$T = 10^{-OD}$

Chapter 3 – Optics (Physiological)

REFRACTIVE STATES

- **Refractive Error**: problems in vision caused by the eye's inability to refract light and focus it clearly on the retina (myopia, hyperopia, astigmatism, anisometropia, and presbyopia)
    - The cornea provides 2/3 of the eye's refractive power, acts like a +43D lens
    - The lens provides 1/3 of the eye's refractive power, acts like a 20D lens
- **Emmetropic eye:** cornea and unaccommodated lens converge light from a distant object to form a clear image on the muscle
- **Myopia** (Nearsightedness): Unaccommodated eye forms the image of a distant object (parallel rays) in front of the retina in the vitreous. At some near object position, the object will be close enough so that the image point is formed on the retina
    - Etiology:
        - **Simple (Correlation Ametropia):** Axial length is too long (most common) and/or the cornea is too steep/lens power too high
        - **Pathologic**: Axial length/refractive power error caused by disease
    - Types
        - **Juvenile Onset**: onset at 8-12 years, common
            - The earlier the onset, the greater the amount of myopia in adulthood
        - **Adult (Late) Onset:** onset between mid-20s to mid-30s, rare
            - Rarely more than -1.00 or -2.00D

	P_{eye}	$Length_{eye}$	Etiology
Refractive Myopia	>60D	=22.6mm	Steep corneal curvature or high lenticular powers
Axial Myopia	=60D	>22.6mm	Too Long. *Every mm of axial elongation causes 3D of myopia*
Refractive Hyperopia	<60D	=22.6mm	Flat corneal curvature or low lenticular powers
Axial Hyperopia	=60D	<22.6mm	Too short.

- **Hyperopia eye** (Farsightedness): Unaccommodated eye does not converge an image prior to the retina so blur points formed. Image is formed "behind" the retina.
    - Compensation for myopia = accommodation
    - Compensation affected by fatigue, illness, mental state, alcohol, drugs, and age
    - Etiology
        - **Simple**: Axial length too short and/or cornea too flat
    - Total Hyperopia = Facultative + Absolute = Manifest + Latent
        - **Facultative**: Amount of hyperopia that can be overcome by accommodation
        - **Absolute**: Amount of hyperopia that cannot be overcome by accommodation
        - **Manifest**: Amount of hyperopia revealed by non-cycloplegic methods of refraction
        - **Latent**: Amount of additional hyperopia revealed with cycloplegics
- **Astigmatism**: most common refractive error. Refractive condition in which a variation of power exists in the different meridians of the eye (principal meridians – greatest and least power)
    - Etiology**:**
        - **Corneal**: Unequal curvature of the cornea. Most common
        - **Lenticular**: Unequal curvature on the surface or in the layers of the lens or the lens is tilted.
    - Types
        - **With the Rule (WTR)**: greatest refractive power is between 60-120°. Correct with minus cylinder lens on Horizontal axis
        - **Against the Rule (ATR)**: greatest refractive power between 30-150°. Correct with minus cylinder lens on Vertical axis
        - **Oblique**: greatest refractive power between 30-60° or 120-150°. Correct with minus cylinder lens on the Oppositve axis. Least common type

- Classification
    - **Simple**: one of the principal refractive meridians focused on the retinal surface and the other meridian NOT focused on the retinal surface
    - **Compound**: both of the principal refractive meridians are NOT focused on the retinal surface
    - **Mixed**: One meridian focused in front of the retina and one meridian focused behind the retina
- **Anisometropia**: difference in refractive errors of the two eyes by at least 1.00D
  - **Antimetropia**: difference in the type of refractive errors between the two eyes (one hyperopic, one myopic)
  - Etiology: **Axial, Refractive, or Pathological** (cataract)
- **Presbyopia**: Reduction in accommodative ability that occurs normally with age. Available amplitude of accommodation insufficient to sustain clear vision at primary working distance. Due to decreased elasticity of the crystalline lens.
  - Types
    - **Beginning, Borderline, Incipient**: caused by medications and UV
    - **Functional**: Partial, Absolute, Premature, Nocturnal

1a. Epidemiology

- **Epidemiology:** The study of the distribution of refractive errors is based upon many studies, using different methods on different populations. Thus general trends have been found.
- **Distribution of Ametropia**: Among adults over 25 two features of the distribution are:
  - The curve is leptokurtic (peaked) showing; most people have low RE's
  - The curve is skewed towards myopia

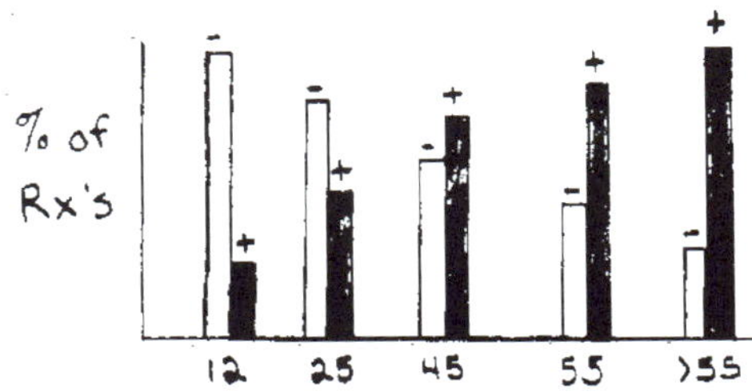

Emmetropization:

- There are several factors that contribute to the refractive status of the eye: axial length, corneal curvature, anterior chamber depth, lens, etc. All of these except axial length are normally distributed. The correlation of all these factors leads to a peaked distribution.
- Most ametropias are due to the components being within normal ranges, but not fully correlating to emmetropia. Only a few ametropia are due to one or more of the factors falling outside normal ranges. The first cases are called **correlation ametropia** and the second cases called **component ametropia.**

Changes with Age: (amount of refractive error changes considerably during the first 5 years of age)

- **Premature infants**
  - High incidence of myopia.
  - Amount of myopia increases as birth weight decreases
  - By age 1, mean RE in premature babies is similar to regular babies
  - Often $\geq$ 2.00D ATR astigmatism
- **Infants**
  - Wide (Normal) distribution of refractive errors at birth, with peak from emmetropic to low hyperopia. Average refractive error is +2.00D
  - Infant cornea is steep, axial length short
  - High rates of astigmatism (usually ATR) in first 6 months that quickly declines
- **Preschool Children**
  - <2% children entering elementary school myopic

- With rapid growth, emmetropization takes place with peaked distribution centered at +1.00 D by age 4
- The earlier myopia appears, the more likely it will progress to higher amount of myopia
- Astigmatism decreases during preschool years

- **School Age/High School**
  - Increasing myopia at the expense of emmetropia with hyperopia remaining about the same. Myopic shift due to elongation of eye
  - >15% of entering high school students have become myopic
  - Corneal curvature stays the same after ~age 2
  - Axial length continues to grow,
  - Decrease in lens power, lens thickness, and lens refractive index in early childhood
  - Lens stops changing in juvenile phase (9-10 years), but the axial lengths continues to grow
  - Teens – slight increase in WTR
- **Younger Adults (Ages 20-40)**
  - Very stable over the mid-adult years. 25% overall prevalence of myopia in adults
  - Slight ATR shift
- **Middle Aged Adults (Ages 40-60)**
  - Hyperopic shift due to lenticular changes.
    - Cortical cataracts cause hyperopic shit (Increased index of refraction in periphery of lens)
  - Increase in ATR Astigmatism.
  - Presbyopia and latent hyperopia becomes manifest

Age	Ametropia
Premature Infants	-Myopia -ATR Astigmatism (≥ 2.00D)
Babies	-Low hyperopia (+2.00D) -High rates of Astigmatism 1st 6 months
Preschool	-Emmetropization -Decrease in Astigmatism
School Age/High School	-Myopic shift -Slight increase in WTR
Younger Adults (Ages 20-40)	-Stable refractive error -Slight increase in ATR
Middle-Age Adults (Ages 40-60)	-Hyperopic Shift -Increase in ATR
Elderly	-Increase in ATR -Refractive error shifts variable depending on lenticular changes and pathologic disease

- **Elderly (>60)**
  - Distributions widen primarily due to lens changes and pathologies. Older lens is thicker and darker. Elderly- small changes due to lenticular changes
    - Nuclear cataracts cause myopic shift (higher index of refraction in the center, which bends light more)
    - Peripheral Cataracts – hyperopic shift
    - Systemic disease (diabetes) may cause myopic shift
  - Average rate of change in astigmatism in adults 40-80 years is 0.25D per decade ATR
- **Gender:** Myopia begins earlier in girls
- **Race**
  - Highest Prevalence of Myopia in Asians (75%)
  - Highest Prevalence of Hyperopia in Native Americans, Africans, Caribbean and South Sea Islanders, and Eskimos
  - Highest Prevalence in Native Americans and Hispanics

Type of astigmatism	
Infants	ATR
Teens, young adults	WTR
Older adults	ATR

Changes in Astigmatism:

- Amount of astigmatism in the first 6 months is greater than in the adult population but quickly declines with time. The prevalence of astigmatism >1.00 DC rapidly decreases by 18-24 months and reaches adult levels by 2.5-5.0 yrs.

- The type of astigmatism, whether "with-the-rule" (WTR) or "against-the-rule" (ATR), varies with age. WTR involves greater power (increased corneal steepness) along the vertical meridian. A correction for WTR astigmatism involves an axis along the horizontal meridian (e.g. "axis 180"). ATR involves greater power (increased corneal steepness) along the horizontal meridian. A correction for ATR astigmatism involves an axis along the vertical meridian (e.g. "axis 090"). The following table summarizes the trend of astigmatism with age.

Etiology of Ametropia:

- Heredity: Twin Studies have shown that the closer the genetic ties the greater the similarity of RE's (positive hereditary influence).

Environment:

- The major argument is that near work contributes to myopia. The observation of pseudomyopia as an acquired myopia due to overaccommodation gives some support to this argument.

1b. History and Symptom Inventory

- The complaint of poor vision needs to be investigated during the history to provide clues as to what may be the cause and what the solution might be. A tentative diagnosis is a goal of the history.
- In most cases ametropia is corrected and the patient and doctor are both happy. However, some ametropia may have further consequences.

Myopia

- Symptoms:
  - Patient complains of blurry distance vision, while near vision is fine.
  - Difficulty when reading signs, looking at the chalkboard, or driving at night.
  - Myopes compensate by squinting. Asthenopia tends to be *rare.*
- Significance:
  - Predisposes the patient to a greater chance of retinal degenerations because the retina is stretched thinner. These include **staphyloma** (bulging of the eye surface that includes part of the uvea into an area of thin, stretched sclera) and **retinal detachments**.
  - Myopia may also be due to increased IOP, especially later in life.
  - Myopic shifts are seen due to nuclear cataracts in the lens.
  - Transient myopia may be due to diabetes (may see posterior subcapsular cataract and/or snowflake opacities).

Pseudomyopia

- This is characterized by the late onset of myopia. Occurs after prolonged near work or with emotional disturbance. Cycloplegic refraction usually reveals hyperopia.
- Symptoms: Asthenopia and temporary blurring of distance vision from ciliary muscle spasm.

Hyperopia

- Symptoms:
  - Patient complains of blurry vision at near, difficulty focusing, abnormally small pupils, the inability to sustain near work, and the avoidance of near work
  - Young hyperopes may be able to see at all distances and their symptoms may be more subtle. The far point of a hyperope is behind the retina, and patients use accommodation at both distance and near to compensate for their refractive error.
  - Individuals who lack that accommodative ability (e.g. presbyopes or a patient who has more hyperopia than accommodative compensation) will experience blur at all distances.
  - Cover test may reveal esophoria at near because of increased accommodative convergence to

maintain a clear image of a near target.
  - **Triad: Hyperopia, Miotic Pupils, Esophoria**
- Significance:
  - In youth, hyperopia can lead to an **accommodative esotropia**.
  - Hyperopes also may have greater likelihood of **angle closure glaucoma** since some have smaller estimated angles on the Van Herrick grading system.
  - Causes of hyperopic shifts include cortical cataracts, intraorbital masses or tumors, and macular elevation including hemorrhage, exudates, and edema.

Astigmatism
- Symptoms:
  - Patient complains of blurry vision at both distance and near, asthenopia or tearing due to the changing of focus between the foci, tilting of the head or reading material, and/or slanting of objects.
  - Oftentimes these patients will complain of "double vision" that is not true diplopia but actually images that are overlapping with one another. → Monocular diplopia
- Significance:
  - Unstable astigmatism may be due to keratoconus, diabetes, ptosis, chalazion, or contact lenses (HCL). High astigmatism may lead to meridional amblyopia early in life if left untreated

Anisometropia
- Symptoms
  - Blocking or closing an eye at different distances, poor depth perception, shifting focus between the eyes leading to eyestrain, reported amblyopia, diplopia, and strabismus.
- Significance
  - This can lead to strabismus and **amblyopia ex anopsia** (amblyopia of disuse- amblyopic eye that has lost form discrimination after central fixation disuse). Occurs if left untreated early in life

Presbyopia
- Symptoms:
  - Eyestrain and focusing problems, having to hold reading material further away, reduced acuity at near, constricted pupils, and drowsiness or falling asleep while reading.
- Significance:
  - Early onset of presbyopia may signal pathology such as glaucoma, diabetes, or oculomotor (III) nerve lesions or disease
- Presbyopia is "a reduction in accommodative ability occurring normally with age and necessitating a plus lens addition for satisfactory seeing at near." Amplitude of accommodation is the difference expressed in diopters between the farthest point and nearest point of accommodation with respect to the spectacle plane, the exit pupil, or some other reference point of the eye. There is a predictable graded decline in amplitude throughout one's life. **Hofstetter formulas** were derived from amplitude data of Donder's, Duane and Kaufman.

Max amplitude	25-0.4 x age
Probable amp	18.5- 0.3 x age
Minimum amp	15 - 0.25 x age

- As a rule of thumb, close work will be comfortable when no more than 1/2 of amplitude of accommodation in used. If it is assumed that close work is done at a distance of 40 cm (2.5D accommodation), then a person with 5D or greater of accommodative ability should not require reading glasses or bifocals. A person having only 3D of accommodation should only have to use 1.50D of accommodation and therefore requires a 1.00D reading add.

- Presbyopia gradually increases over a period of 15 to 20 years and then stabilizes. Many low hyperopes will undergo an increase in hyperopia after reading glasses have been worn several months. By removing stress from the visual system the plus reading lenses are no longer sufficient for near work but are just right for distance vision. This may be referred to as the "hyperopia of presbyopia".
- A gradual decrease in accommodative response to contraction of ciliary muscle is almost entirely due to a decrease in the elasticity, or sclerosis, of the lens. Other arguments that presbyopia may be due to a loss of power of the ciliary muscle have largely been rejected. Fincham (1937) observed a great change in the form of the lens capsule in aphakic presbyopes, evidence that the ciliary muscle was very active in the absence of lens substance to offer resistance to it.
- Symptoms associated with presbyopia:
    - Acceptance of near blur
    - Reduced amplitude of accommodation
    - Increased working distance at near
    - Avoidance of near work
    - Fatigue with near work
- Binocular vision - presbyopes seldom complain of asthenopia even though they tend to be highly exophoric at near while wearing their reading correction. Sheedy and Saladin (1975) compared nonpresbyopes to presbyopes and found greater near exophoria in presbyopes (XP' = 8.7pd) than nonpresbyopes (XP' = 2.8pd) and presbyopes had smaller fusional vergence ranges. However presbyopes had no greater fixation disparity at near than nonpresbyopes. In addition, presbyopic fixation disparity curves had lower slopes than those of nonpresbyopes. Lower slope is associated with efficient and comfortable vision.
- Fry and Jones concluded that the presbyope maintains single binocular vision by nearly unrestricted use of accommodative convergence. Thus they can use accommodative convergence (via the ACA) without getting the reflex occurrence of accommodation. Innervation for accommodation remains intact.

2. Observations and Recognition of Clinical Signs and Techniques/Skills

A. Interpupillary Distance

- **Interpupillary distance:** the distance between the center of the pupils for any given distance
- **Near PD**: At 40 cm, the patient sights the open left eye of the Dr. The Dr. lines up the PD ruler "0" with the temporal limbus of the pt's right eye. The Dr. reads the scale at the nasal limbus of the pt's left eye.
- **Distance PD:** Without moving the PD ruler from the pt's face after taking the near PD, the Dr. now directs the pt. to look towards his right eye. The Dr. again reads the scale at the nasal limbus of the pt's left eye. This is recorded as DPD/NPD, expecting approximately about a 2-4mm difference.

B. Visual Acuity

Snellen Acuity = 1/MAR

- **Visual Acuity**: quantification of the resolving power of the eye
- VA is recorded as the angular size of the gap for the given optotype (eg. letter, Landolt C) that is the smallest gap the patient can resolve: this gap size is the Minimum Angle of Resolution (MAR). Some tests (Bailey-Lovie) specify in terms of Log MAR. The letter size is that distance at which the letter subtends 5 minutes of arc with detail of 1 minute of arc. Snellen (in feet) or the Metric (in meters) use the fraction **Target Distance/Letter Size (TD/LS).** This fraction is the inverse of MAR.
- Some tests use gratings as targets which are specified in cycles per degree. These can be converted to Snellen by the following equation (i.e. 40 cpd converts to 20/15).

"Snellen denominator = 600/cpd"

- Another notation of VA is that used for the S-Chart
- (Landolt C's) which is the Snell-Sterling Visual Efficiency.

- Its relationship to MAR is "Efficiency = 0.836 x 100%." With 20/20 VA, E = 100%.
- S-Charts come in a series of projector slides and each slide represents a difference of 5% from the next in terms of Efficiency score.

Testing Conditions:

1. Chart distance: The chart should be at least 6m away, because any distance short of infinity will lead to overplussing the patient. At 6m the patient is overplussed 1/6m or 0.17D.
2. Illumination: It is recommended that at least 12-20 foot candles be projected onto the screen.
3. Contrast: Standard Snellen contrast is 90%. Below 30% contrast VA drops off quite steeply. Contrast also drops off with cataracts, amblyopes, and retrobulbar neuritis.
4. Letter Size: To calculate how tall a given Snellen letter should be at a known test distance, one should construct a triangle.

Example: *How tall should a 20/200 letter be at 6m?*

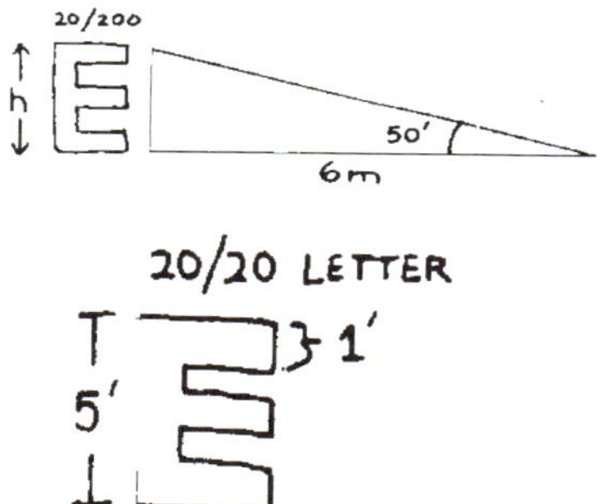

Answer:

Since a 20/200 letter means that its gap size or MAR = 200/20 = 10' and since a standard Snellen letter is 5 gaps tall, then this letter will subtend an angular size of 5 x 10' = 50 minutes of arc. Given the angle and the distance to the letter, the height of the letter is "h = d x tan angle" or in this example,
h = 6m x tan (50/60)degrees = 0.087m or an 87mm tall letter.

Tests of Visual Acuity:

Snellen

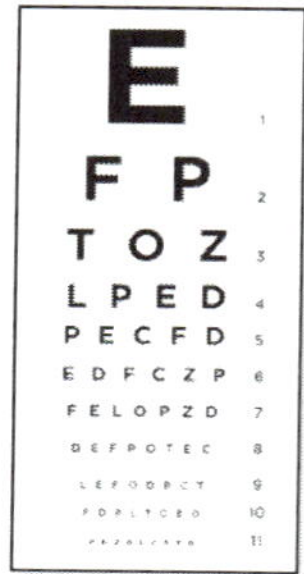

- A letter chart with letters of overall size 5xMAR. The Method of Limits is where the patient goes to the threshold of their ability to correctly identify the letters. Stop and record the line at which the patient misses half the letters. Record the Snellen fraction, plus the number missed/number in that row (eg. 20/40)
    - ADVANTAGE: Fast
- DISADVANTAGE: Task is not constant from line to line
  →different lines have different spacings and different numbers of letters.

Tumbling E

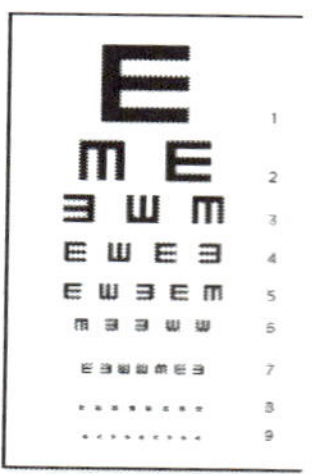

- For non-verbals. The patient identifies the direction of the E. Since chance is 25%, the patient should identify 3 of 4 of the different trials with the same sized E to be awarded that level of VA. E's for Contour Interaction Only

Landolt C

- The patient identifies direction of the gap in the C. Again chance is 25%, so a threshold value must be determined.
    - Eg. Flom Chart (S-Chart)
- Here the 8 C's are presented in a Method of Constant Stimuli and the number correct is plotted. VA is found with the graph depending upon the particular criterion used as threshold. Usually 5 of 8 is considered passing for that level of VA. This represents a 50% value once the score has been corrected for guessing. For the curve below this would lead to a VA of 20/20. Alternately we can assign a Snell-Sterling Efficiency value to the score, as discussed previously.

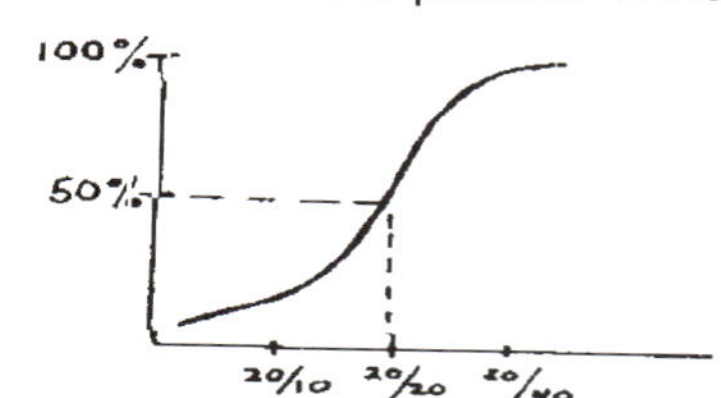

Bailey-Lovie

- ADVANTAGE: Constant task with constant spacings between letters. It can be moved to different distances for low vision patients and the score is easily calculated. A larger LogMAR score is worse VA
- Scoring:

  LogMAR scale is on the right border.
  Each line is a 0.1 difference.
  Each letter is 0.02.
  20/20 is LogMAR 0.0, 20/200 is 1.0, 20/16 is -0.1 (negative is better than 20/20).

LogMAR Score
(Line Score +2) x 0.02/letter

Example: *If a patient gets all except 2 letters on a line, what is their LogMAR score?*

Answer:
(Line score + 2)x 0.02/letter = 0.04.

Changing distances:

- For each 4/5th interval closer to the chart, you add 0.1 to the score. eg. At 16ft you are at 4/5th of the standard 20 ft distance, so if the patient scores a 0.6, you add 0.1 to get a 0.7 corrected score.

Other Visual Acuity Tests

- **Allen preschool Cards** -- these employ figures for kids who don't know letters yet.
- **Broken Wheel** -- The child identifies which of the two cars has broken wheels.

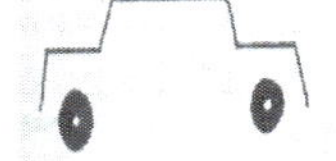
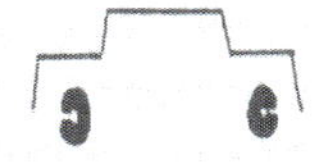

- **Cheerios or Sugar Pellets** -- if the child can see it they get to eat it.
- **Optokinetic Nystagmus (OKN)** -- a striped drum that elicits nystagmus when rotated. This is a very gross measure of VA. Nystagmus signals that the child is seeing the stripes.
- **Preferential Looking (PL)** - the Child is presented two targets: one is a grating while the other is a grey field of equal brightness and equal contrast. The Dr. observes for the child's preferential looking towards the grating,if the grating is detectable as different from the grey field. Reduce the grating size to find the threshold, then interpret this as the level to which the child definitely has good VA. (S)he may be able to see even finer gratings but may not be interested in these targets.

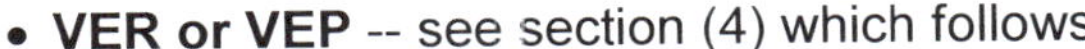

- **VER or VEP** -- see section (4) which follows

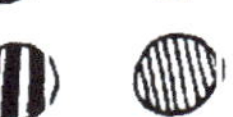
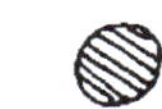

- **Contrast Sensitivity Charts** -- These use both variable contrasts plus variable grating sizes. The task is to identify the orientation of the gratings.
  - ADVANTAGE: This is good for identifying pathologies (i.e. cataracts, glaucoma, retrobulbar neuritis) which cause reduced acuities due to contrast sensitivity losses.
- **Reduced Contrast Snellen Charts** -- These also detect drops in acuity due to pathology, where the sensitivity of a normal 90% contrast Snellen would not be sensitive enough for the patient to see.
- **Lasers** - If we wish to assess potential VA despite degradation due to defects such as cataracts, we need to put a target onto the retina. Lasers can be beamed in past the cataracts such that two beams can interact to create an interference pattern which acts like a grating. The size of the grating can be manipulated until the patient no longer sees any pattern. This can tell us whether the retina has useful vision which will allow the patient to benefit from cataract surgery or if the potential acuity is so poor that such surgery will be of little use.
- **LEA cards** – One of four shapes (apple, house, square, or circle) of various sizes are printed on cards. The cards are held at different distances and the test distance for threshold is measured. The visual acuity is measured by dividing the test distance by the size of the symbol and converted into Snellen units. The clinician may present the cards as forced choice options.

C. Corneal Curvature and Thickness

- **Corneal Measurement** measurements of corneal curvature (K's)

Keratometer

- **Theory:** Mires reflect off the cornea which is shaped like a convex mirror. Knowing the size of the mires, distance to the cornea, and the image location enables us to measure the size of the reflected image. Using the mirror equation the radius of curvature is known. Using an arbitrary index n = 1.3375 (tears), the radius converts to dioptric power
- **Instrument:** 2 vertical apertures act as a Scheiner's Disc so that a single image of the mire is seen only if in focus. 2 horizontal apertures contain prisms to double the image of the mires and allow measurements to be made.

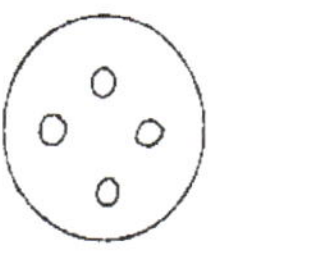

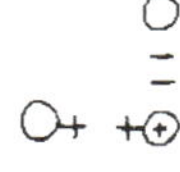

- **Directions:**
  1. Focus the eyepiece
  2. Seat the patient with eye directed towards the center of the tube
  3. Align the cross reticule into the lower right mire, while constantly focusing in order to keep that circle single (focused on the cornea).
  4. Rotate the barrel in order to make the crosses continuous, thus finding the principal meridian
  5. While keeping focus, rotate the left calibrated drum to superimpose the crosses. This drum measures the more horizontal meridian.
  6. Next, rotate the right drum to align the minus signs, thus measuring the more vertical meridian.
- **Interpretation:**
  - Prediction of astigmatism is made using **Javal's Rule**
  - Total Astigmatism (TA)=1.25(K) - 0.50 x090 →Javal's Rule, long method (or + 0.50 axis 180 where K is the corneal toricity)

Javal's Rule (short)
K + 0.50 x 090 (ATR)
Total Astigmatism (long)
TA= 1.25(K) -0.50x090

***Example**: What is the total astigmatism using Javal's Rule of a cornea with the following readings:*
42.00/180 43.00/090

Answer:
ΔK =-1.00 x 180
TA = 1.25 (-1.00 x 180) + 0.50 x 180
TA = -0.75 x 180 (long method)
TA=-0.50 x 180 (short method)

Placido Disc

- A target disc of concentric rings with a peephole for the observer. Reflections off the cornea are observed; large astigmatism (>2.00 DC) is seen as elliptical rings with the long axis of the ellipse as the minus cylinder axis.

Photokeratoscopy

- A placido disc target recorded by photos, which are then measured and the astigmatism found by applying conversion charts.

D. Objective Static and Dynamic Refractive Status, inc. Automatic Refractive Devices

- **Retinoscopy:** This is the primary objective method to assess refractive error. There are two types of retinoscopy: static and dynamic (also called **dynamic skiametry**)

Static Retinoscopy:

- Using plano mirror retinoscope. The patient fixates at distance so accommodation and vergence are relaxed. The principle is to make the far point (Fp) of the eye conjugate to the retinoscope: this is the neutral point. For myopes, since their far point is in real space, it is simply a matter of finding the neutral point where the reflex from the eye is bright and moves infinitely fast. For emmetropes and hyperopes, convex lenses are needed. Motion of the reflex directs what lenses are needed for neutrality.

- If Fp is closer than the working distance, "Against" motion requires minus lenses to neutralize the reflex.
- If Fp is farther than the working distance, "With" motion requires plus lenses to neutralize the reflex.
  -Sources of error:
    - Incorrect working distance: Working closer than calculated causes overplussing.
    - Patient Accommodates: Remind the patient to look at the target and not at the light. If the patient accommodates this leads to overminussing
    - Off Axis: This leads to power and axis errors

Dynamic Retinscopy:

- Begin this procedure with the static retinoscopy or subjective (Dist. rx) in place. Using a fixation target with an accommodative demand at or near the plane of the retinoscope, the observer neutralizes the reflex while moving in towards the patient. In most cases the reflex will be "with," meaning the focus of the eye is beyond the plane of the scope: this is due to the lazy lag of accommodation. Usually it takes +0.75D to neutralize this lag.
- USES
  1. Tentative Add
  2. Measure Rx in young children
  3. Measure of the "full" hyperopia
  4. Distance Rx
- In presbyopes, when neutrality is found, the plus needed is recorded as the tentative add. There is no correction for the working distance. To calculate the distance Rx for a young person based on dynamic retinoscopy, one subtracts the lag from the values in the phoropter. For young children, the Mohindra technique requires the patient to look at the retinoscope. The examiner then neutralizes the reflex usually with lens bars. The neutralizing lens minus 1.25D is the distance Rx.
- Eg. Dist. Rx = NL - 1.25D @ 40cm
- Tips for Mohindra:
  1. Room is completely darkened
  2. Examiner draws child's attention ....
  3. Eye not scoped should be patched

Note: Dynamic retinoscopy is believed to give good results for latent hyperopes, with the Rx approximating the cycloplegic Rx. This is because the accommodative demand involved stresses the system and makes more of the hyperopia manifest.
Note: There are many other variations of dynamic retinoscopy and just as many other applications for them besides determining the Rx (Eg. Acc Ampl, NRA, CAC, etc.).

AMP
Amplitude
Latency
Time

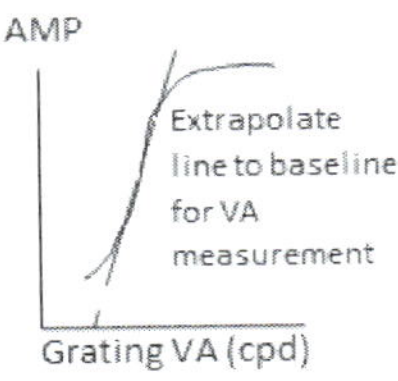

VEP or VER

- Visually Evoked Potentials are responses of the occipital cortex as monitored from scalp electrodes, which provide a trace. Amplitude and latency provide some idea as to the patency of the pathways (e.g. prolonged latency in retrobulbar neuritis). For refractive error,
  1. Lenses can be used before the eye until the best VER is found, or
  2. Computer presented gratings can be shown while VER is recorded and the resulting plot of amplitudes can provide a measure of VA.

E. Standard Subjective Refraction Procedures

Spherical equivalent:

- Purpose: To determine the lenses required in neutralizing the refractive error of the eye without the use of cylindrical (cyl) lenses.
- This is usually done to:
    1. Improve the VA in preparation for determination of the power and axis of the correcting cyl lens
    2. In those cases where the need for cyl lenses will not be attempted, and the best spherical lens for functional vision is to be used
- Procedure:
    1. Determine the patient's best VA.
    2. Place the patient behind the phoropter and occlude the left eye.
    3. Direct the patient's attention to his best VA line and tell him you will be giving a series of choices. Ask patient to report which lens gives the sharper and clearer image or if the image remains unchanged.
    4. With plano in the phoropter, add +0.50 DS. If this improves the VA or the image appears the same, leave the +0.50 DS in the phoropter and add an additional +0.50 DS so that you give a choice between +1.00 DS and +0.50 DS. This procedure is continued until the addition of +0.50 DS blurs the VA line and reduces the patient's performance.
    5. If the first addition of +0.50 DS blurs the VA line and reduces performance, the patient is then given the choice between -0.50 DS and plano. If -0.50 DS appears clearer, the patient should be able to demonstrate an increase in visual acuity (i.e., the patient should be able to read the next line down). Reduce the VA line and repeat.
    6. Continue to bracket the lens power until the addition of minus lenses no longer yields a demonstrable improvement in VA (i.e. do not give any minus unless he earns it).
    7. **Determination of endpoint**: the endpoint is defined as the lens power with which the patient can read the best VA line possible: the addition of +0.25 DS blurs the VA line; the addition of -0.25 DS yields no greater ability to read a smaller line. (i.e., most plus and least minus to read the best VA line).
    8. Continue on for cylindrical refraction to determine the need for astigmatic correction
- A rule of thumb is that there should be an improvement in acuity by one line with every -0.25D added.

Cylindrical Refraction #1: Jackson Cross Cylinder

- Purpose: To determine the power and axis of astigmatism using a Jackson cross cylindrical lens.
- Procedure:
    - Complete a spherical refraction on the right eye.
    - Begin with "best sphere" in place (begin with NO FOG since this is best VA method).
    - Place -0.25 DC X 180 in the phoropter.
    - Place cross cyl in front of the eye and orient the axis so that the white dots and red dots are at 90 and 180 degrees, respectively.
    - Select a line that is 2 lines above their best VA line.
- **Approximate Axis:**
    1. Ask the patient to compare the clarity of the letter with choice one: red dots over 180 degrees; and choice two: white dots over 180 degrees. This is done by "flipping the cross cyl". Ask the patient which gives a more sharp and clear image of the letters. Note the patient's response. Red dots over 180 degrees is an acceptance; white dots is a rejection
    2. Adjust both the phoropter and cross cyl to 90, 45, 135 degrees and repeat step #1 for each of these axes. Note the axis that the patient accepts (i.e. red dots over an axis)
    3. If the patient rejects (white dots over the axis being tested) all four meridians, no astigmatism is indicated and the procedure is terminated
    4. If an axis has been accepted, go to step #7

- **Approximate power**
    5. Place cross cyl over axis of acceptance, aligning dots with phoropter axis. Have the patient indicate if letters are "sharper and clearer" with red dots over axis or white dots over axis
    6. If patient accepts red dots, more power is indicated. Increase the power to -0.50 DC in the phoropter and repeat
    7. The procedure is repeated in -0.25 DC steps until the patient rejects power. At that point, the power in the phoropter is dropped back to the previous cyl power (or to that power which gave the last acceptance). This is your approximate cyl endpoint, utilizing the bracketing technique
    8. As you are adding minus cyl power, for every -0.50 DC, add +0.25 DS to keep the interval of Sturm centered
- **Exact axis** (if retinoscopy is good, enter cross cyl at this step)
    9. Rotate cross cyl to "split the axis". This is done by straddling the white and red dots on either side of the approximate axes. There is a mark on the cross cyl to indicate this position
    10. The cross cyl is again flipped and the patient again indicates which is clearer. The key to this step is to follow the red dots.
    11. When a choice is made, the position of the red dots with respect to the axis in the phoropter is noted. For example: if the red dot is on the clockwise side of the phoropter axis. Move the phoropter axis clock-wise 10 degrees and the split mark of the cross cyl is also moved 10 degrees clockwise to straddle your phoropter axis
    12. The procedure is repeated until there is a reversal in the direction of adjustments
    13. Again bracketing is utilized narrowing the steps to 5 degrees and then 2 1/2 degrees. Ideally there is an exact axis which on either side will give a "reversal" response. The sensitivity of the patient will determine how many degrees away from the "exact axis" will give this reversal
- **Exact power**
    14. Place axis of cross cyl over exact axis and repeat power step utilizing the bracketing technique. If you get a rejection, back off -0.25 DC to get the endpoint
    15. Remove cross cyl and refine sphere power
    16. Repeat for LE

Cylindrical Refraction #2: Stenopaic Slit

- Purpose: To determine power and axis of astigmatism using a slit aperture
- Procedure:
    1. Start with "best sphere" in place
    2. Place stenopaic slit and rotate until best acuity is found. The slit is the AXIS of minus cyl in this position
    3. Rotate slit 90 degrees and obtain the best sphere for this meridian
    4. Rotate the slit back and obtain the best sphere again
    5. Place these spheres on a lens cross and you have the Rx

Cylindrical Refraction #3: Fan Dial

- For a patient with astigmatism, a line oriented along the meridians of poorest focus will be seen as being sharper than lines at other orientations. This effect provides a subjective method of determining the axis and power of a correcting cyl.
- Procedure: (room illumination should be dim for projected target, bright for printed target)
    1. Occlude one eye
    2. Complete a spherical refraction which yields "best sphere" (at this point interval of Sturm is straddling the retina). No cyl in place
    3. Add +0.75 DS fog to relax accommodation and to place interval of Sturm in front of retina.

4. Ask the patient which lines are darkest and sharpest. Have the patient name the hour corresponding to the darkest line
5. Instruct the patient to continue to look at the sharpest and darkest lines. Add plus sphere till that sharp line first begins to blur. This insures that the interval of Sturm is in front of the retina
6. Ask the patient to compare the darkness and sharpness of the sets of lines on either side of the darkest set of lines. The relationship of these lines must remain constant until the astigmatism is corrected.
7. Calculate and set the axis of the minus cyl by multiplying 30 times the indicated hour and fractional hour
8. Add minus cyl in -0.50 DC steps to bring foci together
9. With each step ask the patient to identify the darkest lines
    a. If the axis is exact, the patient will continue to report the same relationship until:
        i. All the lines appear equal to the endpoint, or
        ii. A line perpendicular to the original appears darkest. This reversal brackets the endpoint
    b. If the axis is not correct, the patient will report a shift in the relationship set in step #6. Adjust the axis to re-establish the initial relationship. Usually this requires moving the axis a small amount towards the new "clearer" meridian

        Example: if it was 1:00 o'clock or 30 degrees and suddenly it became 2:00 o'clock or 60 degrees, move from 30 to 60 degrees to re-establish the initial relationship, but do not go past 45 degrees since you already narrowed the location to closest to 30 degrees
10. The endpoint is found by bracketing
    a. The amount of cyl which makes the lines most equal
    b. If the reversal is from one line to another with -0.25DC, the endpoint is the lower cyl

Cylindrical Refraction #4: Paraboline Slide Procedure:

- The AO Paraboline test for astigmatism is conducted while the patient is slightly fogged. About +0.50 DS more plus than the net spherical retinoscopy finding is usually adequate.
- With no cyl in the phoropter, and the fogging lens in place, project the astigmatic chart on the screen.
- Ask the patient which line or group of lines stands out sharper and blacker than the others. If the patient reports that the lines all look equally black, there is no significant amount of astigmatism present as determined by this test.
- If the patient reports that one line or group of lines appears sharper and blacker than the rest, use the knob at the top of the slide to rotate the pointer until it points to the line (or center of the group of lines) that the patient reports as standing out sharper and blacker. Leave the pointer at this setting and move the slide in the Project-O-Chart until the Paraboline Dial is projected on the screen. The Paraboline Dial is automatically positioned for the refinement of axis test as it is geared to the astigrnatic chart pointer.

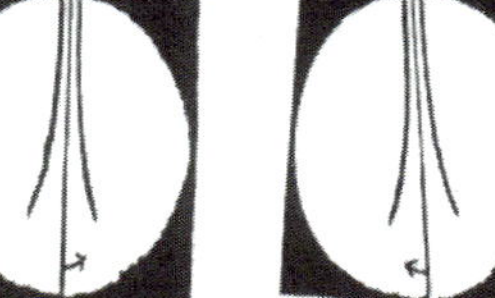

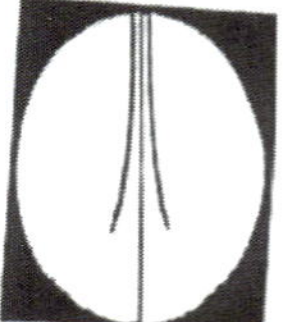

- The exact axis position is obtained by rotating the Paraboline Dial until the patient reports that both limbs near the top of the arrow-like figure appear equally clear of black.
- In this position, the dashed line (which may appear continuous) bisecting arrow head will appear more distinct that the one perpendicular to it. Insert minus cyl power at the axis indicated by the projected SIDE pointer until both dashed lines appear equally clear. (In this position, the original more blurred line will become clearer as minus cyl is added until it appears as clear as the original clear line).

Duochrome (Bichrome) Technique and Balance

- In the eye, short wavelength light (blue-green) focuses closer to the cornea than the long wavelength light (red). This chromatic interval provides a way to identify the spherical endpoint.
- Procedure for **Monocular** Endpoint ONLY: (very dim room)
  1. Complete a monocular sphero-cylindrical refraction
  2. Project a target one or two lines larger than threshold
  3. Put the red-green filter in place
  4. Optional: fog by +0.75 DS
  5. Ask the patient, are the letters on the red background or the letters on the green background sharper
  6. If the patient reports that the letters on the red background are sharper, add minus sphere. If the letters on the green are sharper, add plus spheres
  7. The accepted endpoint is the least minus which makes the letters on the green background slightly sharper than those on the red

Note: This monocular endpoint technique does not represent a balance. However, the duochrome technique can be used in conjunction with the prism dissociation balance (von Graefe). This can make the balance less dependent on equal acuities.

- Procedure for **Binocular** Balance: (very dim room illumination). Use if vas are UNEQUAL monocularly. This technique does NOT work well for hyperopes.
  1. Complete the monocular sphero-cylindrical refractions
  2. Open both eyes
  3. Red-green letters two lines above threshold. Optional: fog by +0.75 DS
  4. Introduce base up and base down prism to obtain diplopia
  5. Direct your patient's attention to the upper image. If green, add plus spheres
  6. Direct your patient's attention to the lower image and follow steps #4, #5, and #6 above. If red, add minus spheres
  7. Recheck the upper image
  8. The refraction is balanced when the conditions described in step #6 occur simultaneously for both images. Green or equal is endpoint (green means slightly over minused)

Von Graefe Binocular Balance

- Purpose: To balance the accommodative stimuli to the two eyes. This comparison test achieves its goal only if the monocular acuities are equal. If VAs DIFFER by more than one line, do NOT use the von Graefe balance.
- Procedure:
  1. Add +0.75 DS to both RE and to LE to fog
  2. Place 3 prism diopters base up before RE and 3 prism diopters base down before LE
  3. Isolate 20/30 or 20/40 line or approximately two lines above threshold
  4. Indicate to the patient that there are two fuzzy lines of letters. Ask whether the letters appear to be equally fuzzy or if one line appears more clear. (The task is to equalize both eyes)
  5. If the patient indicates one line is more clear, add +0.25 DS to the clearer image and repeat comparison
  6. Plus power is added to the clearer image until a reversal is noted. The endpoint is when the two images are equally blurred
  7. If equality is indicated at the beginning, add +0.25 DS, then -0.25 DS to see if there is a reversal
  8. When endpoint is reached, remove prisms and binocularly reduce plus power until the addition of minus power no longer yields an increase in VA

Non-Pharmaceutical Relaxing of Accommodation (for Hyperopes)

Cyclodamia: (meaning ciliary control).

- Done right after retinoscopy. Record retinoscopy leaving work lenses in place. If latency is suspected, slowly reduce plus in +0.25 DS steps encouraging the patient to read the 20/20 line. Record maximum plus giving 20/20. Try to relax accommodation with fog by pushing plus. This is Rx-able.

Sudden Fog

- After subjective, push plus by fogging to relax accommodation. If it clears even for a second, you give it to them as a high manifest.
    1. After subjective, increase the plus until the best acuity line is just readable. Some blur needed.
    2. Insert working lenses suddenly and encourage patient to read best acuity. Leave in for 15 to 30 seconds
    3. Suddenly remove the working lens plus and ask if the line has cleared, even momentarily
    4. If it did, repeat the technique with +0.25 DS OU addition until acuity line no longer clears perfectly after removal of the working lens. Record maximum plus giving best acuity (this is the high manifest). This is Rx-able but takes some time to get used to. Get more plus than with cyclodamia

Modified Peckham Technique:

- Relax accommodative spasm through CA/C. BI prism leads to fusional divergence and this causes a relaxation of accommodative convergence in order to get more divergence, but it will blur as the patient relaxes accommodation. Use this technique particularly when there is a BI to blur point at distance or when monocular best acuity is not obtainable binocularly except through reduction of plus.
    1. Add maximum BI prism OU at distance without producing diplopia. This acts through the CA/C ratio to relax some accommodation.
    2. Slowly add maximum plus until best VA line blurs
    3. Alternately apply steps a and b. Record the maximum plus lens power giving best VA.

Modified Updegrave Technique:

- Slow plus at near because patients need to release spasm accommodation
    1. Combine results of a slow maximum plus NRA and the subjective. Place in a trial frame
    2. Instruct the patient to read at 40 cm until the print clears and try to read clearly beyond this distance. If necessary move print in until clear, then slowly push away (so the patient is relaxing his accommodation to clear it). May take up to 10 minutes
    3. Add +0.50DS to the Rx after the patient has cleared the print (i.e. push plus as the accommodative spasm is relaxed).
    4. Repeat procedure until print no longer clears, substract out the NRA plus, and the remainder is usually close to the total hyperopia. (The NRA is substracted because it is the amount of plus needed at near, but we want a distance Rx).

Pin Hole Retinoscopy

- The pin hole increases the depth of focus and opens the loop to accommodation. As one eye fixates through a pin hole, scope the other eye on axis. Add maximum plus. Alternate between the eyes. Take 10 to 15 minutes.

F. Binocular Subjective Refraction Procedures

Humphriss Binocular Refraction or Balance

- Purpose: This is a binocular refraction or balance in which the eye not being tested is fogged by +0.75 DS. The rationale is that peripheral fusion is still being maintained while centrally the fog provides a physiological septum
- Procedure:
    1. Following the monocular subjective, add blur to one eye and complete the cyl refraction on the other. Refine the sphere
    2. Now switch the blur and perform a spherocylindrical refraction on the second eye
    3. Fog OS by +0.75 DS again
    4. Isolate the threshold VA line
    5. Reduce the fog -0.25 DS binocularly until the patient can see threshold clearly

Note: when performing the Humphriss balance, only the sphere is refined.

TIB Binocular Refraction or Balance

- When a monocular refraction is performed, the patient's visual system is in an abnormal state. It has been shown that more reliable information about the accommodative state, cyl axis position, and VA results when binocular refraction techniques are used.
- Binocular vision can be achieved by presenting a target which is common to both eyes. A stick is positioned between the patient and the chart so that a small portion of the chart is blocked for each eye. This small portion of the chart is seen exclusively by the other eye. There is a physical septum, but there is NO FOG
- Procedure: (very dim room illumination)
    1. Begin with retinoscopy results corrected for working distance. Check the patient's VA
    2. Project a line large enough to be seen by the poorer eye. Any line can be used, but if the chart has a symmetrical portion, use it to set up the stick
    3. Instruct the patient to tell you how to move the stick so that it is exactly in the middle of the line
    4. Determine which characters are seen only by the RE or LE
    5. Direct your patient's attention to the characters seen only by the RE. Patient has to concentrate on letters seen only by that eye. Complete a sphero-cylinder refraction
    6. Bracket the endpoint to achieve the best VA with the least minus
    7. Repeat steps #6, #7, and #8 for the LE. Again, patient concentrates on letters seen by that eye only. Recheck the spherical endpoint on the RE
    8. Remove the septum and binocularly refine the endpoint.

Note: The end result of this technique is a subjective refraction with the accommodative state balanced in the two eyes. Some practitioners use this technique only to balance two monocular subjectives. Unlike the von Graefe technique, this T.I.B. (Turville Infinity Balance) can be used for patient's with unequal acuities.

AO Vectographic (Polaroid) Binocular Refraction or Balance

- Each eye sees different letters due to polarization, while peripheral fusion is intact. Procedures are similar to T.I.B. Be sure to direct the patient's attention only to those letters seen by the eye you are refracting.

G. Cycloplegic Subjective and Objective Techniques

- Definition: Pharmaceuticals which block the Peripheral ANS (accommodation and miosis) muscarinic action of ACh, thereby paralyzing the ciliary muscle, (cyclospasm) and also the pupil constrictor muscle resulting in mydriasis.
- Indications:
  - **Latent Hyperopes**: Patient with focusing problems, difficult sustaining reading.
  - **Children:** Any kids with signs or symptoms of uncorrected RE.
  - **Accommodative Esotropes**: To assess how hyperopia contributes to the squint.
- Drugs:
  - **Atropine:** Used only for kids under 5 with possible accommodative esotropia. Use: Apply 1 drop or ointment once/day for 3 days prior to examination.
  - **Tropicamide:** For all ages, however, does not fully uncover all hyperopia. Use: 1 or 2 drops (0.5 to l.0%).
  - **Cyclopentolate:** Used for those under 20 where hyperopia is suspected. Use: 1 drop (1%).
- Methods:
  - **Subjective:** Methods are similar to non-cycloplegic refraction. It is important to keep patient in the Plus to prevent any residual accommodation from being used.
  - **Objective:** Retinoscopy: May be the only test done with uncooperative patients. Because of dilation, neutralize only the regular reflex seen centrally.
- Notes:
  - **Time:** For cyclopentolate and tropicamide, tests should occur at the 30 minute mark and end within 15 minutes to avoid recovery problems which can confuse the findings.
  - Muscle Balancing, Nearpoint Tests, Binocular Balances are not valid under cycloplegia (accommodation and therefore AC/A is out)
- Prescribing: Prescribing tactics differ between practitioners. Since excessive plus causes blurring and can result in rejection of the Rx, it is often useful to give an intermediate Rx between the cycloplegic and non-cycloplegic. In the case of accommodative esotropes, however, it is best to give the full amount; perhaps using a bifocal. At follow-ups, if the patient seems to accept the plus, more can be added.

H. Amplitude of Accommodation

- The **Near Point of Accommodation (NPA)** is the point representing the maximum dioptric stimulus the eyes can accommodate in the presence of convergence
- The **Far Point of Accommodation (FPA)** is the point representing the minimum dioptric stimulus the eyes can accommodate in the presence of convergence
- **Accommodative Amplitude (AA)** – Maximum focusing ability of the visual system. It is the dioptric difference between the far point and near point of accommodation

Push Up Technique

- Procedure
  - Hold target 40-50cm away and move towards patient until first sustained blur (endpoint)
  - Measure the distance from the spectacle plane to the target (cm) and convert to diopters
- The angular size of the target increases as the target is moved closer to the spectacle plane causing magnification. Proximal vergence also causes accommodation. Thus, push up often results in an overestimation of the AA

Minus Lens Technique (Monocular Test)

- Procedure
  - Hold target (one above threshold) 40 cm from the eye and add Minus lenses until the first

sustained blur (endpoint)

- Amplitude of Accommodation = Total amount of Minus Lenses + 2.50D (working distance)

  Example. If -3.00D minus lenses are added for sustained blur, what is the amplitude of accommodation? AA= 3.00D +2.50D = 5.50D

- The minus lenses cause ~~magnification~~ min of the target and results in an underestimation of the AA. *Some clinicians suggest adding 0.50D to the dioptric equivalence of the WD to compensate*

I. Trial Lenses

- **Trial lenses**: This procedure of placing the tentative add in a trial frame tests the physical ranges in proportion to working distance. Morgan recommends that the add should leave 3/5 of the clear range beyond the working distance.

J. PRA/NRA

- **PRA/NRA**: Positive and negative relative accommodation are measured binocularly at 40cm with threshold acuity letters. For the presbyope, start with the tentative add in place. Plus to blur (NRA) is done first since it is a relaxing test.
- **NRA**- add plus power binocularly until the patient reports blur. Note this change in power as the NRA result relative to the tentative add. Since 2.50D of accommodation is stimulated at the 40cm test distance, the NRA finding should not exceed +2.50. If greater than that amount, the subjective refraction is suspect and the patient may be overminused.
  - As plus lenses are added during the NRA test, a reduction in the stimulus to accommodation occurs which in turn relaxes accommodative convergence. To avoid diplopia positive fusional vergence is required. As long as positive fusional vergence is available, accommodation and accommodative convergence can be relaxed but when the limit of PFV is reached, no further accommodation is relaxed, and blur is reported. Thus, NRA is a test of positive fusional vergence.
  - An NRA finding of less than +2.00D may indicate:
    - Positive fusional vergence is severely limited or
    - Patient was overplussed on the subjective finding.
- **PRA**- reduce the add binocularly until the patient reports blur. Note this change in power as the PRA result relative to the tentative add. As minus lenses are added (plus reduced) the stimulus to accommodation increases. Accommodative convergence also occurs and to avoid diplopia negative fusional vergence must be used. Therefore, the minus lens to blur test is considered a test of the limit of negative fusional vergence.
  - A finding below normal for PRA may indicate:
    - Low amplitude of accommodation or
    - Limited negative fusional vergence.
- To adjust the tentative add using PRA/NRA method, balance the ranges in relative power found so the absolute value of PRA = NRA. Example: tentative add = +2.00, NRA=+0.75, PRA = -1.25. Therefore the adjusted tentative add = +1.75.

  Adjusted tentative add = TA – [abs(NRA) + abs(PRA)]/2

K. Add Powers

- **Retinoscopy**: One method of directly estimating a near point Rx is retinoscopy. With the patient's distance Rx in place have them fixate a near target then add plus until neutralized. The additional plus estimates the near add.
- **Crossed cylinders**: This test may be performed monocularly or binocularly. Near target is the cross cylinder grid. Jackson cross cylinders are placed before each eye, minus axis at 90, and fogging lens of +1.00 over the expected near finding are in place. Patient initially should report vertical lines clearer than horizontal. Then as you add minus (take away plus) patient should report a reversal where horizontal lines are clearest.

- Interpretation: Crossed-cylinder test for a prepresbyope indicates:
  - Lag of accommodation
  - Latent hyperopes who could benefit from a near add or
  - High ACA cases are exposed on the basis of gradient phorias.
- For presbyopes the binocular crossed-cylinder provides a tentative add that may be too high for a beginning presbyope but is usually within 1/4D of the final add for established presbyopes.

Rules for Prescribing Presbyopic Adds:

- Keep half of the amplitude of accommodation in reserve. In other words, for most visual tasks, the patient should not be required to use more than half the amplitude of accommodation. This rule necessitates the accurate determination of the patients habitual preferred working distance.
- Determine an add by balancing the PRA/NRA finding.
- Patients previous prescription or "effective add".

Example:

Distance Rx currently wearing	-0.75D
Rx current subjective	- (-0.25D)
Dist Rx difference	-0.50D

Current Rx addition	+1.25D
Dist. Rx difference	-0.50D
"Effective add" =	+0.75D

- **Subjective visual symptoms:** Patients complain that they must hold near work further away than they would like indicates increased plus power is needed at near. However, large power changes when patients are satisfied with a previous prescription may cause potential dissatisfaction, regardless of the fact that the change may be indicated by a rule of thumb.
- Index of near add with patient age: Zadnik gives general guidelines.

Zadnik's Age vs. Add (Working Distance 40cm)	
Age	Add
40	0.00
45	1.00
48	1.25
50	1.50
52	1.75
55	2.00
60	2.25

- **Spectacle lens options**:
  - Half eyes,
  - Readers
  - Bifocals
  - Trifocals
  - Blended bifocals
  - No line progressive addition adds.
- Contact lens options include:
  - Monovision-one eye corrected for distance and the other for near
  - Bifocal contact lenses-pupil is centered in the top portion for distance vision and moves into the lower segment area when the eyes are turned downward. The lens must be stabilized on the eye by means of truncation, prism ballast or both. Seldom more than 50% success is achieved in fitting bifocal contact lenses even with practitioners reporting 90 to 95% success in fitting single vision lenses
  - Non-bifocal contact lenses which provide an optically perfect secondary curve to function as a bifocal segment. The lens remains centered for distance vision and lags upward when the patient looks down for near vision.
  - Aspheric surface lens designs have been introduced as well but with limited success.

L. Refractive Correction Applications (e.g. LASIK)

- **Objective Types**: The most modern of these employ infra-red (IR) beams to measure the eye and the analysis is aided by computers. The patient is aligned and fixates, the operator pushes a button, and an Rx is generated. All are different in operation but are based on 3 principles:
    1) the IR automated retinoscope;
    2) the Scheiner's Disc
    3) the Lensometer.
- Regardless of which principle the machine is based on, they all beam in IR and analyze how it leaves the eye in order to come up with the eye's refractive error.
- **Subjective Types**: (Patient responds). There are only a few and the better known one is the Humphrey Vision Analyzer. This is an elaborate apparatus which performs binocular refractions without any lenses being in front of the patient. Instead, variable lenses are in the projection apparatus which places targets onto the patient's eye while the other eye is open but dissociated. The lenses affect the target and not the patient's eye. Another model is the AO SR IV, which also has continuously variable powered lenses operated by the patient with a knob.
- **Problems:**
    - Controlling the patient's accommodation.
    - Proper alignment in the machine.
    - Irregular astigmatism.
    - Poor media (Problem of the objective types).
- **Advantages**: Fast, good for large patient loads and impressive pieces of technology.
- **Disadvantages**: Quite expensive, difficult to operate, requires training, accuracy no better than standard retinoscopy and refraction.
- **Lasers:** A laser pattern is shown to the patient so that the patient can observe it for movement. Hyperopes will see a WITH motion as they move their heads. Myopes will see an AGAINST motion. Emmetropes will see NO movement. The doctor manipulates lenses until the patient reports no movement of the laser pattern. (Subjective WITH or AGAINST motion).
- While laser refraction is accurate, it has no advantages. Its disadvantages are that the equipment is expensive and it cannot be used without some expertise; thus, it is not commonly used.

ANOMALIES OF REFRACTION

1a. Epidemiology, History and Symptom Inventory of Aphakia/Pseudophakia

- Before the 18th century "couchers" pierced the cataractous eye with a sharp instrument to push the opaque lens out of the way and got out of town fast before complications set in.
- 18th century Daviel discovered how to remove cataracts through an incision in the limbus. This is **extracapsular surgery** meaning the cataract is removed but the posterior capsule is still intact.
- 1930's risk of complications of extracapsular extraction was decreased by doing **intracapsular extractions**, meaning that the whole lens was removed
- In 50's and 60's intracapsular procedures were improved but still had complications- the methods of extraction include **erysiphake** (suction) and more commonly **cryoprobe** (freeze pencil)

1b. Epidemiology, History and Symptom Inventory of Aniesikonia

- **Aniseikonia** = condition in which the ocular images are unequal in size and/or shape (Dr. Schor's definition = perceived differences in ocular images).
- **Etiology:** Optically induced- from magnification differences in anisometropia (the refractive error of one eye differs from that of the other, generally by a difference of 1D or more) or high astigmatism.
- **Neurosensory:** stretching of the retina or edema, different distribution or spacing of the retinal elements, differences in the distribution of nerve fibers in the cortical path.

- **Incidence:** Duke-Elder estimates that 20-30% of spectacle wearers exhibit a measurable degree of aniseikonia. Schor reports that 2-5% of population affected by aniseikonia.
- **Symptoms:** Headaches, asthenopia, eyestrain, photophobia, perceptual distortions, diplopia or vertigo in large amounts of aniseikonia.

2. Observation and Recognition of Clinical Signs/Phenomena Associated with Aphakia and Pseudophakia

A. Magnification

- When the crystalline lens is removed the eye performs all its refraction at the cornea and so the principle planes of a new spectacle lens/cornea are shifted in front of the cornea. Because this happens, there is an increase in focal length which is directly related to image size. As the lens approaches the cornea the principle planes of the lens eye system also approach the cornea and the secondary focal length gets shorter. Magnification increases the further the lens is from the eye. For this reason contact lenses give much less of a magnification problem than do spectacle lenses. Although objects appear both larger and nearer than they really are the patient can learn to respond to a new set of size and distance clues. If the patient is a unilateral aphake however, adaptation to the magnification difference is not possible.

Example:. *Gullstrand's exact schematic eye has a refracting power of +58.64D and an anterior focal length of 17.05mm. Gullstrand's aphakic schematic eye has a refracting power of +43.05 D and an anterior focal length of 23.23mm. Find:*

A) The power of the correcting lens at a vertex distance of 12mm
B) Find the equivalent power of the spectacle lens and the corneal power.
C) Find the retinal image compared to an emmetropic eye
D) Find the magnification resulting from the lens thickness.
E) Find the total magnification

Note: The magnification for an aphakic wearing spectacles is between 25-35% and only 7 to 8% with contact lenses.

Answer:

A) The far point conjugate to the retina is 85.0 mm behind the cornea.
1/ (0.085m + 0.012m) = +10.31 D
B) $P_e = P_1 + P_2 - d\ P_1\ P_2$
$= 10.31 + 43.05 - (0.012)(10.31)(43.05)$
$= +48.03$ D
C) 58.64/48.03 = 1.22 or 22% larger image size
D) $M_{shape} = 1/(1-t/nP_1)$
$= 1/\ (1-0.006/1.5x12)$
$= 1.05$
E) M_{total}=(1.22) (1.05) = 1.28 or 28% larger

B. Field of View

- The decreased field of view is due to the fact that the high plus lens induces base-toward-the-center prism power. The base in prism also results in a ring scotoma between the outer extent of the field through the lens and the field beyond the edge of the lens. The term jack-in-the-box phenomenon is used to refer to the confusion experienced by the patient when objects jump into and out of the ring scotoma.

Example: *Find the field of view to the outer edge of a frame with the following parameters:*

Vertex distance =14mm
Spec. lens power= +14.00 D
Entrance pupil is 3mm behind cornea
Eye size = 50mm (1/2 = 25mm)

Answer:
Field of view to outer edge of frame:
$\tan a = \frac{25}{17} = 56° \times 2 = 112°$

Where is the image of the entrance pupil? Since it's a 14D lens we can image the entrance point of the pupil through the lens.

Spectacle Plane

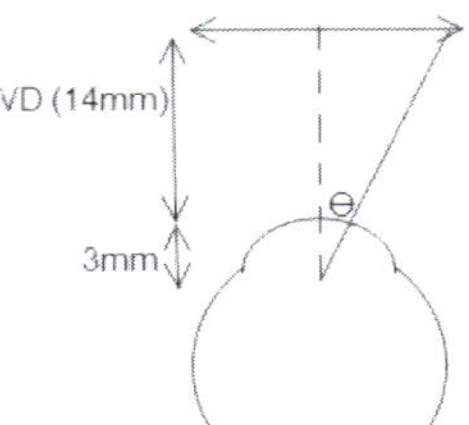

EP= Entrance Pupil
VD= Vertex Distance
3mm= distance from cornea to entrance pupil

> ***Answer:***
> V = U+P
> u= -0.017 meter
> V = 1/-0.017 +14
> v= -22.3 mm

This means the image of the entrance pupil through the lens is not at 17mm where the object is but, further back at 22.3mm. What is the field of view through the lens?

> ***Answer:***
> $\tan \alpha = \frac{25mm}{22.3} = 48.27° \times 2 = 96.5°$

- When an aphake wears a +14 lens in a 50mm frame eye size, there is a wider field of view limited *by* the frame than the field of view limited by the optics of the lens. The result is (112-96.5 =15.5/2= 8°) ring scotoma on each side of the lens. The peripheral field of view is smaller for a contact lens with 7mm diam. than for a spectacle lens of 50mm diam.

C. Spatial Distortion

- Distortion occurs when a stop -such as the pupil of the eye-is placed at some distance behind a lens. The only rays for an off-axis object point that can be included in the image are those entering the periphery of the lens. These rays are subject to prismatic effects which increase as the distance from the lens pole increases. The amount of distortion, therefore, increases with lens power and lens diameter. For a positive lens the distortion causes a square object to suffer pincushion distortion. Peripheral lines appear to bow towards the observer. The eye encounters a gradual increase in magnification when the eye looks further away from the lens center. These distortions can be minimized with more steeply curved aphakic lenses.

pincushion effect of a square through plus lens

Spherical Aberration:

- Spherical aberration and coma occur only for large aperture systems. Most aphakic patients have small pupils are are affected very little by these aberrations. However, off axis aberrations such as oblique astigmatism and curvature of image (power error) need to be addressed in lens design.
- Sph. Aberration is ordinarily neutralized by the lens of the eye but in the aphakic eye the caustic (focal concentration of light along the convergent bundle of rays) becomes longer and narrower
- If the pupil is small, the caustic is reduced in size, but the pinhole effect of the pupil then helps the acuity
- If the pupil is larger, the caustic is increased in size

D. Convergence Demands

- Even though the segment poles are correctly centered for the patients near PD the wearer will be subject to prismatic effects at near due to the power of the distance lenses. Although the induced prismatic effect is negligible for low powered lenses, for an aphakic correction it will reach significant amounts.

Example: *If an aphakic patient requiring a distance prescription of +13.00-1.00x090, is fitted with bifocal adds of +2.50 O.U. and a segment inset of 2mm. What is the amount of induced prism in each eye?*

> ***Answer:*** Since the -1.00 DC manifests its power in the 180 meridian, the power in that meridian is +12.00D and so the amount of induced prism for each eye is:
> P=dF = 0.2(+12)= 2.4Δ

- Since the distance lenses are decentered outward with respect to the near PD, the prism is in the base out direction and is a total of 4.8Δ base out for the two eyes. If the wearer were esophoric at near, the 4.8Δ base out would be an advantage; however, most aphakics, like presbyopes, are exophoric at near, so the induced base out prism may place undue strain on fusional vergence. To help compensate for the strain the PD could be decentered inward but only a small amount since displacement of the optic axis from the line of sight induces a change in both spherical and astigmatic powers.

E. Sensitivity to Glare

- Aphakic patients complain of glare because often times the posterior capsule is left in the eye and it contains small opacities that reflect light and bounce around leading to the glare. Also the quality of the incoming light is different in that more blue light is reaching the retina of the aphakic eye than an eye with a lens.

F. Techniques and Skills for Determining, Evaluating, and/or Verifying

Types and Characteristics of Intraocular Lenses

- **Iris clip lenses** were the most popular lenses in the world between 1977 and 1982.
  - One part of the lens goes behind the iris and another part goes in front of the iris and the patient is put on pilocarpine so the constricted pupil holds the lens in place.
  - DISADVANTAGES: 1) They can flip forward and bang against the endothelium → the incidence of post-op aphakic bullous is high. 2) After ten years a high number of patients end up with corneal transplants.
    - The treatment for patients who have a dislocation of this type of lens is to put them on their back and get them to an ophthalmologist so they can be dilated and have the clip moved back behind the iris.
- **Posterior chamber lenses** are the most popular IOL in the world today.
  - The entire lens goes behind the iris. Probably 99% of implants in the US are posterior chamber lenses.
  - These lenses have a 7mm diameter optical portion which produces the least amount of glare/reflection symptoms.
- **Anterior chamber lenses** are used by choice in secondary implants (meaning pt had cataract removed some time ago without putting in an IOL and now wants an IOL implanted)
  - The anterior chamber lens is also the lens of choice in a situation where the posterior capsule is broken during extra capsular surgery and some of the vitreous is lost.
  - They sit entirely in front of the iris
- IOLs can be made of PMMA or prolene, and there are silicon lenses out on the market now.

Types and Characteristics of Aphakic Spectacles

- The simplest form of aphakic lens is a full-diameter **glass lens** having a fused bifocal segment. Due to the excessive weight of glass and the presence of aberrations, these lenses are now used very little except for temporary lenses to be worn after surgery until the eye stabilizes.
- The development of **plastic aspheric lenticular lenses** was begun about 25 years ago, and at the present time each lens manufacturer has available a lens of this style.
  - Typically, the powered portion of the lens has a diam of 40mm, the back surface has a power of

about -3.00 or -4.00 D, and the aspheric curve is on the front surface.
    - The 40mm diameter of the powered portion allows a significant decrease in both center thickness and lens weight.
    - The field of view is limited compared with that of a full diameter lens but this is not a serious handicap: the oblique aberrations of astigmatism curvature of image, and distortion are at their greatest when the eye rotates sufficiently to look through the peripheral portion of a full diameter aphakic lens.
    - If lenticular lenses are fitted as close to the eyes as possible, not only does the angular field of view increase, but image mag. is held to a minimum.
- Two manufacturers have developed full aspheric lenses having an exaggerated amount of asphericity, or drop, in the periphery.
    - **Welsh 4-drop lens** is made by Cataract Lens Laboratories
    - **HyperAspheric lens** is made by Signet Optical Company.
    - When plano back surface curves are used the wearer encounters more spherical error, astigmatism, and distortion than would be the case if -3.00 or -5.00D back curves were used. In addition, flat lenses suffer more from reflections than meniscus lenses do.
- DISADVANTAGES: 1) Lens weight, 2) Lens thickness, 3) Magnified appearance of the wearers eye, 4) Lens aberrations, 5) Decreased field of view, and 6) Increased retinal image size.
    - All of these problems can be avoided if contact lenses rather than spectacles are fitted. If spectacles are fitted however, the center thickness of an aphakic lens can be reduced by using a lenticular lens consisting of a powered central portion about 40mm in diam. and a plano carrier.
    - Lens aberrations can be minimized by the use of an aspheric front surface, along with careful selection of base curves.

Types and Characteristics of Aphakic Contact Lenses

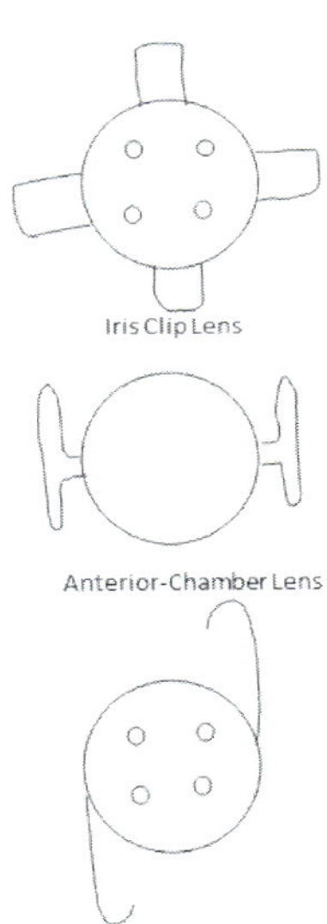

- Three types of contact lenses are available for aphakic patients
    - Rigid contact lenses-PMMA or gas permeable
    - Soft contact lenses
    - Extended wear contact lenses (hydrophilics, silicone and silicone acrylate)
- Aphakic contact lenses differ from those for myopes or low hyperopes in their 1) Increased thickness, 2) Increased weight, and 3) Shape of the edge.
    - A minus lens edge has prism with the base toward the edge orientation and is usually held up nicely by the upper lid
    - A high plus lens edge has prism with the apex toward the edge orientation and tends to be pushed downward by the upper lid.
- Soft contact lenses in the powers required for aphakic eyes are sufficiently rigid so that the lens may fail to conform completely to the corneal surface. As a result, a **negative tear lens** may be formed underneath the apical portion of the lens, requiring more plus power than one would predict on the basis of objective or subjective refraction corrected for vertex distance.
    - As an additional consequence of the failure of the lens to conform to the corneal surface, an aphakic lens may be found to eliminate a moderate amount of astigmatism.
- Polse recommended the following lens dimensions:
    - Lens diam. 8.4 to 9.2 mm
    - Optic zone diam 6.5 to 7.5 mm
    - Minimum center thickness 0.30 to 0.38 mm
    - Minimum junction thickness 0.13 to 0.15mm
    - Edge thickness of minus carrier approx. 0.22mm
    - Radius of front lenticular curve 1.0 to 2.0 mm flatter than radius of base curve
- **Extended wear** lenses for aphakia are of real benefit to older aphakes who, because of arthritis, unsteady hands or senility are unable to handle daily wear lenses.

- The advantages of contact lenses concerning lens weight and lens thickness are obvious.
- The magnified appearance of the wearer's eyes is basically eliminated with contact lenses, since the spectacle magnification is reduced to about 6 or 7 percent (compared to 30 percent or more with spectacles). The lens aberrations of oblique astigmatism and curvature of image are of little concern to the contact lens wearer since he fixates only through the center of the lenses.

Intraocular lens power

- IOL's are available in a wide range of powers, the average lens being +20D
- In 1977, IOL power for emmetropia was estimated by adding +19.00D to the pre-cataractous refraction.
- In 1987, being within ± 1.00D of the target refraction was still reasonable
- Formulas used for calculating IOLs have been constantly evolving. Current standard IOL formulas are in the 3rd and 4th generation theoretic formulas, including the **Hoffer Q, SRK/T,** and **Holladay II**.
- Corneal Power is used directly to predict the postoperative refraction in the vergence calculation
- Corneal Power is alwso usedto predict the effective lens position (ELP) – the depth of IOL relative to the cornea.
- Refractive surgery alters the corneal curvatures and introduces error in measurement of corneal power and ELP prediction, leading to an underestimation of the required IOL power in eyes that had previous myopic refractive surgery and an overestimation in eyes that had previous hyperopic refractive surgery

Special Refraction Techniques

- Patient may not be better than 20/50 post-op but put up a pin hole to assess the VA potential. Also do retinoscopy (behind the phoropter for a psuedophake and in free space for an aphake using hand held lenses or a trial frame.)
- For an aphake, the refractive error is going to be on the order of +12.00 to +14.00 DS so it is helpful to use a +13.00 DS lens in a trial frame to do the retinoscopy. Look at the quality of the reflex as well as the power. Place the trial frame as close to the pts eyes as possible.
- **Keratometry:** Record the readings and the clarity of the mires. Corneal astig./irregularity from the surgery will show up on clarity of the mires. Recording the readings now is important so that when you're ready to Rx you will know when the cornea has stabilized.
- **Visual Fields:** This is done initially to rule out any major defects after the surgery. Confrontation visual fields using your hands and fingers is good enough at this point.
- **IOP:** If the cornea is not disrupted during surgery you can use Goldman tonometry otherwise, use McKay-Marg for the most accurate results.
- **Slit Lamp:** look at tear film for any disruption post-op; look for epithelial staining- some is normal due to manipulative reasons of surgery; look for deposits on endothelium, and examine the cells-they should look the same as before the surgery; check for cells and flare in the aqueous; check the posterior capsule for any deposits; check to make sure that none of the sutures are working their way up through the conj.
- **Fundus:** On initial visit a detailed look at the fundus isn't needed unless medically indicated i.e. endophthalmitis- an infection from the operating room that is associated with iritis, hyphema, and decreased VA in which case this pt must get back to the ophthalmologist or lose the eye within 24 hours.
  - On later visits the pt should be checked for CYSTIOD MACULAR EDEMA and RETINAL DETACHMENT. These are two of the most common problems post-op for the cataract pt. About 1.5-2% of all uneventful cataract surgery will go on to retinal detachment.
- The actual refraction for the aphake should be done in free space using a trial frame, placing the largest plus power closest to the eye and using hand held Jackson Cross Cyl for the best VA. The subjective steps should be offered in large enough steps for the patient to be able to make a choice. The vertex distance is very important since the power of the aphake spec. lenses is so high. The vertex distance should be as MINIMAL as possible.

Aphakic Lens Prescriptions

- Usually 4 - 6 weeks after surgery, (maybe 2 - 3 months if conservative), the patient is ready for an Rx. When 2 refractions and 2 K readings, spaced 10 days apart, are basically identical, the pt's vision is stable
- The distance from the back of the spec lens to the apex of the cornea must be the same as for the trial lenses through which the refraction is done. Again the vertex distance must be as MINIMAL as possible.
- The frame selection is also important because the pt needs a geometrically centered lens, therefore, the BOX SIZE + BRIDGE = PD.
- A plastic lens will be much lighter weight than a glass lens.
- A lenticular lens is aspheric and has decreased weight but is very unattractive.
- A single cut lens is much more attractive for the patient and if you request the plastic ground to a minimum thickness the weight is not such a problem.
- A lens tinted pink #1 helps with the cosmesis of the lens.
- The bifocal seg. height should be set high.-between lower lid and lower edge of pupil in a Flat top style to help deal with the exophoria induced.
- Give instructions at time of dispense that it will take time to adjust to the distortions, ring scotoma etc. of the lenses and that the pt. should be patient.
- The refraction should remain stable after the initial 4-6 weeks post-op. If there are changes in the VA then diabetes or macular edema should be suspected and investigated.

3. Observation and Recognition of Clinical Signs/Phenomena Associated with Aniseikonia

A. Detection of Aniseikonia

- Pt. reports different sized images of a dime when asked to judge the size of the dime monocularly.
- Symptoms unrelieved by refractive or orthoptic means.
- Sudden change in refraction, unequal base curves or thickness of lenses.
- Can be symptomatic when have as little as 2% difference. Many times, more symptomatic with smaller differences since larger differences are suppressed.
- Binocular tasks present discomfort.

B. Measurement of Aniseikonia

Standard Eikonometer

- Pt. views a polarized target with polarized filters and full refractive correction. Pt. must be binocular.
- The magnification units of the target size are altered to get equal sized images for the two eyes and the overall, vertical and horizontal aniseikonia is measured. Oblique aniseikonia cannot be measured.

Space Eikonometer

- Measures the rotations of the observed field as affected by binocular clues alone.
- Able to measure overall, vertical, horizontal and oblique aniseikonia.

Leaf room

- A visual environment devoid of empirical clues for the perception of space.

Keystone cards

- Stereograms in graded series representing various errors, the card which looks normal gives estimate of error.

C. Diagnosis, Management, and Treatment with Spectacle and Contact Lenses

- Treatment depends on the cause of aniseikonia. Can minimize aniseikonia by spectacle lens design (base curve, lens thickness, vertex distance) or by using contact lenses instead.
- Two types of anisometropia:
  - **Axial**: differences in the axial lengths of the eyes (may see a myopic crescent indicating axial condition)
    - Correct with spectacles, no need for adjustments in lens design.
  - **Refractive:** lens or corneal power too high (if corneal, keratometry readings will differ by more than 1 D).
    - Correct with contact lenses; if correct with spectacles, then need to adjust lens design.
- Rule of thumb, if the ametropia is less than + 4 D, then it is refractive, if it is more than + 4 D, then it is axial.
- **High Astigmatism OU**
  - Generally due to cornea, so correct with contact lenses
  - **Axis is important**: if both eyes have same axis, spectacle correction works well. If axis very different between the eyes (more than 20 degrees), spectacle correction causes the retinal image shapes to be oriented differently, maximizing aniseikonia.
- **Spectacle Lens Design:**
  - Can alter spectacle magnification (SM) by analyzing the formula:

    P_1 = front vertex/base curve (D)

    t = lens thickness (m)

    P_v = back vertex/lens power (D)

    d = vertex distance (m)

    n = index of refraction
  - When SM > 1, magnification
  - When SM < 1, minification

Spectacle Magnification (SM)

SM= $M_{Shape} \times M_{Power}$

$M_{shape} = 1/(1-t/nP_1)$

$M_{Power} = 1/(1-dP_v)$

- ✱✱✱ All plus lenses magnify and all minus lenses minify
- Shape magnification factor:
  - Always > 1 since always have a positive base curve with ophthalmic lenses.
  - Increases with front surface power (more so with plus than with minus lens).
  - Increases with lens thickness.
  - Decreases with increase in index of refraction of lens material.
- Power magnification factor:
  - Always > 1 for plus lens (magnification) ....
  - Always < I for minus lens (minification).
  - Increases with increase in plus lens power.
  - Decreases with increase in minus lens power.
  - Decreases with decrease in vertex distance with plus lens.
  - Increases with decrease in vertex distance with minus lens.

Note: it is better to change magnification by increasing the base curve or the vertex distance than by increasing thickness.

1. Dioptric Components

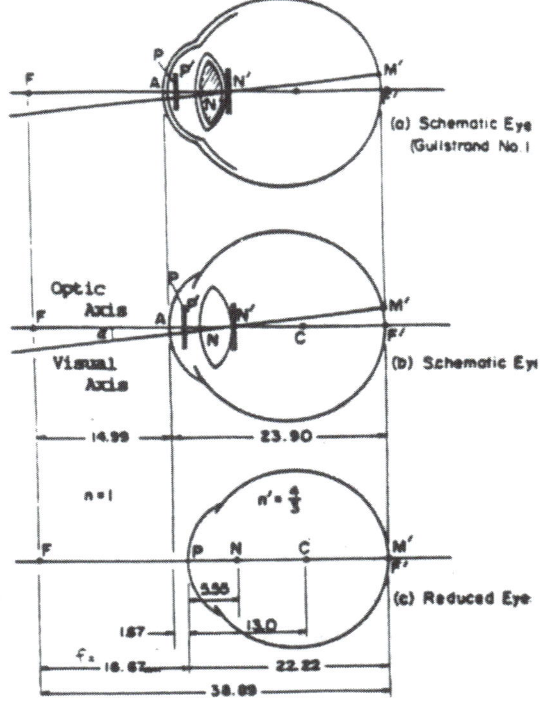

Exact Eye-Gullstrand 1

- The Gullstrand 1 "exact" eye model is the best representation of the real eye. For most purposes, however, the precision of this "exact" eye does not justify the cumbersome calculations it requires. There are six refractive surfaces and four indices of refraction in the crystalline lens. The **six refractive surfaces are**:
  - Anterior cornea
  - Posterior cornea
  - Anterior cortical lens
  - Anterior nuclear lens
  - Posterior nuclear lens
  - Posterior cortical lens
- The **four indices of refraction** are:
  - Cornea (n= 1.376)
  - Aqueous and vitreous humors (n = 1.336)
  - Cortical lens (n = 1.386)
  - Nuclear lens (n = 1.406)

Simplified Eye-Gullstrand 2

- In the Gullstrand 2, the lens is assumed to have a uniform index of refraction (n = 1.416). The posterior surface of the cornea is ignored and the radius of the anterior corneal surface is increased from 7.7mm to 7.8mm. The corneal index of refraction is ignored, and the index of the aqueous and vitreous are taken as n = 1.333.
- Thus there are three refractive surfaces and two indices of refraction for this eye model.

The Reduced Eye

- This eye is treated as an optical system with only one refracting surface and one index of refraction, since the Gullstrand eyes in the relaxed state have their two principal points as well as their two nodal points only 0.30mm apart. The single refracting surface has a power of 60D. The surface separates air from water (n = 1.333) and is situated 1.67mm behind the Gullstrand eye's anterior surface.

2. Cardinal Points, Entrance, and Exit Pupils

Cardinal Points

- There are six points of an optical system. They include the primary and secondary principal points (H, H'), the primary and secondary focal points (F, F'), and the primary and secondary nodal points (N, N').

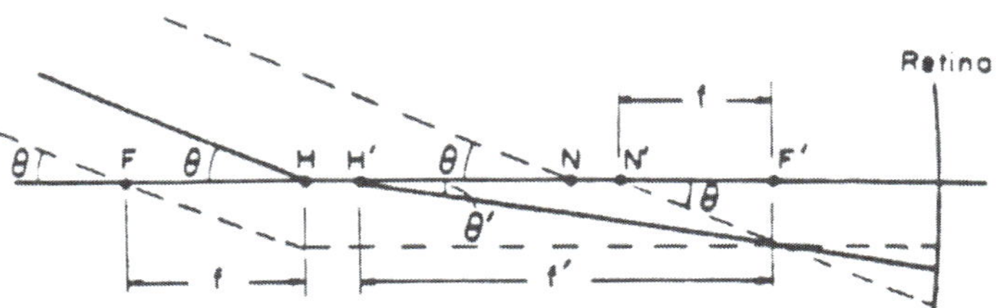

  - F is the axial object point. An object at this point will produce an image at infinity.
  - F' is the axial image point. An infinitely distant object will have its image projected here.
  - H is the point on the optic axis where the optic axis and the

primary principal plane intersect. This plane is the location where a ray from the point F (or its imaginary extension) intersects the image ray emerging parallel to the optic axis (or its extension).
    - H' is similarly defined for a ray leaving or passing thru F'
- There is also a ray that is unbent by the optical system. This is the nodal ray. N is the point where the nodal ray intersects the optic axis. N' is the point on the optic axis where the outgoing nodal ray emerges unbent through the system. N' may be displaced on the optic axis from N because H and H' are not the same position. The incident and emergent nodal rays are always parallel to each other. Planes passing through the nodal points that are perpendicular to the optic axis are called the nodal plane

Entrance Pupil

- The entrance pupil is the image of the aperture stop through the optical elements preceding the stop. If there are no lenses preceding the aperture stop, the aperture stop is the entrance pupil. A ray which lies outside the bundle of rays defined by the entrance pupil can enter the optical system and reach the image plane. In the human eye, the entrance pupil is the image of the human pupil through the cornea (as we see it when we look at one's eye from the outside).

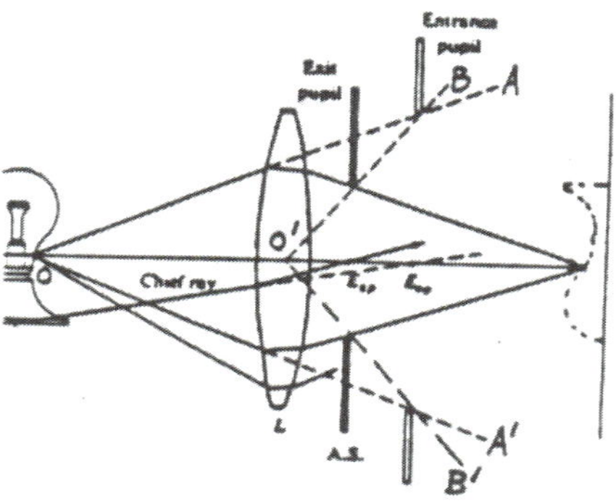

Exit pupil

- The exit pupil is the image of the aperture stop thru any optical elements behind it. No ray outside the bundle of rays defined by the exit pupil can leave the optical system and reach the image plane. If there is no lens behind it, the aperture stop itself is the exit pupil. In the human eye, the exit pupil is the image of the pupil through the crystalline lens and vitreous if we were standing on the retina and looking at the human pupil from the inside.

The Reduced Eye

- In the reduced eye model, H and H' both coincide with the vertex of the cornea. This is because for a single surface refracting interface (SSRI), the nodal points coincide with a single point, the center of curvature. Hence, there is only one nodal point (i.e. N and N' are at the same location). The exit pupil is the pupil of the eye itself, since no refracting elements follow it. The entrance pupil is the image of the pupil as formed by the cornea.
- Since the actual pupil lies on the first principal plane, the exit pupil must lie on the second principal plane. However, the two principal planes coincide; hence the entrance pupil and the real pupil coincide also. Note, however, that even though the two pupils coincide, the real pupil lies in an optical space of index n= 1.00 (air), and the exit pupil lies in a space of index n= 1.333 (aqueous).

3. Ametropia: Far Point, Near Point, Correction

- **Far point:** where an object is placed relative to the eye for it to be in focus with accommodation relaxed. The far point for an emmetrope is at infinity, behind the eye for a hyperope, and in front of the eye for a myope.
- **Near point:** where an object is placed relative to the eye for it to be in focus with accommodation engaged
- **Myopia**: Corrected with Minus Power
- **Hyperopia**: Corrected with Plus Power

4. Accommodation

- An individual can only use half of their accommodative amplitude comfortably.
- Myope accommodates less than emmetrope.
- Hyperope accommodates more than emmetrope.

A_o=accommodation

Accommodation
$\mathbf{A_o=U_{fp}-U_x}$

U_{fp}=far point incoming vergence=how much vergence is needed to focus an object on the retina
U_x=incoming vergence from object

Example: *A -5.00 D myope is looking at an object 12.5 cm away. How much does he need to accommodate to view the object clearly?*

Answer:
u=-0.125m
U_x=-8.0D
U_{fp} = -5.00 D
A_o=(-5.00)-(-8.00)= +3.00

5. Astigmatism

- **Astigmatism:** refractive condition in which a variation of power exists in the different meridians of the eye so that no point focus is formed because of the unequal refraction of light by the eye.
- The total astigmatism is the sum of the corneal astigmatism and lenticular astigmatism.
- Cylindrical correction is needed to allow a pinpoint of light to focus on the retina instead of multiple focus points that result in blur.

6. Retinal Image Size, Spectacle Magnification, and Relative Spectacle Magnification

- Anisometropic prescriptions produce problems with image size differences.
- Spectacle magnification: type of angular magnification that represents retinal image size relative to the optical lens. Product of power (M_p) and shape component (M_s).
  - t=lens thickness
  - n=refractive index
  - P_1=lens front curve
  - d=distance between lens back pole and entrance pupil =stop distance
  - P_v=back vertex power

Spectacle Magnification
M_p=1/[1-(t/n)(P_1)]
M_s=1/[1-(d)(P_v)]
M_T= (M_p) (M_s)

DIOPTRICS OF THE EYE

1. Characteristics of Ocular Components

Curvature

- Cornea
  - Anterior radius = 7.8 mm
  - Anterior surface has 43 D of power, due primarily to the air/tear layer interface.
  - Posterior radius = 6.5 mm
  - Posterior surface has little power due to the small difference of the indices between the cornea and the aqueous.
- Lens
  - Anterior radius = (10 mm to 5.33 mm)
  - Posterior radius = (6mm to 5.33 mm)

  (The first, larger values in parentheses are for the lens in its non-accommodative state).

Thickness

- Cornea
  - 0.52 mm at the center
  - 0.67 mm at the limbus
- Lens
  - 3.5 to 4.0 mm in the young adult, which increases with age up to about 5.0 mm at age 90.

Separation

- The cornea is separated from air by the tear layer
- The crystalline lens is immersed in the aqueous humor in front and the vitreous behind.
- The corneal vault (from the posterior surface of the cornea to the anterior surface of the lens) = 2.6mm.

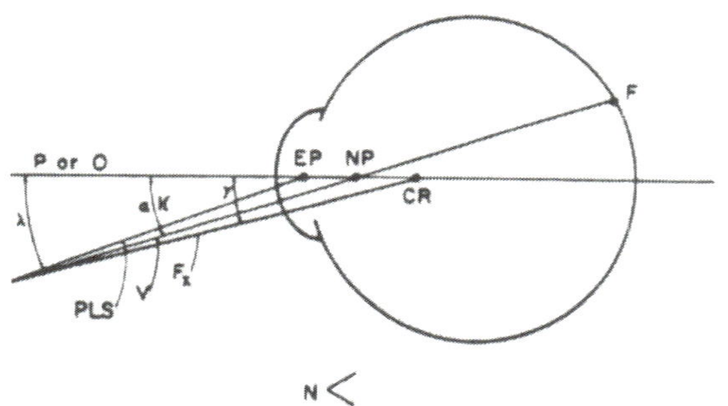

P	Pupillary axis	PLS	Primary line of sight
O	Optic axis	V	Visual axis
EP	Entrance pupil	F_x	Fixation axis
NP	Nodal point	λ	P and PLS
CR	Center of rotation of eye	a	V and O
F	Fovea	γ	O and F_x
N	Nose	K	V and P

Refractive indices

- Tear layer n = 1.336
- Aqueous n = 1.336
- Vitreous n = 1.336
- Cornea n = 1.3376
- Lens n = 1.416

Axial length

- For the emmetropic eye, the axial length (the distance from the corneal apex to the fovea) is approximately equal to 24 mm.

2. Reference Angles and Axes

Axes

- **Optic axis:** connects the centers of curvature of the cornea and lens
- **Pupillary axis:** passes thru the center of the entrance pupil and perpendicular to the center of the cornea
- **Visual axis:** extends thru the fixation point, nodal point and the fovea.
- **Primary line of sight:** from the point of fixation to the center of the entrance pupil.
- **Fixation axis:** from the point of fixation to the center of rotation.

Angles

- **Alpha** (a) between the visual and optic axes
- **Kappa** (k) between the visual and pupillary axes. Measured in the clinic (monocularly) to detect eccentric fixation.
- **Lambda** (λ) between the primary line of sight and the pupillary axes. Clinically, angle λ is equal to angle k.
- **Gamma** (γ) between the fixation point and the optic axis.

An easy method to remember the reference axes and the angles between them is

Reference axes:

F O V P PLS

Reference Angles:

γ a k λ

- The first line of letters represents the first letter of each of the axes.
- The second line represents the 1st letter of each angle and is the angle formed by the two axes located above each angle letter.

3. Catoptric (Purkinje) Images

No.	Derivation	Characteristics	Brightness
1	Ant. Cornea	Virtual, erect, small	1
2	Post. Cornea	Virtual, erect, small	0.01
3	Ant. Lens	Virtual, erect, larger than 1, badly defined due to stippled surface	0.008
4	Post. Lens	Real, inverted, largest	0.008

Note: the first three images are virtual, erect, and minified because they are derived from surfaces that serve as convex mirrors. Image four is derived from what is essentially a concave mirror. "Brightness" refers to relative brightness of the images. Order of size from largest to smallest: III, I, II, IV.

When light strikes a refracting surface, part of the light will pass through the surface and part will be reflected. The fraction of light reflected is given by Fresnel's Formula

Reflectance

$$\mathbf{R = \frac{(n2 - n1)^2}{(n2 + n1)^2}}$$

where n1 and n2 are the refractive indices of the media at the boundary. This law is true only for rays incident perpendicularly to the surface. The equation clearly shows that both refraction and reflection must occur at every interface of two transparent media with different indices of refraction. In the human eye, this gives rise to the four purkinje images, which are summarized above.

4. Retinal Image Size

- Our perception of the size of an object depends not only on the size of its image on the retina, but also how far away we perceive it to be. The angular size of the retinal image is the angle subtended at the secondary nodal point. The law states that perceived size is proportional to perceived distance, for a given retinal image size, is known as Emmert's Law.

5. Optical Function of the Pupil

- **Increase depth of focus (DOF):** A decrease in pupil size for an out-of focus eye tends to result in increase visual acuity because the depth of focus (DOF) is increased.
- **Reduce Aberrations**: The pupil decreases peripheral rays, therefore decreasing spherical aberration, chromatic aberrations, and oblique astigmatism.
- **Adjust amount of light that reaches the retina:** The pupil also functions optically to limit the amount of light falling on the retina. In fact, if the pupil decreases from an 8 mm diameter to a 2 mm diameter, the area of the pupil decreases from approximately 50 mm^2 to 3 mm^2. Thus, the pupil can decrease the amount of light falling on the retina by a factor of 16.

ENTOPTIC PHENOMENA

---

1. Characteristics and Origin of Various Phenomena

Corneal

- Tear droplets and mucus on the cornea acts as a convex lens and they appear as bright spots surrounded by a dark margin. During a blink, the movement of the lids causes them to move upward on the cornea, causing them to appear to float down.
- Striae across the field are due to transient wrinkling of the lacrimal fluid and appear as bright bands with a darker area. Folds, scars, and wrinkles produce similar visual phenomena.

Lenticular

- Opacities in crystalline lens appear dark if the opacity has a lower index of refraction than the lens.

- Small round discs seen with a bright center and a dark border (or vice versa) are called the "Pearl Specks of listing" and are mucus in the liquor Morgagni.
- Small opacities in the lens capsule appear dark.
- Radiating bright patches near the middle of the field are located in the anterior capsule membrane.
- Fine, dark, radiating lines are seen because the refractive index of the cement substance within the laminated structure of the lens is different from the refractive index of the lens fibers.
- Dark lines radiating inwards are shadows on the retina cast by lens opacities.

Vitreal

- Objects in the vitreous media cast a shadow on the retina. If opaque, they cast a black shadow. If semi-transparent but denser than the media, they cast a bright area surrounded by a darker rim. If they are semi-transparent but less dense, they cast a shadow with a darker center then the rim.
- Muscae Volitantes (a.k.a. "floaters") are pale cells, debris of cells and fibers, persistent embryonic cell structures, and remnants of primary vitreous suspended in the vitreous gel. Because they have a certain freedom of movement, those with a specific gravity less than the vitreous move upwards. The majority is located 1/3 mm to 4 mm in front of the retina and cast a sharp shadow on the retina. These are most common in myopes and older individuals who have liquefied vitreous.

2. Vascular and Circulatory Phenomena

Purkinje Tree

- Visualization of the vascular tree of the retina by trans-illumination is a commonly used clinical test of retinal function. The retinal vessels cast a shadow on the rods and cones because the vessels lie anteriorly to the photoreceptors. The shadow is not normally perceived because of local adaptation. To prevent this adaptation, a small flashlight or trans-illuminator is lightly placed against the eyelid near the lateral canthus or directly on the conjunctiva and oscillated in position. Most subjects readily visualize the vascular tree.

Capillary Circulation

- This can be perceived best when one looks at a background of monochromatic light in the region from 350 to 450 nm (hemoglobin absorbs light in this region of the spectrum). Shadows of white and/or red corpuscles are perceived. It is controversial which color is seen. This phenomenon is connected intimately with the circulation of blood. The particles move in more or less definite paths, having the arrangement of capillary loops, and the movement is pulsatile and shows marked acceleration when the heart speeds up.

3. Phenomena associated with Central Vision

Maxwell's spot

- When light is transmitted thru a purple (red plus blue) filter and into the eye, a reddish entoptic spot is seen as a result of the absorption of blue light by the macular pigment. Maxwell's spot is seen at the point of fixation if the subject is foveally fixating. This is used clinically to detect eccentric fixation or to check the integrity of the foveal area.

Haidinger's Brush

- A transient entoptic phenomenon is observed when polarized light-blue light from a large homogenous surface is viewed. It consists of a pair of yellow or blue brush-like shapes which appear to radiate from the point of fixation, believed to be due to variations in absorption by Henle's nerve fiber layer and macular pigment in the fovea. Clinically a shape similar to an airplane propeller or a bow tie is seen. Since the effect is caused by nerves oriented in front of the photoreceptor layer, any process that upsets this orientation, even though it does not disturb the photoreceptors themselves, may lead to disappearance of the brushes. Therefore, the test for Haidinger's brushes may show early changes in the macula, such as edema, before they reach the point of interfering with visual acuity. Haidinger's brush, much like Maxwell's spot, is used to assess eccentric fixation.

4. Phenomena associated with Retinal Distention or Other Retinal Activity

Moore's lightning streaks

- Described by Moore in 1935, they are flashes of light frequently likened to lightning seen in the peripheral of the eye in the vertical direction. These streaks are either accompanied or followed by dark spots before the eyes. This phenomenon is probably the result of vitreous detachment as the vitreous shrinks forward toward its base. Traction on the retina can produce phosphenes (see below). For the patient who reports lightning streak, a good look at the peripheral retina and ora serrata is in order. Fortunately, most persons who report phosphenes do not get a retinal detachment, but some do.

Blue arcs of the retina

- If an observer in a dark room monocularly fixates a point slightly to the temporal sides of a small light source (any shape or color), he will see two small bands or arcs of blue light, radiating from the stimulus toward the blind spot. These arcs are always in the horizontal plane and appear almost as soon as the stimulus is turned on. If the upper edge of the source is fixated, only the lower arcs appear and vice versa. Fixating the nasal side of the source produces a blue haze between the previous regions where the arcs appeared that has been referred to as the blue spike. The cause of the blue arcs is still unknown, but secondary electrical excitation of neighboring retinal nerve fibers or neurons by active nerve fibers is the probable origin of the phenomenon.

Phosphenes

- A phosphene is a subjective visual sensation of luminous spot or an area in the external visual field, arising from mechanical or electrical stimulation of the eyeball.

IMAGE QUALITY

---

1. Aberrations

- Aberrations can be subdivided into lower and higher order depending upon the complexity of the shape of the wavefront emerging from an eye: the more complex the wavefront shape, the higher order the aberration
  - **Lower Order Aberrations**: aberrations that are fully correctible with corrective lenses, also known as spherical and cylindrical refractive error such as myopia, (positive defocus), hyperopia (negative defocus), and astigmatism
  - **Higher Order Aberrations:** aberrations that are not correctible with spherocylindrical lenses.
    - A distortion acquired by a wavefront of light when it passes through the eye with irregular refractive components (tear film, cornea, aqueous/vitreous humor, and the crystalline lens
    - Abnormal curvature of cornea and lens may contribute to the distortion
    - Serious higher-order aberrations can be caused from corneal scarring from eye surgery, trauma, and/or disease
    - Most higher-order aberrations are identified by **Zernike polynomials** (mathematical expressions).
- Common higher-order aberrations include coma, trefoil, and spherical aberration.
  - **Coma**: When rays at one edge of the system are focused before the center and opposite edge, causing an image point that represents a comet's tail or tear drop.
    - Clinically seen in patients with keratoconus and tilted-grafts
  - **Trefoil**: Rays are focused as a three-axis astigmatism
  - **Spherical**: Peripheral rays focus in front of the central rays
    - Clinically seen in post-LASIK and post-PRK patients, it causes night myopia
  - For details on spherical, chromatic, coma, curvature, oblique astigmatism, and distortion, see Chapter 1

- **Wavefront** – imaginary surface joining all points in space that are reached at the same time by a light wave propagating through a medium.
- **Huygen's Principle**: All points on a wavefront can be considered point sources for the production of secondary wavelets, and at a later time the new wavefront position is the envelope (or surface of tangency) to these secondary wavelets
- **Wavefront aberrometry** is a technology that measures higher and lower aberrations due to corneal and lenticular changes. It is used to determine the causes of visual disturbances (aberrations) and to program ablations in wavefront-guided laser eye surgery procedures
- **Aberrometer**, a machine that uses wavefronts to objectively measure overall refractive error.
- There are 3 different types of wavefront aberrometry
  - **Hartmann-Shack**
    - Most popular. Quick. Repeatable, high-resolution.
    - Projects a single infrared laser light point image on the retina. The point source is reflect back through the entrance pupil and passes through a **lenslet array** (small lenses in a specific pattern) made up of between 200-1400 lenses depending on instrument. The emerging wavefront represents the optical properties of the eye.
      - If the eye is optically perfect all the individual rays will exit the eye simultaneously so the wavefront is straight or perfectly curved
      - If the eye has aberrations, the individual rays will exit the eye at different times and the wavefront will have irregularities to it
    - Light passing through an individual lenslet is focused on a charged-coupled device (CCD) array at the center position for the lenslet and then recorded by the computer.
      - CCD- grid of photon absorbing medium that collect and measure electrons released by a material when light hits it
  - **Tscherning**
    - Projects a grid (fixed pattern of spots) onto the retina and the cameras record the image distortion by finding the location of the spots with respect to the expected location. The changes in the shape of the pattern correlate to the eye's aberrations.
  - **Ray Tracing**
    - Consecutive measurements over several sampling points (in ms). Can detect large magnitude errors of reflection
    - Multiple rays of laser light are projected onto the retina. The exiting location of each individual ray is compared to the known entry point and aberrations are calculated using polynomials.
- Aberrometers vary in degree of accuracy, dynamic range, pupil diameter maximums/minimums, analysis, and compatibility.
  - Accuracy – number and spread of points measured. The higher the number of points the better, but spread must be even
  - Dynamic Range – ability to detect higher and lower ranges and subtleties in variations
  - Less precise wavefront sensors may not detect keratoconus, corneal scarring, and severe high order aberrations
- Aberration Calculations
  - Eye's aberration = Ideal Wavefront- Actual wavefront
  - Calculated in microns
  - Positive values: actual wavefront travels further than ideal wavefront
  - Negative values: ideal wavefront travels further than the actual wavefront

2. Diffraction

- See Chapter 2: Wave Optics

3. Stray Light

- **Stray light** – any unwanted light in an optical system. Stray light is caused by light from a bright source shining into the front of the system and reaching the image as unwanted light

- Stray light reduces the contrast of an image and is commonly manifested as either ghost images (veiling glare) or scattered light.
- **Veiling Glare**: When multiple reflections from optical component surfaces cause the object scene or entrance pupil to be "ghosted" onto the detection plane (retina).

4. Point and Line Spread Functions

- Due to diffraction and aberration, the image of a bright point by an optical system is not a geometric point in the image plane, but is a light distribution. The image consists of a bright core surrounded by a less bright halo.
- **Point Spread Function (PSF):** Is the modulation transfer function of a point object. It describes the light distribution of a point source, where the peak of the distribution has the greatest intensity.
    - If the peak of the point spread function for one point source coincides with the point spread function of a second point source, then the two point sources will be resolved as two separate objects. This situation meets Rayleigh's criterion.
    - The PSF of a patient's eye can be measured with a wavefront sensor to "see" what the patient sees. This diagnostic tool allows the optometrist to simulate potential treatments for a patient and see how the treatments would affect the patient's PSF.
    - The interplay between diffraction and aberration is characterized by the PSF
        - The narrower the lens aperture the more likely PSF is cominated by diffraction, and angular resolution (resolving power) of the system can be estimated by Rayleigh's criterion
- **Line Spread Function:** Is the modulation transfer function (MTF) of a line object. It describes the light distribution of two lines. It is used in infrared imaging.

5. Resolving Power

- **Resolving Power:** the ability of an eye (optical imaging system) to separate/resolve points of an object that are located at a small **angular distance**.
    - The resolving power can be limited either by aberration or diffraction which causes image blur
- In terms of spatial gratings, resolving power is the highest spatial frequency grating (most number of bars) that can be seen by the system.
- **Minimum Angle of Resolution (MAR)**: the angle the smallest detail makes. It is the threshold or resolving power of the eye. Units are minutes of arc

Resolving Power of the Eye
MAR=1/VA

6. Modulation Transfer Function (Fourier Optics)

- **Optical Transfer Function (OTF)**: the true measure of resolution that an imaging system is capable
- **Modulation Transfer Function (MTF)**: the magnitude of the OTF. Describes the ability of adjacent pixels to change from black to white in response to patterns of varying spatial frequency, and thus the actual capability of the optical system to show fine detail with full or reduced contrast.
    - MTF can be represented by a graph of light amplitude (brightness) vs. Spatial frequency (cycles per picture width)
- The method of analysis consists of comparing the modulation (also called visibility or contrast) in the object to the resulting modulation in the image

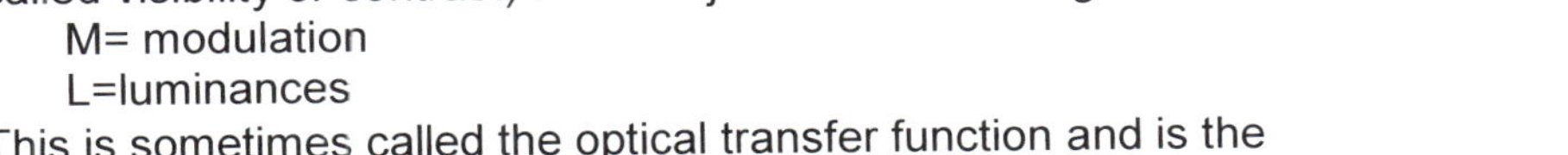

M= modulation
L=luminances

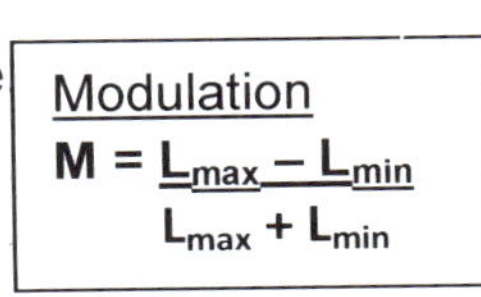

Modulation

$$\mathbf{M = \frac{L_{max} - L_{min}}{L_{max} + L_{min}}}$$

- This is sometimes called the optical transfer function and is the ratio of output modulation to input modulation
- **Fourier Analysis**: a mathematical process. The visual system is considered to be a Fourier analyzer (deconstructs the retinal image into its spatial frequency components.

RADIATION AND THE EYE

1. Radiometry

- **Radiometry**: the measurement of the power produced by a source electromagnetic radiant energy.
- The **watt (W)** is the basic unit of radiometry and is a measure of radiant power

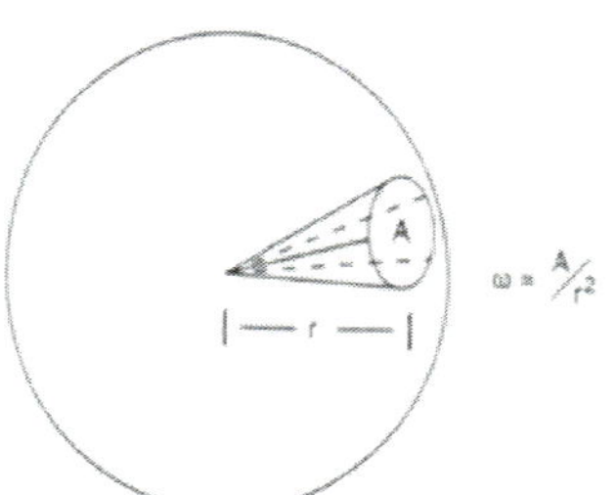

Units

- **Radiant Flux (P_e)** :the radiant energy emitted per unit time (Joules/Sec=Watts)
  E=energy
  t=time
- **Steradian (ω)** – (See picture) the solid angle subtended at the center of a sphere of 1 meter radius by an area of 1 meter squared of the sphere surface.
  A = surface area of sphere
  r = radius of sphere
- **Radiant intensity (I_e)** – the total energy emitted from a source in a given direction. I_e = Watts/steradians
- **Irradiance (E_e)** – the energy incident on a surface at some distance from a source. E_e = Watts/m^2
- **Radiance (L_e)** – the energy emitted from a unit area of a surface. L_e = Watts/steradians x m^2

Radiant Flux
P_e = E/t =J/sec=W
Steradian
$\omega = A/r^2$
Radiant Intensity
I_e=W/ω
Irradiance
$E_e = W/m^2$
Radiance
$L_e = (W/\omega)\ m^2$

2. Photometry

- **Photometry:** Light measurement and its effect of light on the visual system.
- The **lumen** is the basic unit of photometry, and is a measure of luminous power
- Measurement of light by physical instruments is meaningful only if the amount of energy measured corresponds to the quantity which would evoke a response in the eye.
  - The **photopic luminosity curve V(λ)** indicates that certain wavelengths are more efficient at stimulating the visual system than others
  - Two stimuli may have the same power (10 watts for example) but have different effects on the visual system because they have differing luminous efficiencies (400nm=0 Lumens, 600nm=4216 Lumens)
- **Luminous Power/Flux (F_v)**: total amount of light power produced by a source (Lumens)
  - **Lumens (L_m)** = A candela gives off a lumen of 555nm light (peak photopic sensitivity). For converting photometric flux (lumens) to radiometric flux (watts) we use a conversion factor **K_m**

  P_1 = radiant power or radiant flux at 1 (watts).
  V_1 = relative photopic luminous efficiency (CIE) for a given wavelength
  L_e = radiance of extended source
  ω = steradians
  cd = Candela
  (In practice, the range of wavelengths over which integration takes place is 380-750nm.)
- **Luminous Intensity (I_V)** : light power produced (emitted) in a solid angle by a
- point source (Lumens/steradian or Candelas)
- **Luminance (L_v)**: Luminous intensity per unit projected area of an extended source (Candelas/m^2 or Foot-lamberts). Quantifies the amount of light coming off of a surface. Perceptually attributed as "brightness"

Luminance Power
$F_V = 680(P_1)(V_1)$
Luminance
$L_v = (Lm)/\omega m^2$
Illuminance
$E_v = (Lm)/m^2$
Conversions
K_m= 680 Lm/Watt
Lm= K_m (V_1)(L_e)
cd =Lm/ω

- Both luminance and brightness remain constant as the distance from the surface increases because the area of the image decreases at the same rate as does the number of candelas contained within the image (Ratio of candelas:image surface remains constant, so luminance and brightness do not change)

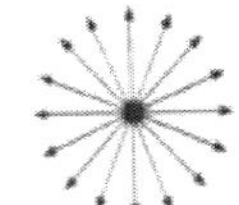

- **Illuminance (E_v)**: Luminous power falling on a surface (Lumens/m^2 also known as "lux" or Lumens/ft^2 also known as "foot-candles"). Illuminance is not affected by the surface on which light falls
- Radiometric and photometric concepts parallel each other, being mathematically related by the relative luminous efficiency curve of the "standard observer" -1924.

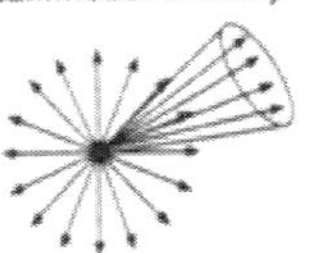

Note: Because individual eyes differ in their spectral sensitivity curves under the same photopic conditions, an international CIE standard observer curve has been established (1924). This curve is called the luminous efficiency curve (V1). The sensitivity characteristics of a physical receiver (such as the eye) should be the same as the V1 curve. The term "efficiency," as applied to visible radiant energy (light), is dimensionless, having a maximum value of 1.0 at 555nm.

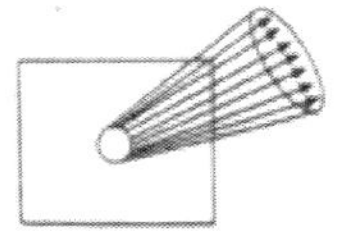

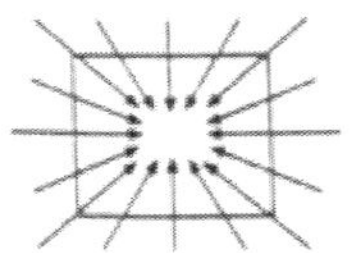

Note: For convenience in developing a system of light units and terms, it would have made sense to arbitrarily define 1 watt of radiant power at 555nm, all other wavelengths being less than 1 lumen per watt by their relative luminous efficiency. However, light has been specified for thousands of years, certainly long before 1924, and the original units of light intensity were based on the very practical use of a candle which was said to emit 4p lumens. In short, 1 watt at 555nm does not equal 1 lumen, but rather 680 lumens.

Photometric Term (Units)	Radiometric Equivalent (Units)
Luminous Power *(Lumens)*	Radiant Power *(J/sec=Watt)*
Luminous Intensity *(Lumens/Steradian) or (Candelas)*	Radiant Intensity *(Watts/Steradian)*
Luminance *(Candelas/m^2) or (Foot-lamberts)*	Radiance *(Watts/Steradian/m^2)*
Illuminance *(Lumens/m^2) or (Lumens/ft^2 = Foot-Candelas)*	Irradiance *(Watts/m^2)*

Example: *What is the luminous power of 10 watts at 600nm?*

> ***Answer:***
> To convert 10 watts at 600nm to lumens, we consult the V1 curve and see that luminous efficiency at 600nm is equal to 0.63.
> Then Luminous power = (10)(680)(0.63) = 4280 lumens.

Lambertian Surfaces

- A **specular surface** like a mirror has varying luminance depending on the direction at which it is measured
- A **Cosine Surfaces** also known as **Lambert, Perfectly Diffusing, or Matte Surface** shows the same luminance regardless of the angle at which the luminance is measured.
- A cosine diffuser is a surface (i.e. matte surface) where light is reflected from a given point in all directions, all with different intensity. If the intensity of each ray reflected from the point is a vector, the longest vector, or most intense ray (I_{max}), is the ray that is normal to the surface. The reduction in intensity of the other rays is proportional to the cosine of the vector angle. If the tips of a given point were connected, they would form the shape of a sphere.

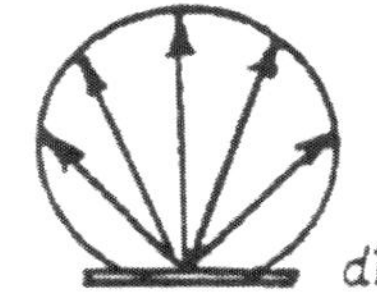

- The main simplification in the Lambert system is the relationship of luminance (L) in foot-lamberts to illuminance (E) in foot-candles. If you take a piece of paper and illuminate it and measure the luminance coming off the paper, the luminance and illuminance are related by a reflection factor (r) which is nondimensional and has no units.

> Luminance of a Lambert Surface
> **L=rE**

Example: *If the illumination of a surface with a 0.05 reflectance factor is 100 foot-candles, what is the luminance of the surface?*

> ***Answer:***
> $E = 100\ lm/ft^2$
> $r = 0.05$
> L = 0.05 x 100 = 50 foot-Lamberts.

- **Inverse Square Law**: As a surface is moved away from a point source, the number of lumens falling on it decreases with the square of the distance, resulting in a decrease in its illumination. This assumes that the surface is normal to the light source.
  - E=illumination falling on the surface
  - I= intensity of the point source
  - d= distance from the point source to the surface

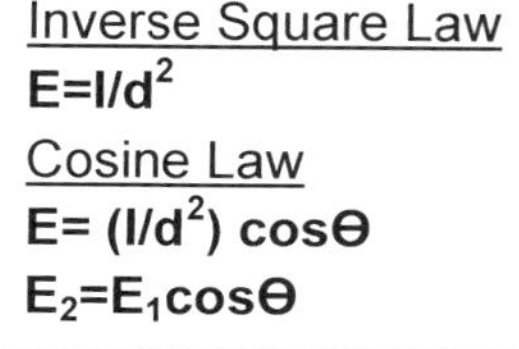

Inverse Square Law
$E=I/d^2$
Cosine Law
$E= (I/d^2) \cos\Theta$
$E_2=E_1\cos\Theta$

- If the surface is tilted, less lumens fall on it resulting in a decrease in illumination, which is proportional to the cosine of the angle of tilt of the surface (Θ). This is the **Cosine Law of Illumination.**
  - Θ= Angle of tilt of the surface
  - E_1= Illumination falling on the surface when normal to the light source
  - E_2= Illumination falling on the tilted light source

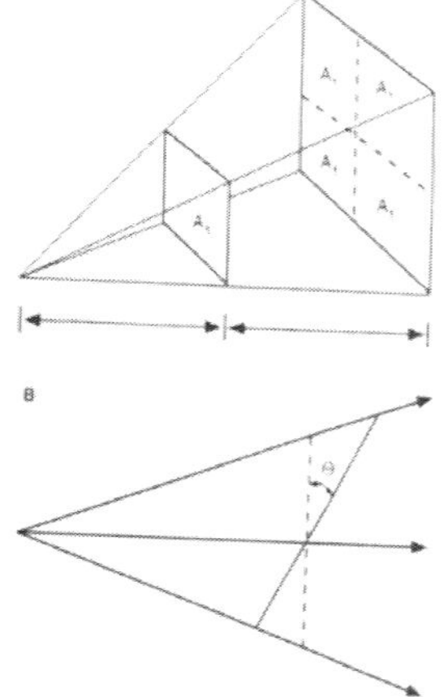

Note: Luminance does not change with the angle because luminance is a function of the source not the viewing angle or distance from the source.

- Most objects emit a polychromatic radiation, not monochromatic. The luminous power for this stimulus is determined by calculating the number of lumens produced by each wavelength and adding the values together, this is known as **Abney's Law**.
- **Abney's Law of Additivity**: The total luminance contributed by a complex spectral radiation is equal to the sum of the luminances of the component monochromatic radiations.
  - Luminances estimated by heterochromatic flicker photometry and minimally distinct border are additive.

Note: Brightness matching is not additive.

Example: *What is the total luminance of an object that emits 5W of 475nm, 4W of 555nm, and 3W of 600nm light?*

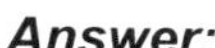

> ***Answer:***
> 5W of 475nm: (0.1)(680Lm/W)(5W) = 340 Lumens
> 4W of 555nm: (1.0)(680Lm/W)(4W) = 2720 Lumens
> 3W of 600nm: (0.62)(680Lm/W)(3W)=1265 Lumens
> Total= 340 +2720 +1265= 4325 Lumens

3. Spectral Transmission of the Ocular Media

- The atmospheric scatter and absorption eliminates the majority of the sun's radiation. The remaining electromagnetic radiation is absorbed by ocular media to protect the retina. Short wavelength light has more energy than longer wavelengths and its blockage is more important.
- The **cornea** absorbs short UV-C radiation. Excessive UV-C radiation (skiing) can lead to corneal inflammation and **solar keratitis**
- The **lens** absorbed most of the UV-A and UV-B radiation. Over time excessive UV absorption leads to **cataracts**
    - Excessive exposure to long IR radiation can lead to "**glass blower's cataracts**"
- **Summary of UV wavelength absorption:**
    - Cornea = 200-290nm
    - Lens = 290-365nm
    - Retina = >365mn

4. Retinal Illuminance

- **Retinal Illumination (T)**: the amount of light falling on the retina. This is pupil size dependent. Units are Trolands (td)
  L= luminance of the surface that is viewed
  A=pupil area
- The retina is sensitive to the flux density (illuminance) of light falling onto it. In daylight conditions, and for all but very small or briefly presented objects, the visual sensation is more or less proportional to the retinal illuminance produced by that object.
- Luminances in object space can be related to illuminance at the retina:
  E_r = Retinal illuminance (lumens/m^2)
  L = object luminance (cd/m^2)
  g = pupil radius (m)
  t = ocular transmittance
  cos q = displacement from the primary line of sight
  k = 0.015

Retinal Illumination
T=LA
or
$E_r = (L)(g^2)(t)(\cos q)/ k^2$

- It can be seen that individuals with different pupil sizes or different transmission characteristics may have significantly different visual effects from identical objects. These individual variations must be considered when predictions of visual behavior are made solely from luminance descriptions of the scene.

5. Effects of Incoherent (IR, Visible, UV) Radiation on Tissue

- **Mechanisms of Damage**
    - Electromagnetic radiation can transfer energy to atoms and molecules in the cellular structure, making the electrons jump to higher energy levels, putting the atoms and molecules into ionized or excited states. These excitations and ionizations can cause injury to living tissues by:
        - Producing free radicals
        - Breaking chemical bonds
        - Producing new chemical bonds and cross-linking macromolecules
        - Damaging molecules that regulate vital cell processes (DNA, RNA, proteins)
    - At low doses, calls can repair certain levels of cell damage. But at high or prolonged doses, cell death can result and tissues can fail to function
    - Absorption of energy by (UV especially) by double bonds in nucleic acids leads to molecular fragmentation. The new molecules may induce inflammation, transform neoplastic cells, or affect the immune system
    - Pigmented molecules (such as melanin) absorb light, causing unstable states and free radical (superoxide) generation, which disrupt cell membranes, mitochondrial membranes, nucleic acids, and destroy tissues.

- While only small amounts of UVA and UVB can reach the inner eye, the ocular tissues are highly sensitive to the damaging effects of **Ultra-Violet radiation** and cumulative exposure makes UVR clinically significant
- Greatest concern with **Infrared Radiation** is the heating (thermal) effects to the lens and retina
- **Visible light** can damage the retina when emitted from high intensity sources (projector bulbs, spotlights, and floodlights) because visible light is focused (concentrated) on the retina by the front of the eye

- **Wavelength, Energy Levels, Threshold for Reaction**
  - Incoherent radiation is classified as UV (100-400nm), Visible (380-780nm), and IR (780nm-1mm) radiation. UV and IR can be subdivided into:
    - UV-A (315-380nm) IR-A(780-1400nm)
    - UV-B (290-315nm) IR-B (1400-3000nm)
    - UV-C (200-290nm) IR-C (3000nm-1mm)
  - **Cornea**: Absorbs UV-B, IR-C, most IR-B
  - **Lens**: Absorbs most UV-A, some IR-A
    - UV-A can penetrate deeper into the eye and damage the retina
  - **Iris**: Absorbs 53% to 95% of IR- A (750-900nm) depending on pigmentation
  - **Retina**: Absorbs most of remaining IR-B and IR-C

Summary of the Biological Effects of Incoherent Radiation on Ocular Tissue			
Ocular Tissue	**Biological Effect**	**Wavelength**	**Radiation**
Skin (Eyelids)	Basal Cell Carcinoma Squamous Cell Carcinoma Sebaceous Carcinoma Malignant Melanoma	280-400nm	UV-A, UV-B
	Erythema	200-400nm	UV-A, UV-B, UV-C
	Erythema → 3rd Degree Burns (thermal)	1400nm-1mm	Visible, IR (rare, laser-induced)
Conjunctiva	Pterygium Pinguecula Squamous Cell Carcinoma	280-400nm	UV-A, UV-B
	Thermal Injury to cornea	1400nm-1mm	IR-C (pulsed laser)
Cornea	Photokeratoconjunctivitis aka Photokeratitis (sunburn of the cornea) Snow blindness Welder's Flash	180-400nm	UV-A, UV-B, UV-C
	Blue Light Photoretinitis aka Solar Retinitis aka Welder's Maculopathy	400-550nm	Visible Blue Light
	Thermal injury of cornea	1400nm-1mm	IR-C (pulsed laser)
Anterior Chamber/Iris	Swelling/inflammation of iris, Hyperemia, papillary miosis→ aqueous flare	780nm-1mm	IR
Lens	Cataracts Nuclear Sclerosis	295-325nm	UV-A, UV-B (chronic exposure)
	Thermal Cataract	800-3000nm	IR-A, IR-B
Vitreous	Aphakes can get shrinking of vitreous gel and denaturation of collagen network	200-400nm	UV-A, UV-B, UV-C
Retina	ARMD	315-400nm	UV-A
	Thermal injury (edema, burns, depigmentation)	400-1400nm	Visible, IR-A (laser)

- **Protective Measures**
    - External barriers to electromagnetic radiation: brows, orbital bones, lids, and lashes
    - Additional Protection:
        - Filters in IOLs (filter out wavelengths <400nm)
        - Avoidance of outdoors
        - Hat/visor
        - Contact Lenses (Silicone hydrogel)
        - Sunglasses (Polarized, Transitions, Wrap-around, 100% UVA/UVB treated lenses)
- **At risk groups**
    - Children
    - Elderly
    - Lightly pigmented individuals
    - Aphakia/Pseudophakia
    - Photosensitizing drugs (oral contraceptives, phenothiazines, 8-methoxypsoralen, allupurinol, tetracyclines)

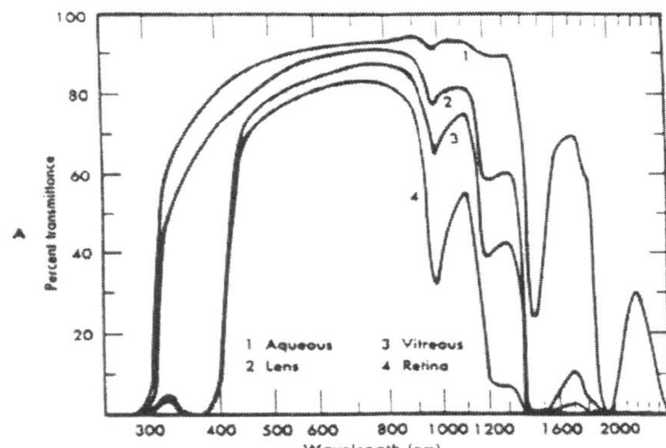

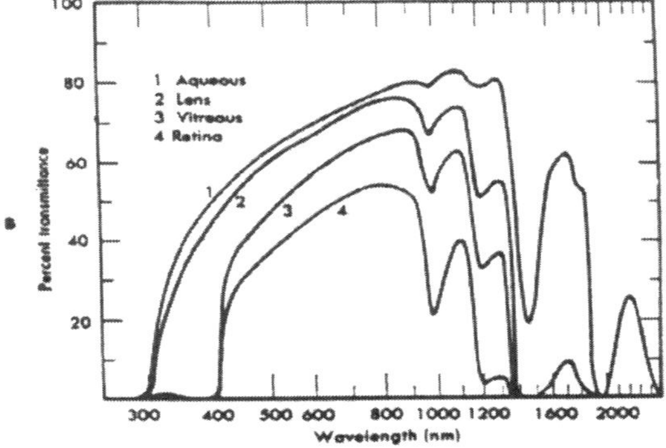

Transmission of visible light and near infrared by ocular media. A, Total transmittance through entire eye. B, Direct transmittance through entire eye. (From Boettner, E. A., and Wolter, J. R.: Invest. Ophthalmol. 1:776-783, 1962.)

6. Effects of Coherent (Laser) Radiation on Tissue

- **Mechanisms of Damage**
    - Health risks from lasers are related to wavelengths and exposure levels
    - **Coherent:** radiation formed by charges within the sources oscillate in unison. Coherence (low divergence angle of laser light) allows for the light to be concentrated into extremely small spots on the retina
    - The majority of injury from lasers is caused by thermal effects
    - Thermal damage (burn) occurs when tissues are heated to the point where denaturation occurs
    - Photochemical damage occurs with short-wavelength and UV light and can accumulate over the course of hours
    - Laser pulses <1 us can cause a rapid rise in temperature
    - Most of the visible and near-IR light is absorbed by melanin in the RPE and causes burns in the retina while UV <400nm is absorbed in the cornea and lens

- **Wavelength, energy levels, thresholds for reactions**

<table>
<tr><th>Type of Laser</th><th>Principal Wavelength(s)</th><th>MPE (eye)</th></tr>
<tr><td>Excimer (Argon-Fl)</td><td>193nm</td><td>3.0 mJ/cm^2 over 8 hours</td></tr>
<tr><td>Argon</td><td>488, 514.5nm</td><td rowspan="5">3.2 mW/cm^2 for 0.1 sec
2.5 mW/cm^2 for 0.25 sec
1.8 mW/cm^2 for 1.0 sec
1.0 mW/cm^2 for 10 sec</td></tr>
<tr><td>YAG</td><td>1064nm</td></tr>
<tr><td>Helium Neon</td><td>632.8nm</td></tr>
<tr><td>Krypton</td><td>568, 647nm</td></tr>
<tr><td>Holmium</td><td>2.1um</td><td>100 mW/cm^2 for 10 seconds to 8 hours, limited area
10 mW/cm^2 for t>10 sec for most of body (skin)</td></tr>
</table>

MPE=maximum permissible exposure limits for commonly used surgical lasers

Summary of Biological Effects and Symptoms from Laser Radiation		
Laser	**Wavelength**	**Biological Effect/Symptoms**
Nd:YAG 1064nm Helium Neon 1150nm	Near IR (IR-A) 780-1400nm	Deep Retinal coagulation, may involve choroid Possible involvement of Lens/Vitreous Rapid onset of scotoma w/o light flash
Holmium 2060nm (pulsed laser)	Far IR (IR-B) 1400-3000nm	Corneal Opacity Cataract Pain, Blepharospasm, Visual Loss
Argon	Visible 488, 514.5nm	Intense blue or green flash without pain or shock After-image may be a complementary color followed by a scotoma – long term insidious loss of cone function -Photochemical, thermal mechanism
Krypton	530, 586, 648nm	Green, yellow, or red flash -Photochemical, thermal mechanism
Helium Neon	632.8nm	Intense red flash

- **Ophthalmic applications**
  - **Argon Laser**: filled with argon gas, which produces blue and green wavelengths that are absorbed by cells that lie under the retina and by the hemoglobin in blood. It acts through photocoagulation
    - Uses: Treatment of diabetic retinopathy, retinal detachment, angle closure glaucoma – laser iridotomy, macular degeneration (destroys abnormal blood vessels), trabeculoplasty
  - **Excimer Laser**: a pulsed gas laser that emits **UV** light, which vaporizes tissues by breaking down molecular bonds in a target area (photoablation). It is considered a "cold" laser because it does not produce harmful heat effects to the surrounding tissues (does not damage adjacent cells).
    - Uses: Laser vision correction surgery (LASIK, PRK)
  - **YAG (yttrium-aluminum-garnet)**: a short-pulsed, high energy light beam that cuts, perforates, and/or fragments tissue. Also known as a neodymium-YAG or nd-YAG laser
    - Uses: Vaporization of posterior capsular opacification post Cataract extraction (posterior capsulotomy).
  - **Holmium Laser**: an infrared light that reshapes the cornea by causing the tissue to constrict (does NOT remove or ablate tissue)
    - Uses:Refractive surgery LTK (laser thermal keratoplasty) to correct mild to moderate hyperopia
  - **Helium Neon (HeNe)** – laser producing light of a visible wavelength used as an aiming beam for ophthalmic surgical lasers that operate at invisible wavelengths
  - **Krypton** – photocoagulating laser used to treat the deeper choroid in macular degeneration
- **Protective Measures**
  - Eye protection – required by OSHA and ANSI Standards
    - Spectacles or goggles with appropriately filtering optics to protect eyes from reflected or scattered laser light

Chapter 4 – Ophthalmic Optics/Spectacles

OPHTHALMIC AND OPTICAL INSTRUMENTS

1. Lens Clock

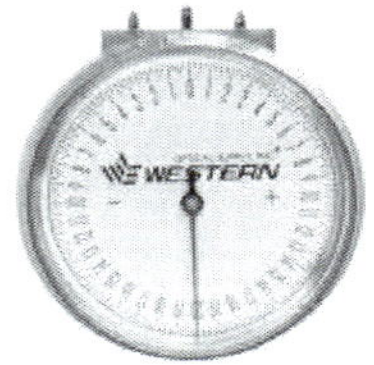

- **Lens clock** aka lens measure aka lens gauge. Often used to determine the base curve of the back surface of a spectacle lens.
- Has three pins: the two on the outside are fixed and the one in the middle is movable and spring-loaded. The position of the center pin in relation to the outer pins indicates the surface sagitta.
- Physically measures the sagittal depth/height of a refracting lens surface (lens sag), which is the distance between a point on a circle to the midpoint of a chord of the circle. The reading on the lens clock reading is in power (diopters), with an assumed index of refraction of n=1.53 (Crown Glass)

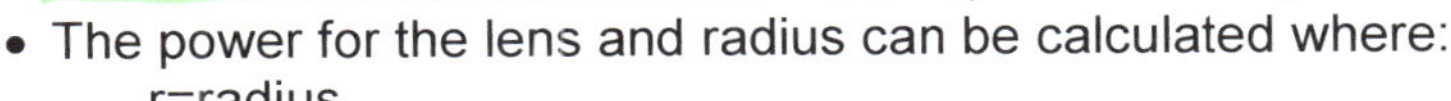

- The power for the lens and radius can be calculated where:
  - r=radius
  - y=chord length
  - s= sagittal height
  - P_{true}= True power of the lens
  - P_{clock}= Power reading of the lens from the lens clock

> Sag Formula
> **$S=y^2/2r = Ph^2/2\Delta n$**
> Single Refracting Surface Power
> **$P_{true}=P_{clock}\ (n_{true}-n_{air})/\ (n_{clock}-n_{air})$**

Example: *What is the true power of a 1.66 index lens that measures -10.00DS by a Geneva lens clock?*

> ***Answer:***
> P_{true}= (-10.00)(1.66-1)/(1.53-1) = -11.32DS

2. Lensometer

- The **focusing system** is based on a **Badal lens** system and contains a light source, a cross hair target, a standard lens, and the lens stop. The target is at the primary focal point of the standard lens and is focused by the power wheel. The light source is behind the target, and the lens stop is at the secondary focal point of the standard lens
- The **observation system** creates a **Keplerian telescope** (without inverting prisms) by making the secondary focal point of the objective lens coincident with the primary focal point of the eyepiece.
- When there is no lens in place and the target is in focus, the target is at the anterior focal point of the standard lens. The light rays diverge from the target onto the standard lens and emerge parallel. This parallel light is incident on the observation (telescope part) of the lensometer creating an **afocal system**, so that parallel light emerges into the observer's eye.
  - The **target** is at the anterior focal point of the standard lens and can move.
  - The **reticule** is at the secondary focal point of the objective/anterior focal point of the ocular and cannot move.
  - P_{std} = power of standard lens; usually + 20.00D → Range of lensometer usually -20 to +20D

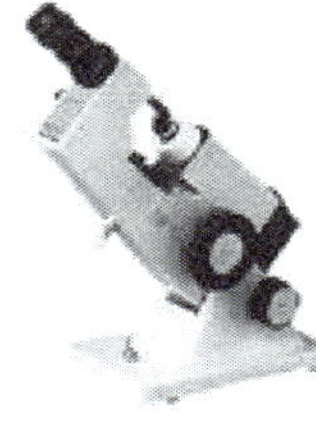

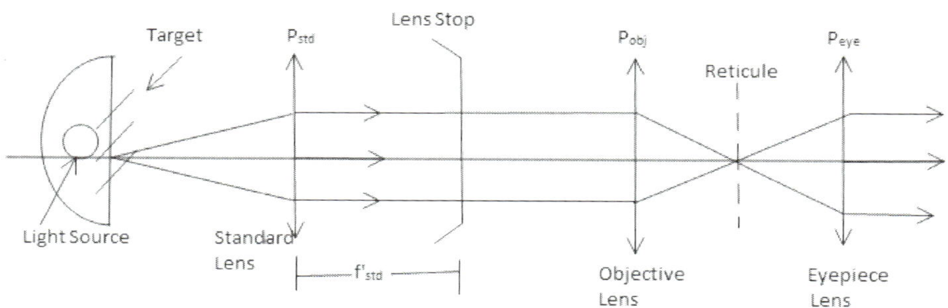

3. Lens Caliper

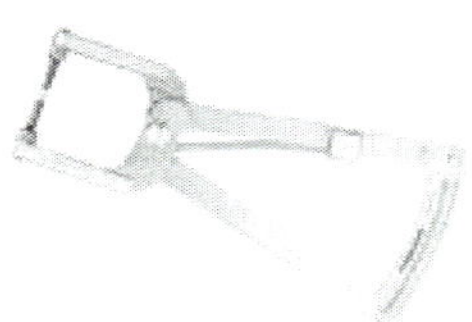

- A **lens caliper** measures lens thickness. Some have a single scale, other calipers have 2 scales – one representing millimeters and the other tenths of a millimeter

---

POLARIZATION

---

1. Linearly Polarized Light

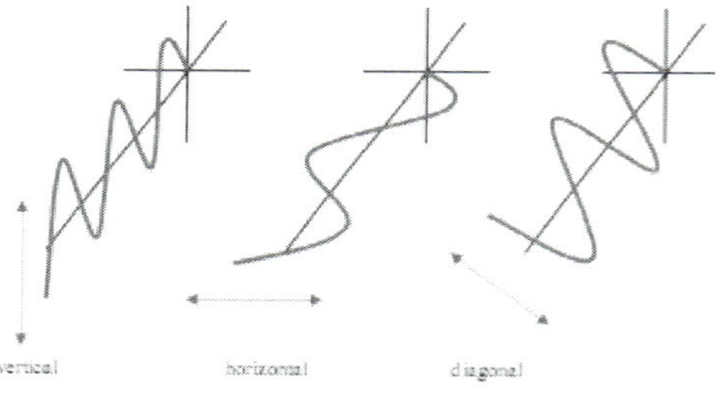

- The electric energy of a polarized beam acts in a specific direction that is perpendicular to the direction of the propagation of the light.
- Polarization arises whenever radiated energy, or light, comes from an excited oscillating dipole molecule oscillating in one direction.
- In the natural environment, these dipoles are oriented randomly and each dipole shifts its orientation over time so normal light is unpolarized. To polarize light, one can:
    - Pass unpolarized light through a polarizing filter
    - Reflect unpolarized light off an appropriately tilted surface
    - Scatter unpolarized light in a specific direction from small particles

2. Circular and Elliptical Polarization

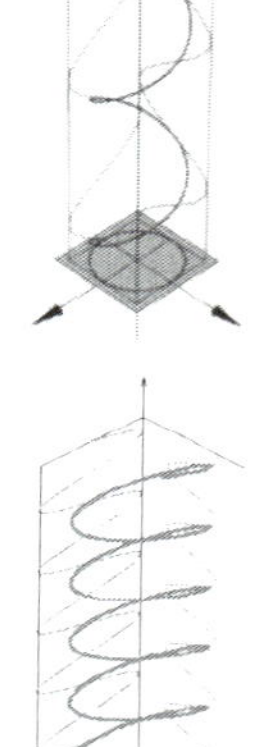

- **Circular polarization** of electromagnetic radiation is a polarization such that the tip of the electric field vector, at a fixed point in space, describes a circle as time progresses. The electric vector, at one point in time, describes a helix along the direction of wave propagation.
- A circularly polarized wave may be resolved into 2 linearly polarized waves, of equal amplitude in phase quadrature (90 degrees apart) and with their planes of polarization at right angles to teach other.
- **Elliptical polarization** is the polarization of electromagnetic radiation such that the tip of the electric field vector describes an ellipse in any fixed plane intersecting, and normal to, the direction of propagation.
- An elliptically polarized wave may be resolved into two linearly polarized waves in phase quadrature, with their polarization planes at right angles to each other. Since the electric field can rotate clockwise or counterclockwise as it propagates, elliptically polarized waves exhibit chirality

3. Polarization by Reflection (Brewster's Angle and Glare Reduction)

- When light normally reflects perpendicularly from a surface, the amount of light reflected is equal to **R= (n'-n)/(n'+n)**. As the angle of incident changes, the amount of reflected light depends on the polarization. If one orientation of polarization reflects more than the other, then the reflected light would be partially polarized
- The angle at which light of only one polarization reflects is called **Brewster's Angle**, which depends on the index of refraction of the reflecting surface

> Brewster's Angle
> **Θ_B=acrtan (n'/n)**

- An oblique reflection can create polarized light
  - Unpolarized light that is diffusely reflected is generally not polarized because it is reflected at all angles. But unpolarized light that is specularly reflected does have some polarization
  - Specular reflections are mirror reflections
  - Polarized sunglasses relieve off-axis specular reflections. 50-60 degrees is not an uncommon angle to see specular reflections. So for activities like driving, boating and skiing, polarized sunglasses can help reduce a good amount of glare. If the transmission axis is vertical, one minimizes the amount of horizontally polarized light that reaches the eye and makes these activities more comfortable.

4. Effects of Scattering on Polarization

- **Birefringence** is the dependency of index on the direction of polarization and gives rise to double refraction. A material is birefringent if a light beam passing through it experiences two refractive indices
  - In crystals, the structure is **anisometropic**, meaning that when the atomic lattice that makes up the molecules is looked upon from different orientations, the lattice itself looks different. The electrons within the lattice will vibrate differently depending on the direction, so light of one polarization will encounter a transparent material with a different refractive index than the other component of polarization.
- Birefringence is often found in crystals (Calcite crystal) but it is also found in ordered arrangements of molecules. In the latter case, it is called form birefringence. The cornea is an example of a tissue that has form birefringence as the lamellae in the stroma comprise of anisotropic collagen strands that are oriented for an overall birefringence. The actual index of refraction difference between the two polarization components is 0.001 (small).
- **Dichroism** is when a crystal absorbs one of the polarization directions more than another. Examples include polarizing filters in sunglasses.
- The eye has dichroic crystals near the fovea (macular pigment granules) which give rise to a selective absorption of some orientations of polarizations. When you rotate a polarizer in front of the eye, you see a corresponding rotating pattern (**Haidinger's Brushes**).

5. Transmission through Successive Polarizers (Stress Analysis/Malus' Law)

- Rules for polarized light: The number of units of intensity that gets through is proportional to the square of the cosine of the angle between the orientation of the incident polarization and the transmission axis of the polarizer.

> Intensity of Polarized Light
> **$I = I_0\cos^2\theta$**

I_0 = 100 units

I = intensity

Io = incident light intensity

Θ = angle b/w orientation of incident polarization and transmission axis

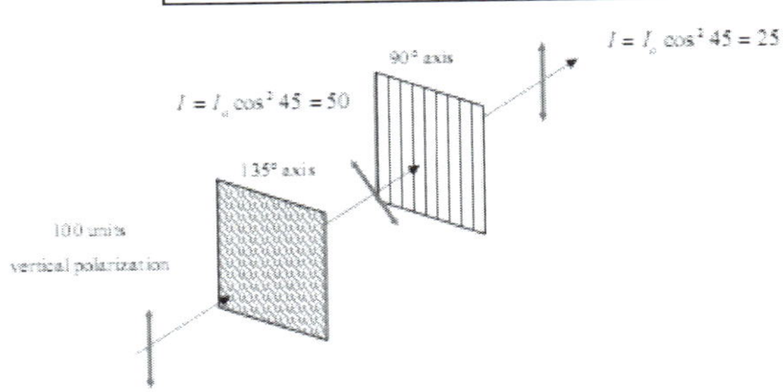

- The orientation of the emergent light is always the same as the transmission axis of the polarizing filter preceding it.
- To create a polarizer, thin wires (on the order of wavelength) allow electrons only to oscillate in one direction and only that orientation of polarization is *absorbed*. The component of polarization in the orthogonal direction will *transmit*.

- Polarizers are described by the orientation of their transmission axis, not the orientation of the conducting wires.
- The intensity of the horizontal and vertical components are characterized by **Malus' Law**, where

  I_x= Intensity in the horizontal direction
  I_y= Intensity in the vertical direction
  A= Amplitude of the wave
  θ= Angle between the orientation of the light and the horizontal component

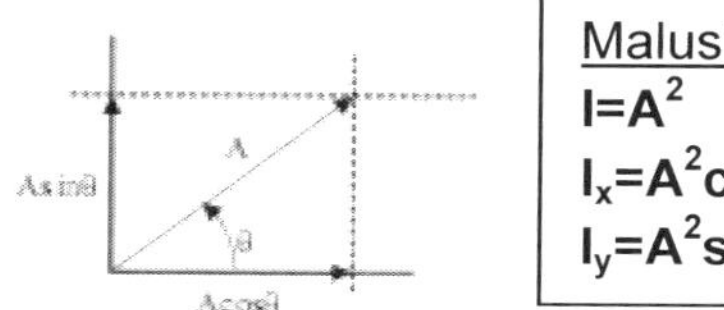

Malus' Law
$I=A^2$
$I_x=A^2\cos^2\theta$
$I_y=A^2\sin^2\theta$

- Polarizers can be used in **photoelastic stress analysis**.
  - Photoelastic materials exhibit birefringence only when there is an application of stress.
  - By passing plane polarized light through a transparent photoelastic material (plastic/glass), the light separates along two principal stress directions relative to the phase retardation between the two waves. A **polariscope** brings the waves together and creates a fringe pattern due to optical interference which characterizes the invisible points of stress in the material.
  - The magnitude of the phase retardation can be determined using the **Stress Optic Law**, where:

    R= induced retardation
    C= stress optic coefficient
    t=specimen thickness
    σ_{11}= first principal stress
    σ_{22}= second principal stress

Stress Optic Law
$R=Ct(\sigma_{11}-\sigma_{22})$

  - This process is used in injection molding, extruded sheets, and cast plastics.

PHYSICAL CHARACTERISTICS OF OPHTHALMIC LENSES

1. Geometry of Lens Surfaces

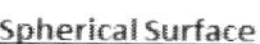

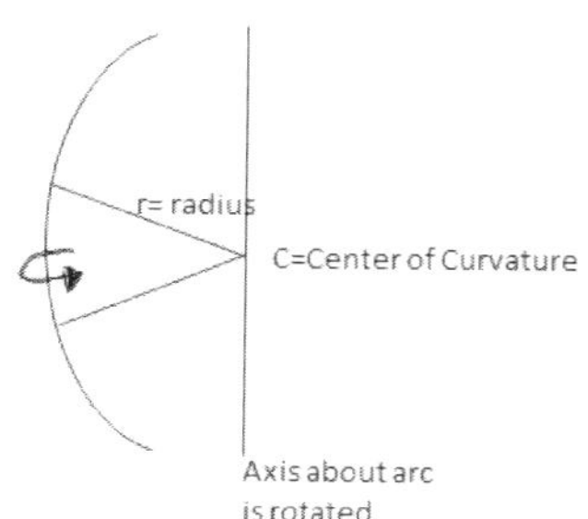

- **Spherical Surface:** a surface created by rotating an arc about one of its diameters resulting in identical power in all meridians
- **Cylindrical Surface:** does not mean that a lens has a cylindrical surface; it means there is a cylindrical component in the lens (i.e., the lens has different powers 90 degrees apart); formed by rotation of a line about another line. This is a special case of toric surface.
  - 2 meridians
  - Axis meridian
  - Power meridian
  - Always perpendicular to each other
  - Principal meridians of the cyl lens.

Cylindrical Surface

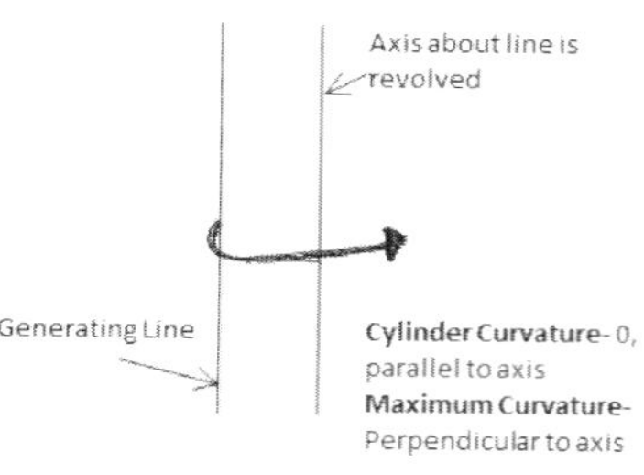

- **Toric *Surface***: a surface created by rotating an arc about a plane that does not pass through the center of curvature; lens having different curvatures in the principal meridians
  - 2 principle meridians
  - Maximum curvature – cross curve (steeper)
  - Minimum curvature – base curve (flatter)
- **Aspheric Surface:** an optical surface which departs slightly from a fixed radius of curvature and hence is free from or has reduced spherical aberrations.
  - Gradual surface power change from lens center to lens edge (rotationally symmetric)
  - Power change different in tangential and sagittal planes, creates astigmatism
  - Power change along a given plane not constant

- At the center, a small sphere
- Away from center, a changing toric surface
- Types:
  - Plus lens – front surface curvature flattens as one moves from the lens center towards the edge
  - Back spheric on plus lens – back surface curvature steepens
  - Minus lens
    - Front surface aspheric, steepens toward edge
    - Back surface aspheric, flattening towards edge; result is flatter and thinner lens (more effective thinning)
  - Progressives
- Pros:
  - Less aberrations
  - Better cosmetics
- Cons
  - More aspheric=smaller sweet spot of good optics
  - More aspheric=flatter=may touch eyelashes
  - More aspheric=flatter=may be more reflective

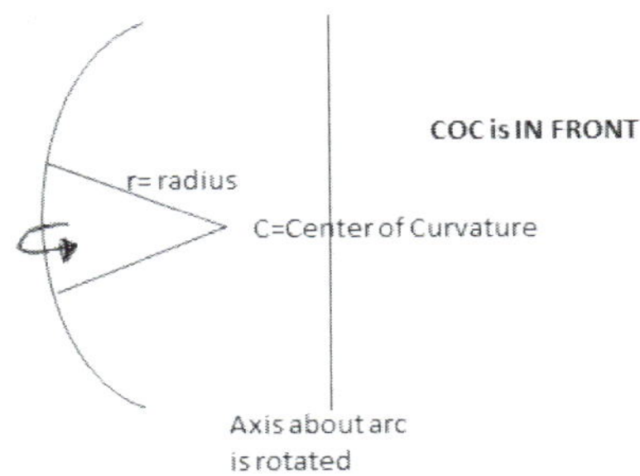

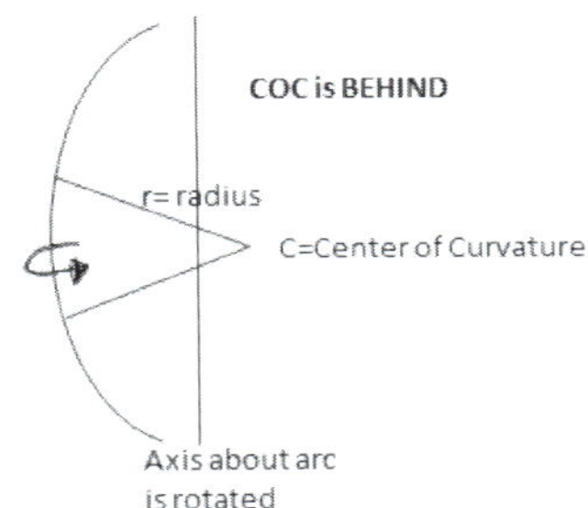

2. Base Curves

- **Base curves (BC)** (used to designate the lens form): a standard curve for a series of lens powers as determined by a manufacturer. It is selected based on criteria to minimize power error and unwanted astigmatism in the final product.
  - Base curve can vary for different ranges of power and for the same ranges of power among different lens manufacturers
  - For every Rx, there is an optimal base curve.
- For Spherical (single vision) lenses: BC is the weaker/flatter of the two curves. It will be located on:
  - Concave (back) side of a plus lens
  - Convex (front) side of a minus lens
- For Cylindrical (single vision) lenses: BC is the weaker/flatter of the two curves on the side opposite in which the cylinder is ground (minus form) or on the same side as the cylinder is ground (plus form)
  - **Plus Cylinder Form:** cylinder is ground on the front surface, BC is the flattest curve on the front side
  - **Minus Cylinder Form:** cylinder is ground on the back surface, BC is on the front spherical side
- Since most lenses are designed in a minus cylinder form, manufacturers
- identify their lenses in terms of the front curve
- For Multifocal lenses: BC is on the spherical side containing the reading segment
- **Vogel's Formula** dictates what the ideal base curve of a corrected curve lens should be

Vogel's Formula
Plus Lens: SE + 6.00
Minus Lens: SE/2 +6.00

3. Lens Thickness

- Lens sag is the distance between a point on a circle to the midpoint of a chord of the circle. It is also the difference between the lens center and edge thickness OR the difference between the center and some point between the center and edge thickness (**strap thickness**)

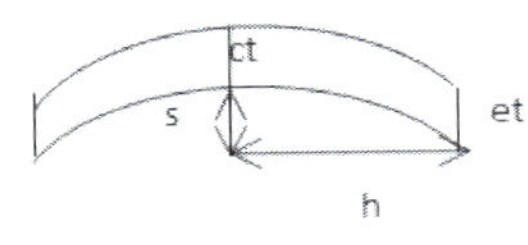

- Sag of lens increases with increasing lens diameter
  - The smaller the radius (contact lens) the larger the sag, and the larger the radius (spectacles) the smaller the sag. Sag is an indirect measure of curvature.

↑ Sag <-> ↑ Diam

- Sag formula is the basis for calculating thickness changes across a lens surface

  s = sag of surface measured with lens gauge

  h = distance between end and middle prong

r = radius of surface lens
P = power of lens
ct= center thickness
et= edge thickness

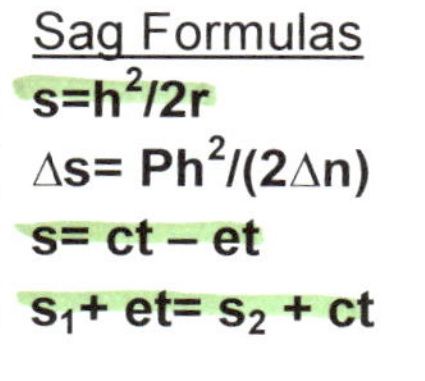

Sag Formulas

$s=h^2/2r$

$\Delta s= Ph^2/(2\Delta n)$

$s= ct - et$

$s_1+ et= s_2 + ct$

- Change in thickness is dependent on lens power and not the shape of the lens.
- To reduce the thickness of a lens you can increase n' of the lens or decrease h by using a smaller lens size. The calculated change in sag is calculated from the pole of the lens.

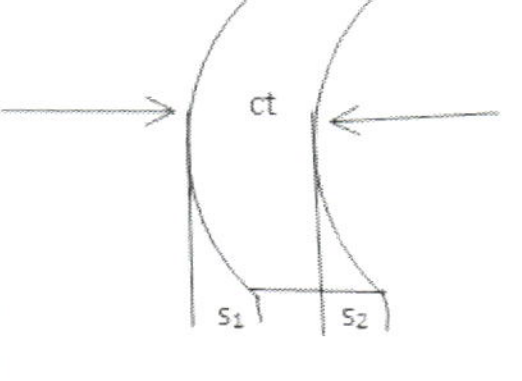

***Example**: A lens is 54mm round and has a center thickness of 2.0mm. The Rx is -4.00DS, index 1.498, what is the edge thickness?*

P=-4.00DS
h=27.0mm
n=1.498
ct=2.0nn

Answer:

$\Delta s=[(-4.00)(0.027)^2]/[2(1.498-1.00)] \times 1000 = -2.93mm$

$et=ct-\Delta s = 2.0-(-2.93mm) = +4.93mm$

According to ANSI Z87.1 (2010)

- Most **Prescription Safety Lenses** must have a **minimum center/edge thickness of 3.0mm** for glass, plastic, and polycarbonate.
  - For high plus lenses over +3.00DS, edge thickness may be reduced to 2.5mm if it meets the impact test
- For **Plano Safety Lenses** thickness can be no less than 3.0mm and no more than 3.8mm
- For **Plano Polycarbonate Lenses** a 2.0mm thickness is allowable.
- For **Dress Eyewear** center thickness is not specified

4. Specification of Lens Size and Shape

- **Datum System**: take the vertical dimension and split it in half, then draw a horizontal line across the frame at the halfway point (called the 180 line or fitting line). Measure eye size and bridge size long this datum line. Measurements are taken between the bottoms of the eye-wire grooves on frames or between the peaks of the bevel on lenses.
- **Boxing System**: The A dimension is the measurement from the farthest nasal point to the farthest temporal point of the lens. This is called the lens size or eye size. The B dimension is the measurement from the farthest superior point to the farthest inferior point of the lens. The difference between the B and A dimension is called the frame "difference."

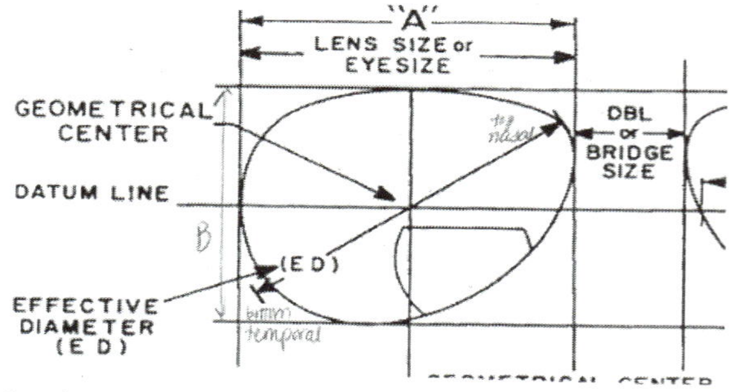

  - **DBL:** the shortest distance between lenses that is often noted as bridge size.
  - **Geometric Center (GC):** Point of intersection of the 2 diagonals of the box enclosing the lens.
  - **Frame PD:** the distance from geometric center of one lens to geometric center of the other; equals to **A + DBL**
  - **Effective diameter (ED)**: the longest dimension of the lens. It is used to calculate the minimum diameter of the lens blank
  - **The Minimum Blank Size (MBS)**: the equal to the ED plus twice the single lens decentration.

Minimum Blank Size

MBS=ED+2(single lens decentration)

- **Lens size**: defined as the effective diameter of 2X the longest radius. Also described by A and B measurement.
- **Lens shape:** the shape of the lens when it has been cut to fit a frame. The shape is defined as viewed perpendicular to the front surface.
- Lens size and shape becomes a factor in high minus and high plus lenses.
  Factors to consider are:
  - Use a strong frame with adjustable nose pads
  - Fit as tight a frame as possible to control vertex distance
  - Avoid excessive decentration. Pick a frame with frame PD that most closely matches the patient's PD
  - Pick a frame shape that allows as close to a round shape as possible. Oblique astigmatism and distortion become more of a factor in the periphery of odd-shaped lenses.
  - Keep the eye size as small as possible using the minimum effective diameter. This minimizes the edge thickness and prismatic effect.

5. Materials

- **Refractive Index (n):** ratio of speed of light in vacuum vs. media; measure of how much the speed of light is reduced inside the medium. The value is >1, but <2
- The index varies depending on what reference wavelength you are using: Helium D (587.56nm) line reference (USA and UK), Mercury E (546.07nm) line reference (Europe).
  - Normal index: n≥1.48 but <1.54
  - Mid index: n≥1.54 but <1.64
  - High index: n≥1.64 but <1.74
  - Very high index: n≥1.74
- **Abbe Value:** represents the index of refraction variance across aspectrum for a given material, i.e. how easy it is to change white light into chromatic spectrum. It is a gauge of the propensity of a lens material to disperse light. The higher the Abbe value, the lower the dispersion (relates to lateral chromatic aberration). Values usually between 25-60
  - Low dispersion ≥45
  - Medium dispersion ≥39 and <45
  - High dispersion <39
- **Specific Gravity:** ratio of density of a substance to the density of a standard substance, usually water or hydrogen, measured in air. (standard reference, 1cc of water, 1 gram)
  Note: high index does not necessarily equate to light weight.
- **Impact resistance/hardness**: regulation set by FDA with reference to minimum standard for dress and occupational safety lenses.
- **Glass**
  - Composed of various **inorganic** oxides (silicon, calcium, sodium, potassium, lead, barium, titanium, and lanthanum).
  - **Ophthalmic crown glass**: silica (60%), soda, lime.
  - Tint with metallic oxides.
  - **Spectralite Glass** has a high index of refraction, making it lighter per dioptric power, but has a lower *nu* value, giving it a large amount of chromatic aberration
  - ADVANTAGES
    - Low reflectance
    - Good optics
    - Chemical (solvents, detergents, oils) Resistant
    - **Scratch resistant**
    - Optimal material for selective tint filtering and ARC
    - Tempering will make lenses more impact resistant
  - DISADVANTAGES→ Heavy
- **Plastic**
  - Composed of **organic** compounds

- There are three main types of plastic: thermoset, thermoplastic, and quasi-thermoset

	Thermoplastic	Thermoset
aka	Thermolabile	Thermostabile
Material	-Cellulose nitrate (flammable) or cellulose acetate → NOT cross linked -Material in pellets, sheets, or granular form -Heated, stretched, pressed and molded- no chemical structure change -Injection molding -Soft, abrasion sensitive	-Liquid monomer, cross-linked (more rigid) -Heated and polymerized in a mold casted process -Solidifies through heat and pressure
Effects of Heat	-Will soften when heated and harden when cooled	-Will not soften significantly when heated after it is made -Once cured cannot be softened -May decompose under high heat -Hear resistant
Impact Resistance	-Very impact resistant because non-cross linked molecules slide past each other	-Less impact resistant than thermoplastics
Examples	-Polycarbonate, Plexiglass, PMMA	-Optyl or CR39, most mid to high index plastics

- Thermoset (aka Thermostabile)
  - **CR39** is impact resistant without being treated, but has the disadvantage of scattering more light at the surface and being more easily scratch than glass
  - **Hi-Index** plastic has good UV properties; tinting variability; softer material – requires scratch resistance coating
- Thermoplastic (aka Thermolabile)→ Polycarbonate, majority of lenses
  - **Polycarbonate** is the most impact resistant material used today in ophthalmics (although **Trivex** is considered comparable); it is 10X stronger than CR-39
- "Quasi-Thermoset" → Trivex
  - Is partly cross-linked, but not completely. Impact resistance comparable to polycarbonate, less scratch resistance than CR-39

Summary of Lens Materials				
Material	Index of Refraction (n)	Abbe Value (nu)	Specific Gravity	Impact Resistance
CR-39	1.49	58	1.32	Good
Crown Glass	1.523	59	2.54	Poor
Polycarbonate	1.586	30	1.2	Excellent
Trivex	1.53	46	1.11	Excellent
Spectralite	1.54	47	1.21	Poor
Mid-Index Plastic	1.55-1.60	34-39	1.17-1.42	Good
Hi-Index Plastic	1.66-1.701	32-36	1.36-1.4	Good
Very Hi Index Plastic	1.74	33	1.46	Good

MIRRORS

1. Planar and Spherical Reflection

- Reflecting surfaces are like refracting surfaces except that the reflected rays travel in the same medium and in the opposite direction as the incident rays. So $n_2 = -n_1$.
- **Law of Reflection**: The angle of incidence (A) is equal to the angle of reflection (a')→Incident angle = Reflected angle
- **Planar mirrors:** The image is virtual (located the same distance away from the plane mirror as the object, but on the opposite side), erect, the same size as the object (magnification is +1), and reversed left to right

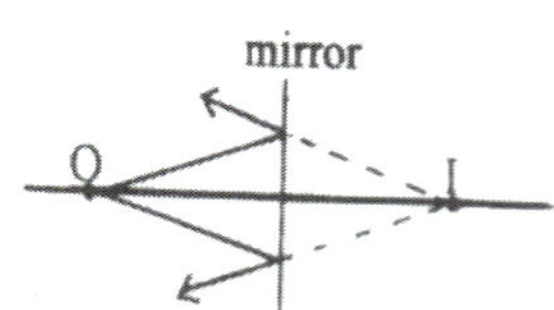

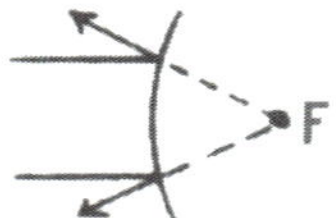

- **Spherical mirrors:** like planar mirrors, spherical mirrors with real objects also give reversed (L-R) virtual images
  - A convex mirror diverges light
  - A concave mirror converges light

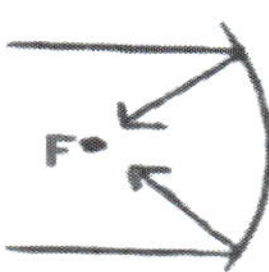

2. Proportion of Light Reflected from a Surface (Fresnel's Law)

- Fresnel's Law: **% reflected = $(n_2 - n_1 / n_2 + n_1)^2$ x 100%**

Note: the % of light reflected is the same, no matter which medium the light originally came from

3. Focal Power, Focal Length, and Curvature

- **Focal power: $P = (n_2 - n_1)/r$** where r = radius of curvature
- Since $n_2 = -n_1$, then $P = (-n_1 - n_1)/r = -2n/r$
- Thus, in air, **$P_m = -2n/r$**
  - Convex Mirrors: P is negative (r is positive)
  - Concave Mirrors: P is positive (r is negative)
- **Focal Length** of a curved mirror is always ½ its radius of curvature (f=r/2)
  - F = focal point
  - C = center of curvature
  - Convex Mirror, focal point to the right of the mirror
  - Concave Mirror, focal point to the left of the mirror
- **Curvature: R=1/r** where r is the radius of curvature in meters

<u>Fresnel's Law</u>
% reflected = $\frac{(n_2 - n_1)^2}{(n_2 + n_1)}$ x 100%

<u>Focal Power</u>
$P_m = -2n/r = 1/f_m$

<u>Focal Length</u>
$f_m = r/2$

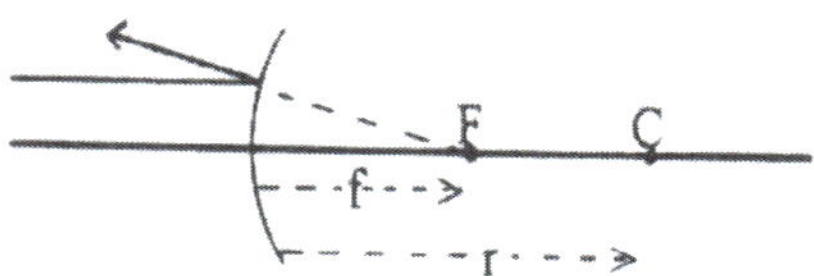

For convex mirrors:
r is positive
P is negative

C
r= (+)

For concave mirrors:
r is negative
P is positive

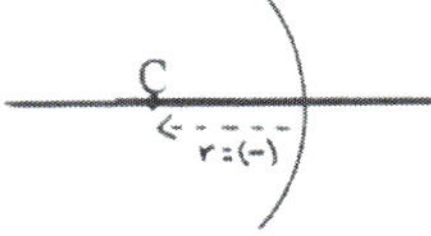

4. Object-Image Relationships

- Convex mirrors form virtual images on the opposite side of the object
  - They add negative vergence like minus lenses
- Concave mirrors form real images on the same side as the object
  - They add positive vergence like plus lenses
  - When an object is located closer to a converging mirror than its focal distance, the image will be virtual and erect (not real and inverted). This principle applies to a concave mirror like a shaving mirror
- Plano mirror add no vergence

Example: *If an object lies 1m in front of a concave mirror whose radius of curvature is 50cm, where is the image vergence?*

Answer:
f=r/2=0.5/2=0.25m
P_m=1/f=1/0.25m= +4.00D
u=-1m, so U=-1D
V=U + P_m= -1.00 + 4.00D = +3.00D
The image is real and lies 33cm in front of the mirror

5. Magnification (Transverse/Lateral)

- Magnification is the ratio of the image size to the object size:
  - If m is positive, the image is erect.
  - If m is negative, the image is inverted.
  - If |m| > 1, then the image is larger.
  - If |m| < 1, then the image is smaller.

> Transverse Magnification
> **m = U/V = v/u = I/O**

6. Lens/Mirror Systems

- If you silver the back surface of a thin lens, light will refract through the front surface, reflect off the back surface, and refract again through the front surface. The total power of the system is the sum of the two refractions and one reflection where

  P_1 = front surface power of the lens
  P_m = power of the mirror

> Lens/Mirror System
> $\mathbf{P_t = 2P_1 + P_m}$

Example: *What is the power of a lens mirror made of a +4.00D biconvex glass lens (n = 1.523)?*

P_1 = +2.00D
P_2 = +2.00D

> ***Answer*:**
> -Solve for $r_2 \rightarrow P_2 = (n_2-n_1)/r_2 \rightarrow r_2 = (n_2 - n_1)/P_2 = (1 - 1.523)/+2.00 = -26.15$cm
> -Calculate $P_m \rightarrow P_m = -2n/r = -2(1.523)/-0.2615\text{m} = +11.65$D
> -Solve for $P_t = 2P_1 + P_m$
> $P_t = 2(+2.00\text{D}) + 11.65\text{D} = +15.65\text{D}$

7. Ray Tracing

- **3 Predictable Rays (Mirror):**
  - Ray 1: a ray parallel to the axis reflects through the focal point (F)
  - Ray 2: a ray going through F reflects parallel to the axis
  - Ray 3: a ray passing through the center of curvature (C) reflects back through C (**nodal ray**)
- 3 Predictable Rays (non-mirror)
  - Ray 1: a ray in parallel to the lens, out through F2
  - Ray 2: a ray in through F1 to the lens, out parallel
  - Ray 3: Nodal ray: any ray passing through the optical center of a thin lens passes straight through without bending

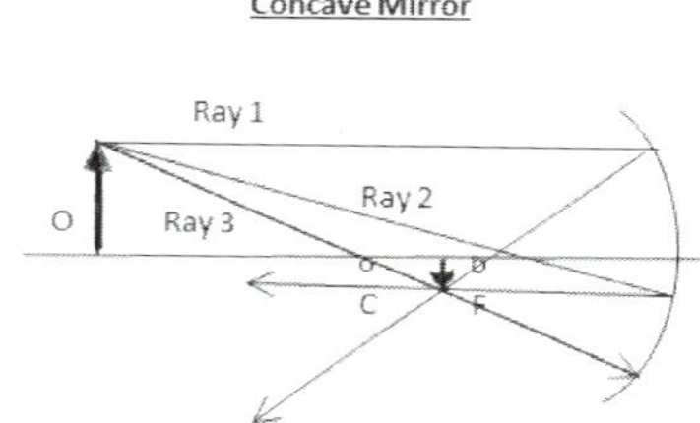

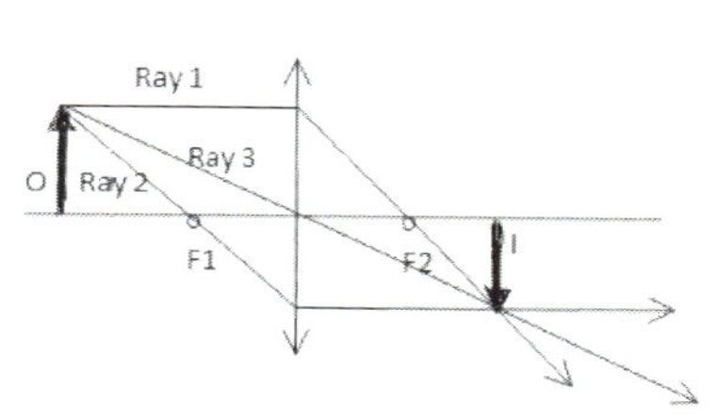

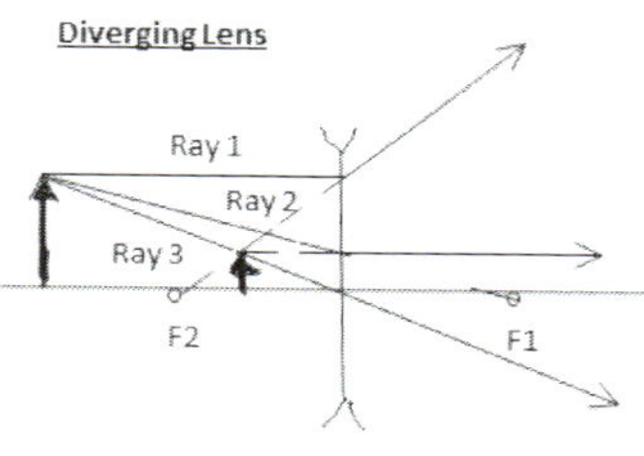

OPTICAL CHARACTERISTICS OF OPHTHALMIC LENSES

1. Locations and Relationships between the Optic Axis, Optical Center, Geometric Center and Major Reference Points

- **Optic axis**: the line joining the centers of curvature of front and back surfaces of a lens and normal to both surfaces (connects anterior and posterior poles of a lens)
- **Optical center**: point on optic axis intersected by a path of light incident on the front that is parallel to the path after refraction on the back side.
- **Major Reference Point** (MRP, now an obsolete term): the point on the lens through which the visual axis (or line of sight) passes. It is also the point at which the proper refractive and prism power has been incorporated, or the point on the lens with the indicated prismatic effect. Where no prism power is required, the lens optical center is MRP.
- **Geometric Center**: this is the center of a box drawn to contain the lens. It is the point of intersection of two diagonals drawn from the corners of the box.
- **Decentration = (Frame PD – IPD)/2**
- IPD = interpolar distance, i.e. the distance between the poles of the lenses. This is NOT intrapupillary distance.

2. Principles of Corrected Curve Lens Design

- **Chromatic aberration**: Short wavelengths are refracted more and focus closer to the lens than do long wavelengths. Chromatic aberration is directly related to dispersive power.

  n_f = index of 486 nm

  n_c = index of 656 nm

  n_d = index of 589 nm

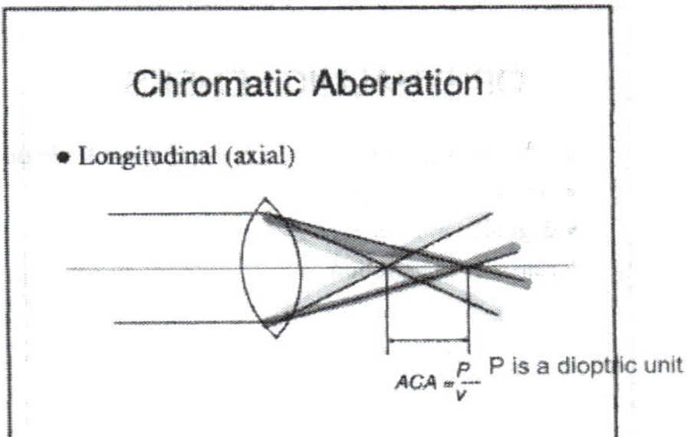

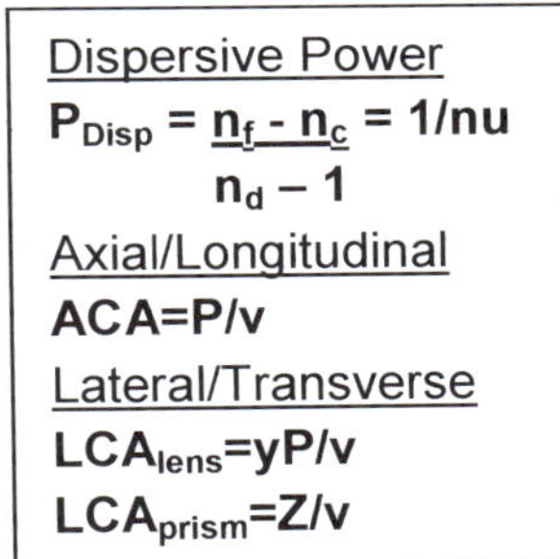
Dispersive Power

$P_{Disp} = \frac{n_f - n_c}{n_d - 1} = 1/nu$

Axial/Longitudinal

ACA=P/v

Lateral/Transverse

$LCA_{lens} = yP/v$

$LCA_{prism} = Z/v$

- Types:
  - **Axial/longitudinal (ACA):** dioptric separation b/w red and blue focus
  - **Lateral/transverse (LCA)**: difference in magnification, size difference
- Reduced with:
  - **Achromatic** system (**doublet**): composed of 2 different materials to produce equal but opposite dispersions; secondary CA remains
  - **Apochromatic** system (**triplet**): to eliminate secondary CA

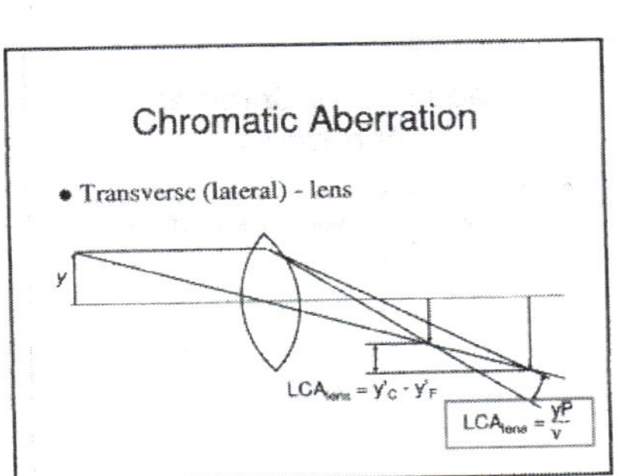

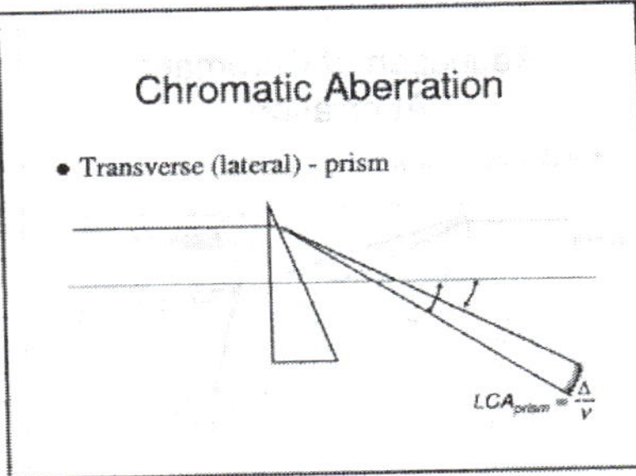

- Controlled with lens material
- **Monochromatic aberration:** comes in 2 categories:

- 1. **Image degradation**
  - **Spherical aberration**: peripheral rays focus sooner than axial rays;
    - Longitudinal
    - Transverse
    - SA reduced with achromatic (doublet) systems composed of 2 different materials to produce equal but opposite dispersions. Apochromatic systems use triplet materials to eliminate secondary CA.
  - **Marginal/oblique/radial astigmatism**: the inability of a lens (spherical) to form a point image of an oblique point object; difference between tangential and sagittal foci in diopters; caused by oblique, paraxial rays; In general, we want the Far Point Sphere to straddle the sagittal and tangential loci. The loci are also sensitive to the location of the aperture stop. Therefore, if the aperture is located at the center of curvature, you eliminate radical astigmatism.
    - **Variable factors**: viewing distance, lens material, and aperture stop location
    - **Tscherning ellipse:** relationship between surface power and back vertex power of a thin lens for which oblique astigmatism is eliminated
  - **Coma:** variation in magnification between peripheral and paraxial rays. Factors affecting coma are the size of the aperture and angle of obliquity.

Spherical Aberration

- Longitudinal SA

aperture

LSA

– depends on *square* of aperture

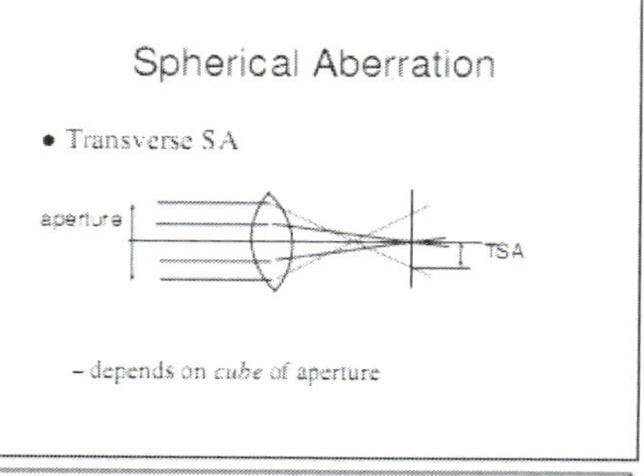

MARGINAL ASTIGMATISM

- also radial or oblique
- important, paraxial rays obliquely
- similar to sphero-cyl imaging (spherical lens)

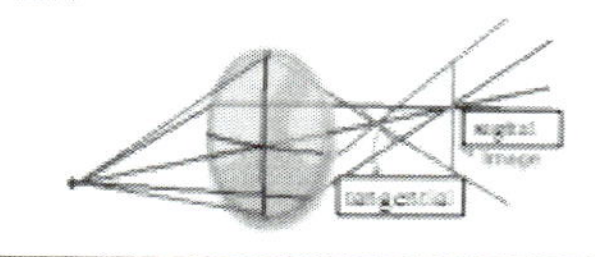

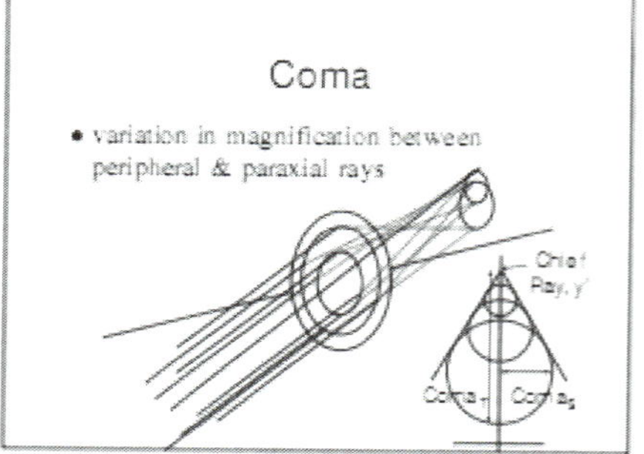

- 2. **Image deformation**
  - **Distortion**: inability of lens to form an image of the same shape as the object; depends on the placement of stops in the optical system
    - **Barrel:** from minus lens; magnification decreases toward periphery
    - **Pincushion:** from plus lens; magnification increases towards periphery
  - **Curvature of field**: Inability of a lens to form a plane image of a plane object.

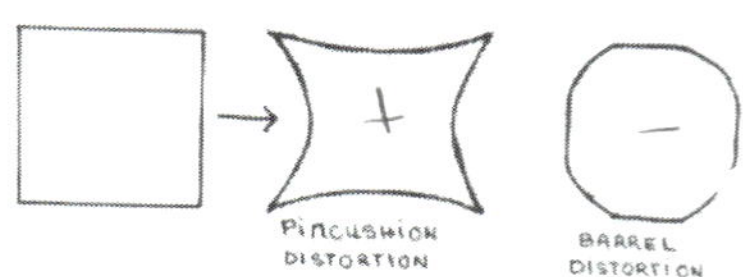

- The two most critical aberrations in lens design is Marginal astigmatism and curvature of field.
- Corrected curve or best form lens philosophies:
  - **Point focal lens:**
    - Reduces oblique astigmatism completely (MOP approx = Pv)
    - Leaves power error uncorrected (MOE ≠ 0)
  - **Percival lens form**
    - Eliminates power error (curvature of field) so that $P_t+P_s/2=P_v$ (MOE=0)
    - Leaves some residual astigmatism, produces a flatter lens
- It is not possible to eliminate all aberrational errors simultaneously. One must find a balance between cosmetics and optics

3. Verification of Lens Prescriptions

Lensometer: is used to measure the secondary focal length of a lens to give the back vertex power. It is comprised of a focusing system and an observation system (See Chapter 4-Ophthalmic and Optical Instruments).

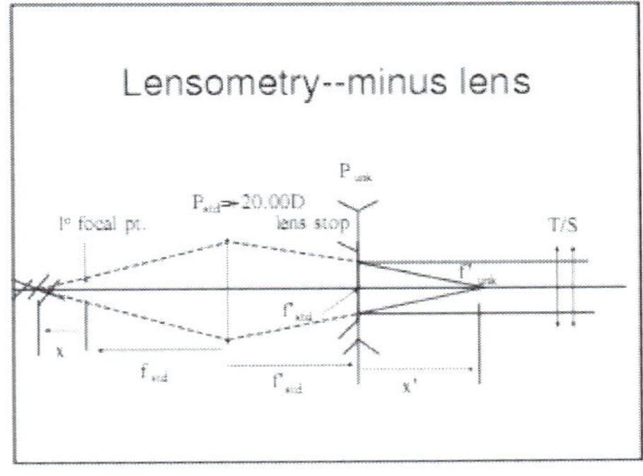

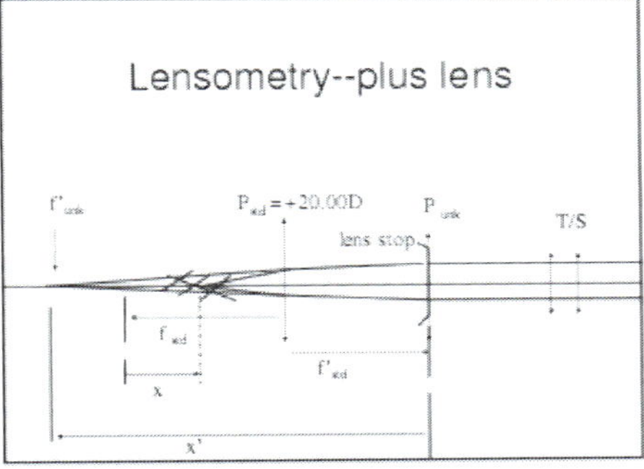

- With an unknown lens at the lens stop, light emerging from the standard lens must be directed toward the secondary focal point of the unknown lens to make the system afocal.
- For a **Minus Lens**, light going into the standard lens must be LESS divergent, so the target is moved **away (to the left)** from the anterior focal point of the standard lens
- For a **Plus Lens**, light going into the standard lens must be MORE divergent, so the target is moved **toward (to the right)** the anterior focal point of the standard lens
- The Equivalent power of the system remains constant regardless of the power of the unknown lens placed on the lens stop because image size is constant.
  - $P_e = P_{std}$ regardless of the power of the unknown lens
- Using **Newton's Equation for Conjugate foci** ($xx'=ff'=1/P_{std}P'_{std}$) we know there is a linear relationship between target movement and power of the unknown. This can be simplified to the equation boxed to the right where the equivalent power of the system is equal to the equivalent power of the standard lens.

  x=distance the target is moved (m)
  P_{unk}= power of the unknown lens
  P_{std}= power of the standard lens.

Equivalent Power of the System
$\mathbf{x=P_{unk}/(P_{std}P'_{std})}$ or
$\mathbf{x=P_{unk}/(P_{std})^2}$

Note: (-)x= target moves AWAY from the observer, behind the anterior focal point, to the left of f_{std}
(+)x= target moves TOWARD the observer, in front of the anterior focal point to the right of f_{std}.

Lens Gauge: By comparing the center pin to the outer two pins, the lens gauge can measure the sag of a lens over a given range, which equates to the lens surface power.

- If the center pin is above the outer pins it is a convex lens, read the black numbers (+)
- If the center pin is below the outer pins, it is a concave lens, read the red numbers (-)
- The pin separation (h) of a standard lens gauge is 10.4mm (20.8mm separation of the two outer pins)
- The lens gauge converts the sag of the lens to the dioptric surface power of the lens using the sag formula $P=(2s\Delta n)/h^2$ where h represents the distance between the lens gauge pegs, and $\Delta n = n_c-1$
- The lens gauge assumes an index of refraction of n_c=1.530. If the true index of the lens (n_t) is less than n_c, then the true surface power of the lens (P_t) is less than the measured surface power by the lens clock (P_c) and vice versa:
  - If $n_t<n_c$ then $P_t<P_c$
  - If $n_t>n_c$ then $P_t>P_c$

Lens Gauge Surface Power
$\mathbf{P_t= P_c \frac{(n_t-1)}{(n_c-1)}}$
$\mathbf{P_c=0.523/r}$

Example: *What is the true refractive power of a CR-39 (n=1.498) lens, if a lens gauge calibrated for 1.53 reads -6.00DS?*

Answer:
P_t= -6.00 (1.498-1)/ (1.53-1) = -5.64D (true refractive power)

- The total power of a lens is equal to the sum of the dioptric power of the two lens surfaces (front and back).
- For cylindrical lenses, measure the lens surface power in two principal meridians and put the numbers on a lens cross to convert to standard Rx form.

Hand neutralization: accomplished by making the secondary focal length of the known lens equal to the primary focal length of the unknown lens by placing the back pole of the known lens on the front pole of the unknown lens.

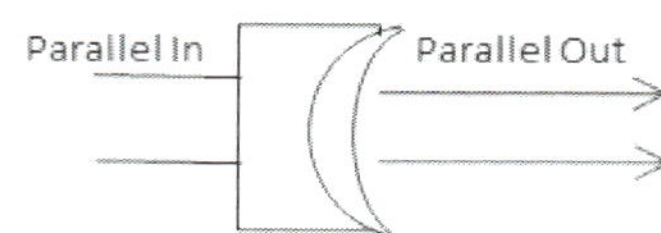

- This method reveals the front vertex power of the unknown lens.
- In the diagram, the left lens is known, and the right lens is the unknown lens.
- Based on principles of linear motion and rotational motion
    - Linear motion
        - Minus lenses – with
        - Plus lenses – against
    - Rotational motion: used to locate axis
        - With – minus axis
        - Against – plus axis

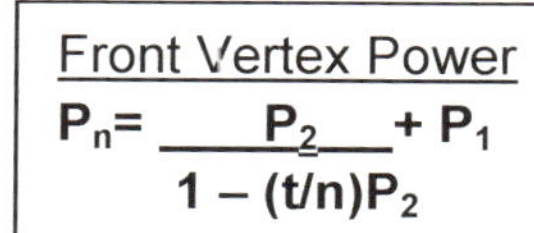

Front Vertex Power

$$P_n = \frac{P_2}{1 - (t/n)P_2} + P_1$$

4. Writing and Transposing a Lens Prescription

- **Writing**: The sphere power is always written before the cylinder power. Most lenses are written in the **Minus Cylinder Form** in Optometry e.g. +1.00 -2.00 x 180 and in the **Positive Cylinder Form** in Ophthalmology e.g. -1.00+ 2.00x 090
- **Transposition:**
    - Add sphere and cylinder power
    - Change the cylinder sign, but not the amount.
    - Change the axis of the cylinder by 90 degrees

Example: *Transpose +2.00 - +3.00 x 135 into minus cylinder form.*

Answer: +5.00-3.00 x 045

- **Crossed Cylinder** form is when you transpose a lens into having a front surface with positive cylinder and back surface with minus cylinder, with axes 90° apart. A **Jackson cross cylinder** is an example of this form, and is usually ±0.37 or ±0.25D in phoropters.
    - The spherical equivalent of crossed cylinder lens is 0.
- **Transposition to cross cylinder form**:
    - Determine the power of each meridian. Separate into front and back powers so that the sphere power for the front and back surfaces is Pl.

Example: *Transpose the Minus Cylinder Form +1.00-2.00x180 into Cross Cylinder Form:*

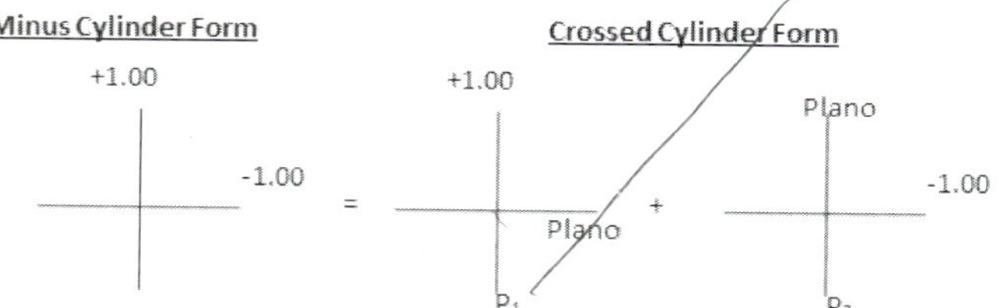

Answer:
Power @ 180=+1.00
Power @ 090= -1.00
Cross Cylinder Form=
+1.00x090 with -1.00x180

5. Effects of Lens Tilt

- When a **spherical** lens is tilted, the optic axis of the lens no longer passes through the center of rotation of the eye, which can induce astigmatism. The greater the tilt and greater the sphere power, the greater the induced power and greater the difference between the real and desired prescriptions. A plus lens will induce plus cylinder, a minus lens will induce minus cylinder
    1. **Pantoscopic tilt** induces minus cyl **axis 180**
    2. **Facial Wrap** induces minus cyl **axis 090**

- **Martin's Formula** allows the calculation of the new sphere power and the cylinder power that is induced due to tilt. The axis of the final prescription is 180 if pantoscopic tilt and 090 if facial wrap

  P_o= original sphere power
  P_{ns}= new sphere power
  P_c= cylinder induced
  α= angle of tilt

Martin's Formula
$P_{ns} = P_o [1 + (\sin^2 \alpha/2n)]$
$P_c = P_{ns} \tan^2 \alpha$

***Example**: A+8.00DS lens has 20° of pantoscopic tilt, what is the new power if n=1.523?*

> ***Answer:***
> P_{ns}=+8.00 [1+(sin^2(20)/2(1.523)]= +8.31DS
> P_c=+8.31 tan^2(20) = +1.10DC
> New lens power: +8.31 +1.10x180

***Example:** A -10.00DS lens has 10° of face-form tilt, what is the new power if n=1.523?*

> ***Answer:***
> P_{ns}=-10.00 [1+(sin^2(10)/2(1.523)]= -10.10DS
> P_c=-10.10 tan^2(10) = -0.31DC
> New lens power: -10.10 – 0.31 x 090

Note: Every frame has a pantoscopic tilt of about 10-12°

- When a **spherocylindrical** lens is tilted, the original cylinder power must be incorporated into the meridian of rotation. The following steps will make this calculation simpler
  1. **Transpose** the spherocylindrical prescription **to 090 if pantoscopic tilt** is being induced or **to 180 if face-form tilt** is being induced. Set the cylinder value aside for later
  2. Using ONLY the sphere power from the original Rx, calculate the new lens power from tilting the spherical part only.
  3. Add the new lens power from the spherical tilt to the original cylinder value that was transposed in step 1. This is your true new spherocylindrical power.

***Example:** What is the new power of a +7.00-2.00x180 lens that has a 17° pantoscopic tilt and n=1.523?*

> ***Answer:***
> Original Rx:+7.00 -2.00 x 180 w/ pantoscopic tilt → +5.00+2.00 x 090
> Set Pl +2.00x090 aside for later.
> P_{ns}=+5.00 [1+(sin^2(17)/2(1.523)]= +5.14DS
> P_c=+5.14 tan^2(17) = +0.48DC
> Lens power from tilting sphere: +5.14 +0.48x180
> Original Cylinder: Pl+2.00x 090 → +2.00-2.00x180
> Add lens power from sphere lens tilt to cylinder
> New lens power: +7.14 -1.52x180

- To get the lens optical axis to intersect the center of rotation of the eye, the optical center must be adjusted for the pantoscopic tilt.
- The **Efmm** is the linear displacement of the optical center due to the effect of pantoscopic tilt.
- The OC must be lowered 1mm per 2° pantoscopic tilt for lens optical axis to intersect C_r of the eye

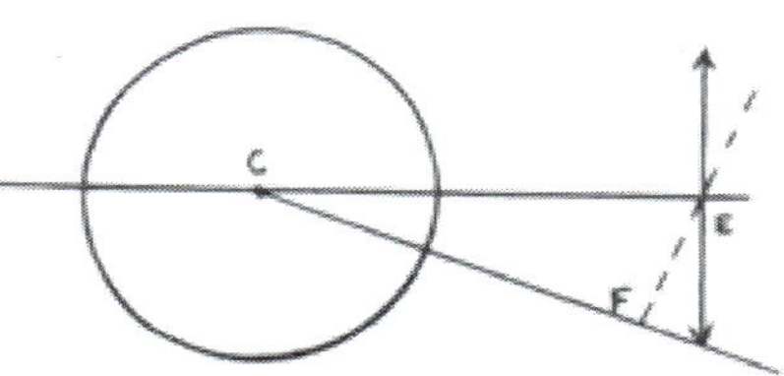

6. Effective Power

- **Effective Power** is the lens' ability to focus parallel rays at a specified plane.
- If one moves the correcting lens closer to or farther away from the eye, the secondary focal point of the lens is no longer conjugate with the patient's far point. There needs to be a different power of the lens for each vertex distance from the eye.

  P_{eff}= Effective power of the lens at the new position
  P= original power of the lens
  d= CHANGE in lens position
  d is + when the lens is moved toward the eye
  d is – when the lens is moved away from the eye

Effective Power
P_{eff}=P/(1+dP)
VD Compensation
P_{vd}=P/(1-dP)
CL Power
P_{CL}=P/(1-dP)

- When moving the lens toward the eye:
  - Plus lenses undercorrect with less plus (become less effective)
  - Minus lenses overcorrect with more minus (become more effective).
- When moving the lens away from the eye:
  - Plus lenses overcorrect with more plus (become more effective)
    - This is why presbyopes where there readers further down their nose
  - Minus lenses undercorrect with less minus (become less effective).

Note: The effective power formula is NOT the same as the vertex distance compensation formula used in contact lenses. The effective power formula calculates the effective power of a lens when it is moved towards or away from the eye. The vertex distance compensation formula calculates what power of a contact lens would be needed to correct the patient due to the increase/decrease in the effective power of a lens when you move it towards or away from the eye.

Example: *What is the effective power of a -10.00DS lens moved to the corneal plane (13mm toward the eye)? What contact lens power would be needed to compensate for the change in vertex distance?*

> ***Answer***:
> P_{eff}=-10/[1+(0.013)(-10)] = -11.49DS
> P_{vd}=-10/[1-(0.013)(-10)] = -8.85DS

This implies that the -10.00DS myope requires a -8.85DS contact lens at the corneal plane. When the -10.00DS spectacle lens is moved towards the eye, it becomes more effective, overcorrecting the patient by 1.49DS.

7. Spectacle Lens Processing

- **Surfacing:** The laboratory surfaces the concave side of a semi-finished lens blank with the proper compensating curves and thickness to provide the requested prescription. The proper lens blank size is selected based on the frame size and location of the lens optical center relative to the frame geometric center
- **Finishing:** After the lens is surfaced, the lab will edge or cut the lens to the shape of the frame. The optical center is placed in the proper location with respect to the frame's geometric center. The other steps involved in the finishing phase are layout, edging, safety beveling, lens insertion, and a final inspection. During the layout process, the lens is positioned to achieve the proper cylinder axis. After the lens is edged to achieve the correct shape, a safety bevel is added to smooth out the concave and convex edges.

8. Spectacle Magnification

- **Spectacle Magnification**: the retinal image size without relative to the optical lens, either spectacle or contact lens. It is a form of angular magnification
- **Relative Spectacle Magnification**: retinal image size in corrected ametropia relative to emmetrope retinal image size.

- The total spectacle magnification of a lens (M_T) has two components the magnification from its shape (M_s) and the magnification from its power (M_P), which is the major component.
    - Note that a lens does not have to have any power to cause magnification (M_S).
- **Exact Method** for determining M_T is the product of both components, while the **Approximate Method** is the summation of both components.
    - The power component causes most of the magnification and is a function of the BVP and vertex distance
    - The shape component is a function of lens thickness, index of refraction and base curve

Shape Component
$M_s = \frac{1}{1-t/nP_1}$
Power Component
$M_P = \frac{1}{1-t/nP_v}$
Spectacle Mag: Exact Method
$M_T = M_S \times M_P$
Spectacle Mag: Approximate Method
$M_T = M_S + M_P$

- **Aniseikonia**: the images the brain perceives from each eye are not the same. This may be due to differences in the size of the optical images on the retina or may be anatomically determined by a different distribution in spacing of the retinal elements.
- **Clinical aniseikonia** can be caused by anisometropia, monocular pseudophakia, monocular PKP, retinal detachment surgery, monocular ocular surgery and posterior staphyloma
    - Commonly aniseikonia is associated with **correction of anisometropia with spectacles** → the difference in magnification by each spectacle produces different sized retinal images.
    - The perception of an image size disparity between the two eyes is due to the images on the retina not falling on corresponding retinal points.
    - The differences in size may be overall (spherical lenses) or meridional (spherocylindrical lenses)
- When prescribing aniseikonic lenses, the size and shape of the final image does not matter, only the images of what each eye matches is important.
- **Iseikonia**: when perceived images are the same size
- **Iseikonic Lens designs** are prescribed for aniseikonic patients with astigmatism
    - Axial ametropia: try to equalize shape component
    - Refractive ametropia: try to equalize power and shape component
    - To equalize shape component, can alter base curve or thickness (shape nomograph).
    - Polaski's factor; for image size difference induced by spectacles for refractive error. Relative spectacle magnification = 0.1%mag/mm vertex dist/diopter bvp
    - For aniseikonia caused by small differences in RSM, Rx equal base curves and equal center thickness
    - For aniseikonia caused by larger differences in RSM, start with the eye that did not need magnification and keep it as thin and flat as possible and steepen and thicken the lens that needs magnification.

9. Methods of Remedying Reflections and Ghost Images

- **Reflections** can be caused by the sky, sand, snow, natural lights, and artificial lights. There are 5 main reflections from lights (See Next Page)
- In general, methods of remedying reflections and ghost images include:
    - Change the **material** – higher index materials have greater reflections
        - Fresnel's equation – reflection is material index of refraction dependent.
    - **Base curve** (flatter or steeper) – shifts the reflections, can compromise corrective curves
    - Increase **pantoscopic tilt** or increase **face-form tilt** – shifts the reflections
    - Decrease the **eyesize** – less area for reflections
    - Add a **tint** – reduce internal reflections
    - Add an ARC

Types of Reflections:

1. Light from behind the lens reflects off the back surface of the lens. This can cause a **ghost image**
    - Remedy: Increase face form, decrease vertex distance, decrease eye size
2. Light from behind the lens reflects off the back of the front surface of the lens. Can cause haze, not particularly bothersome

3. Light from the front reflects off the back surface, reflecting off the front surface, causing a double reflection and bothersome **ghost images**. This is the most problematic reflection.
   - Remedy: Add prism (shift ghost image elsewhere), change base curve or vertex distance
4. Light from the front reflects off the corneal surface, reflecting off lens back surface and into the eye. Causes **veiling glare**
   - Remedy: Change pantoscopic tilt, base curve, and vertex distance
5. Light from the front reflects off the corneal surface, reflecting off the lens front surface and into the eye

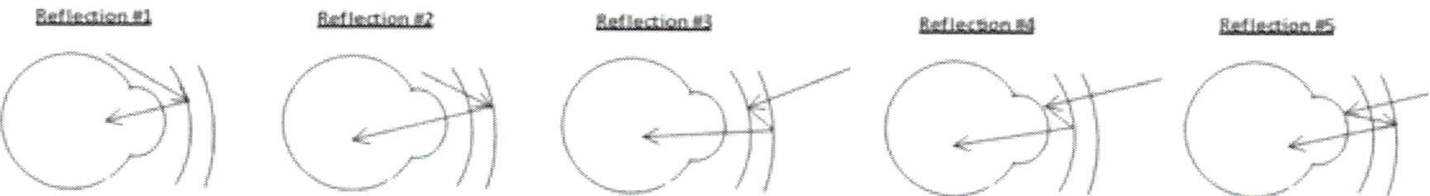

OPHTHALMIC PRISMS AND PRISMATIC EFFECTS OF LENSES

1. Thickness Differences Across a Prism

- Whether fabricated by surfacing or by decentering a lens, prism is prism regardless of how the laboratory achieves the prismatic effect.
- Thickness increases or decreases uniformly across a prism and can be calculated with the following values:

  Z=prismatic power (Δ)
  h=full length of the lens (mm)
  n= index of refraction
  t= thickness (mm)

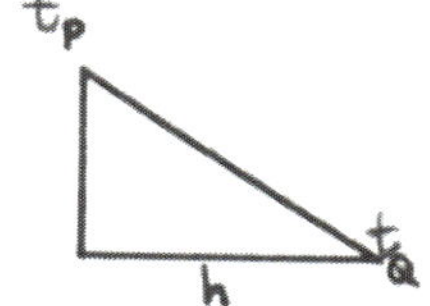

Prism Thickness

$$t_p - t_q = \Delta t = \frac{Z(h)}{100(n-1)}$$

Example: *A 55mm round OD lens is made with 2BI. If the temporal edge is 0.5mm thick, what is the nasal edge thickness if it is made of CR-39 (n=1.498)?*

Answer:
$\Delta t = 2(55) / [100(1.498-1)] = 2.209$mm
$et_{nasal} = \Delta t + et_{temporal} = 2.209 + 0.5 = 2.709$mm

2. Prismatic Effects in the Periphery of a Lens

- Since a lens varies in thickness, it can act as a prism. Plus lenses act as two prisms base to base and minus lenses act as two prisms apex to apex. Prismatic power follows Prentice's Rule, so the farther from the optical center (OC) of the lens one travels and the higher the power of the lens, the greater possible prismatic effect can occur in the periphery. Prism directly relates to decentration and power of the lens

  h = distance from point of concern to optical center (cm)
  P = Lens dioptric power

Prentice's Rule
Z = hP

- Signs are important for Prentice's Rule
  - (-) Z= BI or BD
  - (+) Z= BO or BU
  - (-) h= OC is up/out relative to PRP (prism reference point)
  - (+) h= OC is down/in relative to PRP
- At edge of a plus lens, an object may be out of view (ring scotoma)
- At edge of a minus lens, a double image may be seen.

Example: *What is the prismatic effect when viewing a -5.00DS lens 10.0mm above the OC?*

> ***Answer*:**
> Z=(1.0)(-5)=-5 or 5Δ BU

3. Decentration (Prism from Decentration, Decentering to obtain prism, IPD)

- **Decentration** is done to either move the optical center so that it lines up with the eyes (patient's IPD) to avoid inducing prism, or to induce a desired prismatic effect by intentionally moving it away from the patients pupils.
  - Decentration is the displacement of lens OC from the frame GC.
  - If OC=GC, lens is geometrically centered
  - If OC≠GC, lens is decentered
- Frame PD (FPD) is the distance between the geometric centers of each lens
- Distance IPD (DIPD) is the interpolar distance between the lens optical centers for the patients distance prescription
- Near IPD (NIPD) is the interpolar distance between the lens optical centers for the patient's near prescription (segment Rx for multifocal)
- Distance Decentration is the distance between the distance OC and the GC of the frame per lens
- Segment Decentration is the distance between the distance OC and the near OC per lens
- Total Decentration at near is the distance between the GC and the near OC per lens.

> Frame PD
> **FPD = A + DBL**
> Distance decentration
> **(FPD-DIPD)/2**
> Segment decentration
> **(DIPD-NIPD)/2**
> Total decentration
> **(FPD-NIPD)/2**

Example: If you need 3Δ BI with a +6.00 lens, how much must the lens be decentered and in which direction?

> ***Answer*:**
> Z=hP→ h=Z/P= -3/+6 = -0.5 cm
> h is negative, so the OC is OUT relative to PRP or OC has been decentered 5mm OUT temporally

4. Correction of Vertical Prism Effect

- Usually if there is anisometropia in the 090° meridian, there is an induced prismatic effect upon down-gaze. Prism imbalance is a consequence of the major lens, not the add.
- Vertical prism is of greater significance due to lower amplitudes of vertical fusional ranges → usually 3Δ of vertical prism induces diplopia
- The vertical prism imbalance still incorporates Prentice's Rule where:
  Z= vertical prism imbalance
  P= anisometropia (D)
  h= Reading level (cm)
- Vertical Prism Imbalance Compensation (how to correct):
  - Bicentric Grinding aka Slab Off
  - Double Slab Off
  - Dissimilar Segments
  - Conmpensated Ribbon Segments
  - Prism Segments
  - Multiple Corrections (2 pairs of SV glasses)
  - Contact Lenses
  - Fresnel Prism
  - Fresnel Adds

> Vertical Prism Imbalance
> $Z=h_{reading\ level}\ P_{anisometropia}$

Slab-Off (front, back, top, bottom, reverse)

- **Slab-off** aka **bicentric grinding** is the most prevalent method used to compensate for vertical imbalance at the designated (reading) level only. Bicentric meaning the lens has two optical centers.
    - Above the designated level there will be too much prism and below there will not be enough prism. The reading level is usually approximated to be 10mm below the primary gaze position.
- While it is not cosmetically obvious, it is an additional expense and does increase laboratory turnaround time.
- The limit of vertical imbalance compensation is 1.5 to 6Δ
- **Slab Off Line-** across the lens front or back surface usually coincident with the segment top/segment line on segmented MF's (TF or BF line) or 5-7mm below the distance reference point on PALs
- There are two techniques to slab off:
    - **Conventional Slab Off**: Base down is *removed* from the *most minus (least plus)* lens
    - **Reverse Slab Off**: Base down is *added* to the *least minus (most plus)* lens
        - SV lenses do NOT use reverse slab off method. Use only conventional slab off
- The surface of grinding depends upon the lens material:
    - **Front Surface:** SV glass, fused glass, one piece glass with segment on back (Ultex-rare)
    - **Back surface**: SV plastic, CR39 MF, PALs, executive MF (glass and plastic)

Location of Slab Off Line Summary			
Lens Material	Glass MF Lenses	Plastic MF Lenses	Plastic/Glass SV Lenses
Conventional Slab Off	Front Surface	Back Surface	Back Surface
Reverse Slab Off	Front Surface	Front Surface	n/a

- Bottom Slab Off- lens is ground on the bottom part of the lens to produce BU prism in the remaining area (Conventional)
- Top Slab Off- lens is ground on the top making the wedge shape produce BD prism (Reverse)

***Example**: Given OD -4.00-2.00x180 and OS -3.00-0.50x180 +2.00 Add, FT 25, what is the slab-off prism required to eliminate the vertical imbalance at the reading level, 10mm below the distance optical center?*

Answer:
Power in the 090 axis OD: -6.00
Power in the 090 axis OS: -3.50
Power imbalance: -2.50D
Z=hP= -2.50D(1.0cm) = -2.5Δ
For conventional slab off, slab off (remove) 2.50Δ BD from the most minus lens (OD)
For reverse slab off, slab off (add) 2.50Δ BD from the most plus lens (OS)

***Example**: How much vertical prism imbalance does a patient see if they look through a pair of spectacles with -3.00DS OD and Plano OS at a reading level 10mm below the distance OC? If there was 2ΔBD slab-off added to the lens, how much prism would be left at the 10mm reading level? Where is the center (pole) of the slab-off portion?*

Answer:
h=1.0cm to the reading level, $P_{anisometropia}$=-3.00DS
Z=hP= 1.0(-3.00) = -3ΔBD at the reading level
With 2ΔBD slab off, there would be 1ΔBD left at the reading level.
Z=-2Δ (BD prism is negative) $P_{anisometropia}$ =-3.00DS
h=Z/P = -2/-3.00= 0.667cm
If the patient sees 1ΔBD at 10mm below the distance OC with 2ΔBD slab-off, the pole of the slab-off portion (where there is no vertical prism imbalance) is 6.67mm down from the distance OC and 3.33mm up from the near OC (reading level).If the full 3ΔBD were slabbed off, the pole of the slab-off portion would be coincident with the reading level 10mm below the distance OC.

Double Slab-Off

- **Double Slab-Off** or "dynamic stabilization" is a technique in which base down prism is removed from the bottom of the lens and base up prism is removed from the top of the lens, creating thin zones at the top and bottom.
- This method is used in making toric contact lenses to create **prism ballasting**, which allows the eyelids to exert pressure on the lens and hinder rotation.
- Helps to keep the contact lens from rotating on the eye to keep the cylinder axis in the correct orientation. Works best with ATR astigmatism.

Dissimilar Segments

- **Dissimilar segments** is the use of a different segment styles on each eye with different distances from the top of the segment to the near optical center (r-value), thus differing vertical prismatic effects on down-gaze. This technique is rarely used, but a good optical principle.
- Different levels of prism can be induced by a segment. This technique uses the differential prism from the segment to offset the vertical prism induced by the carrier lens.
- Segment with the greatest r-value placed on most plus carrier lens in vertical meridian

Segment	R value
Ultex	19
Round	½ Segment Diameter
Flat Tops	5
Executive	0

Example: *Given OD +1.00DS and OS -4.00-1.00x 090, +2.50 Add, what segments will help compensate the vertical prism imbalance at the reading level (10mm below the DOC) if the segment top is 3.0mm below the DOC?*

> ***Answer:***
> Power axis 090 OD: +1.00 OS: -4.00→ $P_{anisometropia}$: 5.00D
> $Z_{carrier}$ =(1.0cm)(5.00D)= 5.0Δ vertical prism imbalance from the carrier lens
> h=$Z_{carrier}$ /P_{add}= 5.0Δ/2.5= 2.0cm or 20mm
> h= the difference between the segment OCs
> Two segments that would give about 20mm separation would be an Executive segment (r=0) and an Ultex segment (r=19) → 19mm separation.
> The segment with the greatest r value (Ultex) is placed on the most plus (OD) lens.

Compensated Ribbon Segments

- Similar to the principle of dissimilar segments, **Compensated R (Ribbon)** Segments uses displaced ribbon segments (22x14) in each lens (one up and one down), to produce a more cosmetically appealing method to decrease vertical prism imbalance.
- R-9, R-4, R-5, etc. refers to distance from top of the segment to the near (segment) optical center.
- For bifocal adds, the near optical center represents the base of the "prism," and the reading level represents the apex.
- The maximum separation between the segment OCs of both lenses is 6mm → where the reading level is 4mm below the segment top in one lens and 4mm above the segment top in the other lens
- The most plus lens gets the segment with the greatest r value

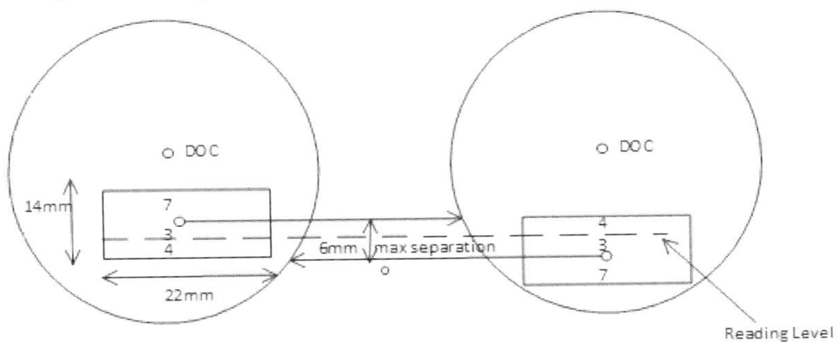

***Example**: Given OD -1.00-0.75x180 and OS +1.00-0.75 x 180 with +2.50 Add on a 46x40mm lens with a segment height of 18mm, what R-compensated segments would leave the patient with a residual vertical prism imbalance of 1Δ if DOC=GC, and the RL is 10mm below the DOC?*

> ***Answer:***
> Power axis 090 OD: -1.75DS, OS: +0.25 → $P_{anisometropia}$: 2.00DS
> Z=hP= (1.0cm)(2.00DS) = 2Δ total imbalance. If want 1Δ residual, $Z_{carrier}$=1Δ
> $h_{segments}=Z_{carrier}/P_{add}$= 1/2.50 = 0.40cm or 4mm. The difference in ribbon segment OCs is 4mm so the following options would work:
> a) r-4:r-8 b) r-5:r-9, c)r-6:r-10 with the highest r-value segment on OS.

Prism Segments:

- **Prism segments** are for people requiring near prismatic corrections when no prismatic correction is needed at distance, or when a different prismatic correction is needed at distance. Thus, prism can be ordered for the segment only. This, however, is usually not a good idea as it is usually a special order requiring a 4 to 6 week delivery.

Multiple Corrections:

- Multiple corrections or multiple pairs of SV lenses (one pair for distance and not for near) can be considered when prismatic correction is needed at distance or near, but not both, or when different prismatic corrections are needed at distance and near or when anisometropic prescriptions cause vertical prism imbalance. A common prescription is a pair of glasses for near only that incorporates near prismatic correction, the patient having no refractive error or heterophoria at distance.
- For anisometropic prescriptions, one might have to decenter the near OC if the patient reads in down gaze rather than tilting their head down to read through the OC.

Contact Lenses

- Since contact lenses are on the cornea, there are no prism induced problems.
- There may be possible image size differences, depending on the type of ametropia (axial vs. refractive)
- This is usually the best option for anisometropic patients

Fresnel Prisms

- A **Fresnel prism** is a temporary solution, where a Fresnel membrane vertical prism is adhered to the back lens surface. Like slab-off, add BD prism on the eye with the least amount of minus.
- A Fresnel prism is actually a series of prisms of equal value and size. A large single prism is effectively made into a sheet of several very small and equal prisms.
- Advantages include substantially reduced weight and thickness with the ability to put the prisms anywhere and in any orientation desired.
- Disadvantages are that the prisms are cosmetically undesirable and acuity tends to fall ½ to 1 line when wearing the lenses.

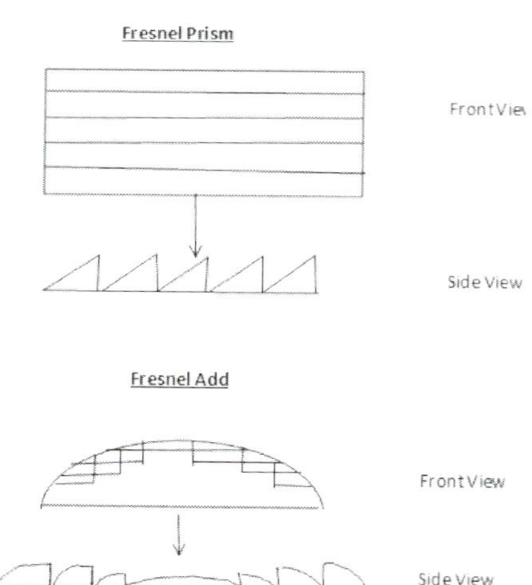

Fresnel Adds

- **Fresnel adds** are a series of arcs cut out from a sphere and lowered to a membrane. The arcs are of equal power and size. The lenses are recommended when high powers are needed

MULTIFOCAL LENSES

1. Types

- Bifocals are made in two different ways: fused and 1-piece lenses.

Fused Multifocals (Glass Only)

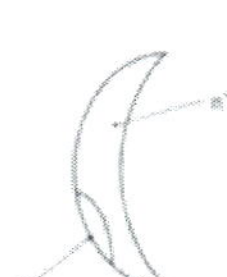

- **Fused** lenses are made with two different types of glass (different indices of refraction) fused together, with the segment button having a higher index of refraction than the carrier lens.
- The curvature is the same between the distance portion and the near portion, so the front has a spherical curve.
- The add of a fused multifocal can NOT be determined by a lens gauge
- The base curve is on the side with the segment
- Segment Types: A (upside down flat top), B (ribbon segment), C (small flat top), and D (flat top)

1-Piece Multifocals (Glass and Plastic)

- **1-piece** lenses are made from one piece of glass or plastic (index of refraction constant). The lens is ground with two different curvatures with the carrier lens having a longer radius of curvature than the segment.
- The curvature is different from the distance portion and near portion, and can be physically felt on the lens.
- The add of a 1-piece lens can be determined by a lens gauge.
- The base curve is always on the front
- Segment Types: Ultex, Executive, Flat Top, Round

Multifocal Types Summary			
MF Type	Glass Fused	Glass 1-Piece	Plastic 1-Piece
Base Curve	Front	Front or Back	Front
Segment Types and Sizes	Panoptic Kryptok FT- 25, 28, 35 RT-22, 25 Curved Top Ribbon	Executive Ultex -38 FT-22,25,28,35	Executive Ultex- 42, 48 FT- 25, 28, 35, 45 RT-15, 22, 24, 25, 28, 35, 40 Curved Top 28

Blended Lenses (Plastic Only)

- Blended/No Line/Invisible Lenses are round segments where the transition between the distance and near lens is blended.
- The blend zone (annulus) is an unusable area with an induced astigmatic error. It is power dependent, so the higher the add power, the larger the blend zone.
- Increasing the zone of blend will decrease the induced astigmatism but increase the unusable amount of the lens.
- This is a 1-piece concept lens and NOT considered a progressive lens because there are only two focal points.
- Advantages include cosmesis, less costly than progressives, and no noticeable image jump.
- Disadvantages include the blend zone, unwanted astigmatism, and only two focal points (distance and near).

Progressive Additions

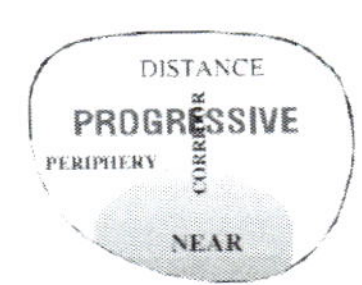

- Progressive additions (PALs) are not a bifocal lens but have a true progression of optics with a gradual increase in curvature based on a 1-piece concept lens.
- Advantages include cosmesis, continuous vision with multiple focal points to mimic "natural vision" and no image jump

- Disadvantages include an optical compromise due to inherent aberrations, areas of defocus, adaptation, cost, and a narrow corridor (smaller viewing zone).

2. Methods of Producing Add Powers

- Change in index (fused) – glass only, MF
- Change in curvature (1-piece) – glass and plastic, MF, PAL, Blended
- **Effective power**: Recall that increasing the vertex distance increases the effective plus power of a lens. So one can increase the add power by sliding a frame with a positive prescription (add) down one's nose.

3. Segment Center Location

Segment Decentration
(DIPD-NIPD)/2
Total Decentration
(FPD-NIPD)/2

- The segment optical center (SOC) is the optical center of the segment itself
  - For flat top bifocals, SOC is usually 5mm below the segment line.
  - For round segment bifocals, SOC is located a distance equal to ½
  - segment diameter from the segment top.
- SOC can be horizontally displaced relative to DOC
  - Normally inset 1-2mm in (OD and OS) for the NIPD
  - May be decentered more to induce prismatic effect from segment
  - Major lens may have induced prismatic effect.
- Segment Decentration is between DOC and SOC
  - Distance Decentration is between frame GC and DOC
  - Total Decentration is between frame GC and SOC
- With a stronger add, the working distance is closer, causing the eyes to converge more to see the target. This high convergence causes a normally inset bifocal (2mm in OD and OS) to induce BO prism, requiring even more unneeded convergence. Thus, the SOC needs to be decentered in to avoid inducing BO prism. In general, the required near PD can be calculated using the following formula where:
  - x= the theoretical inset for the near PD
  - C_{rot}= center of rotation of the eye, usually 27mm
  - u= working distance

Segment Decentration

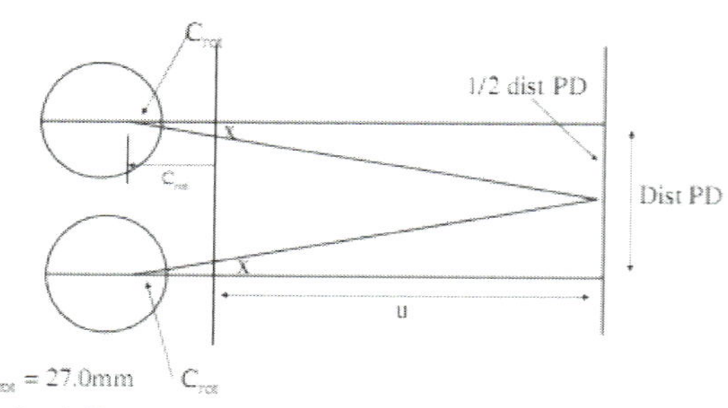

- **Another Rule of Thumb:** – for each diopter of add, there is 1.5mm total decentration. Thus, add 1mm to total decentration if the distance PD is large (greater than 68mm).

Add	Total Decentration (add 1mm for large PD)
+3.00	4.5mm
+4.00	6.0mm
+8.00	12.0mm
+10.00	15.0mm

Segment Decentration
(Using Similar Triangles):

$$\frac{x}{C_{rot}} = \frac{\tfrac{1}{2}\,DIPD}{C_{rot} + u}$$

or

$$x = \frac{DIPD\,(C_{rot})}{2(C_{rot} + u)}$$

- Fitting high adds:
  - Maximum adds for multifocal lenses:
    - Flat Top: +6.00
    - Round Top: +30.00
    - PALs: +3.00
  - **Bailey's Approximate Formula:** multiply every power of add by 1.5mm; IF DIPD >65, add 1mm; subtract finding from DIPD to get NIPD.
  - **Fonda's Approximation:** for every diopter of add, give 1 Δ of BI prism. (Gives patient the least prism)

Bailey's Approx. Formula
$NIPD = DIPD – 1.5(P_{add})$
Fonda's Approx. Formula
1ΔBI per +1.00D P_{add}

Example: *If the desired add is +5.00D with a DIPD of 64mm, what is the NIPD if you were to use Bailey's Formula and what amount of prism should you add according to Fonda's Formula?*

> ***Answer:***
> NIPD= 64- 1.5 (5) = 56.5mm
> 5Δ BI

4. Differential Displacement (Image Jump)

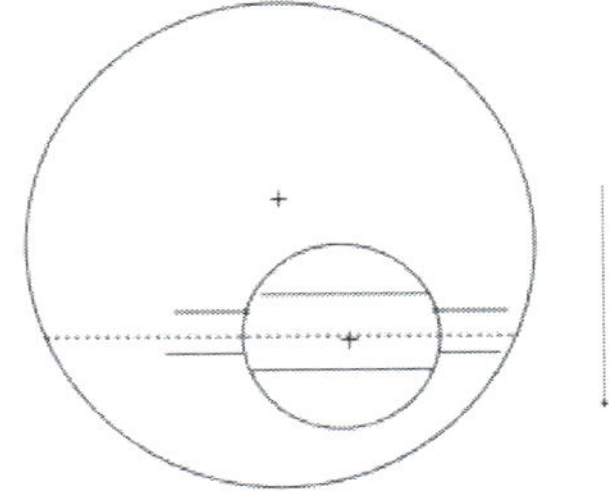

- **Image Jump** is the difference in prismatic effect between the segment and major lens at segment top. It causes a noticeable "jump" in the image for the patient when they move their gaze from the carrier to the segment part of the lens.
- Prismatic effect at the segment top (Base Down)
- Distance from SOC to seg top (r-values) can help you calculate prism at segment top
  - If r=0, there is no image jump → Executive MFs and PALs have no image jump
  - As the r value increases, the image jump increases
- Dependent exclusively on the add power, Independent of distance Rx
- Use Prentice's Rule, $Z=h_{cm}P_{add}$ where h is the r value in cm.

Example: *What is the image jump for the following segments (FT-25, Ultex A, RT-22, and Executive) with the following Rx: OD +2.00DS, OS +2.00DS, Add +2.50?*

> ***Answer:***
> -FT-25; r-5mm; Z=(+2.50)(-0.5)= -1.25Δ BD
> -Ultex A; r=19mm; Z=(+2.50)(-1.9)= -4.75 Δ BD
> -RT22; r=11mm; Z=(+2.50)(-1.1)= -2.75 Δ BD
> -Executive; r=0; Z=(+2.50)(0)= 0

5. Total Displacement, Horizontal and Vertical Imbalance

- The **Total Differential Displacement**, is the prism effect at the reading level. It is dependent on and the summation of both the prismatic effect from the distance Rx at the reading level and the prismatic effect from the add power at the reading level.
- Differential Displacement at the Reading Level due to the add power is different from Image Jump. It is the prismatic effect at the reading level (RL) due to displacement of the reading level and the segment OC. It is also calculated using Prentice's formula, but h is the distance between the RL and the SOC.
  - If SOC=RL there is no displacement at the reading level
  - If RL is above SOC base down prism is induced
  - If RL is below SOC base up prism is induced.
- Differential Displacement at the Reading Level due to the distance Rx is calculated using Prentice's formula, where h is the distance between the DOC and the RL
  - Minus lenses induce base down
  - Plus lenses induce base up

> Total Differential Displacement
> $Z_{total}=Z_{carrier} + Z_{add}$
> $Z_{carrier}=(h_{DOC \to RL})P_{Distance}$
> $Z_{add}=(h_{SOC \to RL})P_{add}$

Example*: What is the total differential displacement if the DOC is 5.0mm above the segment top and the reading level is 10mm below the DOC, given the following Rx: -2.00DS OU; Add: +2.50OU, RT25*

> ***Answer:***
> Displacement from carrier lens: $Z_{carrier}$ = (1.0)(-2.00) = -2.00Δ BD
> Distance b/w reading level and SOC: 7.5mm (r=12.5 for RT25)
> Displacement from segment: $Z_{segment}$ =(+2.50)(-0.75) = -1.875 Δ BD
> Total differential displacement: -2 + -1.875 = -3.875 Δ BD

Note: It is not possible to eliminate image jump and differential displacement at the same time.

Horizontal and Vertical Imbalance

- Since a minus lens can be considered a minus lens as two prisms placed apex to apex and a plus lens as two prisms placed base to base, one can use Prentice's Rule to calculate the horizontal and vertical prism imbalance that can be created when decentering a lens optical center (GC) from the patient's pupil at distance (DOC) or near (SOC).

  ***Example**: What is the vertical prism induced when a patient looks 10 mm below and 5mm in from the distance optical center of a +4.00 –1.00 x 090 lens?*

  > ***Answer:***
  > $Z_{vertical}$ =hP = 1.0 (+4.00DS) = 4Δ BU
  > $Z_{horizontal}$= hP= 0.5 (+3.00DS) = 1.5Δ BI

6. Placement of Distance and Multifocal Optical Centers

- **Placement of the DOC** so that it is in, out, up, or down from the patient's PD creates prism.
  - Use Prentice's rule to determine how much prism is created.
  - To determine base direction, consider a plus lens as two prisms laid base to base and a minus lens as two prisms laid apex to apex.
- The SOC is horizontally displaced relative to DOC
- **Placement of SOCs**: (by varying the segment inset), can induce lateral prism in the near portion only. Insetting the segment more than it needs to be (that is, insetting more than that indicated by the near PD) creates BI prism, and insetting the segment less than it needs to be creates BO prism.
  - Vertical placement: ideal segment height location is from the pupil center to the lower lid margin
  - Horizontal placement: ideally place SOCs to correspond to near PD, unless desire prism
  - Segment decentration is dependent on:
    - Distance PD
    - Distance between eye's center of rotation and lens back pole
    - Fixation distance
    - Distance Rx in horizontal meridian
  - Segment decentration can be calculated using Prentice's rule where h is the amount of inset in or out from the near PD and P is the power of the add.

7. Optical and Physical Characteristics of Segments

Standard Bifocal

- Noted for their visibility and wide field of view.
- Because cosmesis can be the primary factor in your selection, there may be times when these need to be avoided. The flat top is noticeable because of its thick flat edge. The executive is the most noticeable because the segment line goes all the way across the lens. Round segs are the least noticeable because of the knife edge.
- **Fused Bifocals:** Exhibit more chromatic aberration from the differences in indices. The fused bifocal cannot be felt on the outside of the lens because the add is created by increasing index of refraction and leaving the front curve constant.
- **1-piece Bifocals:** creates the add by changing the curvature of the front surface.

Flat Top Bifocals

- Ideal reading level position, minimal jump, good cosmesis, ideal for general wear
- Total displacement same as SV lenses
- Decenter for near prism
- Available in glass, polycarbonate, CR49, Hi-Index
- Many segment sizes: 25, 28, 35, 45

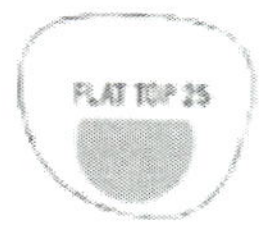

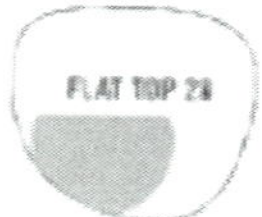

- Add power availability: +0.50 to +6.00D
    - Not in all sizes, materials. Most common add power: +0.75 to +3.00D
    - Most common Hi-Index sizes: 25, 28 and add power: +1.00 to +3.00D
- FT 25 most widely used BF worldwide
- FT 28 mist widely used in the US

Executive Bifocals

- NO image jump
- Very obvious segment line, reflections from segment line
- Large viewing area
- Thicker, heavier lens
- Difficult to get distance/near IPDs
- Careful with plus lens, thin inferior edge
- Available in glass, plastic, polycarbonate
- Add power availability: +0.75 to +3.00
- Note: beginning to be phased out

Blended Bifocals

- The transition between the distance and near portions is blended to take away the sharp bifocal line and make it invisible. It is made from a one-piece bifocal, and therefore a bump can be felt after blending occurs. The goal was to make a bifocal more cosmetically appealing, but there are several problems with this lens:
    - The area that is blended can no longer be used optically. It is a blurred zone, and therefore the area of near vision is diminished.
    - The curvature changes cause an induced astigmatic error that is equal to the amount of the add power. To decrease the zone of blend would cause an increase in astigmatic error, but to reduce astigmatic error would spread out the blend width.

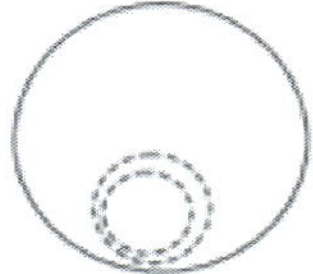

- Distance and near have spherical optics, blend zone has astigmatic optics
- Near segment sizes available – 22, 25, 28mm
- Narrow Blend Zone: Concentrated astigmatism, larger usable area
- Wider Blend Zone: less astigmatism, smaller usable area

Progressive Lenses

- A gradual change of curvature is used to obtain a distance and near lens. The goal is to give a zone in the lens with minimal aberrations and a gradual increase in plus power. To do this, the aberrations must be spread out into other parts of the lens.
    - The lens has a corridor of slowly increasing plus power ending with the add power prescribed near the bottom of the lens. On either side of the corridor are areas of high astigmatism or aberration.
    - The advantages of progressive bifocals are its cosmetic value (no-line bifocal) and its infinite range of focuses as one looks down the corridor.
    - The major disadvantage is the zone of aberrations. How much aberration or astigmatism is created? If a power changes a certain amount, say 1D vertically, then if you move the same distance horizontally from the center of the corridor, you would have approximately 2D of astigmatism, depending on design.
- Design goals: Large stable viewing area, continuous vision with wide channel. Minimal peripheral distortions, no segment boundaries, patient acceptance
- **Corridor Length**: the vertical drop from the fitting cross to the nominal add power
    - Short→ reach the full add quicker, more unwanted astigmatism
    - Long→ greater eye depression to reach full add, less unwanted astigmatism
- **Corridor Width**: defined by the acceptable limits of unwanted astigmatism (0.50DC)
    - Unwanted cylinder increases laterally from the center. There is no unwanted astigmatism in the center of the corridor (umbilicus)
- **Channel Power Function (CPF):** how fast the power changes along the corridor

- Linear: equal power change
- Nonlinear: variable power change. Power change slower at top of corridor
- Corridor shape may predict CPF

- Design Concepts
  - Hard vs. Soft

Differences	Hard	Soft
Zone of Clear Optics	Large	Small
Zone of Concentrated UA	Small	Large zone of low level UA*
Corridor	Shorter, Narrower	Longer, Wider
Concept	BF	TF
Asphericity	Less	More
Adaptation	More difficult	Easier

*Low level UA – easier to interpret

  - Mono vs. Multi
    - **Mono Design**: linear relationship between corresponding points, predictable design within a series of add powers
    - **Multi Design**: design varies with add power nonlinear relationship between corresponding points
  - Add based vs. Need based
    - **Add Based**: Design varied by add
    - **Need Based**: Design based on patient's need (emphasis on intermediate/distance/near)
  - Design by prescription
  - Symmetric vs. Asymmetric vs. Horizontal Symmetry
    - Location of unwanted astigmatism can be equal temporally and nasally (**symmetric**) or more nasally than temporally because of where cut the lens blank (**asymmetric**)
    - **Horizontal Symmetry**: Make temporal and nasal unwanted astigmatism the same only if the OD and OS lens are the same power due to induced prismatic effects when patient looks off of the segment OC. If OD/OS powers are the same, then prism will be the same in magnitude but opposite in direction and thus, cancel.
  - Position of wear (panto tilt 8-10° in spectacles, vertex distance 12-14mm)
    - Atoric PALs
  - Free form processing
    - Integrates free form, atoricity and position of wear
  - Prism thinning
    - Aka **equi-thin design**: increase lens center thickness to account for thin edge thickness in high plus lenses. By shaving off the top side to induce base down to cancel out induced BU prism in higher plus carrier lenses

- PAL Surface Characteristics: Multiple design types

Combinations		
Front Surface	Back Surface	Comments
Spheric-Spheric	Spheric -Conventional	Very old technology: Patient notices a "swimming effect"
Spheric-Aspheric	Spheric- conventional	Old technology
Aspheric	Spheric-conventional	
Aspheric	Atoric- free form	
Spheric	Atoric- free form	PAL power on back surface only
Aspheric	Aspheric	PAL power on back and front surface- Most sophisticated

*Atoric- a toric surface where each principle meridian has been made aspheric

8. Specifying Multifocal Height, Size, Shape, and Location of Segment

Multifocal Height:

- For first time bifocal wearers, textbooks suggest that the seg top be placed at the position of the lower lid margin. Seg height is then measured to the bottom of the eyewire. Most errors are made by setting the segment line too high.

- For blended and progressive lenses, dot the center of the pupil with the patient in primary gaze, and measure to the bottom of the eyewire. Generally, for PALs, this measurement should at least be 22mm or the B dimension of the frame at least 38mm. However, some newer design PALs allow for fitting heights as low as 14mm.
- Round bifocal segments must be fitted higher than straight-top bifocals because the widest and most useful part of the segment is lower. Occupation, head position, and many other factors are important in determining the segment height. In general, the more time spent reading or doing other close work, the higher the segment should be.

Multifocal Size:

- **Segment width:** widest horizontal measurement of the segment. Indicated in mm, after bifocal style. i.e. FT-22, FT25, FT28, FT35. For flat tops, the width is measured 5mm below the segment. For round and Ultex segments, the width is the diameter of the circle.
- Bifocal segments have grown larger and larger in recent years. The smaller segments were designed to infringe as little as possible on the wearer's distance field of vision, whereas the larger segments now in use were designed with the desk worker in mind.
- It can be shown that a 22mm wide segment provides a 35cm wide field of fixation at a 40 cm working distance. Even though a 22mm wide segment is considered wide enough for most everyday near tasks, many patients whose entire working day involves near work may benefit from the Executive-style bifocal.

Multifocal Shape:

- One of the only advantages of selecting a round fused segment is that it is less visible than a straight-top fused segment.
- A ribbon segment should be considered for sports players, carpet layers, mail carriers, tractor drivers, or anyone who must have occasional near vision available.
- An important factor in the selection of a shape of bifocal is the style of bifocal that the patient is currently wearing. If the patient is satisfied with his present bifocal, the best procedure is not the change its shape.

Location of Segment:

- Depending upon the individual patient's needs, bifocal segments may be placed in a variety of locations. For the average person, the segment is placed with its optical center corresponding to the patient's near interpupillary distance.
- The number of locations for segments that may be designed is only limited by the patient's needs and the practitioner's imagination.

Selection of multifocal lenses for vocational/avocational use

- Cosmesis: when cosmesis is important, select an Ultex or Kryptok because their round knife edges are difficult to see. A round fused bifocal with a slight tint is very difficult to see when someone is wearing it.
- **Double bifocal:** two segments, one at the top and one at the bottom. Useful to prescribe for people who do over-head work. Potential candidates include mechanics, pilots, painters, electricians, plumbers, librarians, dentists, surgeons and carpenters.

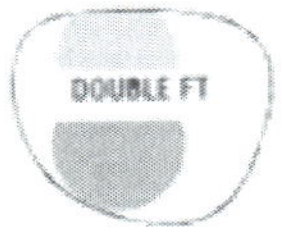

DOUBLE FT

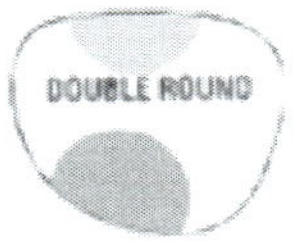

DOUBLE ROUND

Fitting techniques for multifocals

- Height of the patient: taller patients look lower to read and, therefore, need the segs set lower
    - Occupation: patients that do a lot of near work should have the seg fit higher
    - Reason for prescribing: for children the seg top should be at the center of the pupil to force the child to use his/her bifocal.
- **Trifocal height:** most failures occur when the seg is set too low
    - Occupational uses: fit close to the bottom of the pupil
    - Non-occupational uses: fit 1-2 mm below the pupil margin

- The difference between bifocal seg top and trifocal seg top is usually 6 mm. This number corresponds to the width of the intermediate zone.

PHYSICAL CHARACTERISTICS AND BIOLOGICAL COMPATIBILITY OF FRAME MATERIALS

- Frames are fabricated with one of the following materials:
  - Cellulose acetate or zylonite (zyl)
  - Optyl
  - Cellulose propionate
  - Nylon
  - Co-polyamide or Polyamide
  - Carbon fiber
  - Polycarbonate
  - Rubber
  - Metals: Gold, aluminum, stainless steel, monel, beryllium nickel, titanium, trilam.
- Predominant frame material in current usage is made of some type of metal while some 15-20% is made of plastic
- **Cellulose acetate**
  - Material derived from wood flakes and cottonseed fibers or pulp
    - Plasticizers and stabilizers are added to the raw material during the formation of zylonite sheets.
  - Ways to create sheet stock acetate
    - **Block method**: colors hand laid onto a sheet then pressed with heat and pressure
    - **Extrusion method**: extruder machines melt down the colored resins and it is fed to a dye. The dye regulates the flow of the color to make an overlay or any other pattern
    - **Laminate Method**: laminates sheets made by the block/extrusion method together
    - **Ceblox Method**: forms sheets by compression molding
    - **Injection molded**: resin is melted and forced into a mold, then cooled to frame shape
  - Pantographic Procedure: Frame components are cut from the sheets of pre-colored blocked cellulose acetate. These are then polished and tumbled in a tumbler for high luster
  - Unlimited styles, colors, ease of handling, adjustments hold well
  - Fades when exposed to heat or the sun, yellowing and discoloration due to contact with skin acids, and oils, material becomes brittle with age
- **Optyl**
  - Epoxy resin plastic coated and cured with polyurethane
  - Hypoallergenic, weighs 30-40% less than zyl
  - Made from dye-cast process
  - Known as the "frame with a memory"
    - When heated, frame returns to manufacturer's original molded shape
  - Does not fade or discolor with age, more resistant to abrasion, can withstand higher temperature than cellulose acetate
  - Longer adjustment time, possible breakage if bent cold
- **Propionate**
  - Hypoallergenic, light but not as strong as other two materials
  - Made by injection molding
  - Frames have high luster, polish well
  - More heat sensitive, possible fading
- **Nylon**
  - Material is very durable and heat resistant
  - Makes lens insertion or adjustments much more difficult
  - Material gets brittle with age
- **Polyamide or Co-polyamide**
  - Relatively strong material, maintains shape well, flexible, has good impact resistance
  - Vulnerable to high temperature – use air blower

- **Carbon Frames**
    - Made from carbon and nylon
    - Brittle, tends to break on impact or when exposed to cold weather
    - Difficult to adjust due to heat resistance
- **Polycarbonate**
    - Recreational and safety type eyewear
    - Significant impact resistance and adjustments are difficult
- **Metals**
    - Tend to be made from several alloys
    - Coloring of frames usually an inlay or plating
    - **Gold** - Heavy, expensive, rarely used except for metal-allergy patients
    - **Aluminum** - Light weight, hold adjustment well
    - Most frames are stainless steel, monel, titanium, or some metal alloy frame
    - Lower quality frames contain more nickel - patients with metal reaction tend to react to frames with nickel → consider using plastic, nickel-free or pure titanium frame
    - **Stainless Steel**- lightweight, durable, anti-corrosive, anti-allergenic
        - Usually 17% chromium, 8% nickel, 0.05% carbon, 2% manganese
    - **Monel**- combination of nickel, copper, and iron.
    - **Pure titanium** – lightweight, strong, more expensive

FITTING, ADJUSTMENT, SPECIFICATION, AND NOMENCLATURE OF FRAMES

1. Frame Nomenclature

- **Frame front** – entire frame minus the temples
    - **Eye wire** – the portion of the frame which encircles and holds the lenses in the grooved rims of the eye wire
    - **Bridge** – the part of the frame which fits over the nose and connects the left and right eye wires. Bridges of zyl frames are usually fixed and classified as keyhole or saddle.
        - Saddle: rests on the bridge of the nose. It is made for large noses 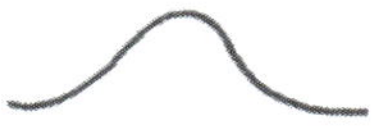
        - Keyhole: this was made for smaller noses and rests on either side of the nose bridge 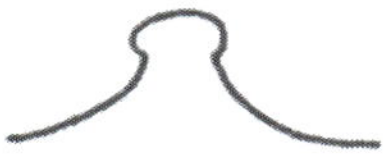
    - **Guard arms** – with most metal frames, a short, thin piece of metal, known as the guard arm is soldered to the inner nasal portion of the eye wire; it supports the nosepad. The domestic type is called the gooseneck and can be adjusted in the x, y, and z plane.
- **Nose pads** – support and distribute the weight of the spectacles on the nose and are made of plastic or silicone
- **End piece** – the area that forms the connection between the eye wire and the temple
    - Monoblock
    - Wrap-around
- **Temples** 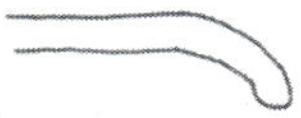
    - Skull temple: most common 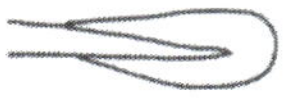
    - Library temple: those go straight back for people who take their glasses on and off constantly. 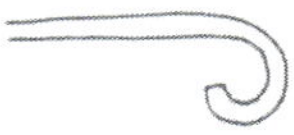
    - Comfort cable/riding bow: usually only on metal frames, made of a spring type loop that goes around the ear. Plastic covers the loop to avoid alloy irritations with the skin.

2. Frame Adjustment and Fitting

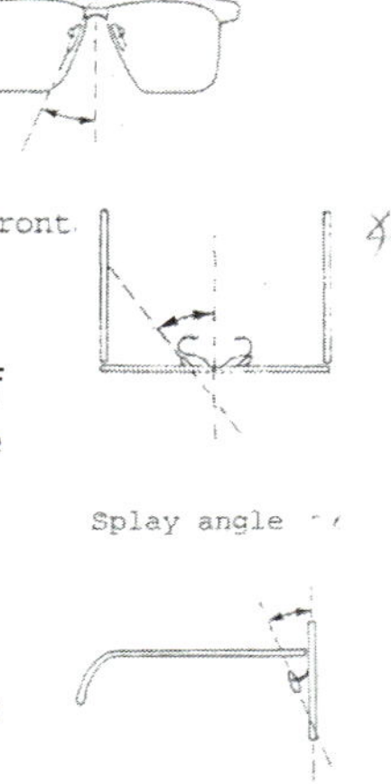

- Consider the fitting triangle – the 3 points of the fitting triangle represents the points of contact between the eyewear and the skull (2 temples and 1 nose bridge)
- Adjust the bridge
  - **Frontal angle** – how the nose angles outward from the midline; best viewed from the front
  - **Splay angle** (traverse angle) – the angle between a line through the center of the bridge and the face of the nose; represents how the nose widens from the front to back or the angle from the center of the bridge back towards the cheek. In general, Asian and Afro-American bridges are relatively flatter, so the bridge splay angle is greater; best observed from the top
  - **Vertical angle** – applicable to adjustable nose pads, this is the angle from the top edge of the nose as seen from the side; this is adjusted by moving the guard arms up or down

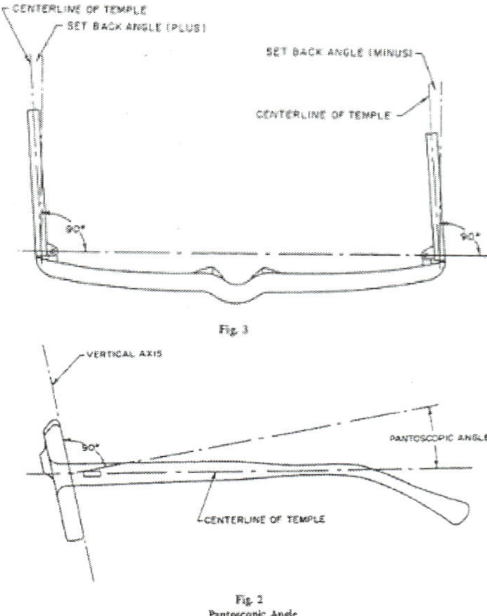

Fig. 3

Fig. 2
Pantoscopic Angle

- Pad adjustment – move closer together to push frame up. Spread pads apart to move frame down
- Front or side angling
  - X-ing: lenses not in the same plane
  - Set back angle: angle at the end piece made between the frame front and the center line of the temple. When the angle is >90degrees, it's a positive set back angle. When the angle is <90degrees, it's a negative set back angle. Generally, the 2 set back angles will be minus.
- End piece adjustment: changes panto or retroscopic tilt.
- Concepts of fitting and adjusting
  - If one lens is situated higher on one side: increase the pantoscopic tilt on the low side or decrease the pantoscopic tilt on the high side.
  - If one lens is farther from the face: adjust the temple angle so that it is greater than 90° on the side furthest from the face (means the current angle is probably <90degrees, and pushing the frame out on that side)

3. Frame Specification

- Most frame manufacturers will imprint on the frame the specifications (eye size, bridge size, temple length, color, frame manufacturer and name of frame
- There is no universal standard as to the location of where this information must appear on the frame
- The "CE" notation found on most frames refers to "Conformite Europeenne" French for European conformity to the European Union Safety Requirement
- If frame measurements are designated as 54□16, then the manufacturer used the OMA's Boxing system. If the measurement is designated 54/16 or 54-16, the measurements are taken along the Datum Line

OPTICAL AND FRAME CONSIDERATION OF HIGH POWERED LENSES

- **Frame Shape** – the larger the A and B dimensions of the frame, the larger the minimum blank size of lens and heavier the resultant cut lens will be.
  - Exotic frame shapes (e.g. harlequin, aviator) require larger MBS than round or oval frame

1. <u>Spheric Lenses</u>

- High powered spectacle lenses (Prescription powers stronger than ±4.00DS) have increased optical and mechanical issues.
  - The fit and design of the lens become more critical due to the sensitivity of the higher powers to changes in lens design or position.
- When fitting and dispensing high-powered lenses, consider:
  - **Magnification** of plus lenses results in a **small FOV** and results in an unappealing "bug-eye" appearance. → Decrease the vertex distance, use a flatter, aspheric lens design to minimize magnification and its related effects
  - Thick edges of high minus lenses produce **internal reflections (power rings)** → use an ARC
  - High powered lenses are subject to **greater optical aberrations in the periphery** including oblique astigmatism and chromatic aberration → select correct base curve, use high Abbe value lens material
  - As the **vertex distance** changes, the power of the lens as perceived by the patient changes (effective power effect). If the fitted vertex distance of the actual frame is different from the refracted vertex distance, the power of the lenses must be adjusted.
- Patients with high powered prescriptions have frame selection issues, consider using disposable CLs

Optical Problems with High Powered Spherical Lenses	
High Plus	High Minus
-Decreased FOV (ring scotoma) -Increased aberrations -Increased convergence and acc. demands -Cosmesis (eyes look huge) and weight -Larger Retinal Image Size	-Edge reflection -Edge thickness -Decreased convergence and acc. demand -Weight

- Solutions in order of effectivity

High Plus	High Minus
1. Decrease eye size 2. Aspheric lens 3. Increase index	1. Decrease eye size 2. Increase index 3. Decrease center thickness 4. Aspheric Lens

2. <u>Aspheric Lenses</u>

- An optical surface that has a gradual power change from lens center to lens edge
  - Minus lenses get steeper in the periphery
  - Plus lenses get flatter in the periphery
- Rapid change results in greater surface astigmatism
- Problems with aspheric lenses
  - Too much asphericity
  - Lens sits too close to the eye
  - More reflections
  - Peripheral optics
  - Cosmetic appearance
- Aspheric lens fitting
  - Monocular PD's
  - Vertical OC placement – 1mm drop per 2° of tilt
  - No decentration (prism)
  - Vertex distance considerations (FOV) – no greater than 12-13mm
- The use of aspheric surfaces allows for flatter more cosmetic lenses that do not compromise the optical performance. Aspheric lenses provide equivalent vision (not better) in a flatter, thinner,

and lighter lens. For high power prescriptions (>+8.00DS) aspheric lenses can actually provide considerably better vision than any spherical base curves in any form

3. High Index Refractive Lenses

- High index materials can make high prescription lenses thinner and lighter.
- Refractive index is associated with the thickness of the lens, abbe value is associated with the optics of the lens and density is associated with the weight of the lens.

ABSORPTIVE LENSES

---

1. Specifications of Lens Tints and Absorptive Coatings

- Glass lenses can be tinted solid or surface coated.
    - **Solid glass tints** are lenses with permanent metallic oxides within glass melt.
        - ADV: They do not fade, reduce internal reflections, are scratch resistant, takes coatings well, are optically correct with less distortion and have good uniformity.
        - DIS: With high Rx's the tint is not uniform giving a bull's eye or raccoon effect, comes in limited colors (gray, brown) is difficult to match, and the tint cannot be removed
    - **Surface-Coated Glass Tints** are lenses with a thin film of inorganic material deposited onto the concave side.
        - ADV: They have a uniform density (no raccoon/bulls eye effect), can be applied to previously through and through tints, is chemical resistant, and can be de- or re-coated.
        - DIS: Tint has limited colors, is time consuming, more expensive, may scratch/peel off with time, and increases surface reflections
- **Tinted Plastic Lenses** are tinted by surface absorption (not through and through). The lenses can be CR39, polycarbonate, or high index plastics.
    - ADV: They are light weight, impact resistant, quick and easy to tint, thickness independent, and come in many colors.
    - DIS: They tend to fade over time, have poor IR absorption, are not as scratch resistant as glass, and tints can be difficult to predict/control
- **Indoor Tints** (Cosmetic tints) have similar transmittance to clear lenses, come in a lighter rose/pink tint in glass or plastic.
    - ADV: blocks out blue light → recommended for photophobics, fluorescent lighting conditions, computers (reduces brightness), low myopes (decreases ghost images), and patients with internal reflection problems. Can also be used to make bifocals less visible
- **Outdoor Tints** (true sunglasses) have selective absorption across the specrum.
    - ADV: overall reduction in light intensity (minimizes veiling and discomfort glare)
    - DIS: more expensive
    - True sunglasses: less than 67% transmittance
- **Blue-green filters:** created by ferrous oxide added to the batch in glass lenses. Examples include Calibar (A.O.) and Rayban (B&L)

Spectral transmission curves

- Spectral transmission curves indicate what wavelengths are absorbed and what wavelengths are transmitted by the lens. The x-axis represents the wavelength (nm) and the y-axis represents the % Transmission where 0% transmission indicates 100% absorption and vice versa. Lens transmittance and reflectance are characteristic of their lens color. The dashed line represents the relative luminous efficiency curve and the solid line is the transmission curve of the lens.
- Infrared - usually produces thermal effects; the most effective wavelengths are 800 - 1200nm. These wavelengths produce immediate effects like solar burns, coagulation of protein, sun blindness, iris atrophy, corneal opacities and cataracts.
- Visible – 380 - 760nm. The light of maximum intensity that we are exposed to is 560-590nm, and this corresponds to the wavelengths of greatest sensitivity. There appears to have been an evolutionary adaptation process.

- Ultraviolet – this is known as ionizing radiation, and it causes delayed tissue damage. Out of the 200 – 380nm UV range, 265 –280nm are the most effective. UV is absorbed mainly in the anterior of the eye, hence in aphakes the retina is at risk.

Spectral Transmission of Colored Tints:

- **Pink Lens** – Both glass and plastic have 100% UVB and 80% UVA protection
    - Note that tinting the plastic lens does not change the characteristics of the UV absorbant properties of the lens
- **Gray Lens** –does not specificially attenuate a certain band of wavelengths across the spectrum, absorbs equally across the spectrum.
    - Oxide- nickel mixture, possibly cobalt and iron
    - Decreases overall brightness, limits color distortion
    - Noted difference between CR39 and glass curves
- **Green Lens**- blocks more blue light and red, suggested for golfers
    - Oxide- ferrous oxide, chromium oxide, or iron
    - Good UV, IR absorption for glass
    - Some noted color distortion
    - More IR wavelengths are transmitted in CR39 than glass
- **Brown Lens**- Blocks out more blues and yellow light
    - Oxide- Nickel
    - Some color distortion
    - Good UV absorption
    - Preferable in cloudy, hazy conditions

PINK LENS TRANSMISSION (GLASS)

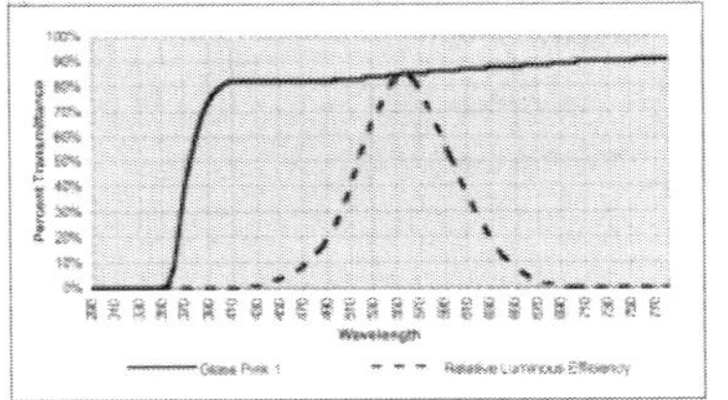

PINK LENS TRANSMISSION (CR-39)

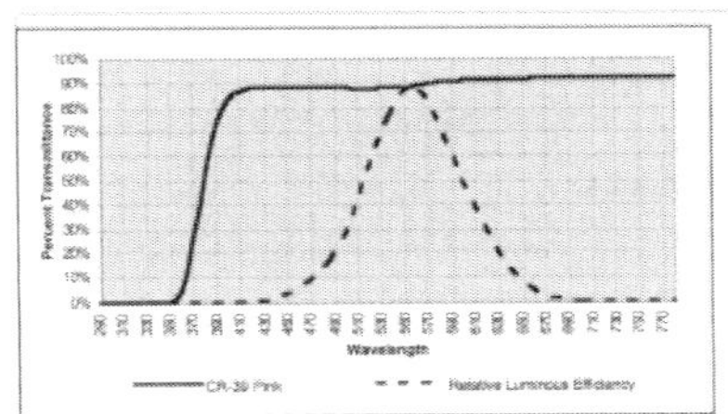

GRAY LENS (GLASS)

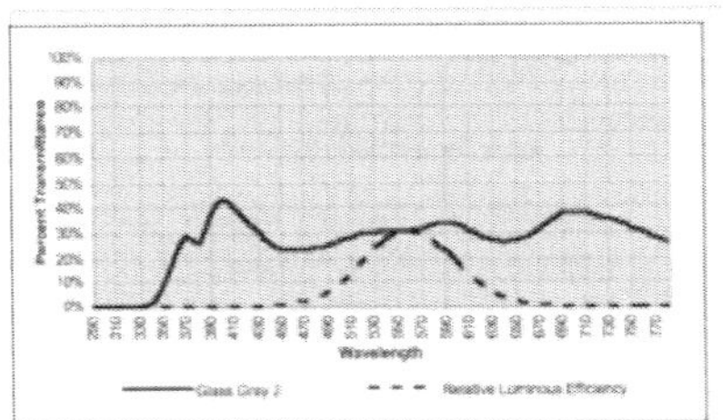

*courtesy of Darryl Meister, Sola Optical

GREEN LENS (CR-39)

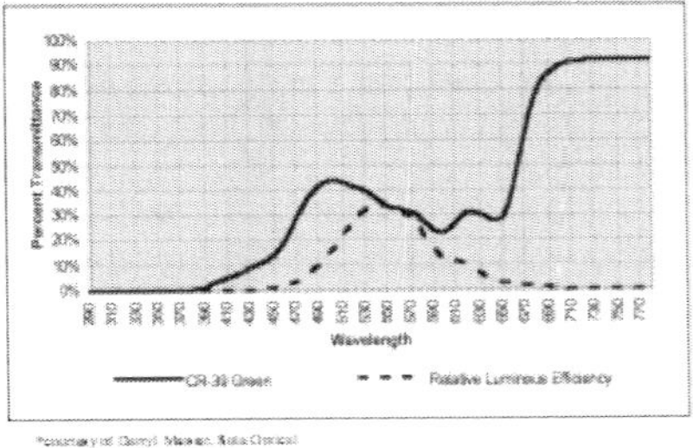

*courtesy of Darryl Meister, Sola Optical

GREEN LENS (GLASS)

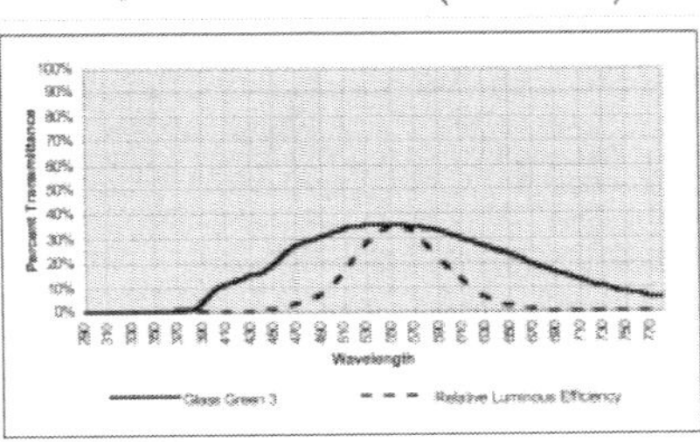

*courtesy of Darryl Meister, Sola Optical

GRAY LENS (CR-39)

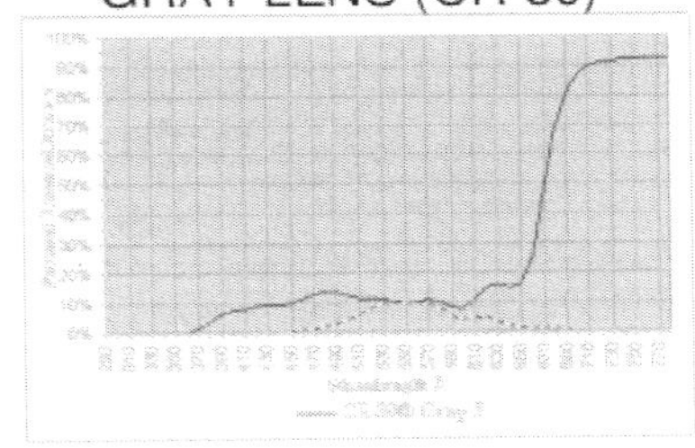

courtesy of Darryl Meister, Sola Optical

BROWN LENS (GLASS)

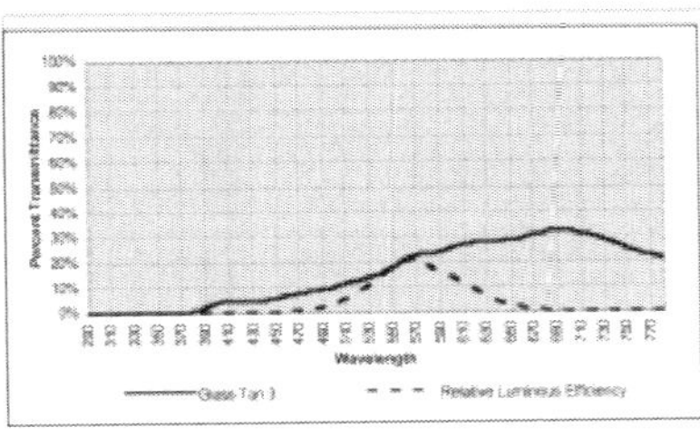

BROWN LENS (CR-39)

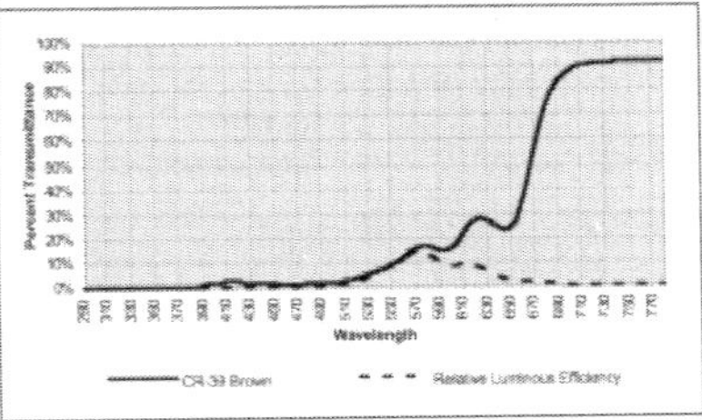

*courtesy of Darryl Meister, Sola Optical

- **Yellow Lens**- Blocks out blue light
    - Oxide- Uranium, cadmium, sodium
    - Good UV and blue light filtration
    - Reduced scattering of light and veiling glare
    - Increased contrast
    - Preferable for hunters, shooters, hazy weather, and skiers
    - Brings absorption up to 450nm
- **Blue Lens**- filters out in 500-650nm range, lets in more UV range
    - No noted functional benefit, more cosmetic
    - IR transmission
    - VisionEase- makes a blue lens called Unisol for glass blowers cataracts
- **Didymium**- smoke blue or rose brown in color
    - Oxide- cerium with didymium
    - Designed primarily for glass blowers to filter out Na light,filtering out the yellow flame
    - Absorbs in the 570-590nmrange
    - Dichroic: rose (fluorescent light)/ greenish-blue (incandescent light)
    - Others: green didymium (dark: shades 4 and 5) designed for welding

YELLOW LENS (GLASS)

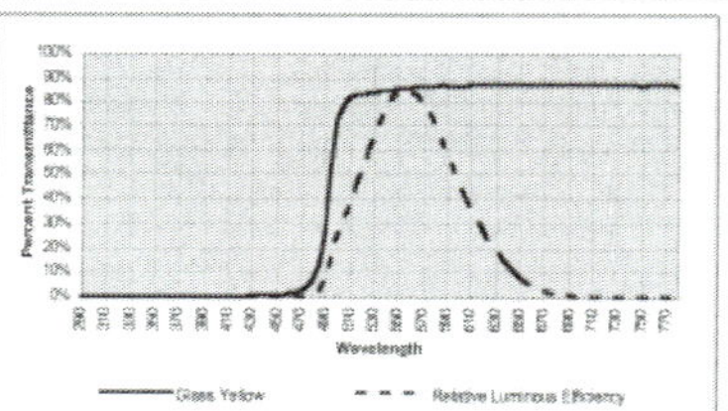

YELLOW LENS (CR-39)

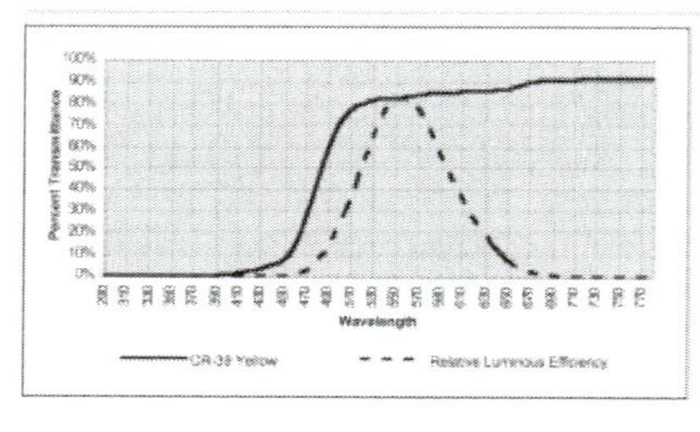

DIDYMIUM

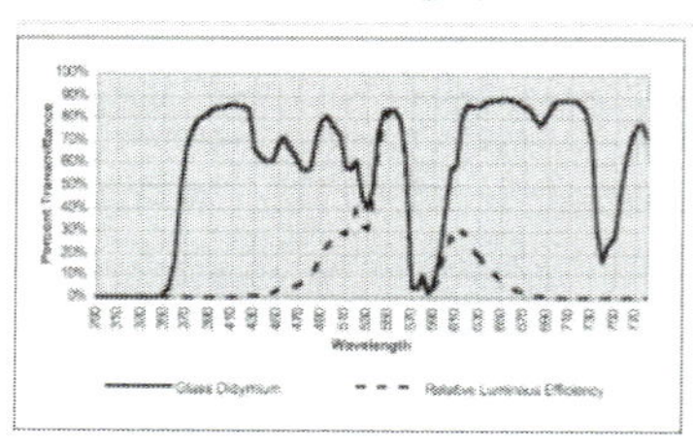

UV Absorptive Lenses

- Glass, clear: 100% UVC, 85% UVB, 15% UVA
- CR-39, clear:100% UVC/UVB, 85% UVA
- Polycarbonate: 100% UVC/UVB/UVA
- Trivex, clear: 100% UVC/UVB/UVA
- Glass coated UV400 lenses
- CR-39 UV400 treated lenses
- CR-39 380 lenses (newer)
- Hi-Index plastic lenses
- Melanin lenses (polarized or unpolarized, green)
    - Melanin in the plastic material, provides all of the UV coverage and some polarization
- **Note:** color of the lens is not an indicator of UV absorptive properties

Coatings

- **Scratch Resistant**
    - Functional purpose to reduce hairline surface scratches, superficial → not designed to eliminate all scratches
    - Inorganic or organic coating
    - Reduces impact resistance of lenses
- **Anti-Reflective**
    - Increases visual performance, resistant to dirt, dust, water
    - Use with all high index lenses, plus lenses (double reflections), Rx sunlenses, photochromic and polarized lenses
    - Ideal for professional drivers, pilots, night drivers, elderly
    - Lenses must be tinted prior to ARC application

2. Characteristics of Photochromic Lenses

- Temperature dependent: darker in cooler temperature, lighter in warmer temperature; works the best in temperature between 65-85F
- Lens thickness: thicker parts have more silver halide crystals, hence darker with glass
- Tempering method: darker with heat tempering
- Illumination: bright days→darker lens; fluorescent lighting may darken a lens; inside a vehicle, may not be as effective
- Breaking in period: all photochromic lenses require a certain number of days use to reach full efficiency.
- Glass (inorganic or mineral): ophthalmic glass with light sensitive silver halide (300-400nm) microcrystals; radiation causes the micro-crystals to dissociate into silver particles, forming a silver colloid; when light is removed, silver colloids split apart into silver and chloride ions; This process is reversible, indefinitely.
    - Photogray II: range of transmission: 88% to 40% (phased out)
    - Photogray Extra: range of transmission: 85% to 22%
    - Photobrown Extra: range of transmission: 85% to 25%
    - Photosun II: range of transmission: 40% to 12% (phased out)
- Plastic photochromic lenses (organic): must use an organic compound (ISN – indolino spironaphthoxaine, oxazines, fulgide derivatives, or napthopyran); UV stimulates molecular structural change; absence of UV or heat results in lens fading; Do not get as dark as glass or last near as long
    - Transition Plus – range of transmittance: 80% to 30% (72F) ; darkens in about 15 seconds; fades to bleached state in 15 minutes (68%)
    - Transitions III – similar Transition Plus – truer gray; darkens quicker and darker than Transition Plus; range of transmittance - 85% to 25% in 15 seconds (72F); fades to 69% in 15 minutes.
    - Transition Extra Active – essentially Transitions Plus, but tinted; range of transmittance – 75% to 15% (72F) {75% to 25% at 95F}

3. Relationship between Lens Thickness and Spectral Transmission

- Optical density changes from the center to the edge in a glass lens. It becomes noticeable around four diopters. Plastic lenses will solve this problem since the transmission is independent of penetration.
- Transmission
    - Equation for total transmission (T) through lens where:
      R_f= reflection at front
      I_f= incident at front
      q=transmittance factor
      x= units
    - If I_f=1, then $T= (1-R_f)^2 q^x$
    - Equation for amount of transmitted light (I_x) where:
      q=transmittance factor
      x= number of units of equal thickness having a transmittance factor q
      I_o= amount of light passing front surface (reflection not yet considered)
      I_x= amount of transmitted light

> Optical Density
> **$\log_{10} T = -OD$**
> **$T=10^{-OD}$**
> Transmission
> **$T=[(I_f-R_f)q^x (1-R_f)$**

Example: *Given a glass lens 2mm thick, n = 1.523, 30% transmission. If the lens is made 3.5 mm, what is the % transmission?*

Hint: Define the surface densities using Fresnel's equation: Then find the surface densities, media density per unit, and total density before converting to Transmission.

$$R_f = \frac{(n_f - n_o)^2}{(n_f + n_o)^2}$$; generally $n_o = 1$

Answer:

R_f = $\frac{(1.523 - 1)}{(1.523 + 1)}$ = 0.043 [(1 – 0.043) x 100] = 95.7%

log 1/T = log 1/.957 = 0.0191 (one surface)
0.0191 x 2= 0.0382 (surface density of front and back surface)
If T=30%, total Density = log 1/T= 1/0.30=0.523
0.523-0.383 (surface density) = 0.4848/2mm thickness = 0.2424/mm
If have 3.4mm, media density = 3.5 (0.2424)= 0.8484
Total density = 0.8484 +0.382 (surface density)= 0.8866
T=$\log^{-OD}$=$\log^{-0.8866}$= 12.98%

4. Special Occupational Requirements

Optical Density
OD= 3/7 (Shade #-1)
Shade Number
Shade #= 7/3 OD +1

- Shade number
  - Used with many safety Rx
  - UV and IR absorption
  - Higher shade #, darker lens
  - Recommended shade # for viewing sun's eclipse
- Shade numbers 1.5 to 3 look like regular sunglasses and are used b[...] welding, but not actually welding themselves.
- #5 is for light gas cutting – light electric spot welding
- #6 – 7 are for gas and medium gas cutting or for arc welding less than 30 amps
- #10 is for 70 to 200 amps arc welding
- #12 is for 200 to 400 amps arc welding
- #14 is for greater than 400 amps arc welding
- Didymium is often used for glass blowers or welders

IMPACT RESISTANCE

---

1. Degrees of Resistance of Ophthalmic Lens Materials

- **Impact resistance**: the ability of a lens to resist fracture or breakage when the lens is subjected to impact by some particle. Does NOT mean the lens wont break
- Factors which influence impact resistance
  - Lens material physical characteristics
  - Lens coating
  - Lens thickness
  - Lens surface characteristics (scratches or flaws)
  - Size of object or particle impacting lens
  - Velocity at which object impacts the lens
  - Lens prescription and sphericity/cylinder of Rx
  - Lens support (Rimlon vs. Rimless vs Rim)
- Rigidity- the more rigid the material, their ability to stand up to stress is not as great (less flexible). When an object hits a flexible lens, the energy gets dissipated. In a rigid lens all energy on impact is on one point of the lens which leads to fracture
  - Glass- Rigid
  - CR-39- soft, flexible
  - Mild and High Index- softer than CR-39, as flexible as CR-39
  - Polycarbonate- softest, extremely flexible

- Lens impact resistance is regulated by the FDA, therefore it is a requirement and not voluntary. However, an impact resistant lens does not mean it is unbreakable.
    - Dress ophthalmic lenses: no center thickness requirement; only needs to pass FDA's Drop Ball Test according to Z80.1
- Generally, the impact resistance of various materials are polycarbonate>CR-39>chemically tempered>heat tempered>untreated lens

2. Methods of Rendering Materials Impact Resistant

- Tempering is available for *glass* lenses:
- In chemical tempering, a finished lens is placed in a salt bath solution and heated. The smaller ions (Na+) in the lens are exchanged for larger (K+ for crown glass; Li for photochromics) ions in the salt bath. This is known as stuffing action.
- In heat tempering (aka air or thermal tempering/toughening), the lens is heated to near melting point (650°C), then both surfaces are rapidly chilled by blasts of forced air. The lens must be at least 2.0mm center thickness or 1.0mm edge thickness.

Method	Pro	Con
Chemical	-No lens warpage -May temper many lenses together -1-2x more impact resistant than heat	-Greater turnaround time -Salt bath must be changed periodically
Heat	-Short turnaround time	-Lens warpage -May only process a few lenses at a time -Less impact resistant than chemical

3. Methods of Verifying Impact Resistance

- **Drop Ball Test**
    - The standard or "referee" test
    - Lens must be able to withstand the impact of a 5/8" (15.875mm) steel ball weight 0.56 oz (15.88gm) dropped from a height of 50" (1.27m) onto the horizontal upper surface of the lens
    - May use any test considered superior to the DBT
    - No thickness guideline
    - Lens shall not break on impact
- **Ballistic Testing** – a small, high velocity projectile fired at the lens
- **Static Testing**- apply energy load to lens front surface continuously until it breaks
- Chemically tempered lenses will exhibit a glow at the lens edge (ring) when dipped into glycerin and the observer looks through a polarizing lens
- Heat tempered lenses will show a maltese cross pattern when looked at through a polariscope or colmascope.

HT--pattern

4. Performance of Materials Upon Impact and After Impact

- Lens Fracture Mechanism (Glass)
    - **Hertzian Failure**: result of low mass, high velocity objects' typical of BBs, a front surface failure, upon impact a flaw is created and fracture occurs, subsequently propagating to read surface (cone shaped)
    - **Rear Surface Fracture:** moderate mass, moderate velocity object: due to lens flexure, stress transferred from point of impact to back surface, more likely fracture mechanism on DBT with minus lenses
    - **Edge Fracture:** large mass, low velocity objects, lens flexure causing lens to flatten, fracture at lens edge, plus lenses

HERTZIAN FAILURE

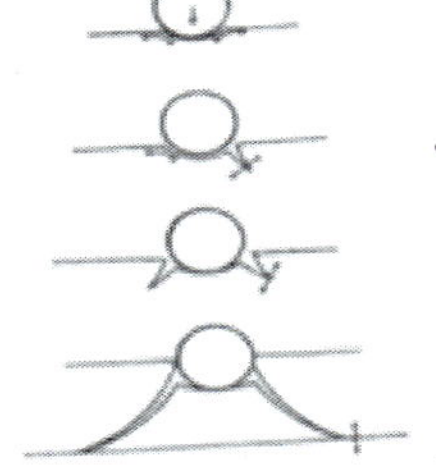

- **Elastic Wave Reflection**: high velocity, low mass objects, point of impact starts fracture at a peripheral flaw
- Glass: Glass breaks into long, sharp slivers that tend to spray toward the eye
- CR-39 fracture usually starts at lens edge
- CR-39 breaks into large, dull pieces, with edges not as sharp as glass
- Uncoated poly up to 22x greater impact resistant than CR-39
- Other factors
  - Coatings reduce lens impact resistance as a result of reduced tensile stress by the coating
  - AR coated lenses mean fracture energy 63% less than uncoated lenses
  - SR coated lenses mean fracture energy 57% less than uncoated lenses.
  - scratching the surface of a glass lens has the effect of reducing the surface compression and therefore reducing the impact resistance

REAR & EDGE FRACTURE

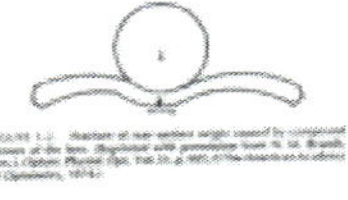

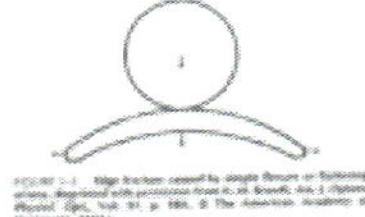

ELASTIC WAVE FRACTURE

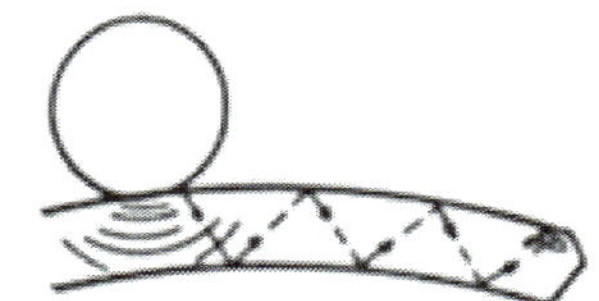

5. Specifications of Occupational Safety lenses

- Basic impact: lens shall not break when 1" steel ball dropped from 50" onto lens horizontal surface
- High impact: CT must be at least 2mm; will be denoted with a + mark, meaning the lens passed a high velocity impact test, where a ¼" steel ball was shot at the lens at 150fps
- Lens markings
  - Non-Plano Basic Impact lenses do NOT need to be marked with a "+", 3.0mm thickness requirement
  - Non-Plano High Impact lenses must have the "+" mark, 2.0mm thickness requirement
    - Plano High Impact lenses have no thickness requirements
- If tint prescribed, must meet Z87.1 standards for minimum and maximum visible light transmittance and maximum UV and IR radiation transmittance
  - Absorptive lenses must absorb both UV and IR radiation, and lenses must be marked with the shade #

OPTICAL TOLERANCES AND PHYSICAL REQUIREMENTS OF OPHTHALMIC LENSES AND FRAME MATERIALS

- Regulations are enforceable and required by law
  - FDA (impact resistance requirement)
  - OSHA (Occupational and Safety and Health Act)- Safety in industries
- Standards are NOT enforceable by law
  - ANSI (American National Standards Institute) is a private organization with voluntary membership that sets optical standards and publishes them.
  - Currently there are 10 ophthalmic related standards revised every 5-10 years.

ANSI Z80.1 – Prescription Ophthalmic Lenses – Optical Tolerances

- Power tolerances is on highest power meridian
- Power (Spherical)
  - $\pm$ 0.13D up to 6.50D
  - $\pm$ 2% above 6.50D
- Power (Spherical) - PALs

- ± 0.16D up to 8.00D
- ± 2% on powers >8.00D

- Power (Cylinder)
  - ± 0.13D up to 2.00DC
  - ± 0.15D between 2-4.50DC
  - ± 4% > 4.50DC
- Axis (Cylinder)
  - ± 14° up to 0.25DC
  - ± 7° >0.25 to 0.50DC
  - ± 5° >0.50 to ≤ 0.75 DC
  - ± 3° >0.75 to ≤ 1.50DC
  - ± 2° >1.50DC
- Prism imbalance (mounted lenses)
  - Vertical: 0.33Δ (0 to ± 3.375D), 1mm variance between lenses if ≥ 3.375D
  - Horizontal: 0.67Δ (0 to ±2.75D), max 2.5mm variance if > ± 2.75D (For SV and MFs)
    - For PALs, power limit is ± 3.375D
- IPD: ±2.5mm
- Base Curve: ± 0.75D
- Warpage: 1D
- Center thickness: ± 0.3mm
- NIPD: ± 2.5mm
- PAL fitting cross: ± 1.0mm of specification (horizontal and vertical)
- Segment height: ± 1.0mm of specification
- Segment size: ± 0.7mm
- Add power: ± 0.12 up to 4.00D: ± 0.18> 4.00D
  - Vertical: 0.33Δ (0 to ± 3.375D), 1mm variance between lenses if ≥ 3.375D

ANSI Z87.1- Practice for Occupational and Educational Eye and Face Protection

- Lens thickness
  - Most prescription safety Rx: 3.0mm ct/et for glass/plastic
  - For high plus >+3.00DS, et may be reduced to 2.5mm
  - Plano prescription safety eyewear no less than 3.0mm thick or more than 3.8mm thick
  - Plano polycarbonate- 2.0mm thickness
  - Prescription polycarbonate – 3.0mm thickness
- Lens Impact
  - 1" steel ball dropped 50" onto lens horizontal surface, lens shall not break
- Lens Retention Test
  - Lens must not be displaced from frame
- Lens Impact (Basic/High)
- Side Shields
  - Side shields required when there is hazard from flying objects
- Frame
  - Must have "lip" behind lens to prevent lens displacement towards patient.
  - Lenses must be inserted from the front
  - Must meet high mass/low velocity test, low mass/high velocity test, and flammability/corrosion standard

OSHA

- OSHA regulates industries. States all industrial eye and face protectors will meet requirements of Z87.1 as should spectacle frame and lens.
- Industrial lenses in a dress frame or dress ophthalmic lenses in an industrial drame do NOT meet the standard
- Requirements of Employer
    - Perform work hazard assessment
    - Equipment selection
    - Proper training on use of personal protective equipment (PPE)
    - Proper size, use, and PPE
- Protective eyewear must protect against
    - Flying particles
    - Molten metal
    - Liquid chemicals
    - Acids or caustic liquids
    - Chemical gases or vapors
    - Injurious light radiation

FDA

- Oversees the release of safe and effective products for consumer use in timely fashion
- Monitors products for continued safe use over time
- Regulates medical devices (contact lenses), food, drugs, biologics, cosmetics, and readiation omitting products

Chapter 5 – Contact Lenses

OPHTHALMIC AND OPTICAL INSTRUMENTS

1. Radiuscope

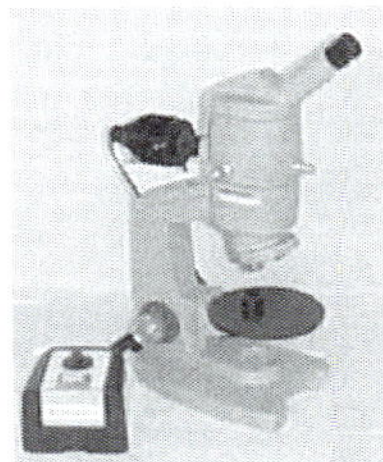

- Functions to measure the radius of curvature of contact lenses
- Most often used and most accurate in the measurement of the base curve of GP lenses and can also be used to measure soft contact lens center thickness
- The instrument consists of a compound microscope in which a target is projected along its axis. An image of this target will be seen through the microscope when it is focused upon a reflecting surface, such as a contact lens. The image will also be seen when the microscope is focused at the center of curvature of the concave or convex surface due to light being reflected back along its path. The distance between the two positions, where an in-focus target image is seen, equals the radius of curvature.
- A warped contact lens can be determined by checking the base curve on the radiuscope
- When in the zero position, one is able to see debris and scratches on the posterior (ocular) surface of a GP lens. This is helpful clinically when the patient is symptomatic due to deposits on the posterior surface

2. Videokeratography

- Method for measuring the major portion of the corneal contour in a single capture
- Operates similar to a keratometer except the two sets of mires are replaced by a multiple object target consisting of 16 to 24 concentric circles, which allow a large number of measurements over a greater corneal area
- Video camera takes a video of the image reflected off of the cornea and uses a **frame grabber** to electronically capture a single picture of the video image, which is then processed
  - First, the computer scans across all of the rings to find the image distances for each ring, which are converted into radius values
- Most popular display is the **corneal map**, which shows zones of equal radius, to give an overall impression of the corneal contour in very rapid time
  - The **relative scale** is determined by the maximum and minimum radius values, and then the isoradian zones are divided into 12-14 steps of approximately equal difference for the display
    - The values for the various colors may change form one keratogram to another
  - The **absolute scale** provides an absolute value to each color, which is consistent for each keratogram. This allows the operator to associate the radii without referring to the scale, but the large number of colors can sometimes cause confusion

3. Keratometry

- Measures the radius of curvature of a spherical reflecting surface. Used to measure corneal curvature and the curvature of contact lenses as well as the base curve, comes with a rigid gas lens holder and calibration set
- The **keratometer** has two sets of mires which are reflected off the cornea/contact lens and the observed notes the image.
- The size of the mire image and distance between the reflection points is a function of the radius of curvature of the reflecting surface since the object size and object distance are constant for a given type of keratometer.
- The keratometer only measures the central 4 to 5 mm of the "corneal cap"
- The range of the instrument is typically 35 to 50D, but can be extended to 61 DK by placing a +1.25 DS trial lens or to 31DK by placing a -1.00 DS trial lens in front of the telescope objective

4. Reticule Magnifier

- A **reticule magnifier** measures the total diameter of the contact lens, and one can visualize the posterior optic zone diameter, and the width of the peripheral and secondary curve systems
- Reticule (also called magnifier or contact lens loupe): for measuring total diameter and optic zone diameter, estimating amount of blending at curve junctions, evaluating edge contour of rigid gap permeable lenses, inspection of lens surface quality, the lens is held concave side down on the flat side opposite of the ocular

5. V-Channel Gauge

- For rigid gas permeable lenses
- For measuring total diameter, allow the lens to slide into the channel by gravity, the diameter is read from the scale adjacent to where the lens stops

6. Lensometer

- To measure back vertex power of soft and rigid gas permeable lenses, pat soft contact lens dry (only an estimate of power), place the concave side of the lens on the lens stop, prism is measured by quantifying the amount of mire decentration using the concentric rings in the ocular lens

7. Thickness Gauge or Caliper

- To measure the center thickness of rigid gas permeable lenses, center and place the lens concave side up between the rod and the plunger, the center thickness is read directly off the scale

8. Lens Clock

- To measure center thickness of rigid gas permeable lenses, place lens on a flat surface convex side down, place the middle pin of the lens clock at the center of the rigid gas permeable lens, 1D on the plus scale = 0.1mm of center thickness

OPTICAL CHARACTERISTICS OF CONTACT LENSES

1. Surface Characteristics of the Lens and the Cornea

- The cornea is aspheric, getting flatter as one goes out to the periphery.
- Contact lenses are usually spherical; this can induce spherical aberration when put on the eye.
- Features of corneas: toricity (WTR, ATR, oblique), asphericity, apex location, local anomalies (e.g. tight eyelids), tear production

2. Specification of the Lens (Power, Base Curve, Thickness, and Edge Characteristics

- **Power:** the lens power of a contact lens is indicated in the same form as if ordering glasses (back vertex power).

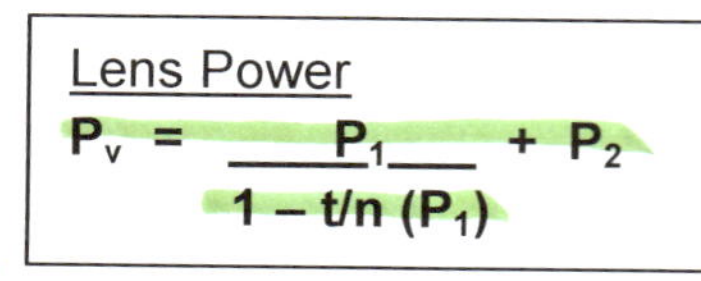

- **Base curve**: the base curve for contacts is always the radius (mm) of P2 (back surface) in the central zone of the contact. To get the desired base curve, take the K readings and calculate the radius of P2 using the adjusted index value of 1.3375. Although the base curve needs to be specified to the manufacturer, the particular value chosen is for fit rather than optics.
- **Center thickness**: measured in mm
- Once these three parameters are specified, the manufacturer decides what P_1 should be. It is obtained from the vertex power.
- Edge characteristics: traditionally, rigid gas permeable lens edges should have an even thickness with an apex closer to the back surface than to the front surface

Example: *BC = 8.00 mm, Pv = -3.00 D, CT = 0.2 mm and P_2 = -61.5 D. What is P_1?*

> ***Answer:***
>
> $P_1 = \dfrac{P_v - P_2}{1 + t/n\,(P_v - P_2)} = \dfrac{-3 - (-61.25)}{[1 + .0002/\,1.49\,(-3-(-61.25))]}$ - +57.80D

3. Effective Power Considerations of Contact Lenses

- Same as for spectacles.
- The effective power of a contact lens considers the vertex distance, or distance from the spectacle plane to the cornea, so that the actual power of the contact lens is equal to the refractive power of the spectacle lens. Where
  - P1: spectacle correction, in D
  - P2: effective power of the contact lens, in D
  - d: vertex distance, in meters

> Effective Power
>
> **P2=P1/(1-dP1)**

- For minus power contact lenses, a reduction in power is needed to maintain the same effective power.
- For plus power contact lenses, an increase in power is needed.

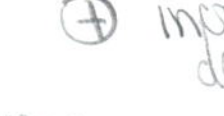

4. Tear-Lens Optical Considerations

- The tear-lens is can have plus power if the rigid gas permeable is fit steeper than the cornea, or minus power if the rigid gas permeable is fit flatter than the cornea
- The in-situ system describes the optics of a contact lens on a cornea without dividing the interfaces with a layer of air. We will assume that the interface between the tears and cornea remains constant (i.e. both curvatures remain constant and the cornea is not changing shape).
- Therefore, only two surfaces need to be considered: the air to front surface of contact lens, and the back surface of contact lens to tears surface.
  - **P_1 (air) + P_2 (tears) = K's + ocular refraction**
- Assumptions used in rigid lens problems:
  - Rigid contacts n = 1.49
  - Keratometer calibrated n = 1.3375
  - Cornea n = 1.376
  - Tears n = 1.3375
  - Tear radius = cornea radius

Summary of n values	
	n values
Cornea	1.376
Tear	1.3375
Keratometer calibration	1.3375
RGP	1.49

Example: *spectacle Rx = pl -1.00 x 180°, BC = 44.00 D (r = 7.67 mm), K's = 44.00 @ 180° c 45.00 @ 090°. What is the power of the front surface in both meridians? What is the radius of the front surface?*

> ***Answer:***
>
> P_{tears}= (0.3375-0.49)/ 0.00767 = -19.91
>
> K_{180}= +44 Rx_{180}=0
>
> K_{090}= +45 Rx_{090}=-1.00
>
> P_{180}=+63.88
>
> The power of the front surface=63.88D in both meridians
>
> The radius of the front surface is:
>
> $\dfrac{1.49 - 1.00}{63.88}$ = .00767m = 7.67mm

5. Prismatic Effects

- Often BD prism is added to toric lenses for balancing. This helps the lenses to position in the desired way for the correction of astigmatism. Vertical prism can also be added when the prescription calls for it but lateral prism cannot be added.
- BD prism can be added to stabilize the contact lens – **usually 1 to 1.5$^{\Delta}$**

6. Fabrication, Inspection, and Verification

- **Fabrication:**
  - Rigid gas permeable lenses come in buttons, for non-lenticulated lenses, a base curve tool, secondary curve tool, peripheral curve tool, and anterior surface tool cut the various curves of a rigid gas permeable lens.
  - **Lenticulation** for rigid gas permeable lenses: an anterior peripheral curve is added to change center thickness or edge thickness to create an anterior optic zone, always for prescriptions beyond -4.00 or +2.00D
  - Soft contact lenses can be made by spin-cast, diamond turning, or molded methods
- **Inspection:** contact lenses can be inspected with a 7X contact lens loupe to check for scratches, edge defects, etc.
- **Verification**
  - **Power:** can be verified with the use of a lensometer.
  - **Diameter:** can be verified with a contact lens loupe.
  - **Base curve:** can be verified with a radiuscope

7. Lens Types and Materials

Lens Types

- Soft Spherical Contact Lenses
  - Central Front Curve
  - Central Back Curve
  - Peripheral Curve(s), anterior or posterior
- Soft Toric Contact Lenses
  - Back toric – most common
  - Front toric – less common, useful for patients with spherical cornea
  - Stability Enhancements:
    - **Prism Ballast** – thin on top, thicker on bottom (2Δ BD)
    - **Dual Thin Zone**- top and bottom of lens are thin so eyelids push the thicker part away, best for ATR astigmatism
- GP Sphere
- GP Toric (Described further later)
  - Front Toric
  - Bitoric
    - CPE
    - SPE

Lens Materials

- FDA Groups
  - Group 1 – low (<50%) water, non-ionic (most deposit resistant)
  - Group 2 – high (>50%) water, non-ionic
  - Group 3 – low water, ionic
  - Group 4 – high water, ionic (least deposit resistant)
- Hydrogels – nearly all HEMA based
  - Various monomers added to affect water content, hydrophilicity, O2 permeability, hardness, strength, and deposit resistance
- Silicone Hydrogels
  - Non-HEMA
  - Water content ranges from 24 to 48%, transmit up to 18x as much O2 as HEMA
  - O2 permeability not tied to water content

8. Optics of Contact Lenses

Curves, Zones, Widths

Anterior Surface of Lens | Posterior Surface of Lens

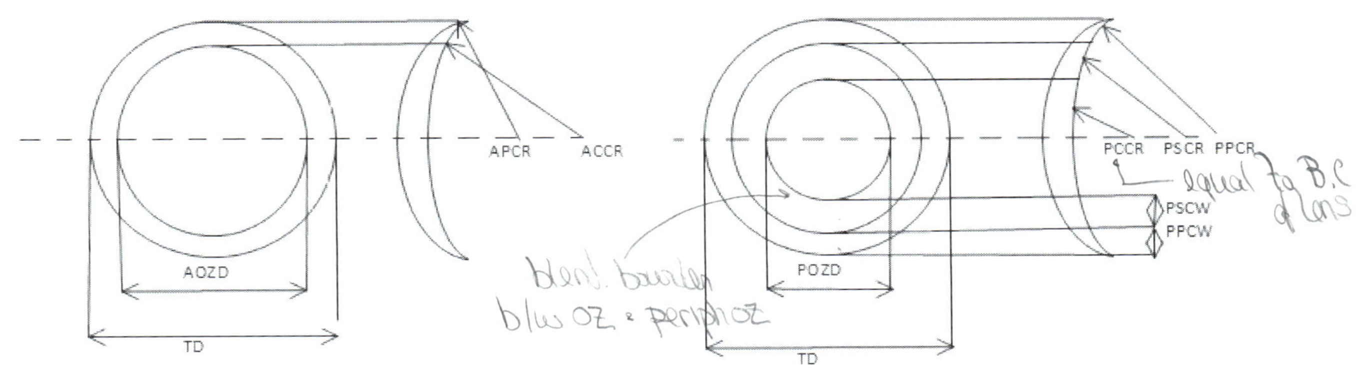

TD-Total Diameter
AOZD- Anterior Optic Zone Diameter
ACCR- Anterior Central Curve Radius
APCR - Anterior Peripheral Curve Radius

TD- Total Diameter
POZD- Posterior Optic zone Diameter
PCCR- Posterior Central Curve Radius
PPCR- Posterior Peripheral Curve Radius
PSCW- Posterior Secondary Curve Width
PPCW- Posterior Peripheral Curve Width

- Base Curve (Radius) – the higher the number, the flatter the lens, the lower the number, the steeper the lens
  - Rarely think of Soft CL base curves in diopters (unlike with GP)
  - Average K is 43.50D or 7.85mm
  - Typical Soft CL BC is 8.6mm or 39.25D
  - GP Base Curve is the PCCR

Base Curve Conversion
BC (mm)= 337.5/ BC(D)
P=337.5/r (mm)

- Zones
  - Contact lenses have zones, the optical zone and the peripheral zones which are present on both the anterior and posterior surfaces
  - Zones are created by using different tools to shave the material off the button (GP lenses)
  - **Optic Zone** – the area of the lens dedicated towards the optical correction of the patient
  - **Peripheral Zone** – typically flatter than the optic zone, utilized for fit of the lens
    - There can be multiple peripheral zones
    - The border between the peripheral and optic zones is called the "**blend**" and can vary in size depending on the manufacturer
- Curves
  - Each zone is consider a lens curve, so a two zone lens is called a bicurve, three zone a tricurve, etc.
  - The zones curve radius and width can be determined through measurements of the lens

Parameter	Soft	GPs
Diameter	13.8 to 15.0mm	8.5 to 10mm
Optic Zone (Anterior or Posterior)	8 to 13mm	7 to 8.5mm
Base Curve (Radius)	8.3 to 9.1mm	7.2 to 8.5mm
Sphere Power	+6.00 to -10.00DS	+8.00 to -15.00D
Cylindrical Power	-0.75 to 2.25DC	
Center Thickness	0.025 to 0.15mm	0.10 to 0.18mm
Water content	24 to 79%	

Tear Lens Effect – GP Optics

- Tear lens corrects cylinder in the amount of ΔK
  - Tear lens is a real lens that refracts light
  - Think of the GP, tear lens, and cornea as separate thin lenses
- If the GP is fit flatter than K= Minus Tear Lens
- If the GP is fit steeper than K = Plus Tear Lens
- Remember:
  - **FAP** (Flat add Plus)
  - **SAM** (Steep add Minus)

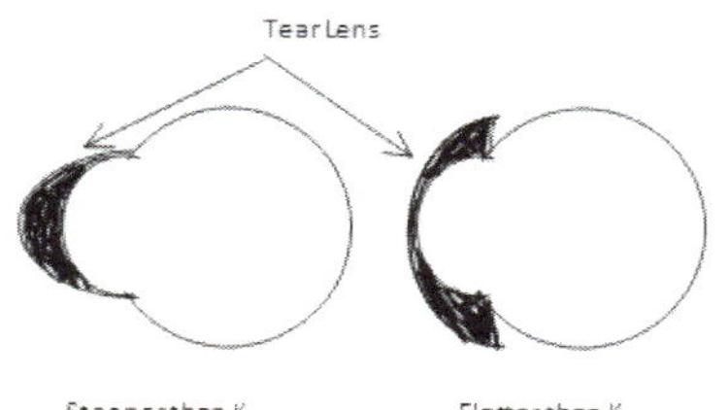

> Power of Tear Lens
>
> $P_{TL}=K_{contact\ lens}-K_{cornea}$
>
> Power of Contact Lens to Order
>
> $P_{CL}=P_{Rx}-P_{TL}$

Example: *A patient has a K of 43.50, Rx -2.00DS. What would the power of the Tear Lens be and the total power of the Contact Lens should be ordered if it were fit a) on K (43.50) b) Flatter than K (43.00) or c) steeper than K (44.00)?*

> ***Answer:***
>
> a) 43.50-43.50 = 0 – $P_{tear\ lens}$
>
> P_{CL}= -2.00DS
>
> b) 43.00-43.50 = -0.50D – $P_{tear\ lens}$
>
> P_{CL}= -1.50DS
>
> c) 44.00-43.50 = +0.50
>
> P_{CL}= -2.50DS

- For toric corneas, a spherical GP will correct the cylindrical power by ΔK.
  - If Δk= refractive cylinder power, then a spherical GP will correct the astigmatism
    - This is only true when the GP is not flexing (forming) to the eye.
    - **Lens Flexure** changes the cylinder power of the tear lens (decreases)
  - If Δk≠ refractive cylinder power, there will be residual astigmatism with a spherical GP
    - All cylinder power is on the back of the GP lens
    - When Δk<cyl, you undercorrect cyl
    - When Δk> cyl, you overcorrect cyl
- For calculating contact lens powers, the following general rules are helpful
  - If Δk= refractive cylinder, ignore the cylinder, and compare the flat K and sphere power to determine the power needed for the contact lens

Example: *A patient has K's of 42.50/44.25/090 and an Rx of -1.00-1.75x180 and is fit with a contact lens of 43.00, what power must the contact lens be?*

> ***Answer:***
>
> Δk=1.75, same as refractive cyl
>
> Flat k= 42.50, CL BC = 43.00
>
> P_{TL}=+0.50 (spherical meridian)
>
> P_{CL} = -1.50DS

Example: *A patient has K's of 44.00/45.00/090 and an Rx of -2.00-1.50x180 and is fit with a contact lens of 43.50, what power must the contact lens be?*

43.50 - 44.00 = -0.50 P_{TL}

> ***Answer:***
>
> Δk=1.00, not the same as refractive cyl
>
> CL BC= 43.50

K_{180} = 44.00	K_{090}=45.00
P_{TL-180}=-0.50 P	P_{TL-090}= -1.50
P_{Rx-180}=-2.00	P_{Rx-090}=-3.50
P_{CL-180}=-1.50	P_{CL-090}=-2.00

> P_{CL}=-1.50-0.50x180

Sagittal Depth

- The ocular sagittal depth of the cornea can be matched by the sagittal depth of the contact lens. If the lens is sitting too flat or too steep, the lens sagittal depth and ocular sagittal depth are mismatched, and the lens parameters can be changed to better the fit
- Contact Lens sagittal depth is:
  - Increased by steeper or larger CL
  - Decreased by flatter or smaller CL
- Ocular Sagittal depth is increased by
  - Corneal diameter
  - Rate of peripheral corneal flattening
  - Central corneal curvature (K's)

Lens Flexure

- Young's Modulus Of Elasticity – for Soft Lenses
  - Resistance to deformation, measured in megapascals (MPa)
  - Higher modulus lenses are easier to hangle but the eye is more prone to mechanical complications
  - The lower the water content the higher the modulus of elasticithy
    - HEMA typically 0.2 to 0.5 MPa
    - SiHy 0.4 to 1.52 MPa
- GP Flexure
  - Lens flexes on the eye, loses spherical shape, tear lens power is decreased by the amount of flexure
  - More common in steep or thin lenses on toric corneas

Asphericity

- Contact lenses have a curve in the periphery to compensate for ocular and contact lens spherical aberrations
- Aspheric lenses do not correct cylinder, but may improve VA when low residual astigmatism is present due to reduced spherical aberrations

Contact Lens	Spherical Power	Toric Power
Spherical Base Curve	Sphere	Front Toric
Toric BC	Warped lens	Bitoric (CPE/SPE)

Toric Designs

- GP spheres won't work when ΔK ≠ refractive astigmatism or when ΔK>2-3DC (due to fit)
- Problems with a spherical lens on a toric cornea:
  - Excessive edge lift
  - Excessive movement
  - Corneal molding → spectacle blur
  - Lens flexure
  - Corneal staining
- Front toric → spherical BC, toric front, use when ΔK≠RE
- Bitoric → Toric BC, toric front, use when ΔK>2-3D, two types:
  - **Spherical Power Effect (SPE)** – lens acts like a sphere, can rotate without visual affect, occurs when BC toricity = CL cylinder
  - **Cylindrical Power Effect (CPE)** – acts like a toric lens on the eye, rotates by the difference in BC toricity and CL cylinder correction
- Ideal cornea to fit is spherical with mild WTR

RE vs ΔK	Match (within 0.75DC)	Mismatch (>0.75DC difference)
ΔK<2-3DC	GP Sphere	GP Front Toric
ΔK >2-3DC	SPE Bitoric	CPE Bitoric

BASIC THEORIES AND METHODS OF FITTING AND CONTACT LENS SELECTION AND DESIGNS

1. Soft Lenses

- Fitting
  - Goals
    - Optimize Vision (VA within ½ line of best corrected spectacle acuity)
    - Optimize Comfort (good limbal coverage, centration, and movement)
    - Minimize risk of complications
  - Determine Patient Use (Wearing Modality)
    - Occasional wear
    - Daytime wear
    - Extended wear
    - Visual needs/activities (distance/near, sports, environment, presbyopes/non-presbyopes)
  - Determine Type of Lens
    - Spherical → patient has less than 0.75 DC
    - Aspheric → patient has greater than or equal to 0.75 DC or cylinder is a major part of the refractive error
    - Toric
    - Multifocal/Monovision
    - Tinted
  - Determine Lens availability
    - Daily Disposable (good for alternative to EW, patients with high risk for ocular allergies, teenagers, patients with history of deposits/GPC, water sports –*Acanthamoeba*)
    - Planned Replacement (2w, 1m, 3m, etc)
  - Select Trial Lens → Parameters
    - Diameter – want the smallest lens that provides the best (0.5-1.5mm) coverage and movement
      - The smaller the diameter the better, with too much overlap you limit tear exchange
      - Consider
        - Visible Iris Diameter
        - Aperture Size (small eye – small lens)
    - Base Curve
      - Less effect on movement than diameter
      - Want the flattest base curve that gives good comfort without excessive movement
      - Flatter lenses move more on the eye (*longer radius is a flatter lens)*
    - O2 transmissibility
      - High Transmissibility (High-water HEMA or SI-Hy) use especially if:
        - High refractive error (thicker lens, want more O2 permeable material)
        - Extended wear
        - History or signs of hypoxia
      - Low Transmissibility (Low-water or non-ionic) use especially if:
        - History of deposits
        - Dry eyes
    - Thickness
      - Want thinner lenses if using HEMA, high refractive error, extended wear, or history/signs of hypoxia
      - Want thicker lenses if patient has difficulty handling or dry eyes
    - Tint
      - Transparent (light eyes) or Opaque (dark eyes)
      - Visibility
      - UV block
      - Functional

- Prosthetic
- Power
  - Reference spectacle power to corneal plane if power is ±4.00D
  - Rule of thumb: vertex power change = $P^2/100$ per cm of vertex distance
    - Consider each meridian separately
    - For minus powers it changes less than this equation predicts, for plus powers it changes more than it predicts

***Example:** What would the contact lens power be for a spectacle Rx of -5.00-2.00x180 with a vertex distance of 10mm*

Answer:
$(-5)^2/100 = 0.25$ → -4.75 x 180
$(-7)^2/100 = 0.50$ → -6.50 x 090
CL Rx: -4.75 -1.75 x 180

***Example:** What would the contact lens power be for a spectacle Rx of +7.00-2.00x180 with a vertex distance of 10mm*

Answer:
$(7)^2/100 = 0.5$ → +7.50 x 180
$(5)^2/100 = 0.25$ → -5.25 x 090
CL Rx: +7.50 -2.25 x 180

- Observations
  - Vision
    - Measure VA with CL and Spherical Over-Refraction (SOR)
    - 20/20 vs 20/15 → 0.50DC uncorrected cylinder possible, if residual astigmatism is unacceptable consider toric or different sphere power
    - Spherocylindrical Over-Refraction (SCOR) useful for Toric lenses
  - Coverage
    - Symmetrical limbal coverage is ideal but perfect centration not necessary
    - Centration more important for opaque tints and high Rx's (optical zone is smaller, might notice glare at night with decentered lens and dilated pupil)
    - No limbal exposure
    - **Lens Fluting (Buckling)**
      - Lens edge does not lie flat on sclera along circumference of lens and sticks on the lower lid – very uncomfortable for the patient
  - Movement
    - Ideally 0.25 to 0.50mm vertical movement in primary gaze, 0.50 to 1.00mm vertical movement in up gaze
    - Often minimal movement with thin lenses
    - **Finger Push Test** – nudge to determine if lens is too tight
      - If lens is too tight, go smaller or flatter (decrease sagittal depth) or thicker to increase movement
  - Comfort – can be affected by:
    - Trapped debris, lens (edge) design, excessive movement, lens inverted, crack or tear in lens
  - Rotation
    - If spherical, slight rotation is tolerated
    - **Rule of 30** – for every 30° of off-axis rotation, residual astigmatism is induced by the total cylindrical power (RA= (rotation/030) x P_{cyl}
    - If toric, rotation affects vision, want rotation to be stable and constant (stable over time, with blink, in different gazes, etc)

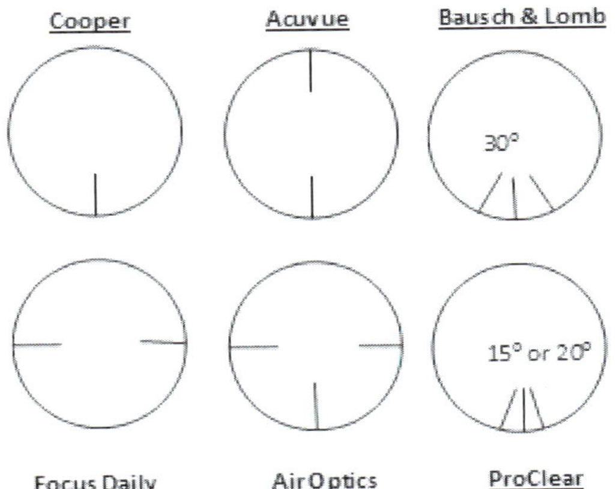

- Markings on a toric lens are used to assess the orientation of the cylinder and do NTO represent the cylinder axis itself
- Marking rotations from the vertical indicates lens rotation. Estimate rotation direction from the bottom of the lens and whether the marking has rotated (to the Doctor's Right or Left/ Nasal or Temporal/ CW or CCW)
- To adjust for lens rotation, use "**LARS**"
    - **L**eft/**A**dd or **R**ight/**S**ubtract amount of rotation to or from the spectacle axis

Example: *If a patient with Rx -6.00-1.00x175 is fit with a contact lens of Rx -5.00-0.75 x 180 for the right eye, which rotates 15° nasally on the eye and is stable there, what is the expected residual astigmatism with this lens (cylinder power, not axis)? If you were to stay with this brand, what power will you select for the next trial lens (assume sphere powers in0.25D steps, cylinder power in 0.50D steps, and axis in 10° steps)*

> ***Answer:***
> RA= (15-5/30) x 0.75 = 0.50 DC
> 15° nasally OD = to the doctor's right – subtract
> Fit -5.00-0.75 x 160

2. GP Lenses

- Fitting
    - Goals
        - Vision
        - Comfort
        - Healthy Response
        - Wearing Time
    - Proper Fit
        - Position – centered well, lid attachment, interpalpebral
        - Movement – needed for tear exchange
            - 1-2mm downward
            - Slow, should not touch lower lid during interblink
        - Lens-Cornea Relationship – even pressure distribution, avoid mid-peripheral heavy touch
            - Minimal Apical Clearance – well centered, lid attachment → idea
            - Apical Clearance – pooling, central bubble → lens is too steep or too tight
            - Apical bearing – central touch, peripheral pooling→ lens too flat or too loose
    - Strategy
        - 1. Diameter
            - Palpebral Aperture Size (PAS) → larger the PAS, larger lens diameter
            - K reading → Flatter K, larger lens diameter
            - Pupil/Cornea Size→ larger pupil/cornea, larger lens diameter
        - 2. Base Curve Radius
            - For a spherical cornea:
                - Larger Diameter (9.6 or >)→ Fit -0.25 to -0.50D flatter than K
                - Smaller Diameter (9.6 or <) → Fit on K
            - For a toric cornea:
                - Increase the BC 0.25D for every 1DΔK
        - Flatter fit will increase bearing/decrease pooling
        - The 2nd curve is 2.0mm flatter than BCR
        - The 3rd curve is 3.0mm flatter than BCR

PATIENT SELECTION AND POST-FITTING COMPLICATIONS

1. Patient Selection

- Contact Lenses are preferable to spectacles when/for:
    - Balancing image size – anisometropia, anisophoria

- Better peripheral vision
- More "natural" form of vision – glasses cause minification/magnification, changes in FOV, prism induction, etc
- Cosmesis (general, occupational)
- Sports/occupation
- Glasses are inconvenient, uncomfortable, hard to keep clean/dry
- Visual benefits (keratoconus, myopia reduction/control
- Changing eye color (tints)
- Therapeutic bandage

- Visual benefits of contact lenses
  - Aberrations
    - Contact lenses get rid of most aberrations except spherical aberration
    - Always looking through the optical center of the contact lens – no off-axis aberrations
  - High refractive error
    - No magnification effects
    - Spectacles – High minus minify, high plus magnify
- Patient History
  - Motivation/reason for interest in CLs
  - Past corrective history
    - Past use of spectacles – full time or partial
    - CL history, past reasons for discontinuing
  - Occupation – hobbies, sports, activities
    - Environment – Dust (soft lenses better), Noxious (GPs better), air conditioning – exacerbate dry eye
    - Visual demands
  - Disease
    - Systemic – thyroid issues increase dryness
    - Ocular – Dry eye, recurrent erosions, etc
  - **Ocular Medications**
    - Since non-hydrogel lenses do not absorb drugs, some topical ocular medication can be administered while the lens is on the eye. However, the epithelium layer may be compromised due to contact lens wear so that the drugs may cause irritation or penetrate the cornea in greater quantities, which may give unwanted side effects.
    - Hydrogel lenses absorb drugs readily and can be used as a drug delivery device in some cases. In normal situations the lenses need to be removed before instilling the drugs.
    - It is contraindicated for glaucoma patients to wear hydrogel lenses during topical epinephrine treatment.
  - **Systemic Medications**
    - Some systemic medications cause dry eye problems resulting in discomfort with lens wear. A number of drugs such as **tetracycline, phenazopyridine, phenolphthalein, and nitrofurantoin**, can cause lens discoloration
- **Hydrogel Lenses for Protecting the Cornea**: Hydrogel lenses can be used as a bandage to protect and lubricate the cornea following surgery or injury, or to occlude the eye in amblyopic or anti-suppression treatment.
- Patient Measurements
  - Refractive Error
  - Accommodation
    - Increased accommodative demand for myopes
    - Decreased accommodative demand for hyperopes
    - Can become an issue for patients approaching presbyopia
  - Binocular status
    - Can correct ~2Δ vertical phoria with prism ballasting
    - Cannot correct horizontal phoria
    - Contact lenses can worsen the phoria
      - High esophoria with high myopia
      - High exophoria with high hyperopia

- Contact lenses can lessen the phoria
  - High esophoria with high hyperopia
  - High exophoria with high myopia

2. Post-Fitting Complications

- Impacts of Contact Lenses on Physiology
  - Hypoxia (greater with extended wear, less with silicone hydrogel)
  - Tear film disruption
  - Mechanical
  - Immunological (response to denatured protein deposits or hypersensitivity to solutions)
  - Microbiological (alteration of flora and host defenses)
  - Chemical (solution toxicity)
- Effects of Hypoxia
  - Epithelium
    - Reduced epithelial adhesion
    - Decreased barrier function
    - Epithelial thinning and edema
    - Decreased corneal sensitivity
    - **Microcysts** – extracellular accumulations of cellular debris in the basal layers of the epithelium, indication eye is not getting enough O2
  - Stroma
    - Edema → striae (4-6% swelling), folds in Descemet's (7-12% swelling), takes 15% swelling to effect vision
    - Acidosis – from increased lactate or CO2
    - Corneal neovascularization – long term indicator
    - Thinning – response to chronic hypoxia and destruction of collagen
  - Endothelium
    - **Blebs** (endothelial edema) – short term indicator
    - **Polymegathism** – change in cell size, long term indicator
  - Other
    - Limbal and conjunctival redness
    - "Myopic creep" 0.50-0.75D myopic change with extended wear
- Mechanical Effects
  - **SEALs (Superior Epithelial Arcuate Lesions)**
    - Epithelial splitting – arcuate band lesions 1-2mm from superior limbus
  - Dimple "veiling"
    - Bubbles that cause dents in epithelium
  - Mucin Balls – more common in high modulus lenses
  - **CLPC (Contact Lens Papillary Conjunctivitis)**
    - Immunological response to denatured protein deposits on the surface
    - Greater with silicone hydrogel extended wear
    - Palpebral conjunctiva show papillae, hyperemia, and mucus discharge
    - Symptoms: foreign body sensation, itching, decreased lens wearing time or asymptomatic
  - **CLPU (Contact Lens Peripheral Ulcer)**
    - Circular peripheral infiltrate (polymorphonuclear leukocytes)
    - Response to exotoxins from gram positive bacteria (Staph) colonizing the lens surface
  - **CLARE (Contact Lens Acute Red Eye)**
    - Patient awakes with pain, lacrimation, and photophobia, commonly in extended wear
    - Circumlimbal hyperemia with focal or diffuse sub-epithelial infiltrates
    - Response to endotoxins from gram negative bacteria (Pseudomonas) colonizing the lens surface
  - **MK (Microbial Keratitis)**
    - Pathogenic organisms, entry point to infection with altered defenses and hypoxia
- Lens Deposits
  - Depend on tear chemistry, wear time ,replacement schedule, care regimen, and compliance

PREPARATIONS USED WITH CONTACT LENSES

1. Solutions in General

- In order to understand the uses, problems, and interactions of the contact lens solutions, it is important to consider individual properties of these solutions.
- The solutions should be tonic with tear film to maintain normal corneal thickness, especially with hydrogel lenses (osmolarity).
- If the solution is too acidic, irritation among other things will occur.
- Contact lens solutions vary from pH 4.2 to 8.6. Buffering is necessary to keep these solutions at a desired pH.

2. Types of Solutions

- **Non-Hydrogel Lens Solutions**
  - Wetting Solutions: Wetting solutions should be used on any hydrophobic surface to provide comfort, good vision, and a good interaction with tear film. Often preservatives and viscosity agents are added to prevent contamination and a surface coating on the lens.
  - Soaking Solutions: Soaking solutions maintain lens hydration and preservatives prevent microorganism contamination. They also help maintain a clean surface by removing lipid and protein deposits.
  - Cleaning Solutions: These cleaners contain non-ionic surfactants in combination with EDTA, which softens the water and enhances the antimicrobial activity of other preservatives (Note: not for use in the eyes).
    - Enzymatic cleaners can be used once a week to enhance comfort and wearing time.
  - Combination Solutions: Combination solutions are used for noncompliant patients. They are convenient but not as effective as a separate cleaner.
  - Lubricating for Re-Wetting or Comfort: Viscosity agents hold the tears on the eyes and alleviate discomfort. None of the off-the-counter artificial tears is FDA approved to be used with contact lenses.
- **Hydrogel Lens Solutions**
  - These lenses are hydrophilic; water and other compounds are absorbed by the lenses. Solutions must be compatible with the eye.
  - Disinfection: Because saline solutions are effective media for bugs to grow, disinfection is a must.
    - Heat disinfection requires no preservatives so toxic or allergic reactions can be avoided. Unfortunately, heat shortens the life of the lens. This system becomes inconvenient for traveling and lenses could be contaminated during handling. It is gradually becoming obsolete.
    - Cold or chemical systems require preservatives so there is the possibility of irritation.

Examples of Agents in Multi-Purpose Solutions	
Cleaners	Isopropyl alcohol Poloxamine (Surfactant) Sodium citrate Pluronic (poloxamer)
Wetting Agents	Tetronic Dexpanthenol Sorbitol
Rewetting Drops (sometimes separate product)	Tetronic Sodium hyaluronate Carboxymethyl cellulose Sodium perborate (NP) Purite
Disinfection	Chemical -Biguanides -Quaternary ammonium compounds -Amiodamine -EDTA Hydrogen Peroxide

- Hydrogen peroxide is a very effective antibacterial and antiviral and helps maintain clean lenses but is toxic to cells. Because of this lenses must be neutralized. It is not effective against the protozoan *Acanthamoeba*.
- Iodine systems are marketed outside of the USA.

- Cleaning Hydrogel Lenses: Surfactant cleaners are the most common used solution. These solutions often contain a nonionic detergent, wetting agent, chelating agent, buffers, and preservatives. These agents lower the surface tension and emulsify lipids and oils. The lens needs mechanical rubbing with surfactants and rinsing with saline.
  - In addition to surfactants, enzymatic cleaners which hydrolyze proteins into polypeptides and amino acids, are required once a week or twice a month to further breaking down protein.
- Rinsing and Storage Solutions for Hydrogel Lenses: All the rinsing solution used with soft contact lenses contain 0.9% saline. It is isotonic with human tears and has a pH from 7.0 to 7.4 to maintain the lenses' properties and the wearer's comfort.
- Lens Lubricants: Lens lubricants contain a low concentration of nonionic surfactant to help keep lenses clean, a polymer to lubricate the lens, and buffering agents. They are used to lubricate and rewet the lens on the eye.

- **GP Solutions**
  - Adds viscosity, cushioning agents to make the solution thicker so that the GP can be coated when inserted into the eye to increase patient comfort
  - Less concerned with uptake of solution into the lens (unlike with soft lenses)
  - Abrasive cleaners can alter the power

3. Preservatives

- Preservatives are used to kill and prevent the growth of bacterial and viral pathogens.
- However, many patients are allergic to preservatives such as thimerosal and chlorhexidine, so some alternatives to preservatives are used. Aerosol sprays and unit-dose packaging help to defend against microorganisms and function as alternatives to preservatives. They are expensive and the unit-dose may be abused by patients.

Most commonly used preservatives:

- **Benzalkonium Chloride (BAK or BAC):**
  - A quaternary ammonium compound and is extensively used in PMMA lens solutions.
  - Its action is to change the cell membrane permeability of the bacteria and it is often used in combination with EDTA, which increases its effectiveness.
  - It can be toxic to the epithelium in high concentrations so you want to use the least amount possible.
  - It is **not** for use in hydrogel lenses because it is absorbed and later released, which is toxic to the cornea.
- **Ethylenediaminetetraacetic Acid (EDTA):**
  - EDTA is a chelating agent that binds metal ions, removing them from the cell membrane allowing increased penetration of other preservatives. It is often used in combination with other preservatives.

Preservatives in CL Solutions
Benzalkonium Chloride (BAK or BAC)
Ethylenediaminetetracetic Acid (EDTA)
Chlorobutanol
Thimerosal
Chlorhexidine
Sorbic Acid
Polyquad
Dymed
Hydrogen Peroxide

- **Chlorobutanol:**
  - Chlorobutanol is used for hard contact lenses only. It is very volatile and is easily lost from solution. It is effective at an acidic pH. Often used in combination with BAC.
- **Thimerosal:**
  - Thimerosal acts by releasing mercury thereby interfering with the respiration of bacteria.
  - It is used in both hard and soft lens solutions in combination with EDTA.
  - It is broken down by light so it should be stored in dark bottles. 25% of the patients who use it develop sensitivities, especially with hydrogel lenses.

- It is now being replaced by other preservatives even though it is very effective against bacteria and fungi.

- **Chlorhexidine:**
  - Chlorhexidine is extensively used in hydrogel lenses but it does bind to the lens so it can cause irritation to the eye.
- **Sorbic Acid:**
  - Sorbic acid is currently popular and used in hydrophilic lens solution because of the low incidence of allergic or toxic reactions.
  - It may cause yellowing of some lenses, especially those containing methacrylic acid.
- **Polyquad:**
  - Polyquad is high molecular weight quaternary compound. The large molecules will be rinsed off by tear, so it can be used for hydrogel lenses without causing toxic or allergic reactions.
  - An example of a solution utilizing polyquad is Alcon's Optifree.
- **Dymed:**
  - Dymed, a brand name for polyhexamethylene biguanide, is from the same family of compounds as chlorhexidine. It can be used at a very low concentration for disinfection.
- **Hydrogen Peroxide:**
  - Hydrogen peroxide is a very effective disinfecting agent for hydrogel lenses. The hydrogen peroxide can be neutralized with numerous methods including a platinum catalyst, enzyme catalase, sodium pyruvate, sodium sulfite, or dilution by multiple rinses with saline.
  - An example of a hydrogen peroxide cleaning system is ClearCare.

Chapter 6 – Low Vision

OPTICAL CHARACTERISTICS OF LOW VISION DEVICES

1. Magnification, Field of View, and Working Distance

- **Magnification** looks at the ratio of the object to the image, whether it be object height (o) relative to image height (i), object distance (u) relative to image distance (v), or incident vergence (U) relative to emerging vergence (V).
- **Relative Size Magnification (RSM)** occurs when the size of the object is increased while the distance remains the same. RSM is equal to the original size of the object (θ_1) relative to the new size (θ_2). For instance, increasing print size would be an example of RSM.
- **Relative Distance Magnification (RDM)** occurs by bringing an object of the same size closer to the eye, so that the size of the imate on the retina is larger. RDM is equal to the original working reference distance (r) in relation to the new working distance (d)

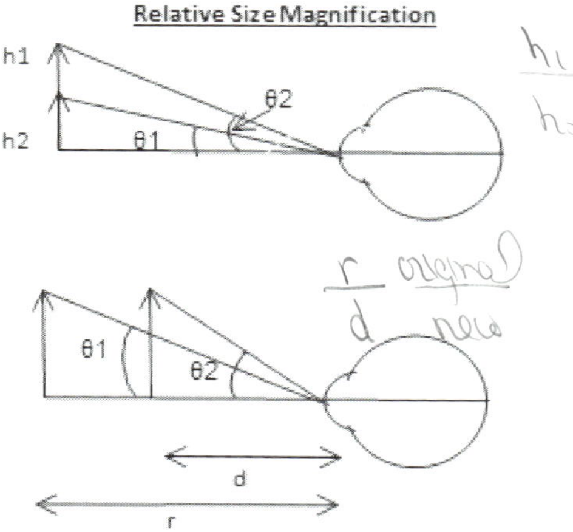

- **Angular Magnification (M)** occurs when an optical system is placed between the object and the eye, while the object remains the same size and distance away from the eye. M is the comparison of the object size without the optical system to the object size with the optical system and is dependent upon the power of the lens system (P) and the distance of the optical system to the eye (d).
- **Axial Magnification** occurs when the object occupies more than one plane (is 3D). It is the distance between two object planes along the optical axis and is proportional to the product of the transverse magnification for the pair of conjugate planes (M1 and M2) at the front and back of the object. If M_1 and M_2 are close in value, axial magnification approximately equals M^2.

> Magnification
> **$M = i/o = u/v = V/U$**
> Relative Size Mag.
> **$RSM = \theta_2/\theta_1 = h_2/h_1$**
> Relative Distance Mag.
> **$RDM = r/d = \theta_2/\theta_1$**
> Angular Mag.
> **$M = dP$**
> Axial Mag.
> **$M_{axial} = M_1 \times M_2 \rightarrow M^2$**

***Example**: A 3cm thick object is placed 10cm in front of a +5.00D lens. What is the axial magnification using the exact and approximate formulas?*

> ***Answer**:*
> The two planes of the object are located 10 and 13cm in front of the lens.
> $U_1 = 100/-10 = -10.00D$ $\quad U_2 = 100/-13 = -7.69D$
> $V_1 = -10 + 5 = -5.00D$ $\quad V_2 = -7.69 + 5 = -2.69D$
> $M_1 = -5/-10 = +0.5x$ $\quad M_2 = -2.69/-7.69 = 0.35x$
> Axial Mag (Exact) = 0.5 x 0.35 = 0.175x
> Axial Mag (Approximate) = 0.5^2= 0.25x or 0.35^2 = 0.1225x
> Notice the Exact Method value is in between the two Approximate method values

- **Field of View (FOV)** is the linear (or angular) width of the field (how much of the target will be seen) from the entrance pupil. The FOV can be determined by using similar triangles to get the angular FOV when using a simple lens.

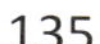

Example: *Given a -4.00DS lens that is 50mm in diameter, what is the FOV (°) assuming the entrance pupil is 17mm from the lens? What would be the FOV if the lens had no power?*

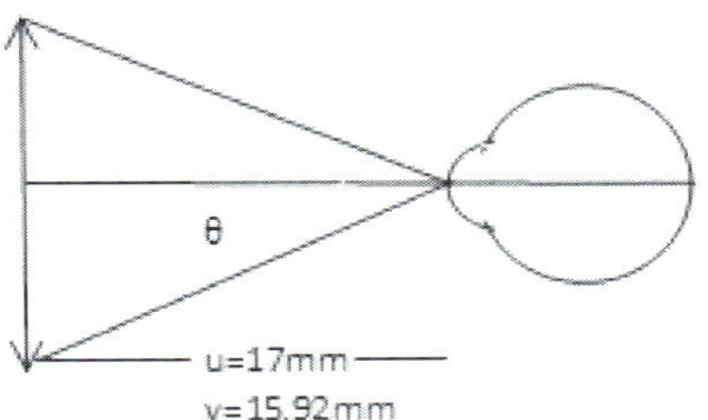

***Answer*:**
U=100/-17= -58.82D
V= -58.82 + -4.00 = -62.82D
v=100/-62.82 = -15.92mm – image distance to the eye
tanθ=25/-15.92 → θ= 57.5°
FOV = 2θ = 115° → with -4.00DS lens
tanθ=25/17 →θ=55.8°
FOV = 2θ = 112° → without power

- The power of the lens changes the FOV. A minus lens increases the FOV, while a plus lens decreases the FOV. Thus, a corrected myope will have a larger FOV than a corrected hyperope or emmetrope.
- The closer the **working distance** the larger the FOV and the larger the magnification.

2. Simple Magnifiers

- **Simple magnifiers** (magnifying glass) are not held close to the eye. They can be held as far away from the eye as necessary for the patient so long as the object viewed is held at the focal point of the magnifier.
- **Stand magnifier** is a hand magnifier with "feet" which maintain a fixed
- Lens to object distance when the feet are rested on the object.
- The magnification of a simple magnifer is equivalent to its dioptric power (P) multiplied by the viewing distance to the eye from the object without the magnifier (u_e)
- The standard definition of the magnification of a simple magnifier (M_r) is for a working distance of 25cm, in which it is noted as M_{25}. The manufacturers calculate the dioptric power of a hand magnifier with a different equation so people think their magnifiers are stronger than they actually are.

Simpler Magnifier's
$M=u_eP$
Standard Definition
$M_{25}=P/4$
Manufacturer's Definition
$M_{25}=P/4+1$

3. Telescopes

- There are two types of telescopes, **Galilean** and **Keplerian**. Both telescopes have a positive objective lens that converges light towards an inverted image, but the Galilean has a negative ocular lens creating an erect image and the Keplerian has a positive ocular lens creating an inverted image.
- Telescopes have a magnifying effect if the power of the ocular lens is stronger than the objective lens.
- Telescopes minify the image by a factor of M, but the image moves closer by a factor of M^2 allowing for a total magnification effect
- An afocal telescope (P=0) generates parallel outgoing light (V-0) with parallel incident light (U=0), so it is designed for emmetropes to view distant objects (u=∞)

	Keplerian	Galilean
Objective lens	(+)	(+)
Ocular lens	(+)	(-)
M_A	(-)	(+)
Image	Inverted	Upright
Ramsden	Real (small)	Virtual (large)
Prisms	Present	Absent
Magnification	High	Low (rarely above 4x)
Length	Long	Short
Compound eyepiece	Yes	No
Field of view	Large	Crisp

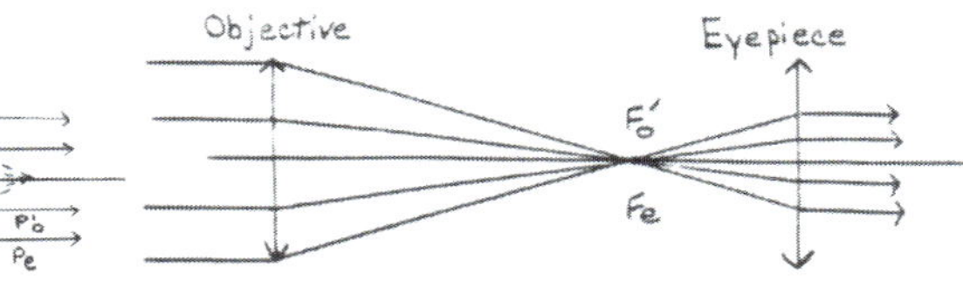

- For an afocal telescope, the secondary focal point of the objective coincides with the primary focal point of the ocular lens.
- The angular magnification of an afocal telescope (M_A) is proportional to the power of the ocular (P_{oc}) and objective (P_{obj}) lenses where d is the length of the telescope (m).

Angular Magnification

M_A=-P_{oc}/P_{obj}

M_A=1/(1-dP_{obj})

M_A=1-dP_{oc}

d=f_{obj}+f_{oc}

- The **Ramsden circle** is the image of the objective lens formed by the ocular. It is a real image with Keplerian telescopes and a virtual image with Galilean telescopes. The radius or diameter of the Ramsden ($h_{ramsden}$) and distance of the ocular to the Ramsden circle ($d_{ramsden}$) can be calculated.

Ramsden Circle

$h_{ramsden}$=h_{obj}/M_A

$d_{ramsden}$==d/M_A

m=1/M_A

- There are three methods to adjust an afocal telescope for an ametrope:
  1. Add a cap to the ocular M_A=1/(1-dP_{obj})
  2. Add a lens to the objective M_A=1-dP_{oc}
  3. Adjust the telescope length, (d) M_A=-P_{oc}/P_{obj}

     Note that borrowing power P'_{oc}=P_{oc}-U_{fp} where U_{fp} is the power of the lens needed to correct for the ametrope's refractive error.

Example: *How would you adjust an afocal Keplerian TS (P_{obj}=+20D, P_{oc}=+60D) for a -10D myope using all three methods?*

***Answer*:**

1) Add a cap to ocular

P_{oc}=-10D (BVP needed to correct RE)

Afocal TS portion has not changed

M_A= -(+60D)/(+20D)= -3X

P_v=-10D

d=(1/+20) +(1/+60) = 6.67cm

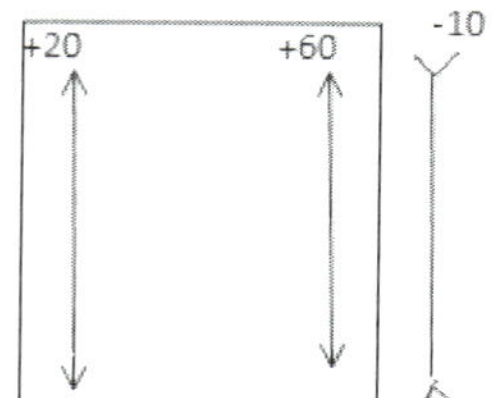

2) Add a cap to objective

P'_{oc}=P_{oc}-U_{fp}= 60- (-10) = +70D

M_A=1-dP'_{oc}=1-(0.0667)(70)= =3.67x

V_{obj}=-70/(1-(-70)) *-0.0667m=19.09D

U_{obj}=V-P=19.09-20=-0.91D

Reading cap =-0.91D to make afocal

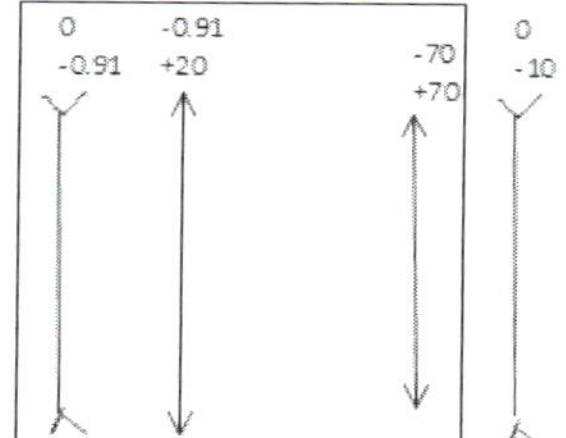

3) P'_{oc} – borrowing power = +70D

d=1/P_{obj} – 1/P'_{oc}= 1/20 +1/70 = 6.43cm

M_A=+70/+20 = -3.5x

4. Loupes

- Loupes (aka hand lenses) are a system of focusing lenses contained in a cylinder. It is a form of a microscope that has a longer vertex distance than what is used for the microscopes found in spectacles.
- There are three basic types in order of lowest to highest amount of magnification: 1) simple lens 2) Galilean, and 3) Prismatic
- Loupes can be mounted on lenses in spectacles and are commonly used in professions that need high magnification for detailed work such as surgeons, dentists, and jewelers.

5. Microscopes

- Bifocals or single vision lenses intended for near vision only (here the term does not mean the laboratory microscope). They are used to view an object, located within the optical system's focal length. They are mounted in a conventional frame with a very short vertex distance. Because of the short vertex distance the lens doesn't need to be large (i.e., weigh a lot) to allow a large enough FOV.

- Characteristics of a microscopic lens:
  - High Add – one piece Bifocal around +20.00, segment on front
  - Any need cylindrical correction on back
  - **M = P/4, M = 1 + P/4**
  - Considered a thin lens
- Manufacturers who make microscopic lenses:
  - Design for Vision:
    - Bifocal 2x to 10x (+4.00 to +40.00) with distance in carrier lens
    - Full-Diameter microscopes 2x to 20x
  - American Optical (glass):
    - Bifocal 2x to 8x (+8.00 to +32.00)
    - Single Vision (Aspheric) 6x to 12x
    - Half Eye – +4.00 to +12.00
- Problems associated with microscopic lenses:
  - Aberrations: Often seen with high powered lenses so need aspheric surfaces
  - Illumination: Reading material is held close to the eye so ambient light is blocked by the head.
  - Centration of lenses:
    - If each eye has a lens, the two lenses need to be closer than the 2mm difference from distance to near pd
    - Total decentration = [27 x(distance pd_{mm})] / [(reading $distance_{mm}$) +27]
    - ***Example***: *if reading distance = 10 cm and PD is 60 mm then total decentration = 12.8*
  - Maintenance of the proper viewing distance:
    - Hard to adapt to the 5cm reading distance of a +20.00 D lens and depth of focus is small so moving a slight difference can greatly blur the image
    - At such a short distance, the depth of focus is small so small changes in reading distance can greatly blur the image.

EPIDEMIOLOGY, HISTORY AND SYMPTOM INVENTORY

1. Epidemiology

- **Low vision** is reduced central acuity (20/100 or less) or contracted visual fields (diameter of 20 degrees or less in any one direction) and is considered legally blind; low vision is usually 20/60 or 20/70. *As of 02/07 The Social Security Administration changed the VA for legal blindness from 20/200 to 20/100.
- **Epidemiology** (prevalence):
  - 1% of population is visually impaired.
  - 0.2% of population is legally blind of which 1/10 became visually impaired in the last 12 months.
  - Of this 0.2%, 85% have some useful vision and 15% do not.
  - 87% of legally blind are over age 60.
  - 27% of people in their 80's are legally blind. Up to age 50 more males (ratio is 55/45), after 50 more females (ratio is 30/70).

Example: *Of 10,000 people: 100 are visually impaired, 20 are legally blind, 2 within last year; 17 have useful vision, 3 do not.*

History and Symptom Inventory

- When taking a case history for a low vision patient ask about:
  - Ocular history
  - Visual performance

- Mobility
- Activities
- Near vision
- Illumination
- Life style
- Education/employment
- Rehabilitation
- Motivation
- Present aids

- Diseases of aging associated with low vision: ARMD, cataracts, glaucoma, vascular conditions, RP, myopic degenerations, retinal detachments and trauma.
- In general, observe patient during the exam for the following: mobility, posture, fixation, cosmesis, physical and psychological factors

OBSERVATION AND RECOGNITION OF CLINICAL SIGNS AND TECHNIQUES AND SKILLS FOR DETERMINING A CORRECTION

1. Visual Acuity

Distance Visual Acuity

- Distance charts should have letters up to 20/700 or 20/800. Gradations should be fine enough to measure acuities in the ranges between 400 and 300, 300 and 200, 200 and 100. Also should be able to hold large charts at 10 feet or closer and to vary the illumination upon them.
  - **Snellen chart**
    - Size sequence is irregular and different degrees of crowding exist. Also, there are no standard Snellen charts and if you vary the distance the score doesn't change as predicted.
  - **AMA VA chart:** has irregular spacing; uses visual efficiency scale where 20/20 is 100% and 20/200 is 20%.
    - Formula: Visual Efficiency (VE) = $0.2^{(MAR-1)/9}$
  - **Sloan chart:** a log progression chart; standardized a group of 10 letters that have equal legibility.
  - **Feinbloom chart:** A low vision chart. 14" x 12" booklet.
    - Advantages:
      - Numbers (easier to read)
      - Range of size is substantial
      - Goes in small steps – psychologically good
  - **Bailey-Lovie chart**: The **ultimate** chart!
    - Advantages:
      - Task and spacing the same on each line
      - Letter spacing is proportional
      - Log progressions- chart decreases in size at a constant rate
      - Contains British standard letters
      - Each row is of equal difficulty
      - Same number of letters on each line
  - **Univ. of Waterloo chart**: Letters are arranged in columns.
- Acuity charts provide a quantitative assessment of visual functioning, **contrast sensitivity** charts provide a qualitative assessment.
  - Contrast sensitivity testing can detect changes when Snellen VA is normal, which can occur with cataracts, glaucoma, corneal disease, and other ocular diseases.
  - It helps predict illumination, contrast, magnification needs, and optical magnification.

Specifying near VA notation for near vision charts:

- **Reduced Snellen acuity**: Poor! Used to specify height of print when it is really an angle measurement.
- **Jaeger**: Poor! No standardization. J1 = pretty small, J10= pretty big
- **Points**: Based on print size. 1 point = 1/72". 8 points = 1M. Block height for 8 point font is 2.82mm (~2M). Lower case is 1M (without limbs). Capitals and numbers are 1.5 x lower case size.
- **N – Notation**: Based on print size read at certain distance, for example N5 at 20 cm. N8 = 8pt; so N5 = 5/8 = 0.625 M.
- **M units**: Specifies print size. M units equal distance in meters at which letters subtend 5' of arc; 1M print subtends 5' at 1 meter. Newsprint is about 1M; also, newsprint is 8 points and 1.45mm. note # of points/8 = M units.

Near charts:

- **Feinbloom:** 4 to 24 point. Poor, numbers are arbitrary.
- **Lebenson**: 2 to 24 point. Unrelated words and numbers.
- **B&L:** 0.4M to 1.1M. Numbers on card = dist. in decimeter so 10 = 1M, 9 = .9M etc.
- **AO CHART:** chart #11970 is 2M to .5M; # 11960 is 13 lines of illiterate e's from 14/14 to 14/224.
- **Lighthouse cards**: pictures for kids, not really used in LV.
- **Sloan:** 1M to 10M. Range not large, no log progression.
- **Birds-fly:** log steps, simple sentences, aka UNC chart (Univ.of North Carolina).
- **Bailey-Lovie chart**: log progression, 17 lines, 40x different from top to bottom. Each row has 42 letters (two 4 letter, 7 letter and 10 letter words, total of six words.) smallest row is 0.25M at 40cm.

- **VA charts for infants to children, by age level:** VEP, pref. looking, cheerios, lighthouse/broken-wheel, tumbling e's, numbers, letters.
  If pt cannot read a VA chart: Measure vision with hand movements and light perception. Finger movements are not preferred though, best to use larger VA charts
- **Useful VA Conversions**: (know how to do these type of conversions): VA , MAR, LogMar, Decimal, VAR, % Visual Efficiency

***Example**: 20/400 = 6/120 = VA, MAR = 20,*
Decimal = 20/400= 0.05,
VAR = 100- 50xlogMar = 35,
Visual Efficiency % = $0.2^{(MAR-1)/9}$ x 100= 3.35%

2. Special Refraction Techniques

- When doing LV refraction use trial frame and lens clips.
- Jackson hand held flip cross for astigmatism.
- Start with best Rx (old Rx or retinoscopy) and give large dioptric differences for choices. Make sure to bracket.
- Encourage patient and promote success.
- Can also use a stenopaic slit which reduces light, channels light, and increases depth of focus. Evaluate illumination. Make sure with new Rx pt can see the improvement

Near Add Determinations:

- **Kestenbaum**: give mar of distance VA and call it diopters. For example, 20/50 MAR = 2.5 add = 2.5 diopters.
- **Wrongly reasoned rule**: Wrong because it does not take into consideration the change in working distance (Kestenbaum also guilty of this). E
  - ***Example**: Dist VA = 20/200 and the near VA desired is 20/40 a 5x increase, now use the equation M= F/4 so 5= F/4 so F= +20.00D, print will be at 5cm.*
- **Bailey's Rule**: consider what size print pt wants to read and at what distance. Several ways:

***Example:** A patient reads 3M print at 10 cm, but wants to read 0.5M. How much closer must the patient be to view this letter size print?*

> ***Answer:***
> This is a 6-fold increase (from 3M to 0.5M) to must alter distance by 1/6 from 10cm to 1.67cm.

Example : Use **Bailey's log scale method**:
6.3 8 10 12.5 16 20 25 32 40 50
If a patient can read 16 point at 25cm, at what distance can he/she read 6 point?

> ***Answer:***
> 10cm. – 4 step difference in print so 4 step change in distance

- General LV near add prescribing tips:
  - Refine near Rx.
  - Check to see if pt appreciates Rx. Encourage good illumination.
  - Near PD is important, recall equations: NPD=DPD - 1.5x add (an approximation),or NPD = DPD x WD/(WD + z) (the exact method)

3. Visual Fields

- The **Amsler Grid** can be helpful to locate and characterize scotomas, as well as in eccentric fixation detection and training
- Types
  - **Central/paracentral:** tangent screen (25-30 degrees). May have to help pt by drawing cross in periphery to hold fixation.
  - **Precise central:** Amsler grid (0-20 degrees).
  - **Peripherial field**: bowl perimeter (beyond 30). Automated and manual fields i.e. Dicon, Humphrey, Friedman.
- Purpose of VF measurement:
  - **Screening**: target should just be seen centrally but not in far periphery
  - **Diagnosis**: small target, trying to detect small pathology
  - **Monitoring**: target same as last time, even if you believe it was done incorrectly the first time do it the same and then do it a 2nd time the correct way.
  - **Functional:** large targets that flash if needed to detect any visual functioning. You are looking for a potential scotoma. Size and extent of scotoma should be explored as well as integrity of macula and para-macular areas.
- Treatment of Field defects:
  - **Fresnel Prisms:** 15 to 30 prism diopters, base away from pupil placed on half of the glasses in which the field defect is present. i.e. R-hemianope with R-eye, place prism on right side/temporal side with BO.
  - **Hemianopic mirror:** mounted 5-10° (towards the eye) on nasal eyewire of the blind eye.

4. Reading Skills

- A scotoma immediately to the right of fixation is more of a problem in reading than one on the left side. Adaptation can be made by turning the material upside down and reading from right to left, or turning the page 90 degrees and reading vertically. If the scotoma is more lateral than vertical, turning the page up to 45 degrees may be easier than a full 90 or 180 degrees. Larger letters and more separation between lines will help prevent confusion and loss of place on the line.
- When training someone to read or assessing reading skills, consider vocabulary, reading level, ability to relate to and understand material, and interest in material.
- According to Bailey, there is always a constant relationship between maximum reading efficiency and maximum resolution

5. Effects of Illumination

- In the normal eye and most types of ocular pathology, decimal acuity for black letters on a white background increases linearly with the log of the luminance up to about 10 Lumens (about 12 foot candles), but remains relatively constant at higher intensities. There are two conditions of ocular pathology where this relationship between acuity and luminance may be quite different:

- **Maculopathies**: A higher than normal luminance is often required to attain maximium acuity.
- **Congential Achromatopsia**: Acuity reaches its maximal value at a low luminance and, with further increase, falls rapidly unless retinal illumination is reduced by partial lid closure or by wearing very dark glasses.

6. Magnification Determination

- **Afocal Telescopes**: (Review)
  - Keplarian (++) and Gallilean (+-).
  - Mag = $-P_{oc}/P_{obj}$ $d = f_{oc} + f_{obj}$
  - Element Separation $t = 1/P_{oc} + 1/P_{obj}$
  - Power mag = $1/(1 - dP_v)$
  - Shape Mag = $1/(1 - t/n\ P_1)$
  - Total mag = (Power mag) x (Shape mag)
  - d = distance from back pole of a lens to the entrance pupil of the eye.
  - Vergence magnification = Freed's Equation

> Freed's Equation
> **V=M x U**

- **Collimating Lenses:**
  - Produce image at infinity when object is at focal point of lens
  - EVP (Equivalent Viewing Power) is power of the lens
  - Magnification is constant, but field of view decreases as you move back from lens. ↓ FOV further from lens

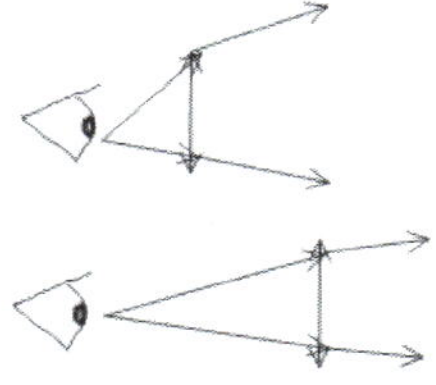

  - Width of field of view can be calculated, where:
    - A - lens diameter
    - f - focal length
    - z - vertex distance
  - Hand held magnifiers with spectacle adds can be calculated, where:
    - P_e - total power
    - P_1 - add power
    - P_2 - Magnifier power
  - Neutral point is one focal length away from the magnifier: at this point P_1 has no significance to the system's power.

> FOV Width
> **$W = A \times (f/z)$**
> HHM Power
> **$P_e = P_1 + P_2 - z(P_1P_2)$**

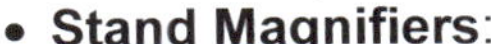

- **Stand Magnifiers**:
  - Object is located between focal length and magnifier;
  - A large divergence enters the lens and a low divergence emerges so that the image is more remote than the object, and the image is enlarged by the magnification $m = l'/l = u/v$

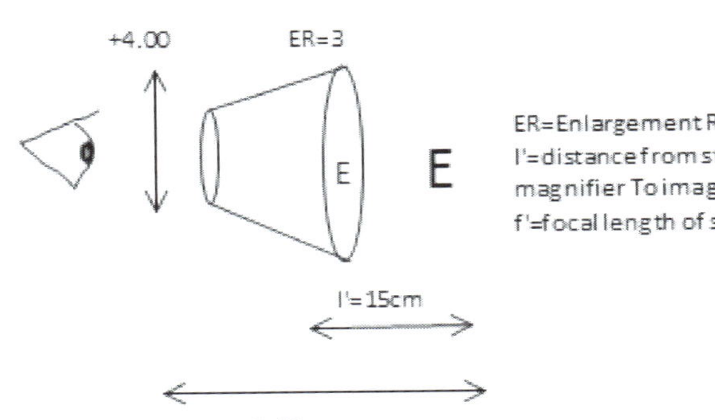

ER=Enlargement Ratio
l'=distance from stand magnifier To image
f'=focal length of spectacles

- **Transverse Magnification (Multac Factor)**:
  - EVD (Equivalent viewing distance) is equal to the eye to image distance (u_{eye}) divided by the transverse magnification (M_t)
  - EVP (Equivalent Viewing Power) is equal to the accommodative demand (AA) multiplied by the transverse magnification
- **Near Vision Telescope**
  - Adding plus add over objective
- **Video Magnifiers**
  - Magnification is 7 to 45x

> Transverse Magnification
> **$M_t = V + P/V$**
> Equivalent Viewing Distance
> **$EVD = U_{eye}/M_t$**
> Equivalent Viewing Power
> **$EVP = AA \times M_t$**
> Near Vision Telescope
> **$EVP = P_{add} \times M_{telescope}$**

7. In-Office Evaluation with Low Vision Devices

- In prescribing and evaluating low vision aids a complete eye exam is necessary Dr. Bailey outlines the following model and emphasizes that the case history is the most important:

- History
- Inspection
- Refraction
- Near vision power
- Near vision aids
- Telescope power
- Telescope aids
- Fields
- Other tests ie, color vision, contrast sensitivity, Amsler Grid
- Deciding recommendation
- Presentation
- Follow-up
- Special attention should be given to the patient→ Patient's needs, wants, chief complaint

- A goal should be set, achieve that goal by confirming the magnification or lens power needed and decide on the appropriate aids that will best meet the patient's needs
  - Diagnosis, management, and treatment of low vision patients, and prognosis.

Note: parts of this section have been discussed in detail in the above section.

- **Needs to Consider**
  - There needs to be analysis and interpretation of personal, social, vocational, and psychological patient needs. Often one device cannot satisfy the majority of the daily needs of the patient
  - A presbyope who has microscopic spectacles with short working distance and narrow field will still have difficulties writing, eating, cooking, locating article in newspaper or finding a bill in a file. An intermediate add (1/3 of microscopic add) must be provided.
  - Many patients require magnification for distances.
  - Compact hand held scopes up to 10x mag are obtainable and useful for reading street signs, house numbers, chalkboards, scoreboards, etc
  - For shaving, applying make-up, combing hair, etc magnifying mirrors may be useful.
  - Many non-optical devices are available which can be helpful for daily tasks; braille typewriters, jumbo playing cards, high contrast backgrounds, etc
  - Social needs.
- **Age-Related Needs to Consider**
  - Adolescence - very self-conscious, very sensitive.
  - Young adult - concerned with independence.
  - Adults - concerned with employment, marriage and family.
  - Elderly - fear of isolation, dependence, won't be able to travel.
- **Vocational Needs**
  - Patient may be limited in their employment abilities encourage other options and possibilities.
- **Psychological Needs**
  - The patient may feel nothing can be done and reject the aids anyway
  - Fitting and adapting to low vision aids may difficult. Can try to promote a successful orientation
  - Good words to use- low vision, partially sighted, aid, can see able, change, unusual.
  - Bad words to use- sub-normal vision partially blind, correction, can't see, unable, deterioration, abnormal
- **Prescribing Low Vision Aids**
  - Set goals
  - Correct the refractive error
  - Test patients abilities
  - Predict changes
  - Verify

Example: *A patient has a 3.00D add and reads 4M at 32cm with a goal to read 1M, at 8cm what add should you expect? Expect =12.50D add*

- **Types of Low Vision Aids**
  - Strong specs

- Hand held magnifiers
- Stand magnifiers
- Near vision telescopes
- Spectacle mounted telescope
- Bioptic telescope
- Distance telescopes
- Closed circuit TV

- **Patient Education and Training**
  - Studies have shown that training programs with low vision pts have had positve outcomes. Some general guidelines are:
    - Train on a regular schedule
    - Set goals that are reasonable and achievable
    - Reinforce progress
    - Start out easy than get tougher
    - Training should carry over to real life.
- **Roles and Relationships With Other Disciplines**
  - Patient can be referred from other optometry offices for additional care and services:
    - Rehabilitation counselors - find jobs, training
    - Psychological counselors/social workers - family & personal issues
    - Teachers - access to educational material orientation and mobility instructors
    - Community services - transportation, ~libraries
    - Medicare
    - Health care workers
    - Daily living assistants
- **Prognostic Factors and Follow-Up Care**
  - Periodic re-evaluations are more essential for low vision patients.
  - Where perception of detail has been curtailed for some time or never developed, it is often found that this ability improves with use and consequently a lower aid may suffice
  - Where old pathology progresses or new occurs, further deterioration of vision may require a higher power aid
  - New demands (as in growing children) may require different solutions.

Log Scale
320
250
200
160
125
100
80
63
50
40
32
25
20
16
12.5
10
8

Chapter 7 – Accommodation/Vergence/Oculomotor Function

EYE MOVEMENTS

1. Purpose and Roles for Vision

- Anatomical Considerations
  - Retinal organization (fovea) requires tracking
  - Location of orbits (forward eye placement) requires vergence
  - Large overlaps of the visual fields permit stereopsis
- Roles for vision
  - Place images on the fovea and permits image tracking (pursuits, saccades)
  - Enhances visual acuity and visibility of interesting objects
  - Reduces retinal image smear
  - Control light level
  - Expand field of view
  - Support stereoscopic depth perception by aligning visual axes to maintain bifoveal fixation
  - Image stabilization during locomotion and with respect to head position (vestibular)
  - Coordination and control of eye movements to achieve normal unification of images from both eyes.

2. Dynamics and Kinematics

- The dynamics will be discussed individually for each type of eye movement.
- Kinematics are determined by the formation of actin-myosin cross bridges characteristic of striated muscle.
- The general range of extraocular muscle length is ±20% of their nominal length (or about ±8mm in length).
- This maintains the extraocular muscles always near maximal tension.
- This allows for eye excursions of ±40deg. Eye excursions are limited by check ligaments.
- The amount of nervous activation rather than the optimal muscle length determines the maximal force of the extraocular muscle.
- Extraocular muscles operate in a time optimal, non-linear fashion.
- Numerous "laws" generalize how eye positions are determined by the nervous system.
  - **Descares-Sherrington's Law of Reciprocal Innervation**: the innervations of antagonist muscle pairs are reciprocal so that as the agonist innervations increases innervations to the antagonist decreases.
  - **Hering's Law**: yoked muscle pairs from both eyes are equally innervated during ocular movements so that they rotate the eyes by the same amount. This ensures bifoveal fixation
  - **Euler's Rule**: there are an infinite number of axes of rotation that can change gaze from one direction to another, however each axis produces a unique torsion. Implying that there is only one axis of rotation that can describe eye orientation in a given direction of gaze
  - **Donder's Law**: each gaze direction has a unique torsional posture, no matter what path the eye took to get there

3. Specification of Direction of Gaze and Ocular Orientation (Torsion)

- Refer to chart of points, lines and angles pertaining to eye and Fick's system on the next page.
- **Center of rotation of the eye:** The eye is like a sphere that only rotates about the three principal axes (vertical, horizontal, and anterior-posterior-axes). This point in the geometric center of the eye would never move as the eye rotates.
    - In reality, when the eye rotates around an axis, small translational movements occur. Because of this, there is no true center of rotation of the eye. The center of rotation of the eye is described as the region that the eye functionally rotates around.
    - The center of this volume is located 13.5mm and 1.6mm nasal to the geometric center of the globe.
- **Primary position** of gaze is when both eyes are looking straight ahead at infinity. The visual axes are parallel. The X-axis is perfectly horizontal, the Z-axis is perfectly vertical and the Y-axis is normal to Listing's plane and pointed at infinity.
- **Secondary position** of gaze is the position that results from a cardinal eye movement. A **cardinal eye movement** is a rotation about either the X or Z axis but not both.
- **Tertiary position** of gaze results from rotations of the eye around both the X and Z axis (equals two cardinal eye movements). A rotation around both X and Z axis can also be described as a rotation around some oblique axis in Listing's plane. This is not equivalent to torsion.
- **Fick's system** employs 3 axes to define ocular orientation.
    - Vertical movements are rotations about the horizontal X-axis.
    - Horizontal movements are rotations around the vertical Z-axis.
    - Torsions are rotations about the Y-axis.
- True torsion of the eye around the Y-axis is not under voluntary control and does not occur except for compensatory torsional movements of the eye in response to labyrinthine and tonic neck reflex areas. These torsional movements work within a small range to keep the sensory vertical raphe of the retina perpendicular to the horizon. If the upper end of the vertical meridian of the eye tilts toward the nose, this is termed incycloduction, and if it tilts toward the temple, excycloduction. With a 30° head tilt, there is a mean incycloduction of the ipsilateral eye of 7.00 ± 3.10° and an excycloduction of 8.36 ± 2.50° of the contralateral eye. Thus torsional movements of the eye compensate for small degrees of lateral head tilt from the erect position and tend to keep the vertical meridians of the retina perpendicular to the horizon.
- Agonist-Antagonist relationships
    - **Agonist** - muscle moving eye in desired direction of gaze.
    - **Antagonist** - muscle in same eye having the opposite action.
    - **Yoked muscles** - are those muscles of the two eyes which simultaneously contract to turn the eyes equally the same direction.
    - Synergistic muscles give the same action in a given eye. Muscles can be synergists for one action and antagonists for another.
    - Evaluation of the synergistic or antagonistic relationship of any two muscles is based upon a muscle's action in primary position.
    - The actions of the EOM's are summarized below. Note that there is some variation between sources; for example some sources state that the primary action of the obliques is torsion and their secondary action n is elevation or depression, while other sources state the opposite.

	Primary	Secondary	Tertiary
LR	Pure abduction		
MR	Pure adduction		
SR	Elevation	Adduction	Intorsion
IR	Depression	Adduction	Extorsion
SO	Depression	Abduction	Intorsion
IO	Elevation	Abduction	Extorsion

4. Reflex Movements, Including Compensatory Movements

- Command, random movements, and involuntary movements toward visual and auditory stimuli are always saccades.
    - **Saccades**: very fast movement that shifts the image in a step like motion to place the image on the fovea. Allows you to shift your attention from one target to another
- Image stabilization during body movements (OKN, VOR) are reflexes because they occur automatically without conscious effort

- **VOR (Vestibulo-ocular reflex)**- compensates for brief head and body rotation. During head movements, the semicircular canals of the vestibular labyrinth signal how fast the head is rotating and the oculomotor system responds to this signal by rotating the eyes in an equal and opposite velocity. This stabilizes the eyes relative to the external world and keeps the images fixed on the retina
- **OKR (Optokinetic Reflex)**: responds when we move about in a visual scene. Unlike the VOR, this reflex requires a visible retinal image. OKR supplements the VOR by responding to constant retinal image velocity caused by constant body rotation or translation. OKR maintains the stabilization and compensates for a damaged vestibular apparatus

- **Bell's phenomenon** is the normal upward and outward rotation of the eyes on bilateral closure or attempted closure of the eyelids. Its absence is seen in 10-50% (depending on source) of normal, healthy individuals.
- The reflex fusion stress test (using prisms of 6pd) measures the latency, velocity, accuracy, and fatigability of the fusional vergence system to an obstacle.
- With an extraocular muscle paralysis or imbalance, head tilts may be manifested to avoid diplopia or minimize its adversity. Compensatory eye movements are required (especially cyclorotations) to maintain single vision.

5. Small Movements Associated with Steady Fixation

- Even without any fixational target error, eye movements spontaneously occur. Some consider it a noise in the system, but other evidence indicates that at least some of the movement is necessary to prevent gray out of the retinal image.
- Three main types of fine fixational movements:
    - **Microsaccades:** moderately rapid eye movements (2-10 deg/sec) with amplitude of 1'-25' arc and durations up to 25msec.
    - **Microtremors:** occur at a high frequency (about 70 Hz) but are of very small amplitude (about 10').
    - **Microdrifts:** composed of smooth pursuit, vergence, and VOR eye movements are slow (0.025%/sec or less). They are of moderate amplitude (about 5' arc).

6. Versional Movements (Pursuits and Saccades)

- When lines of sight maintain the same visual angle the movement is a **version**. Versions are yoked or conjugate eye movements and may be voluntary or involuntary. If one eye is occluded it will move with the fixating eye.
    - In lateral versions, the medial rectus is linked with the lateral rectus of the other eye. **Dextroversion** is a rightward looking. **Levoversion** is a leftward looking.
    - In vertical versions, identical vertical muscles are linked. **Supraversion** is upward looking. **Infraversion** is downward looking.
    - Torsional version require that muscles which produce incyclotorsion in one eye be linked with muscles which produce excyclotorsion in the other. **Dextrocycloversion** is a rotation rightward. **Levocycloversion** is a leftward rotation.
- Smooth **pursuit** is a slow, steady, involuntary type of eye movement that is mediated by a graded response producing a constant velocity.
    - Slow pursuits can be analyzed via a closed loop continuous feedback and monitoring system that can function at speeds up to 40-deg arc/sec.
    - They have a moderate latency of about 125 msec (may be shorter than the latency for saccades).
    - The mechanism is aimed at achieving a stationary image on the retina irrespective of the error of the position of fixation
- **Saccades** are very rapid eye movements that may reach 1000 deg arc/sec initiated via a burst of nerve impulses from each of the neurons in the agonist muscle preceded by relaxation of their antagonist extraocular muscle(s).
    - Refixations generally occur via involuntary saccades following a latency of 120-160 msec.

- The original burst or pulse of nerve impulse which initiate a saccade differs from the step change for a vergence movement and is proportional to the amplitude of the eye movement required.
- A consequence of the multiple pulse saccadic movements are dynamic overshoots.
- The saccadic system operates via a sample-data delay which may result in belated or inaccurate eye movement responses to stimuli briefly presented.

- Position errors are corrected by the Saccadic system and velocity errors are corrected by the smooth pursuit system.

Movement	Velocity	Latency	Amp	Duration
VOR	4 Hz	15 msec		
Microsaccade	2-10 deg/sec		1'-25' arc	25 msec
Microtremor	70 Hz		10'	
Microdrifts	0.025 deg/sec		5' arc	
Saccade	1000 deg arc/sec	120-160 msec		
Smooth pursuit	40 deg arc/sec	125 msec		
Vergence	21 deg arc/sec	160 msec		

7. Vergence Movements

- **Vergences**, or disjunctive eye movements, enable the subject to fixate points at various distances in visual space. This calls for either active convergence or divergence. Vergence movements have a maximum velocity of approximately 21 deg arc/sec, which is much slower than the speed of pursuit or saccadic movements.
- The latency for convergence and divergence is about 160 msec, which is twice as fast as that for accommodation.
- The time constant for convergence, divergence and accommodation (time necessary for two-thirds of the action to be completed) is about 0.33 seconds.
- There is dynamic overshoot in convergence and accommodation, but not in divergence.
- The stimuli eliciting vergence movements are two in number:
  - 1) the change in blur pattern of images on the retinas stimulates accommodative convergence
  - 2) a displacement of the image away from the fovea, that is to noncorresponding retinal points by a change in the real or apparent distance of the object of regard from the observer stimulates fusional vergence.
- In the Maddox classification scheme vergence eye movements are described as tonic, accommodative, proximal, and fusional.
  - **Tonic vergence** represents the tonus within the extraocular muscles, e.g. the physiological position of the rest of the eyes. The clinical correlate of the combination of tonic convergence and the anatomical position of rest of the eyes is the distance phoria through the subjective refraction.
  - **Accommodative convergence** occurs as part of the synkinesis of convergence and accommodation. The AC/A ratio describes the amount of accommodative convergence in prism diopters which occurs when the eye accommodates one diopter
    - For perfect yoking, AC/A=IPD (cm) Norm is 4Δ/1D
  - **Proximal (psychic) convergence** is caused by the awareness of nearness of a given object of fixation.
  - **Fusional convergence** serves to maintain fusion of the two retinal images. The effective stimulus for fusional convergence is disparity, not sensory fusion.
  - The basic assumption underlying Maddox's classical graphical analysis is that the dissociated phoria places a real demand on the system which has to be overcome under normal viewing conditions, not just under dissociated conditions.
  - An alternative model suggests that the vergence demand be considered in light of several compensatory mechanisms.
- Prism adaptation or vergence adaptation may occur to an individual's unique fixation disparity essentially setting a new zero point. Fixation disparity or accuracy of vergence movements shows the error in binocular alignment of eyes while viewing a single target.
- Additionally, proximal and accommodative convergence may further lessen fusional vergence demand which if not considered may result in over-estimation of prism needed for fusion.
- The vergence, accommodative, and papillary systems act together in a **near response** often referred to as the **near triad**. Shifting gaze to a near object involves convergence, positive accommodation, and papillary constriction simultaneously.

8. Vestibulo-Ocular Reflex

- The vestibulo-ocular reflex (VOR), also known as the Doll's Head Phenomenon, allows the eye to be fixed on the object of regard despite head movement. The three semicircular canals sense the position of the head and operate via a 3 neuron arc. A vestibular sensory neuron sends its signal to the vestibular nuclei to an extraocular muscle nuclei and an eye movement is manifested through action of an efferent motor neuron. If VOR worked perfectly, the gain of the eye wouldn't move in space though they would move within the orbit. VOR has more rapid dynamics than the pursuit system. VOR can track at up to 4 HZ. Also, there is a shorter latency of only about 15msec for VOR. The target is acquired quickly under VOR via a fast saccade. There is a longer latency and slower movement of the head to complete the reflex.

ANOMALIES OF EYE MOVEMENTS

---

1. Epidemiology, History, Sign/Symptom Inventory

- To diagnose the deviation, check for comitancy, frequency, direction, magnitude, ACA, variability, cosmesis, eye laterality, and eye dominancy
    - **Underactions** are due to trauma, faulty muscle insertions and ligament abnormalities, innervational deficiencies (III, IV, VI), or infectious disease.
    - **Overactions** can be explained in terms of Hering's law of equal innervations to 2 yoked muscles. For example, if the right lateral rectus is paretic, then it requires abnormally high innervation sent to the left medial rectus, making it spastic.
- It is critical to determine if the onset is recent or longstanding, which can be done with a quality symptom inventory:

Symptom Inventory		
Sign/Symptom	**Longstanding**	**Recent**
Diplopia	Rare	Almost always present
Onset	Generally unknown	Probably sudden
Amblyopia	Common	Rare
Trauma	Not usual	Common
Symptoms	Not usual	Common and extreme
Comitance	Spread of comitance may obscure original palsy	Always incomitant
Abnormal head posture	If present well established and difficult to alter	Can be marked but easy to alter. Covering paretic eye eliminates problem
Past-pointing	Absent	Present
Health	Not usually related	Current health may be a significant issue

2. Techniques and Skills to Test

- **Purkinje Images** – Visual Angles
    - Corneal reflex is one of four images reflected from the four surfaces of the eye's optics. These are called **catoptric** images which means they are reflected.
    - Normally the corneal light reflex is displaced about 0.5mm nasally from the pupil center in an adult and 1mm nasally in an infant
    - **Angle Lambda** – angle formed between the papillary axis and the subject's line of sign
        - **Papillary axis** – a line perpendicular to the cornea that passes through the center of the pupil
        - **Light of sight** – a line passing from the center of the pupil to the object of regard
    - **Angle Kappa** – angle formed between the papillary axis and the visual axis
        - **Visual axis** – a line passing from the fovea through the nodal point of the eye
        - **Positive angle kappa =** normal nasalward displacement of the corneal light reflex from the center of the pupil

    - **Negative angle kappa =** temporalward displacement
    - If you measure unequal angles between the two eyes, it indicates that one eye is not fixating foveally, a condition known as **eccentric fixation**, which commonly accompanies amblyopia
  - **Angle Alpha** – angle formed by the intersection between the visual axis and the optical axis
    - **Optical axis** – a line passing through the nodal point that is normal to the surface of the cornea
  - **Angle Gamma** – angle formed between the fixation axis and optical axis
    - **Fixation axis** – a line connecting the point of fixation to the center of rotation of the eye
- Subjective Measurement of Eye Position and Movement
  - **Cover Test**
    - Unilateral to find tropia
    - Alternate to quantify deviation and find phoria
    - In different gaze positions to determine comitancy
  - **Maddox Rod** – place a distorting filter over one eye and align the image of the distorted line with another image seen by the other eye
    - If the eyes are aligned, the targets appear superimposed
    - If the eyes are not aligned, the targets appear displaced in a direction opposite to the ocular deviation
  - **Hirschberg Test** – evaluates the accuracy of binocular fixation
    - Uses angle Lambda and the corneal light reflection to measure eye position
    - 1mm displacement corresponds to 10Δ
  - Angle Kappa Test – evaluates the accuracy of monocular fixations
  - **Worth dot test**
    - Suppression: patients sees only the red or only the green dots
    - NRC: 5 dots if the position of the lights correspond to the angles of deviation. S=H
    - ARC: 4 dots with a manifest deviation. S=0 red glass test (diplopia test gives opposite result.)
    - Uncrossed diplopia=eso
    - Crossed diplopia=exo
- Objective Measurement of Eye Position and Movement
  - Gross positions of globes
  - EOG (Electro Oculography)
  - Infrared limbal tracker
  - Video pupil tracker
  - SRI eye tracker
  - Pursuit and saccadic observation
- Calculating a vertical deviation:
  - Park 3-Step Method
    - Circle the two possible muscles in each eye capable of causing the hyperdeviation
    - Make a vertical circle in the field of gaze causing the greatest vertical hyperdeviation
    - Make an oblique circle in the direction of the head tilt causing the greatest deviation. Muscle circled three times is the paretic muscle.
    - Ex. A patient has a LHyperT that increases on right gaze and left tilt = LSO paresis.

Comitance

- Comitancy means that the angle of deviation of the visual axes remains the same throughout all positions of gaze.
- Incomitant deviations indicate that the angle of deviation changes in different positions of gaze. There are two main types of incomitant deviations:
  - **Congenital** deviations are due to developmental problems in anatomy or functioning of one of the extraocular muscles or their nervous system. They tend to become more comitant as the patient gets older

- **Acquired** deviations are due to long standing conditions that requires no medical attention, recent trauma, or active disease that could require an immediate medical referral like diabetes, hypertension, multiple sclerosis, thyrotoxicosis, temporal arteritis, or tumour
    - It is critical to determine if the onset is recent or longstanding
- Non-Commitancy: A-V patterns
    - A change in ocular alignment that occurs on up, midline, and down gaze as the eyes move from the primary position. Deviation change must be greater than 5D.
    - **A pattern** is when the eyes are relatively closer together in up gaze.
        - Associated with the overaction of the superior obliques with or without underaction of the inferior obliques.
    - **V pattern** us when the eyes are closer together in down gaze.
        - Associated with overaction of the inferior obliques and underaction of the superior obliques.
    - Best pattern for reading is an A pattern eso or V pattern exo.
    - V eso most common, then A eso, V pattern Exo; least is A pattern exo

Esodeviations

- Esodeviations (phoria/tropia) are a constant or intermittent inward deviation of the eye(s).
- Epidemiology
    - 60% of all strabismus in the West is esotropia
    - 30% of all strabismus in the East is esotropia
    - In the US, children are diagnosed with esotropia on average by age 3, with an age of onset of 6 mos to 7 years.
    - 90% of esodeviations in the US occur by age 5
    - Esotropia is more commonly associated with amblyopia than exotropia or hypertropia
    - 10% of esotropes are fully accommodative, 63% of esotropes have some sort of accommodative component.
- **Accommodative Esotropia**
    - An acquired constant or intermittent esotropic deviation that is corrected or reduced 10 Δ or more after wearing hyperopic spectacles.
    - Most prevalent form of childhood strabismus in the West
    - Associated with overaction of the convergence reflex in its association with accommodation
    - Initially intermittent, later becomes constant
    - Many are high hyperopes (average of +4.50D) and/or have a high AC/A
    - Treatment
        - #1 choice is bifocals to correct the refractive error and relax the accommodation. Use a **centration point add** which is equal to the distance deviation (D) divided by the IPD (cm). for children make sure to bisect the pupil.
        - Vision therapy is an adjunct that leads to a greater success rate
        - Miotics: DFP and phospholine iodine (0.06-0.12%) once a day. The literature says that there is no advantage of this therapy compared to bifocals. 51% develop iris cysts which can be prevented with the use of phenylephrine chloride 2.5%. May get nausea and headaches with miotic use
- **Congenital Esotropia**
    - Aka infantile/essential infantile esotropia
    - A constant non-accommodative esotropia in a neurologically intact child which develop shortly after birth (by 6 months)
    - Angle of deviation is large (usually greater than 30D) with moderate refractive error. Often alternating.
    - If unilateral~40% become amblyopic
    - Make sure to differentiate from abduction limitation syndromes or lateral rectus paresis including Duane's and Mobius Syndrome
    - Signs
        - Overacting inferior obliques (68%)
        - Dissociated vertical deviation (50%)
        - Latent Nystagmus (30%)

        - Cross-fixation
    - Treatment
        - Surgery (only a good prognosis for a functional cure if the surgery is done between 1 and 2 years)
- **Duane's Retraction Syndrome**
    - Fibrosis of the lateral rectus muscles and paradoxic innervation due to anomalous connections at the nuclear level in the central nervous system. As a result, CN III goes to the LR instead of the MR causing it to contract on adduction.
    - Signs:
        - Absence of abduction of one eye in lateral gaze (looks like, but isn't, a lateral rectus paresis) with some restricted adduction and retraction while attempting to adduct that eye.
        - Tend to have small eso deviations (as opposed to huge deviations in LR paresis),
        - Head turn to the affected side.
    - Treatment: Alternate occlusion as treatment for amblyopia before age 1
- **Mobius Syndrome**
    - Congenital bilateral CN VI palsy with bilateral CN VIII paresis
    - Signs:
        - Mask-like appearance, sagging of the lower lids (ectropion).
        - Many systemic assoc. mental retardation, decreased bulk, congenital heart defects.
    - Symptoms: tongue weakness/partial atrophy is the most commonly associated feature.
- **Acquired Non-Accommodative Esotropia**
    - An uncommon deviation that develops after 6 months of age that is not associated with an accommodative effort but has an underlying neurological disease.
- **Abnormal Central Nervous System Esotropia**
    - Esotropic deviation associated with a developmental or neurological disorder including cerebral palsy, developmental delay, Down syndrome, and seizure disorder
- **Sensory Esotropia**
    - An esotropic deviation caused by a unilateral or bilateral ocular condition like anisometropic amblyopia, cataract, corneal scarring, and retinal or optic nerve disorders that prevents normal fusion
- **Microstrabismus**
    - A small angle esotropia that most frequently occurs secondarily to surgery for congenital esotropia
    - Signs
        - HARC equal to the angle of deviation
        - Reduced stereo acuity (100 seconds)
        - Small central suppression scotoma
    - Use the 4BI prism test to check for lack of movement
    - Poor prognosis for improvement, it is usually an end stage condition.

Exodeviations

- Exodeviations (phoria or tropia) are an outward deviation of the eye(s)
- Exotropia tends to occur in older children than with esotropia and is less commonly associated with amblyopia
- **Intermittent Exotropia**
    - An acquired intermittent exodeviation ($\geq 10\Delta$) that is not associated with an ocular, paralytic or neurologic disorder.
    - Most cases are divergence excess esotropia, where the patient has a high AC/A with a distance deviation significantly larger than the near deviation
    - It is associated with normal fusional vergences and amplitudes, no amblyopia
    - Harmonious Anomalous Retinal Correspondence (HARC) when troping, Non-Retinal Correspondence (NRC) when eyes are straight = covariation
    - Symptoms
        - Blurred vision
        - Eyestrain/headaches

        - Suppression if early onset
        - Photophobia
    - Treatment
        - For angles <30Δ vision training is the most effective used concurrently with a minus add in a bifocal at distance
        - For angles >30Δ surgery may be indicated
- **Congenital Exotropia**
    - A constant exodeviation that develops by 6 months of age
    - Rare, but can often result in amblyopia
    - Often associated with neurologic or other disorders
- **Convergence Insufficiency**
    - An exodeviation at near due to inability to converge sufficiently
    - Respond best to vision training, can try a minus add at near
- **Abnormal Sensory Nervous System Exotropia**
    - An exodeviation that is associated with a congenital or acquired developmental or neurological disorder like cerebral palsy and developmental delay
- **Sensory Exotropia**
    - An exotropic deviation caused by a unilateral or bilateral ocular condition like anisometropic amblyopia or cataract prevents normal fusion.

Hyperdeviations

- Hyper and Hypotropias are a vertical displacement of one eye relative to the other
- 25% are associated with CN IV palsy
- Other causes can be primary inferior oblique overaction, Brown Syndrome, and CNS associated Hypertropia
- **Brown's Syndrome**
    - Caused by a restricted action of the superior oblique due to a short and fibrosed tendon sheath
    - Signs:
        - Inability to elevate the abducted eye above mid-horizontal;
        - Eye does not elevate on forced ductions.
        - No positive head tilt test.
    - **Note:** mimics IO paresis.

Diplopia

- Diplopia or double vision is a variable symptom that is difficult for patients to describe. If the patient's fusional mechanism is not overtaxed it could be intermittent.
- Almost all diplopia occurs as a result of an acquired paresis or palsy of one or more extraocular muscles or fusional disturbances
- The following questions can help characterize the patient's diplopic symptoms
    - When/how was the diplopia first noticed? (Trauma)
        - Is there a medical history of trauma, diabetes, hypertension or dysthyroidism?
    - Did one or both eyelids droop- partial/total ptosis? (Myasthenia gravis, CN III palsy, Horner's Syndrome)
        - Any other symptoms that might indicate an ischemic episode? – light-headedness, dizziness, spinning, weakness/tingling in the face, arm or leg, difficulty with speech or swallowing, facial or ocular pain?
    - Did one or both eyelids retract? (dysthyroidism)
    - Are the images side by side (horizontal deviation), one above the other (vertical deviation) or a combination?
    - Is one image tilted? (SO palsy)
    - Is it constant throughout the day or intermittent?
    - Is it worse in the distance (LR palsy) or at near (MR or SO palsy)?
    - Has it been getting worse, staying the same or getting better?
    - Is it monocular or binocular?

- Monocular (ghost image) diplopia is usually the result of opacities/irregularities in the cornea and lens (water vacuole), a high degree of astigmatism, a partially dislocated lens, or macular edema.
- Binocular diplopia can be horizontal, vertical, and tilted. Check to see if it is worse in a specific direction to isolate a muscle palsy.

- **Thyroid Ophthalmoplegia (Ophthalmic Grave's)**
    - Hyperthyroidism causing a hypertrophy of the extraocular muscles by cell infiltrates and mucopolysaccharides, which leads to muscle fibrosis. The inferior rectus is affected first, followed by the medial rectus.
        - **Note:** systemically there may be low, normal, or high thyroid levels
        - Mostly affects older women, 50-60 yrs
        - Progressive disease. May get optic neuropathy in which case decompression surgery is indicated
    - Signs: limited elevation, which leads to symptoms of diplopia.
    - Test for proptosis:
        - **Exophthalmometry** -- most important sign is one eye bulging out more than the other (one eye tends to lead the other in thyroid eye disease). Normal exophthalmometry reading is 10-20 mm
- **Myasthenia Gravis (MG)**
    - A chronic autoimmune disease caused by decreased acetylcholine receptor concentration at neuromuscular junctions.
    - 2x more women are affected than men with a peak onset for women of 20-30 years. For men, no peak age onset.
    - Signs:
        - Ptosis and diplopia becoming more severe as the day goes on
        - Weakness of convergence and upgaze.
        - Weakness in muscles involving facial expression and swallowing.
    - Clinical testing: **Tensilon test**
    - Treatment: cholinesterase inhibitor and immunosuppressants.

Motor Fusion

- Motor fusion is the fusion of the eyes based upon disparity vergence, and it maintains eye alignment.
- Common tests of motor fusion include
    - **Reflex Fusion Test**: where you introduce a 15Δ base out prism over the dominant eye and ensure the patient maintains fixation on a near target. The patient should have a convergence response followed by a divergence of the dominant eye upon prism removal.
    - Amblyoscope
- Motor fusion is needed for sensory fusion and stereopsis
- The presence of good motor fusion is a sign that a successful surgical outcome may remain over time
- Motor fusion may be anomalous in strabismics

Paralytic Syndromes

- Extraocular muscle paresis indicates a muscle is weak to pull, whereas a palsy indicates a complete inability of the muscle to pull.
- An extraocular muscle paresis are commonly caused by three things:
    - Cranial nerve paresis
    - Primary muscle disease.
    - Mechanical limitations on the muscle
        - Scarred or "tethered" muscle tissue preventing transmission of muscle pull to the globe (for instance in a blowout fracture where the IR muscle is entrapped in the orbital floor)
        - Posteriorly displaced rectus muscle ("slipped" muscle)
- Many diagnostic tests can be employed to differentiate the paralytic cause
    - Electromyography to determine if and when muscle neurons are fired
    - Forced Duction test to determine if absence of movement is due to neurological disorder or mechanical restriction

        - Tensilon tests to rule out MG
- **III Nerve palsy**
    - Congenital III Nerve palsy
        - The etiology is unknown but involves the IR, MR, SR and IO (never the intraocular muscles)
        - Signs
            - Unilateral lid ptosis
            - Exotropia with hypertropia (down and out)
            - Intact pupil and accommodative reflexes.
        - Symptoms: no diplopia,
        - Treatment: surgery
    - Acquired III nerve palsy
        - Caused by damage to CN III due to:
            - Brainstem lesion
            - Medial longitudinal facsiculus lesion,
            - Inflammatory disease,
            - Vascular lesions
            - Intracranial tumor
            - Multiple sclerosis
            - Trauma.

CN Review		
CN	**Name**	**Function**
I	Olfactory (S)	Smell
II	Optic (S)	Vision
III	Oculomotor (M)	Lid and Eyeball Movement
IV	Trochlear (M)	Eyeball Movement
V	Trigeminal (M, S)	Chewing Face/Mouth Touch & Pain
VI	Abducens (M)	Eyeball Movement
VII	Facial (M, S)	Facial Expression, Tears &Saliva, Taste
VIII	Vestibulocochlear (S)	Hearing, Balance
IX	Glossopharyngeal (M, S)	Taste, Senses Carotid BP
X	Vagus (M, S)	Senses Aortic BP, Slows Heart Rate, Stimulates Digestive Organs
XI	Spinal Accessory (M)	Sternocleidomastoid & Trapezius Muscles
XII	Hypoglossal (M)	Tongue Movement

        - May be partial or complete, involving the extraocular muscles (IR, MR, SR, IO) and/or the intraocular muscles. (if both, complete progressive external ophthalmoplegia)
        - Signs
            - Sudden onset of unilateral ptosis
            - Exotropia and hypotropia
            - If the intraocular muscles are involved, then there is a fixed dilated pupil with paralysis of accommodation.
        - Symptoms: Most likely no complaints of diplopia unless ptosis is lifted.
        - Treatment: PCP referral for MRI and intracranial angiography. May spontaneously resolve if palsy is caused by ischemic vasculopathy.
- **IV Nerve palsy**-superior oblique paresis
    - If acquired, trauma is #1 cause. Can also be caused by lesions, infarcts, aneurysms, diabetes, hypertension.
    - CN IV palsy is the #1 cause of vertical deviation.
        - IV and VI nerve palsies are the most commonly acquired non-comitant deviations.
    - Symptoms:
        - Sudden onset of vertical diplopia, possibly also torsional and vertical.
        - Worse with down gaze at near.
    - Signs:
        - Head tilt to the opposite shoulder.
        - **Bielschowsky's sign** – hyperdeviation increasing markedly towards the side of the paretic superior oblique with the Maddox rod.
- **VI Nerve palsy**-lateral rectus paresis
    - Usually caused by trauma, diabetes, hypertension, stroke, tumors, or neurological disease
    - Symptoms: Horizontal diplopia, worse at distance.
    - Signs:
        - Esotropia in primary position which increases on attempted lateral gaze in the direction of the involved muscle.
        - Head turn towards the side of the paretic muscle.
        - Chin down to take advantage of physiological exo in upgaze
    - Be wary of secondary contracture of the MR; fibrosis can set in

- Distinguish from infantile esotropia causing pseudoparalysis of the lateral rectus. The vestibular system will activate and the eyes will abduct.
- **Congenital VI nerve palsy**: rare, distinguish from Duane's and Mobius syndrome.
- **Acquired VI nerve palsy:** Most likely due to trauma, hypertension or diabetes.

- **Double Elevator Palsy**
  - Monocular paresis of SR and IO.
  - Etiology: supranuclear disturbance
  - Signs: Hypotropia in primary gaze, and affected eye cannot elevate in abduction or adduction.
- **Parinaud's Syndrome**
  - Most commonly caused by pineal gland tumor.
  - Signs:
    - Paralysis of upward and downward gaze.
    - Associated with absence of convergence and pupillary reaction to light.
- **Marcus-Gunn Jaw-winking Syndrome**
  - Abnormal innervation between motor branches of CN V with the superior division of CN III.
  - Signs: unilateral ptosis and momentary lid retraction of the ptotic eye when the mouth is opened or the jaw is moved towards the uninvolved side.
- **Complete Progressive External Ophthalmoplegia**
  - Progressive paresis of the extraocular muscles innervated by the CN III, thought to be caused by a mitochondrial myopathy. Muscle fibrosis occurs.
  - Inherited autosornal dominant
    - In congenital external ophthalmoplegia the internal muscles are also affected; a rare autosomal recessive disease
  - Signs: bilateral condition. Eyes are down and out with fixed ptosis. The ciliary body and the pupils are not affected
  - Treatment: no available therapy.
- **Internuclear Ophthalmoplegia (INO)**
  - Medial longitudinal fasciculus lesion, disrupting communication between CN III, IV, and VI.
  - Signs:
    - Looks like medial rectus paresis.
    - If lesion is towards the posterior, convergence is intact.
    - If lesion is anterior, convergence will be affected.
    - If bilateral or in a young patient, think Multiple Sclerosis.
    - May be confused with Myasthenia Gravis

Fixation Disparity

- **Aka Retinal Slip, Microstrabismus, Closed-loop error**
- Fixation disparity is a small misalignment of the eyes under binocular conditions that is proportional to the demands on fusional vergence. It is a condition in which the images of a binocularly fixated object are not imaged on exact corresponding retinal points but are still within **Panum's fusional areas**
- Fixation disparity is the difference between the convergence angle under binocular viewing and the angle subtended by the target at the center of rotations. It is reflective of the amount of fusional vergence that is active in the total vergence system.
  - The small vergence error is related to the magnitude of an underlying phoria or misalignment of the eyes
- Fixation disparity if a steady state error under viewing conditions
- Factors that influence the magnitude of fixation disparity
  - Phoria
    - Most patients with exophoria have small amounts of fixation disparity but those with esophoria have large amounts because it is more difficult to diverge the eyes and overcome an eso than it is to converge and overcome an exo
  - Prisms
    - Base out reduces eso fixation disparity but induces exo fixation disparity
    - Base in reduces exo fixation disparity but induces eso fixation disparity

- Lenses
  - Horizontal phorias can be changed with binocular accommodation due to the associated stimulation with accommodative convergence
  - Plus lenses relax accommodation and reduce eso
  - Minus lenses stimulate accommodation and reduce exo
- **Associated phoria** – the amount of prism that reduces the fixation disparity to zero. It is a good index of how much prism to prescribe

Nystagmus

- Classification of nystagmus allows identification of abnormal physiology or causative lesions.
- Nystagmus is categorized by the direction of the fast phase
- Nystagmus can be pendular or jerky
  - In jerk nystagmus, the fast component is towards the side of lateral gaze.
- Caloric testing measures the ability of the pontine gaze mechanism to function when internuclear ophthalmoplegia is suspected (recall "COWS"-cold opposite warm same pneumonic).
- Voluntary nystagmus is a rapid, horizontal, pendular type of benign though fatiguing nystagmus.
- Congenital Nystagmus
  - May be different depending on gaze but is usually a pendular, horizontal nystagmus in primary gaze
  - May have a null point about 10-15° away from primary gaze where no nystagmus is present.
  - Congenital nystagmus can decrease visual acuity and is frequently found with other neurological signs.
  - **Infantile Nystagmus**
    - Usually horizontal and uniplanar
    - Dampens with convergence
  - **Latent Nystagmus**
    - Occlusion of one eye results in bilateral jerk nystagmus with the fast component away from the covered eye.
    - Direction is usually horizontal, some rotary, rarely vertical
    - Usually pendular type. A change in the waveform, for example from pendular to jerk is diagnostic for congenital nystagmus.
    - Constancy changes in frequency and amplitude over with time and with field of gaze
    - Frequency-variable, larger in peripheral gaze
    - The nystagmus decreases on convergence
    - Usually have a null point and head turn
  - **Afferent Nystagmus**
    - Nystagmus due to poor vision caused by sensory deprivation, such as
      - Macular scarring due to toxoplasmosis
      - Macular hypoplasia (ocular albinism, aniridia)
      - Retinal degeneration
      - Optic nerve atrophy/hypoplasia
      - Achromatopsia
      - Congenital cataracts
    - Clinical implications: poor prognosis, severely reduced acuity.
  - **Efferent Nystagmus**
    - Due to ocular motor disturbance such as
      - Pathway lesion affecting the pursuit system
      - Brain stem lesion
      - Idiopathic
    - Clinical implications: fair prognosis, minor visual impairment.
    - Associated conditions:
      - Esotropia (50%)
      - Amblyopia (30%)
      - Moderate to high astigmatism

- 40% have defective VOR and OKN
  - **Spasmus Nutans**
    - A transient form of high frequency, low amplitude nystagmus which starts after birth but resolves by childhood.
    - Nystagmus is fine, pendular, rapid, and is often asymmetric in amplitude between the eyes.
    - Often associated with strabismus and head nodding
    - Spasmus Nutans triad: nystagmus, head nodding, torticollis.
    - Must rule out glioma of optic chiasm with MRI.
- Acquired Nystagmus
  - **Downbeat/jerky nystagmus**
    - Appears on horizontal and down gaze; null point usually in upgaze
    - Jerk nystagmus with rapid downbeat, slow upbeat.
    - slow movement with eyes towards the side of the lesion. fast jerk with eyes away from the side of the lesion.
  - **Vestibular nystagmus**
    - A disease of the vestibular nuclei that can cause horizontal, rotary, and vertical nystagmus
    - Intensity increases with gaze in direction of the fast phase
    - Caused by damage to the VIII nerve or the labyrinth, leading to overstimulation of the VIII nerve
    - Associated with vertigo, nausea, oscillopsia, deafness (if CN VIII involved)
    - Acute lesions usually cause nystagmus whereas slow growing lesions may not
    - COWS- normal response
- Induced Nystagmus
  - **Optokinetic Nystagmus (OKN)**
    - A type of induced nystagmus not dependent on high visual acuity. It is a manifestation of the fixation, and following mechanisms with a fast phase that may either represent foveation or corrective movement.
    - Reflexive tracking of extended movement is the basis of the **optokinetic drum.** The OKN drum is a grid of vertical parallel stripes that move across the observer's visual field. As the stripes move across the observer's field of view, his eyes exhibit a series of reflex oscillations, called optokinetic nystagmus, in which tracking alternates with rapid retrace of flyback movements.

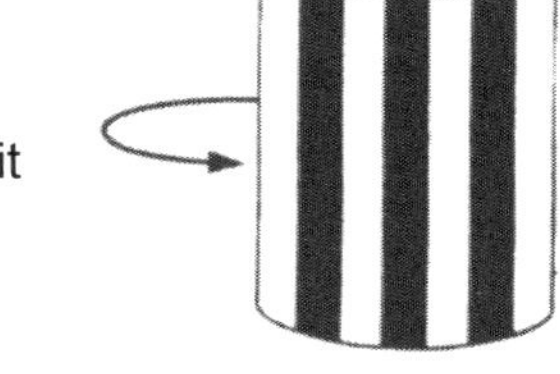

OKN Drum

    - The OKN movements cannot be completely inhibited in the absence of a fixation point.
    - There are two phases of OKN related to fixation.
      - A slow phase velocity (smooth pursuit) which depends on the speed of the stimulus
      - A fast phase which depends on the innate saccadic velocity of the individual.
    - Since angular subtense of the stimulus can be related to visual acuity and since OKN is an involuntary reflex, it can be used to **estimate visual acuity in incompetent or uncooperative subjects.**
    - The most common clinical use of the optokinetic test is the diagnosis of parietal lobe disease.
      - If the patient has a homonymous hemianopsia in the temporal or occipital lobes of the brain, the OKN response is normal.
      - In deep parietal lobe disease affecting the visual radiations, a disturbance of the OKN occurs when targets rotating in the blind field are used.

ACCOMMODATION AND ACCOMMODATIVE VERGENCE

1. Epidemiology, History, and Sign/Symptom Inventory

- **Accommodation** is the ability of the eye to vary its dioptric power in order to focus various distances conjugate to the retina
- According to **Hofstetter's Rule**, the minimum amplitude of accommodation= 18.5 – (age/3) implying that 1D of accommodation is lost every 3 years
- Maddox Components of Accommodation
    - **Blur Driven** Accommodation (Retinal Optical Reflex)– fine adjustment to loss of contrast in fine details of a target
    - **Convergence** Accommodation (Cross Coupled) – increases when the eyes make a fusional convergence movement
    - **Proximal** Accommodation (Perceptual-Spatiotopic) – perception of nearness will stimulate a change in accommodation
    - **Tonic** Accommodation (Intrinsic) – an intrinsic baseline balance between autonomic (sympathetic and parasympathetic) inputs. Resting focus is usually around +1.50 myopic (pseudomyopic) for an emmetrope, reflecting a balance of sympathetic and parasympathetic innervations
- Epidemiology
    - Anomalies of accommodation are commonly encountered in optometric practice
- Symptoms (generally associated with near work)
    - Long-standing blurred vision
    - Headaches
    - Eyestrain
    - Reading problems
    - Fatigue and sleeping problems
    - Loss of comprehension over time
    - A pulling sensation around the eyes
    - Movement of the print
    - Avoidance of reading and other close work
- Drug effects: alcohol increases tonic vergence, decreases AC/A and fusional vergence. THC decreases tonic and fusional vergence.
- **Over Accommodation** (accommodative spasm)
    - Two different types of accommodative spasm
        - Tonic = fixed state of ciliary spasm
        - Clonic = spasmodic cramping of ciliaries
    - Can be caused by physiological (lesions in brain) reasons or refractive error
    - **Latent hyperopia:** amount of hyperopia not revealed by standard refraction.
        - Symptoms:
            - Usually clear distance vision, but occasionally blurring distance and near
            - Sluggish near-focus
            - Blur spasm particularly after reading
            - Headaches
            - Tearing
            - Fatigue
        - Signs:
            - Manifest hyperopia
            - Family Hx of hyperopia,
            - Often a young person under age 15
            - Difference between retinoscopy and subjective refraction of over 0.50 D
            - Eso deviation at near,
            - BI blur point at distance
            - High NRA
            - High dynamic retinoscopy
            - High plus ophthalmoscopy
            - Spasmotic or small pupils, limited near pupil reflex, cornea plana.

- Refractive techniques to relax accommodation: Cycloplegics, sudden fog

- **Pseudomyopia**
    - Symptoms
        - Association with increases in near work
        - Asthenopia when reading, frontal headaches
        - Late onset in life,
        - Spasms of blurred vision
        - Night myopia
        - Stress or tense disposition.
    - Signs:
        - More common in lower amounts of myopia
        - Difference between retinoscopy and subjective
        - Fluctuating refraction
        - Esophoria at near
        - Low accommodative amplitude and facility,
        - High or low plus acceptance on NRA,
        - No lag or lead in accommodation
        - Spasmodic pupil.
    - Testing: cycloplegic or auxiliary refractive techniques to relax an accommodative spasm.

- **Under accommodation:**
    - 3 types:
        - **Accommodative infacility:** problems changing from distance to near and back
        - **Accommodative insufficiency:** decreased amplitude
        - **Accommodative fatigue**: accommodative abilities decreases with time
    - Possible causes of binocular or monocular reduction of accommodation:
        - Functional etiology: Binocular: deficient accommodation due to biological variation in the population, excessive near point work, low illumination, low oxygen level, ocular and general fatigue, convergence insufficiency. Monocular: strong sighting eye dominance.
        - Refractive etiology: Binocular: manifest and latent hyperopia, myopes who do not wear an Rx at near, pseudomyopia, premature and normal presbyopia. Monocular: uncorrected anisometropia, poor distance refractive balance, unequal lens sclerosis.
        - Ocular disease:
            - Binocular: internal ophthalmoplegia, bilateral amblyopia, premature cataracts, bilateral glaucoma, iridocyclitis.
            - Monocular: same as above, but affecting one eye more than the other.
        - Systemic diseases or conditions:
            - Binocular: Hormonal or metabolic: Pregnancy and menstruation, menopause, diabetes, thyroid conditions, anemia, vascular hypertension.
            - Neurologic: Myasthenia Gravis, multiple sclerosis, pineal tumor. Infections: influenza, tuberculosis, whooping cough, measles, syphilis, tonsillar and dental infections, encephalitis.
            - Drugs and medications: Binocular: Residual effects of a cycloplegic eye exam, alcohol neuropathy, many systemic medications.
            - Emotional: usually binocular stress reaction, malingering, hysteria.
        - Lack of accommodation: ciliary muscle involvement or oculomotor nerve as a result of flu, syphilis, diabetes, cerebral disease. Usually accompanied by dilation of pupil.
        - Unequal accommodation:
            - Rare due to unequal sclerosing of lens, III nerve lesion, poor distance refraction

2. Techniques and Skills to Test

Amplitude, Facility of Accommodation

- Duane's Calculation of amplitude of accommodation:
    - Mean = 18.5 - 0.3 (age)
    - Minimum amplitude = 15.0 - 0.25 (age)
- Skills to test:
    - Accommodative Amplitude:
        - Subjective: Push up

- Objective: MEM retinoscopy
  - Normal: small lag of about 0.50D, see fast bright with motion deficiency:
  - Abnormal: greater than 0.75D lag, slow dim with motion spasm:
  - no lag or lead, against motion
- NPA/NPC: check for fatigue on repetitions 5cm break 7cm recovery >10 cm abnormal
- Accommodative facility:
  - Flippers
    - Children: use ± 2.00D flippers at 40 cm and record how many cycles are performed in one minute
    - Adults: use ± 1.50D tippers at 40 cm and record how many cycles are performed in 1 min
    - Means are 12 cycles per min monocularly and 8 cycles per min binocularly

Accommodative Disorders				
Tests	**Insufficiency**	**Ill-Sustained**	**Excess**	**Infacility**
ACC AMP	↓	↓ with repeat PU	Normal	Normal
NRA	Normal	Normal	↓	↓
PRA	↓	↓ slightly	Normal	↓
Monoc/Binocular Flippers	↓ Minus	↓Minus with time	↓ Plus	↓Plus and Minus
MEM	Large Lag	High Normal or Lag	Lead	Normal
Fused X-Cyl	High Plus	High Normal or Lag	Low Plus	Normal
Treatment	Reading Glasses VT	Reading Glasses VT	VT	VT

Analysis of Accommodation and Vergence Relationships

- In cases of accommodative dysfunction, it is not unusual for the phoria to be outside norms
- Accommodative insufficiency can be associated with esophoria. This is because the patient uses additional innervations to compensate and causes additional accommodative convergence causing esophoria.
- **Pseudoconvergence insufficiency** is when a patient has an accommodative insufficiency and underaccommodates relative to the stimulus. Decreased accommodative convergence will measure as a larger exophoria at near. Treatment of the accommodative insufficiency will eliminate the appearance of the exophoria.
- The **Near Response (Triad)** is the term given to the working together of the vergence, accommodative and papillary systems, when the gaze is shifted to near (convergence + positive accommodation +pupillary constriction)
  - The **AC/A Ratio** describes the amount of accommodative convergence (prism diopter) which occurs when the eye accommodates 1D.
    - High AC/A ratios are hard to treat because patient has inability to diverge eyes
    - Lower AC/A ratios are easier to treat because patient can compensate with accommodative convergence. normal 4Δ/1D
    - AC/A Ratio can be calculated by comparing the phoria positions at distance and near
      - Eso deviation (+)
      - Exo deviation (-)
      - D_n= deviation at near (Diopters)
      - D_d= deviation at distance (Diopters)

AC/A Ratio
AC/A = PD (cm) + (D_n-D_d)/2.50

    - AC/A is innate, mostly linear, stable until presbyopia than increases resistant to change through orthoptics
  - The **CA/C Ratio** is the amount of convergence accommodation (D) which occurs when the eye converges 1 prism diopter
    - Divergence relaxes accom
    - Convergence increases accom
    - BI prism causes divergence so accom decreases through CA/C
    - BO prism causes convergence so accom increases through CA/C

Modified Duane White Classifications					
Classification	**Distance Deviation**	**Near Deviation**	**Calculated AC/A Ratio**	**Treatment Option 1**	**Treatment Option 2**
Convergence Insufficiency	Ortho to low Exo	High Exo	Low	VT	BI Prism Readers
Divergence Insufficiency	High Eso	Ortho to Low Eso	Low	BO prism overall or at distance only	VT
Convergence Excess	Ortho to low Eso	High Eso	High	Added plus at near and BO overall if Eso at distance	BO or VT
Divergence Excess	High Exo	Ortho to Low Exo	High	VT	Added Minus at distance or BI
Basic Esophoria	Eso similar to near	Eso similar to distance	Normal	BO prism overall	Added Lenses or VT
Basic Exophoria	Exo similar to near	Exo similar to distance	Normal	VT	BI Prism overall

- Vergence training techniques:
  - Tromboning: eccentric circles or pencil push ups
  - Vergence jumps: fusion circles jumps or jump ductions
  - Sliding vergence: eccentric circles or vectograms
  - Step vergence: red-green circles and loose prism
  - Isometric vergence: hold eyes crossed or use training lenses.
- Clinical wisdom rules:
  - **Exo**: treat 1/3 of angle of deviation, VT works better
  - **Eso**: treat entire angle of deviation, optics work better
  - **Sheard's criterion**
    - compensating reserve is 2x demand; **R >= 2D**
    - **P = 2/3 D - 1/3R**; disregard + and – signs
    - Rx compensating prism, only when + P
  - **Percival's criterion**
    - Does not take phoria into account
    - Center demand line in the center 1/3 of patient's zone
    - P = 1/3G - 2/3L; G & L are greater and lesser blur values on VG
    - Only a (+) P will be Rx'ed
    - Prism is given in direction of greater
    - If phoria is asymmetric in zone, patient can get opposite prism (decompensating)

3. Biomechanics of Accommodative Reflexes

- The **Gullstrand/Helmholtz Relaxation Theory of Accommodation:** The ciliary muscle contracts and acts against a passive elastic restoring force produced by Bruch's membrane and the Zonule of Zinn. The contraction relieves the tension on the Zonule of Zinn, allowing the lens to assume its more natural rounded shape (increasing its refractive power)
  - The overall position of the lens is slightly more forward because most of the changing of the lens is in the anterior surface.
  - Relaxation of the ciliary muscle allows the elastic fibers (zonules) to pull on the lens capsule and flatten it.
- Neural pathway for accommodation
  - The tone of the ciliary muscle is determined by the balance of innervations from parasympathetic and sympathetic inputs
    - Parasympathetic inputs act to contract the muscle and sympathetic inputs act to inhibit the parasympathetic inputs
    - The **ciliary ganglion** (located inside the orbit) contains cells which generate parasympathetic signals for both accommodation and papillary constriction

- The **parasympathetic input** to the ciliary muscles from the **Edinger-Westphal Nucleus** of the oculomotor nucleus.
- Supranuclear control of accommodation has not been studied so little is known about the specific pathway
- The **sympathetic input** to the ciliary muscle follows the same general pathway as for pupil dilation. Axons from the 8th cervical and first two thoracic regions in the spinal cord synapse in the superior cervical ganglion and project to the ciliary body via the **long posterior ciliary nerves**

- Physiological changes that occur during positive accommodation
  - The lens thickens by about 0.5mm along the anterior-posterior axis (3.5-4mm)
  - The horizontal lens diameter is reduced slightly (1mm to 9.6mm)
  - Central anterior radius of curvature (ROC) decreases from 11-5.5mm
  - Choroid is pulled forward, stretching the retina slightly, causing displacement of the blind spot
  - Lens drops slightly under the influence of gravity

PUPILS

---

1. Purposes and Roles for Vision

- Varying the size of the pupil serves three main functions:
  - Modifies amount of light into eye, increasing sensitivity of the eye under bright and dim conditions.
    - Pupil size varies from 2-8mm.
  - Increases depth of focus (during constriction)
    - Minimizes optical aberrations by reducing aperture size.
  - Increases the power of the eye (during accommodation)

2. Dynamics of Muscle Action

- **Iris**
  - Most anterior portion of the uveal tract.
  - Consists of two muscles which are derived from neural ectoderm: the sphincter pupillae and the dilator pupillae.
  - **Sphincter muscle:**
    - When maximally contracted can constrict the pupil down to approximately 1.0 mm.
    - Smooth muscle under parasympathetic control. PS fibers synapse in the ciliary ganglion and continue to the sphincter via short ciliary nerves.
    - Innervation carried by CN III
  - **Dilator muscle**
    - Can dilate the pupil up to approximately 9.0 mm.
    - Fibers of the dilator muscle are in a primitive state and are called myoepithelial cells. They are not true muscle fibers, as are the fibers of the sphincter muscle.
    - Primitive smooth muscle under sympathetic control.
    - Innervated by cervical sympathetic chain, synapsing in the superior cervical ganglion. Post ganglionic fibers enter in the eye through short and long ciliary nerves.
    - The dilator muscle consists of radial extensions of the unpigmented anterior epithelium of the iris.
  - The layers of the iris are: anterior border layer (part you see), stroma (contains sphincter muscle), anterior epithelium and dilator muscle (one cell layer), and posterior pigmented epithelium (also one cell layer).
- **Ciliary body**
  - Consists of smooth muscle in three different orientations:
    - Longitudinal - which arise from the anterior choroid and run to the scleral spur
    - Circular fibers - which form a sphincter around the edge of the ciliary body just behind the root of the iris

- Radial fibers - which form a meshwork between the longitudinal and circular fibers
  - Accommodation occurs via these three types of smooth muscles relaxing tension on the zonule fibers. The meridional fibers pull on the epichoroidal tissue and drag the ciliary body forward. The circular fibers decrease the diameter of the circle the lens is suspended in. The radial fibers perform both of these actions but to a lesser degree.
  - Ciliary body also produces aqueous humor. Pars plana restores mucopolysaccharides important to vitreous pars plicata makes aqueous (mostly H20) via active transport or diffusion from capillaries just beneath epithelial layers of the ciliary body
  - A third function secondary to accommodation is facilitation of aqueous outflow due to stretching of the trabecular meshwork during accommodation

3. Biomechanics of Pupillary Reflexes

- The rods and cones are the receptors for the pupillary response to light as well as for accommodation.
- Pupillary reflexes
  - **Constriction** – light falling on the retina excites the rods and cones which send information up the optic nerve to the pretectal nucleus where a synapse occurs. From here the signal travels to the Edinger-Westphal (EW) nucleus on both sides of the brain where a 2nd synapse occurs (refer to figure on previous page). From the EW nucleus, signals travel down the third cranial nerve on both sides of the brain to the ciliary ganglion in each orbit where a 3rd synapse occurs. Signals enter both eyes through the short ciliary nerves and innervate the sphincter muscle to give rise to both the direct and consensual pupillary light reflex.

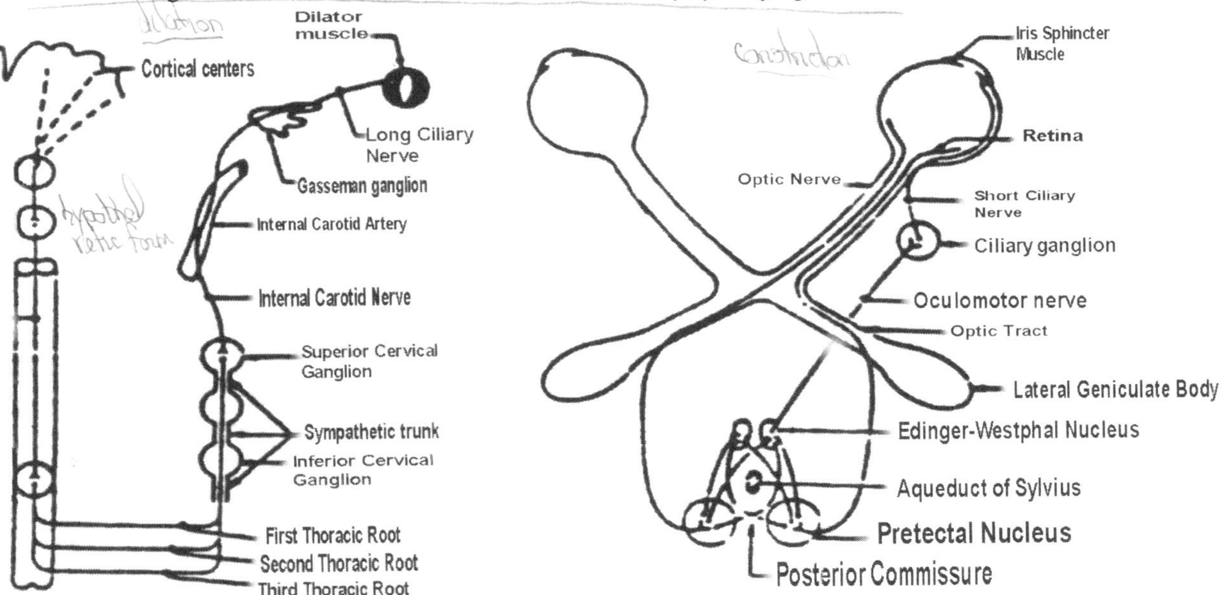

  - **Dilation** – light (or absence of) falling on the retina excites the rods and cones, which send signals up the optic nerve to synapse in the lateral geniculate body. The signal then travels to the cortex and synapses again in the hypothalamus and reticular formation (refer to figure on previous page). From there, the signal travels down the spinal cord to the sympathetic trunk on both sides of the spinal cord to synapse once again in the superior cervical ganglion. From there, the signals travel through the long ciliary nerves to the eye, where they innervate the dilator muscle to give rise to dilation.
  - **Accommodation** – the stimulus to accommodation is foveal blur. This is reported via the optic nerve to higher visual centers. Parasympathetic fibers originating in the EW nucleus travel down the third cranial nerve to the ciliary ganglion in the orbit. The signal is carried to the eye through the short ciliary nerves which innervate the ciliary muscle. Parasympathetic stimulation causes contraction of all three parts of the ciliary muscle resulting in accommodation due to relaxation of the zonules.

4. Interrelationships between Pupillary Changes, Accommodation, and Convergence (the Near Reflex)

- Accommodative Controller sends signals to Vergence Controller producing Accommodative-Vergence or AC/A ratio.
- Vergence-Accommodation or CA/C ratio – vergence producing accommodation is the most common occurrence in normal visual function. When target moves from out to in, the target will be off the fovea causing a large bi-temporal disparity. The accommodative system only works with foveal stimulation. Therefore, the fovea must be aligned with the image before there can be stimulus for accommodation. The foveal disparity drives the vergence system to converge and align the images.
- After convergence puts the target on both foveas, accommodation can correct blur and use blur to drive the accommodative system. If blur falls off the fovea, the accommodative system does not respond. We use the vergence system all the time this way. CA/C = convergence and implicitly stands for divergent accommodation produced by divergence.
- Controller of vergence to controller of pupil - there is a large neurophysiological controversy over what drives the pupil. Both accommodation and vergence drive the pupil. When a target moves near, convergence accommodation drives pupil constriction, the "near reflex". If the target moves away, divergence relaxes accommodation and the pupil dilates.

5. Factors affecting Pupil Size

- Aging – From the second year of life to adolescence, the pupil increases in size and thereafter decreases. The pupillary area at 60 years of age is approximately one-third the size at age 20. Apparently, the muscles controlling pupillary dilation age more rapidly than those controlling contraction. In addition, degeneration occurs in the epithelial cells of the iris as well as in other ocular structures, and the loosened cells may be found on the surfaces of the iris, cornea and lens capsule. These changes tend to increase the scattering of incident light.
- Sleep – constriction
- General anesthesia:
    - Stage 1 - excitatory phase – dilation
    - Stage 2 - light anesthesia – dilation
    - Stage 3 - deep anesthesia – constriction
    - Stage 4 - near death – dilation
- Light/vergence/accommodation – the near triad
- Corneal pain – constriction due to oculopupillary/trigeminal reflex, but prolonged pain activates the sympathetic system and the pupil dilates
- Systemic pain dilation
- Vestibular stimulation dilation
- Psychic stimulation – dilation (i.e. danger, surprise, arousal, etc., stimulate the sympathetic system)
- Hippus – normal spontaneous fluctuations in the pupillary control system

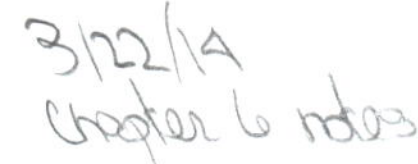

Chapter 8 – Amblyopia/Strabismus

SENSORY ANOMALIES OF BINOCULAR VISION/STRABISMUS

1. Epidemiology, History, and Symptom Inventory

- **Amblyopia** (aka "lazy eye") is a unilateral or bilateral loss of vision due to pattern deprivation and/or a barrier to binocular interaction. It is a reduction in form vision with a retention of normal light perception
  - The loss of vision is not correctable by refractive or surgical means and is not due to structural or pathological anomalies (vision loss is still present even after the pathology has been ameliorated)
- Types of Amblyopia
  - Refractive (Anisometropia, Isometropia, and Meridional)
  - Strabismic
  - Stimulus Deprivation
- Epidemiology
  - Amblyopia affects 6-10 million Americans.
  - Strabismus is the most common cause of amblyopia
  - There is a genetic link
- Symptoms/Signs
  - Strabismus (constant/unilateral is more detrimental)
  - Inability to judge depth correctly
  - History of poor vision in one eye
  - Family history of strabismus and amblyopia
  - Visual acuity is 20/30 or worse, or the interocular acuity difference is greater than 2 lines.
  - Vision is described as indistinct (not helped by pinhole). Strabs especially deny "blur."
  - Visual acuity measurements are heavily influenced by contour interaction. The strongest interference for contours is about 2-2.5 times the unflanked Minimum Angle of Resolution (MAR); while there is no effect for separations of 5 times unflanked MAR.

2. Techniques and Skills to test:

Monocular Fixation Patterns

- Monocular fixation – except the very young, anxious, hyperactive, and inattentive, every patient should be capable of monocular fixation for 10 seconds without any grossly noticeable eye movements.
- Using a monocular visuscope, measure and analyze the
  - Type of fixation: central, parafoveal, paramacular, peripheral
  - Mode of fixation: steady vs. unsteady
- Eccentric fixation is often associated with amblyopia. The further eccentric the fixation pattern the worse the optimum visual acuity in the amblyopic eye will be
- Some examples of monocular fixation disorders of fixation include the following
  - **Ocular flutter** - horizontal oscillations that burst in a spring-like manner, and decrease gradually: may accompany saccades or occur randomly; usually due to cerebellar disease
  - **Opsoclonus** – more advanced form of ocular flutter
  - **Square wave jerks –** rare disorder that can be confused with nystagmus; consist of unwanted saccades that occur at random, interrupting fixation, followed by a corrective saccade
  - **Congenital nystagmus** – the most common type of nystagmus (affecting males twice as frequently as females), present at birth or shortly after birth, can be solely a jerk nystagmus,

pendular, or a combination. The following symptoms may be present: head turns, rhythmic head movements, reduced VA's of varying degree.
    - **Latent nystagmus** – conjugate, jerk nystagmus which Is only evoked by occlusion of one eye. Associations include: strabismus (congenital esotropia, double hypertropia, and amblyopia). Usually have no reported symptoms.
    - **Acquired nystagmus** – should be evaluated by a neuro-ophthalmologist, especially in the case of acquired vertical nystagmus. Patients may complain of vertigo, nausea, and variable oscillopsia.
    - **Spasmus nutans** – characterized by head nodding and pendular, high frequency, low amplitude (usually horizontal) nystagmus; it is most commonly found between the fourth and twelfth month after birth, lasting about 2 years. It affects males equally as frequently as females.

Amblyopia

- **Strabismic** – prognosis is worse with constant, unilateral, and early age of onset.
    - Contrast sensitivity could be reduced
- **Refractive** –
    - *Anisometropic:* unilateral; typically in eye with greatest plus; acuity worsens in proportion to refractive difference; hyperopia > 1.5 D difference; myopia > 3 D difference;
    - *Isoametropic;* bilateral; associated with high, but approximately equal, refractive error; depends on amount and sign of error;
    - *Meridional:* unilateral or bilateral; due to uncorrected astigmatism; in meridian mostly out of focus
- Form deprivation due to: congenital cataract; tumors; ptosis; corneal opacities; occlusion
- Other causes of amblyopia include toxic/nutritional factors and functional visual loss (hysterical or malingering)
- Tests:
    - Visual Acuity: Single optotype visual acuity better then linear acuity (crowding phenomenon)
    - Contrast sensitivity
    - Fixation pattern (eccentric fixation)

Sensory Fusion and Stereopsis

- Sensory fusion can be of color or of form. Color fusion is of lesser importance. Form fusion is of four levels:
    - Simultaneous perception (diplopia) – no fusion occurs
    - Superimposition (first degree fusion) of two dissimilar objects, confusion occurs (rather than true sensory fusion).
    - Flat fusion (second-degree fusion) of two similar objects, resulting in true sensory fusion without stereopsis
    - Stereopsis (third-degree fusion) occurs when there is a disparity between images that results in the perception of a three-dimensional object in visual space.
- Eccentric fixation and strabismus can make stereo acuity reduced

Anomalous correspondence

- Anomalous retinal correspondence (ARC) occurs as a defense mechanism against diplopia, likely during cortical development and is characterized by a lack of correlation between homologous retinal loci with respect to directional values.
- Presence of ARC indicates a difference between the horizontal objective angle of deviation (H) and the subjective angle of directionalization (S), resulting in an angle of anomaly (A).
- ARC can be harmonious (HARC) or, less often, unharmonious (UNHARC), and even more rare

(NRC)	H = S, A = 0
(ARC)	H ≠ S
(HARC)	H = A, S = 0
(UNHARC)	H > S; H > A
(PARC Type I)	A > H; S opposite direction to H (S < 0)
(PARC Type II)	S > H; A opposite direction to H (A < 0)

are the paradoxical types (PARC). The conventions for calculating angles for eso and exo deviations are (+) and (-), respectively.

- Caution is advised in the cases of UNHARC and PARC, and even in large non-comitant deviations, as intensive binocular training in these cases may result in intractable diplopia.
- One study has shown ARC to be present in 45% of strabismics; amongst esotropes, 53% had ARC, and amongst the exotropes 16% had ARC.
- Conditions that make ARC more likely are: infantile strabismus (rather than late onset), constant angles (rather than intermittent), small angles (rather than large), and esotropia (rather than exotropia).

Suppression

- Suppression is a lack of perception of objects in all or part of the field of vision in one eye under binocular conditions. It is attributed to cortical inhibition and can occur especially in amblyopes due to the decreased visual acuity in the amblyopic eye.
- Can occur to a small degree with heterophoria, and to larger degrees in strabismus.
- Classified by size (central or peripheral) and intensity (a gradient between natural/shallow to unnatural/deep).
- Patient may report diplopia under natural viewing conditions; specific fields of gaze; or at specific distances
- **Worth Dot Test**: red-green filters are worn by the patient (convention: red over right). Suppression is assessed in light (natural) and dark (unnatural) conditions. The distance between the flashlight and observer is varied to determine the size of suppression. 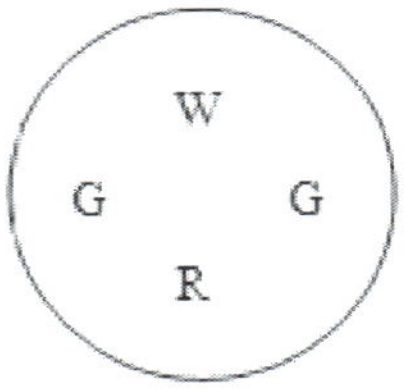
- The major amblyoscope can be used to detect the presence of suppression with first-degree targets which utilize superimposition targets. Suppression size and depth can be assessed with second-degree targets which utilize flat fusion targets. Lack of stereopsis can be assessed by using third-degree targets (stereo-fusion targets) which would also indicate the presence of suppression.

Chapter 9 – Perceptual Function/Color Vision

ANOMALIES SECONDARY TO ACQUIRED NEUROLOGICAL IMPAIRMENT

1. Adaptations to Clinical Techniques and Tests

- Adaptations are needed to allow the assessment of the visual abilities of patients with acquired systemic conditions (CVA, multiple sclerosis, etc) and Traumatic Brain Injury (TBI) which result in neurological impairment and subsequent vision perceptual dysfunction.
- Subtle deficits can be overlooked in the patient with acquired brain injury. These defects may be secondary to trauma, stroke, and cerebral vascular accident. Of particular interest are binocular vision disorders – especially exodeviations, convergence insufficiency; accommodative disorders (including accommodative insufficiency, excess, and infacility); and saccadic and pursuit anomalies.
- Tests that measure each system's ability to maintain performance over time are crucial.
- Patients may report discomfort or nausea during some tests. If normal results are obtained during these tests, they should be repeated multiple times or with extended time limits for facility testing.
- The following side effects of brain injury should be taken into account when testing patients
    - Visual Field loss – Central, Sector, Peripheral, Total, Altitudinal
    - Photophobia
    - Reading disorders – accommodation problems, convergence problems
    - Diplopia – exotropia, esotropia, hypertropia
    - Cranial Nerve Paresis/Palsies – III, IV, VI, VII
    - Small changes in refractive errors, unstable ambient vision
    - Nystagmus
    - Lagophthalmos, dry eye (decreased blink rate)
    - Visual hallucinations, memory loss
    - Anisocoria
    - Eye movement disorders, fixation, pursuits
    - Frequent headaches
    - Disturbances in body image and spatial relationships
    - Right-left discrimination problems
    - Agnosia – difficulty in object recognition
    - Apraxia – difficulty in manipulating objects

Noncomitancy

- Comitancy: variation of deviation in different fields of gaze. Cover tests should be performed at distance in all fields of gaze, as well as at near in the reading position.
- Classified by process:
    - **Congenital:** nerve palsy, forceps injury, hydrocephalus, agenesis of muscle
    - **Acquired:** trauma, acute inflammation (orbital cellulitis, cavernous sinus thrombosis, meningitis), chronic inflammation (syphilis, orbital pseudotumor, thyroid ophthalmopathy, tuberculous meningitis), tumors (glioma, meningioma, acoustic neuroma, orbital tumor metastases), demyelination, vascular (aneurysm, diabetes, hypertension, ischemic cerebral disease, embolism, giant-cell arteritis). degenerative (progressive external ophthalmoplegia)
- The most common non-comitant deviations are sixth- and fourth-nerve palsies. Detailed EOM and pupil testing are essential to rule out sixth nerve palsies. The Parks 3-Step method should be used to detect fourth-nerve (superior oblique) palsies:
    - **Step 1:** Which eye is deviated upward in primary gaze?

- **Step 2:** Is the deviation greater in left or right gaze?
- **Step 3:** Is the deviation greater when tilting the head to the left or right shoulder?

- Because cyclovertical heterophorias are common in patients with a brain injury, the double Maddox rod test should also be performed.

Field loss and neglect

- Detailed field testing should be conducted to determine the presence and location of brain lesions. The clinician should keep in mind the neural anatomy when considering the following ten key points with respect to field defects:
    - Optic nerve-type defects
    - Defects involving the optic chiasm
    - Optic tract or LGN defects
    - Altitudinal separations of the temporal lobe
    - Altitudinal separations of the parietal lobe
    - Central homonymous hemianopia
    - Macular sparing
    - Congruity
    - Optokinetic nystagmus
    - Temporal crescents
- Hemifield neglect may result from damage to the right cerebral hemisphere (in the areas controlling visuo-spatial attention – the PPC, FEF, and cingulate gyrus). The left hemifield is affected, and may appear as a left homonymous hemianopia when testing confrontational fields bilaterally. Unilateral testing will reveal intact areas of the left visual field.

Loss of accommodation

- Loss of accommodation may occur. Suspect it especially in young head injury patients who should not have a loss of accommodation (under age 42).
- Direct measures include monocular amplitudes and monocular accommodative facility testing. Indirect measures include binocular accommodative facility testing, NRA/PRA, and MEM retinoscopy.

Loss of fusion

- Loss of fusion: direct testing includes step vergence and facility testing, near point of convergence, stereopsis testing, and Worth 4 Dot. Indirect tests include NRA/PRA, binocular accommodative facility, MEM retinoscopy
- Patients may have reduced convergence abilities after stroke or head injury

Vision perception-motor deficiencies

- Vision perception-motor deficiencies: eye movement assessments can quickly be made using the developmental eye movement test, or through an objective eye movement recording via the Visagraph.
- Patients may need to relearn reading skills, and may not be able to recognize or manipulate objects
- Depending on the area of brain injury, deficits may cause the inability to integrate the function of the two sides of the body, inability to perceive form and position in space, and visual figure ground.
- Many believe that all of these inabilities can be aided with vision therapy

2. Modification of Optometric Management for the Patient with Acquired Neurological Impairment

- Role of the optometrist in screening, evaluating, managing, and referring patients within the multi-disciplinary rehabilitation team concerning sequelae of neurological impairment. The optometrist should work actively with the rehabilitation team, including physicians, as well as the occupational, physical, and recreational therapists, and speech and language pathologists.
    - In addition to making referrals to neuro-ophthalmologists as necessary, the optometrist should be responsible for the management of:

- Refractive error
    - Binocular vision
    - Accommodative disorders
    - Eye movement disorders
    - Visual field loss
    - Ocular disease
    - Other visual manifestations of acquired brain injury
- Modification of optometric treatment for the patient with acquired neurological impairment
- Lenses and prisms: because small amounts of ametropia can result in seemingly exaggerated symptoms in patients with acquired brain injury, optical correction of ametropia should be the first consideration.
    - Patients with accommodative insufficiency and ill-sustained accommodation may benefit from added plus lenses.
    - The higher prevalence of vertical heterophoria and non-comitant deviations make small amounts of prism crucial in cases of ABI.
- Forms of occlusion (nasal, temporal, full, etc.): if intractable diplopia cannot be eliminated and causes enough distress to the patient, total or sectoral occlusion of the non-preferred eye is recommended. This can be done with rigid or soft contact lenses or with Magic Tape 64 over spectacles.
- Vision therapy: while there are studies that show that patients with acquired brain injury may show spontaneous improvement in symptoms over the course of 6-12 months after the injury, the clinician should still actively work to rehabilitate the patient. The primary differences in vision therapy with patients with acquired brain injury are the prognosis for improvement and the length of treatment. Both are more variable and unpredictable. Factors that affect results are the cognitive and perceptual problems involved, visual fields loss, excyclotorsion, and sensory fusion disruption.
- Counseling and education: patients and their families should be made aware of how the visual problems associated with acquired brain injury may affect daily living activities, such as with reading, writing, shopping, dressing, sports, and driving. Recommendations on modification to the patient's environments should be made to enable the highest possible level of function. These recommendations are best arrived at by working closely with the rehabilitation team

---

SPACE PERCEPTION

---

1. Direction and Depth Discrimination

Monocular cues→ Pictorial

- Pictorial cues are observed in a 2-D representation
- **Retinal image size:** As an object moves toward or away from the observer, the size of the retinal image will vary in the direct proportion to the distance. The larger object appears closer to the observer.
- **Interposition** (or overlap): If an object partially occludes another, the occluded object is perceived to be behind, in back, or furthest away. This is one of the strongest cues to depth. (see figure)

Overlap Figure

- **Lighting and shadow:** Both create strong depth cues since objects with depth usually cast shadows. Shadows are expected at the bottom of an object since the light source is expected to come from above and from a distance.
- **Clarity:** objects that are far away appear less clear or more hazy than objects that are close, thus giving the perception of depth. Objects that are far away also appear bluer in color.
- **Elevation horizon:** Objects higher on the horizon or higher in the field of view appear to be farther away.
- **Linear perspective:** If an object extends in depth toward and away from the observer, the near portions of the objects will be imaged larger on the retina than the more distant portions.
- **Texture gradient:** Created when the spacing between adjacent objects decreases with distance from the observer, as in the case of railroad tracks. The observer assumes that all the objects are the same size and only by being farther away can they appear smaller and more tightly packed together.

- **Contrast:** The lower the contrast ratio, the further the apparent distance.
- **Familiarity:** Based on personal experience, we know how large certain things are, so depth can therefore be deduced or estimated.

Monocular Cues→Kinetic

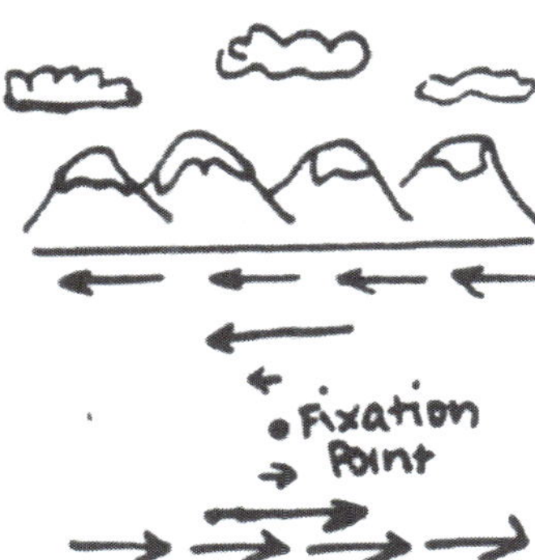

- **Looming:** As an object approaches, its image gets bigger on the retina.
- **Motion parallax** or optical flow patterns: The relative movement of objects at different distances from the observer. For example, if you drive down a road and fixate on the horizon, all objects closer than the horizon will move in the opposite direction. (see figure)
- **Observer motion:** When you fixate on something close and move from side to side, the object stays in place but the background moves. When you fixate on the background, the objects that are closer appear to move.
- **Dynamic interposition:** The observer motion cue gives information on how far an occluded object is behind an anterior object.

Binocular Depth Cues

- At large viewing distances, the monocular cues become more important. Binocular differences in visibility and perspective are due to the lateral displacement of the eyes, giving them different views.
- Convergence: Range-finding information. If the eyes are converged, the object must be close.
- Accommodation: Same mechanism as convergence.
- Situational myopia: The eyes accommodate not on the object but slightly closer as though the eyes were myopic. Four types of situational myopias are night (dark focus), space (empty field), instrument, and accommodative spasm myopia.
- Specific distance tendency: In the absence of depth information, points are perceived at a certain distance, usually around 1.5 meters.
- Binocular disparity: Whenever the relative positions of objects on the retina are different, binocular disparity gives a three dimensional perception.

Oculocentric Spatial Localization

- A monocular phenomenon. It involves localization of each direction in space with reference to the entrance pupil of the observing eye and its angular deviation from the line of sight.
- Every point on the retina has a visual direction associated with it called the local sign.
- The local sign associated with the fovea is called the primary visual direction. All other retinal elements have local signs associated with them called secondary visual directions. The secondary directions are all relative to the primary visual direction. The fact that the secondary visual direction is always relative to the primary visual direction is known as oculocentric visual direction.

Egocentric Spatial Localization

- Localization of an object in visual space with the self as the center of reference.
- Hering's law of identical visual direction states that the two foveae have the same visual perception when both eyes are open.
- When both eyes are open, oculocentric visual direction is no longer used but rather the egocentric visual direction is seen. This direction is relative to the mid-line and is analogous to a cyclopean eye.
- This localization takes place at the cortical level and requires a combination of two oculocentric localizations.

2. Characteristics of Sensory Function

- **Summation**: The cumulative effect of stimulating both eyes simultaneously. The probability of seeing is 75% with two eyes versus 50% with one eye according the formula; p = 1-(1-p)

- **Binocular suppression:** The lack of perception of normal visible objects in all or part of the field of view of one eye when viewing with both eyes. Attributed to cortical inhibition, binocular suppression is often seen in strabismus and amblyopia.
- **Binocular rivalry:** Alteration of perception during stimulation of the eyes with targets of different orientations, colors, or borders.
  - Contrast dependent: If contrast is unbalanced, the eye with the greater contrast will see the image more than the other eye.
  - Attentional factors: Attending only to horizontal lines slows down the rivalry.
  - Spectral sensitivity changes under dominant and suppressed phases: dominant phase – chromatic channels; suppressed phase – active luminous channels.
- **Retinal correspondence:** When stimulated, points in each of the retinas simultaneously give rise to a single percept. These points have common lines of direction.
  - Corresponding retinal points: the visual directions of the two foveae correspond; receptors situated on the same side of each fovea and at the same angular distance have the same visual direction; these are called corresponding retinal points. Images stimulating the two retinas at corresponding retinal points are interpreted as arising from the same visual direction or point in space.
  - Two stages in the single binocular vision process:
    1. The image of each eye must fall on corresponding retinal points.
    2. These points must be relayed to the brain for processing; this is called sensory fusion. The images must be similar for fusion to occur. Within certain limits, stimulation of disparate points will allow for stereopsis. This area is called Panum's Fusional Area. An object that does not lie on Panum's area will be seen as double. (Crossed: image seen by the left eye is on the right field of view. Uncrossed: image seen by the left eye is on the left field of view.)
- **Horopter:** The locus of points in space for which binocular disparity is zero. For a fixed convergence of the eyes, as in point P of the figure, the horopter represents the surface of points where images on the two retinas will be projected at corresponding locations in space. For locations off the horopter but still within the bounds of Panum's Fusional Area (PFA) as shown in the diagram, there will be some amount of retinal disparity, which will be reported as seeing the object with depth perception. Outside of PFA, double images will be reported. This is the basic definition of the horopter. There are a number of different criteria used to determine the horopter.

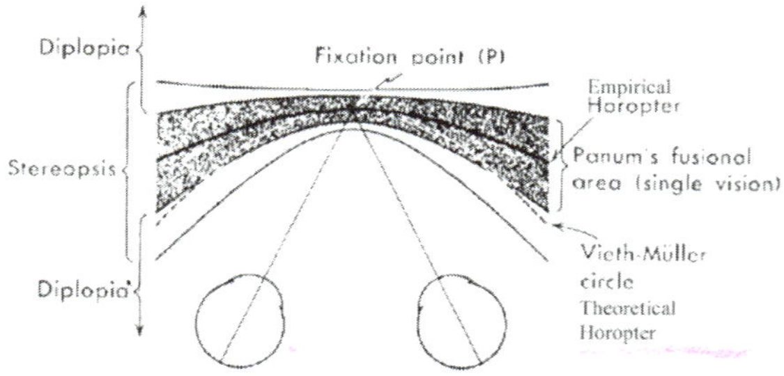

- **New horopter criteria:**
  - **Apparent Fronto-Parallel Plane (AFPP)**: Established when an observer marks points in space perceived as equidistant from the self.
  - **Vieth-Mueller Circle (VMC)**: Defined as the locus of points with zero geometric retinal disparity, based on the fact that the visual angle between the fovea and any other point for corresponding retinal points will be the same; two criteria for the Vieth-Mueller circle to be the horopter:
    - Corresponding retinal points are geometrically related to the fovea in each eye (cover points).
    - The horopter intercepts a horizontal plane that passes through the fixation point and the centers of the entrance pupils.
  - **Empirical Longitudinal Horopter (ELH)**: Horopter determined with vertical wires or rods instead of spatial points.

3. Disturbances of Perceived Direction and Distance

- **Aniseikonia** occurs when there is a significant difference in the perceived size of images. It can occur as an overall difference between the two eyes (i.e. one eye sees a larger image than the other eye), or as a difference in a particular meridian (i.e. in one eye, the image is elongated in one direction compared to the other). Aniseikonia can occur naturally or be induced by the correction of refractive error, usually anisometropia or antimetropia. Meridional aniseikonia occurs when refractive differences only occur in one meridian, as in astigmatism. Aniseikonia can also occur if one eye is aphakic (lacking the crystalline lens), leaving it much more hyperopic than the other eye.

- **Amblyopia** is reduced visual acuity not correctable by refractive means and not attributable to ophthalmoscopically apparent structural or pathological anomalies or proven afferent disorders.
  - *Strabismic amblyopia* – Much spatial uncertainty and regional spatial distortion due to compression and expansion of the perceptual field.
  - *Anisometropic amblyopia* – Moderate spatial uncertainty and little spatial distortion.
- **Contour interaction:** Causes a crowding phenomenon in normal as well as strabismic amblyopia. The greatest effect of contour interactions on decreasing visual acuity occurs when the surrounding letters are 2*MAR away from the test letter.
- **Spatial distortion** due to different retinal image sizes (aniseikonia) was qualitatively studied using the Leaf Room.

Types of Distortion

- Geometric effect: The image of one eye is magnified by a meridional lens (axis 90°) in the horizontal meridian. The floor appears slanted down towards the eye with the magnifier. The ceiling slants in the opposite direction, higher on the side with the magnifier. The wall on the side of the eye with the magnifier appears further away and the opposite wall appears closer. The facing wall appears skewed away from the eye with the magnifier.
- Induced effect: Produced by meridional size lens (axis 180°); produces opposite tilt of geometric effect.
- These two effects are opposite, so people with overall size differences rarely see spatial distortions since the two effects cancel.

4. Sensory-Motor Interactions

- **Fixation disparity**: An inexactness of bifixation, usually +3 to –5 minutes of arc due to Panum's Fusional Area (PFA). Usually larger in the periphery.
  - Crossed disparity – a target nearer than the binocular fixation point is said to be seen with divergent exophoria.
  - Uncrossed disparity – a fixation further than the binocular fixation point is said to be seen with convergent esophoria.
  - Associated phoria is the amount of prism required to reduce the fixation disparity to zero. It is measured with a chart that consists of two polarized lines (one seen only by the right eye, the other seen only by the left eye). The observer moves the lines so they are perceived to be vertically aligned. If they are truly aligned, there is no fixation disparity. The amount of disparity is seen in terms of angular separation.
- **Past pointing:** Pointing too far in the direction of displacement of a fixation object presented monocularly in the field of action of a paretic extraocular muscle. A similar error may occur when an amblyopic eye with eccentric fixation is monocularly fixating.
  - Example: A subject with a paralyzed right medial rectus is placed in a dark room and asked to look at a light and point to it (egocentric task). If the target is to the right, the subject can abduct the right eye and point correctly. If the target is 20° over on the paralyzed side, the brain believes the eye is 20° over even though it is not. The target is still 20° off from straight ahead and the eye overshoots 40°.
- **Visually guided behavior:** Thought to be controlled by the superior colliculus which is the major center for visual control for eye, head, and body movements. Appropriate orientations of the world are maintained even though there may be a change in the orientation of the retinal image.
- **Body posture and perceived orientation:** The vestibular ocular reflex of the cerebellar system seems to be responsible for the adaptation in perceived orientation from prisms and cylindrical lenses. Maintained postural deviations are controlled by the otoliths in the uticles and saccules (inner

ear), while postural movements resulting from acceleration are controlled by impulses from the hair cells in the semicircular canals.

- **Self-motion:** Perception of our own movement during locomotion tasks. Self-motion, otherwise known as vection, is derived from peripheral retinal image motion (>30° eccentricity) and corresponds to background motion, i.e. a person in a rotating room

---

FORM PERCEPTION

---

1. Static Visual Acuity

- Static visual acuity (including test configurations, various acuity tasks, and factors influencing acuity including blur, intensity and contrast); specification of visual acuity
- This is defined as the capacity to discriminate the fine detail of objects in the field of view.

Types of Acuity

- **Minimum visible acuity** = Threshold acuity detection; determines the presence or absence of a target. Involves rod function.
- **Threshold** = 1 arcsec. Test situation can be a bright object against a dark background, a dark object against a light background, or low contrast objects whose luminance is not much different from the background. (The task is actually intensity discrimination)
- **Minimum resolvable acuity** = Snellen acuity; resolution and a recognition task ("is this a 'c' or an 'o'?") to determine presence of distinction between more than one identifying feature on a visible target.
- **Threshold** = MAR (minimum angle of resolution) = 30" to 1' arc.
    - **Resolution**: Response to separation between elements of pattern.
    - **Recognition**: Requires naming test object or specifying the location of some critical aspect of it.
- **Vernier/offset acuity**: Minimum discriminable; a hyperacuity.
    - Threshold 2 to 10 arcsec.
- **Stereoacuity**: Also a hyperacuity. Threshold – 3 to 20 sec arc

Test Configurations

- **Snellen chart**
- **Landolt C**: Gap width and line thickness equal to 1/5 outer diameter of C: visual acuity defined as reciprocal of the angle in minutes subtended by the gap that is correctly identified 50% of the time.
- **Tumbling E**
- **VEP** (Visual Evoked Potential): sine wave luminance gratings used to measure acuity
- **VA** (Visual Acuity): 1/MAR (arcmin) = (testing distance)/(distance at which letter subtends 5 arcmin)
    - "20/20": Numerator is test distance (in feet); denominator is Snellen letter size (in feet).

Factors influencing VA

- **Blur**: Decreases VA. Can be due to refractive error or MAR. Width of point spread function inversely proportional to amount of defocus. Amount of blur – (dioptric error) x (focal length of eye) x (pupil diameter).
- **Pupil size**: VA decreases with pupil larger than 6 mm due to aberrations from lens periphery.
- **Retinal eccentricity**: VA best at fovea.
- **Exposure duration**: VA decreases with decreased exposure time (800ms-1sec).
- **Static vs. moving target**: VA decreases with increasing target speed (>2°).
- **Crowding effect**: Lateral inhibition.
- **Type of letter**: Script; some letters are easier to read than others.
- **Color of chart and/or letters** (chromatic aberration).

- **Contrast**: ΔI/I – (luminance of target minus background)/(luminance of background). The contrast of a printed Snellen letter is 90%. Projected charts are 40 to 50%. Contrast just needs to be 20-30%. VA is independent of contrast at high luminance.
- **Intensity** (ambient light level): acuity improves with illumination as long as it is in the photopic range.

2. Spatial Contrast Sensitivity Function

- The CSF uses sine waves as targets. The spatial frequency is the number of bars in a unit angle expressed in cycles per degree. **Sensitivity = 1/threshold.**
  - At low spatial frequencies, the system differentiates between changes in contrast and is limited by the physiology of the eye.
  - At intermediate spatial frequencies, the CSF is limited by neural pathology. Intermediate objects are what the human eye sees best.
  - At high spatial frequencies, the system integrates contrast.

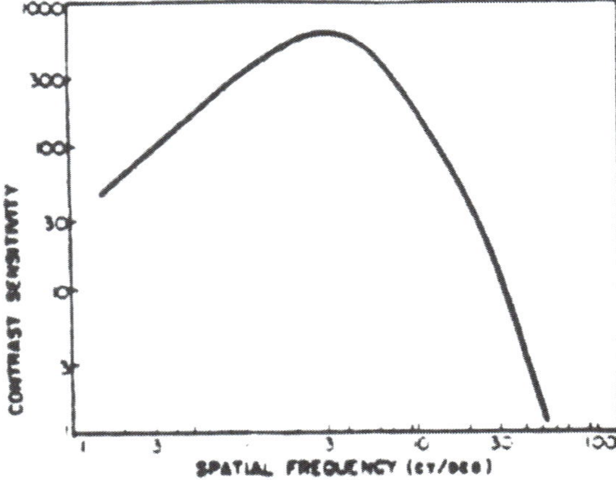

- The CSF is limited by blur and foveal diseases. A general depressing of the curve is due to opacities of the media. Optical defocus is resistant to intermediate spatial frequencies. VA is determined by high frequency cutoff.
- Contrast – defined as the relative difference between the intensities of the target and its surround:

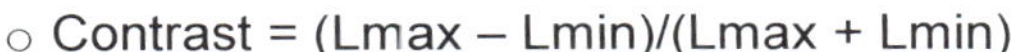

  - Contrast = (Lmax – Lmin)/(Lmax + Lmin)

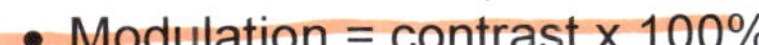

- Modulation = contrast x 100%

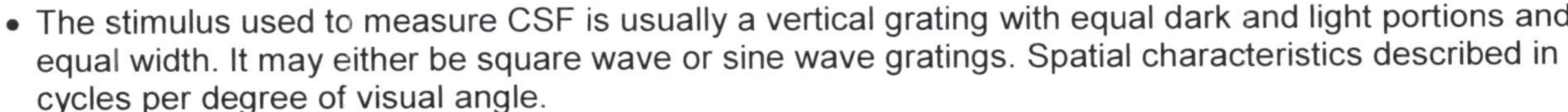

- The stimulus used to measure CSF is usually a vertical grating with equal dark and light portions and equal width. It may either be square wave or sine wave gratings. Spatial characteristics described in cycles per degree of visual angle.
- 1 cycle = 1 light and 1 dark bar
- Greatest sensitivity: 2-3 cycles per degree.

3. Illusions, Constancies, and Figure-Ground Relations

Illusions:

- Ambiguous figures or figures that lead to erroneous perception.
- **1. Corridor illusion** – cylinders of equal size in a linear perspective background appear different in size.
- **2. Ames room** – illusion of size; the perceived distance is constant, but retinal image size varies.
- **3. Hering illusion** – two parallel lines are straight, but appear to bow outwards in the middle due to the distortion produced by the lined pattern in the background, which creates a false impression of depth.
- **4. Wundt illusion** – opposite effect of Hering illusion; two parallel lines are straight, but appear to bow inwards in the middle.
- **5. Necker cube** – an ambiguous wire-frame drawing of a cube in oblique perspective. The picture does not show which corner is in front and which is behind, making the picture ambiguous. When staring at the picture or focusing on different parts of the cube, it will often seem to flip back and forth between two valid interpretations.
- **6. Illusions of brightness** – white dot in center looks brighter than white surround.
- **7. Müller-Lyer illusion** – two lines of equal length appear unequal due to arrowheads in opposite directions.
- **8. Poggendorf's illusion** – if oblique lines are extended across vertical ones as in the figure, the oblique line on the left is in the same straight line with the lower oblique line on the right. However,

the upper oblique line on the right is perceived to be the approximate continuation of the oblique line on the left.

- **9. Autokinetic illusion** – the apparent motion of a small single stationery object when continuously observed in a surrounding dark environment.
- **10. Aubert Fleischl illusion** – an illuminated moving target appears to move more slowly in a dark room if tracked with the eyes rather than the head.

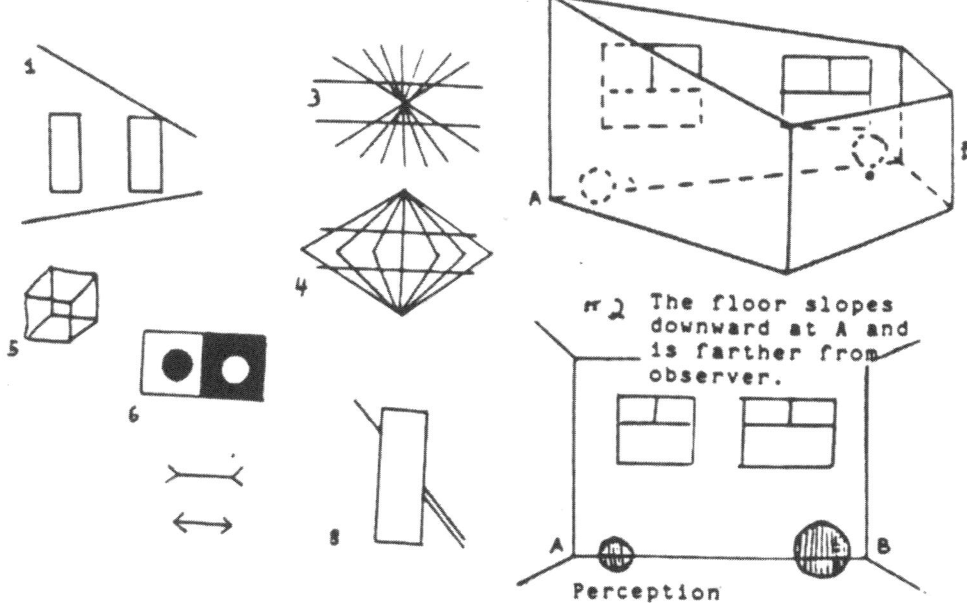

Constancies

- **Lightness constancy**: The ability to correctly perceive a white sheet of paper in dim light as white, or a black cat in bright sunlight as black, even though there may be a thousand times more incident light of the cat. We cannot detect how much incident light is falling on an object, which is the product of incident illumination and the reflectance.
- **Size constancy**: The ability to correctly judge the size of objects despite the differences in retinal images.
    - **Emmert's Law**: An afterimage appears smaller when looking at a near object as opposed to a distant object, though the image size on the retina remains unchanged. With a fixed size of afterimage, its perceived size will be proportional to the perceived distance at which it is located.
    - **Boring and Holway Moon Illusion Experiment** (1941): Provided evidence that when distance cues are impoverished, judgments of size increasingly rely on the size of the retinal image. Later rejected by Boring in 1943 because when he asked people to directly estimate the distance to the moon, they tended to judge it as closer when it was near the horizon than when it was high in the sky.
- **Color constancy**: A large change in the chromatic characteristics of the illumination does not cause much change in perceived color of an object.
- **Shape constancy**: As position relative to object changes, the shape of the retinal image changes, but perceived shape remains constant.

Figure-ground relations:

- The figure becomes a distinct entity that is set apart from the remainder of the scene. A pattern in the figure and ground may exchange roles

4. Simultaneous Contrast and Spatial Interactions (Mach Bands)

- **Simultaneous contrast:** Comparing the amount of light reflected by an object with the amount of light reflected by adjacent regions in the visual field. An object of moderate reflectance should look brighter in front of a black background than it would in front of a white background.
- **Mach bands:** A psychophysical perceptual phenomenon that involves spatial contrast enhancement.
- **Definition of contrast:** $(I_{max} - I_{min}) / (I_{max} + I_{min})$. This defines the change in intensity at the border of two adjacent stimuli. If a stimulus is presented to an observer who is then asked to plot the apparent brightness profile, the resulting plot would look like that shown in this figure. There is heightened contrast at borders and edges.

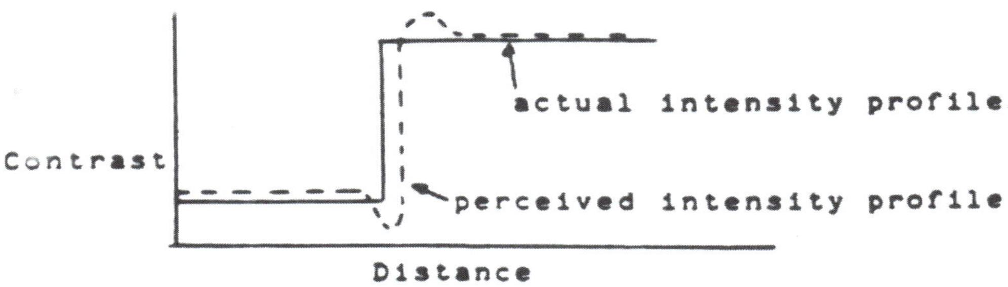

LIGHT PERCEPTION

1. Detection Characteristics at the Absolute Light Threshold

- The experiment by Hecht, Schlaer and Pirenne determined the absolute threshold of the human visual system, which is the minimum stimulus required to evoke the sensation of light in the fully adapted state. They found that one quantal emission (a single photon) in a dark-adapted rod is sufficient to get a signal to one molecule of photopigment, and that 100 quanta simultaneously are necessary to detect light.
- The experiment used a red fixation light (rods are least sensitive to long wavelengths, thus preventing bleaching) on individuals who were dark-adapted for at least 30 min.
- The stimulus was viewed eccentrically at 20 degrees temporally so that light would fall on the region of the retina with the highest concentration of rods. The stimulus was very small (10 min in diameter) to ensure that there would be complete spatial summation of the stimulus, and the exposure time was very short (0.001 sec) so that temporal summation would operate.
- A light of 510 nm (blue-green) was used as the stimulus because of the **optimal scotopic sensitivity** to light of this wavelength. 100 quanta on average were delivered to the front of the eye. About 50% was absorbed by ocular media, 4% was scattered or absorbed, and only 20% of light at most was actually absorbed by the rhodopsin of the receptors, with the rest absorbed by other tissues such as blood vessels. In the end, only 5-14 quanta were left to elicit a response by the receptors. In the 10-min area being stimulated, there are approximately 500 rods, making it highly unlikely that more than one quantum will strike a single rod at threshold levels of intensity.
- Based on this, the experimenters concluded that in order to see, it is necessary for only one quantum of light to be absorbed by a single molecule of photochemical pigment in each of 5 to 14 rods.

2. Brightness Difference Thresholds at Various Adaptation Levels

- **Weber's Law**: As the background brightness is increased, the increment intensity must be increased such that the ratio of the increment intensity (ΔI) to the background intensity (I_B) remains constant for the detection of an absolute difference. Weber's fraction or Weber's constant: $k = \Delta I/I_B$. Increment threshold for brightness discrimination only holds true in photopic region. See Area 3 on figure below.

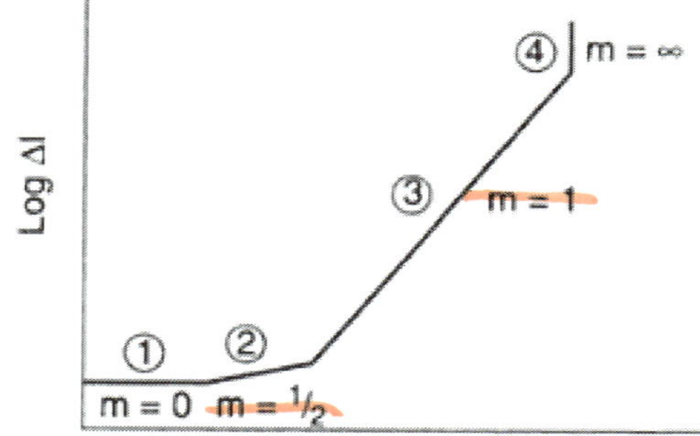

- **DeVries-Rose Law**: Predicts the ideal threshold of a stimulus upon a background. The background is so dim that fluctuations inherent in the light source that produces it play a primary role in determining threshold. It differs from measured thresholds since the eye filters out some of the light. Difference increases with increasing background levels. $k = I/\sqrt{I_B}$. DeVries-Rose law describes a perfect detector. The eye exhibits perfect discriminating behavior when the size of the increment is small and the duration of exposure is brief. See area 2 on figure below.

3. Dark and Light Adaptation Processes and Theories

- **Dark Adaptation**: The adjustment occurring under reduced illumination in which the sensitivity to light is greatly increased or the light threshold is greatly decreased. The process is slower than light adaptation. The figure below shows the results of an experiment by Height, Haig, and Chase (1937) in which a subject fixated on a small red spot of light.

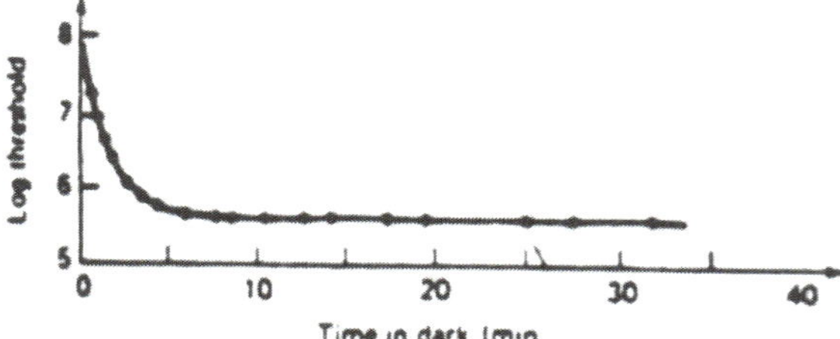

- As the subject remained in the dark after the adapting field was extinguished, threshold decreased. The change was most rapid just after the subject was placed in the dark, and tapered off to a fairly stable threshold level by 5 or 10 minutes. This plateau represents a threshold lowering of about 2 log units, or improvement by a factor of about 100 in the subject's ability to detect the red light. This represents dark adaptation by cones. For the first seven minutes, cones are more sensitive in the dark. However, cones aren't as sensitive as rods in the dark, they just adapt faster.

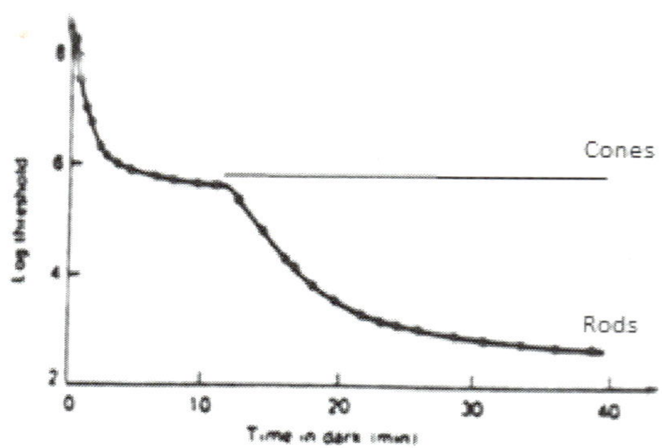

- When testing with a large violet light, there was again rapid movement after the adapting field was extinguished. It gradually leveled off to a new threshold about 1 log unit lower than when a small red light was used. About 8 minutes after the adapting field was extinguished, the threshold plunged again. Over the next 20 minutes, it dropped 3 log units (1000 times) and finally settled at a value much lower than before.

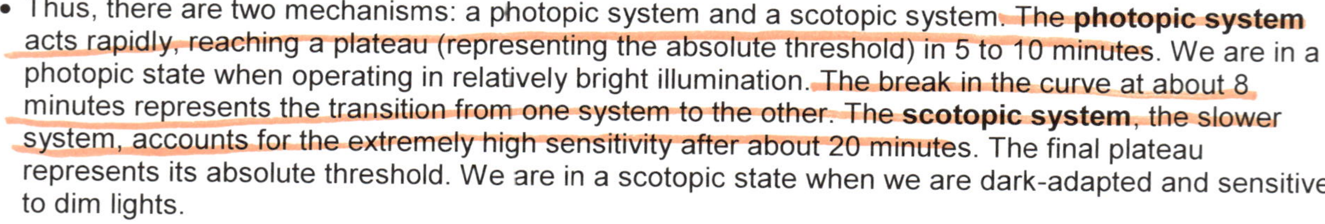

- Thus, there are two mechanisms: a photopic system and a scotopic system. The **photopic system** acts rapidly, reaching a plateau (representing the absolute threshold) in 5 to 10 minutes. We are in a photopic state when operating in relatively bright illumination. The break in the curve at about 8 minutes represents the transition from one system to the other. The **scotopic system**, the slower system, accounts for the extremely high sensitivity after about 20 minutes. The final plateau represents its absolute threshold. We are in a scotopic state when we are dark-adapted and sensitive to dim lights.

- The scotopic system is more sensitive than the photopic system for all wavelengths except the longest. The photopic system is most sensitive at 555 nm (green), but the scotopic system is still more sensitive even at that wavelength. Cones serve the photopic system. Although no single pigment matches the photopic curve, the curve is closely approximated by the combination of three pigments. The scotopic system is most sensitive at 505 nm (blue-green). Rods are the receptors of this system, peaking at 505 nm (the rod pigment, rhodopsin, also peaks at 505 nm). 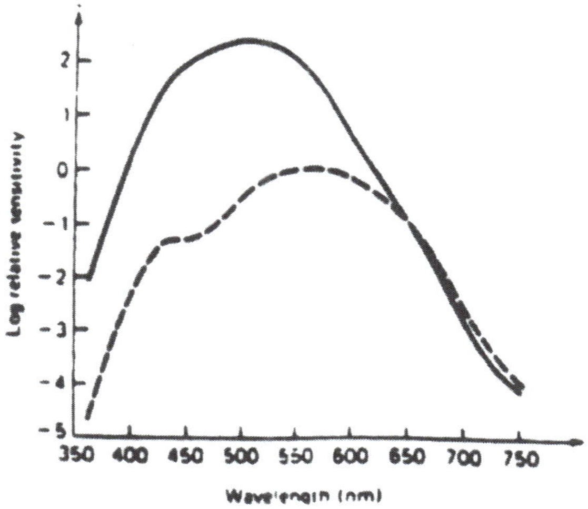
- Rods contain a photopigment called rhodopsin, which is made up of the protein opsin and a chromophore, 11-*cis*-retinal. Visual excitation occurs when 11-*cis* retinal is changed to all-*trans* retinal.
    - Rhodopsin cycle: 11-*cis*-retinal + opsin (protein) → rhodopsin → photon absorbed → isomerization (neural response) → 11-*trans* retinal + opsin → "bleach" → resynthesis → (1) spontaneous reactivation through enzymes (2) supply area with fresh vitamin A through circulation.
    - Once a molecule of rhodopsin is bleached, there is a 50% probability that it will regenerate in 5 minutes. It is not possible to totally bleach all the rhodopsin in the retina because of continued reversing from combined form to partially uncombined form.
    - The eye functions over a 10^{10} range of illumination, which means that the sensitivity of retina is based on a log function and not on the number of molecules of rhodopsin that are bleached.

Comparison of Scotopic and Photopic Systems		
Property	**Scotopic System**	**Photopic System**
Retinal Location for Highest Sensitivity	Outside Fovea	Fovea
Outer Segment Morphology	Separate Disks	Disks are infoldings of membrane
Weber's Fraction	0.14	0.015
Photopigments (Peak Absorption)	Rhodopsin (507nm)	Erythrolabe (565nm) Chlorolabe (535nm) Cyanolabe (430nm)
Maximal Sensitivity of System	507nm	555nm
Chromatic Discrimination	Colorblind (black and white only)	Color discrimination
Sensitivity	Dim lights	Moderate or bright lights
Spatial Resolution	20/200	20/20
Spatial Summation	Excellent	Poor
Temporal Resolution	Poor (20 Hz)	Excellent (70 Hz)
Temporal Summation	Excellent	Poor
Contrast Sensitivity	Low	High
Stiles-Crawford Effect	Minimal	Present

- Cones regenerate 3 times faster than rods. This explains the difference in dark adaptation time. Since cone pigment regenerates faster, cones recover their sensitivity much faster than rods, but their sensitivity is limited.
- **Light Adaptation**: The adjustment occurring under increased illumination in which the sensitivity to light is reduced (or light threshold is increased). When in the light, both rods and cones become less sensitive, and the retina is light-adapted. This is the photopic state. Refer to table on the previous page, which contrasts the properties of the photopic and scotopic states. In the scotopic state, a threshold light is detected by the rods, and color is not sensed. If the light is made more intense, it will soon stimulate cones, and color can be detected.
- The amount of light that must be added to threshold in order to make its color evident is called the photochromatic interval.

4. Spatial and Temporal Summation Characteristics

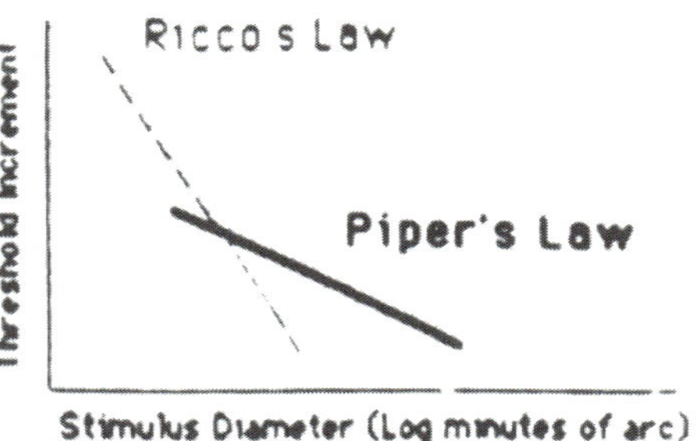

- **Spatial summation:** The combination of the effect of two or more stimuli that impinge simultaneously on different retinal regions. Many more rods than cones communicate with a ganglion cell. This illustrates how the scotopic system sums up information over space to a greater extent than the photopic system.
  - **Ricco's Law (Charpentier's Law):** For stimuli up to 10 seconds of arc in diameter, the total number of quanta necessary for detection is constant. This means that the threshold number of quanta could be delivered in a one second area test spot or spread out over a larger area, up to 10 seconds of arc.

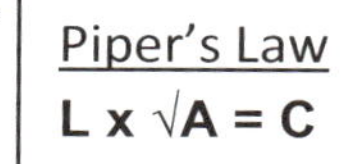

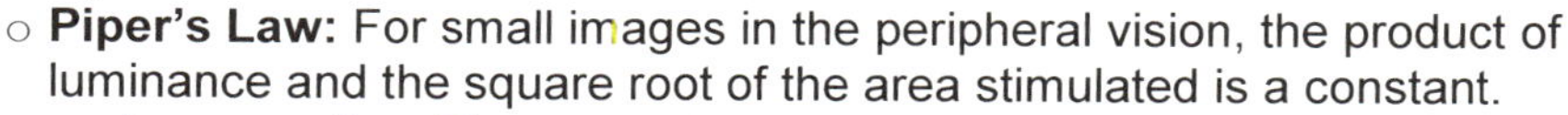

  - **Piper's Law:** For small images in the peripheral vision, the product of luminance and the square root of the area stimulated is a constant.

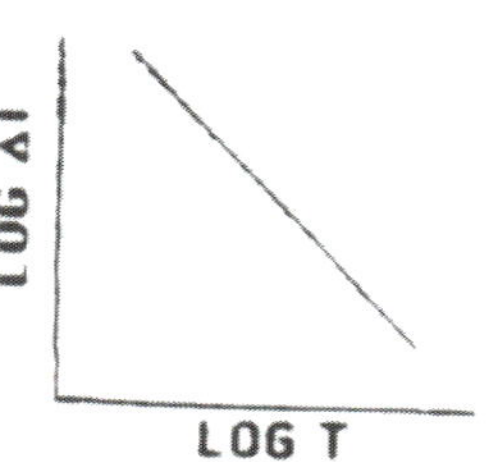

- **Temporal summation:** The scotopic system sums up information over time to a greater extent than the photopic system. However, the photopic system is better able to distinguish two flashes of light separated by a brief interval in time. Therefore, the photopic system has superior temporal resolution.
  - **Bloch's Law:** As long as the threshold number of quanta are delivered within the critical duration (100 msec for rods, 10-50 msec for cones), it does not matter how they are delivered. They could be presented in one or more flashes.

MOTION PERCEPTION

1. Factors Involved in the Detection of Real and Apparent Motion, Detection of Displacements

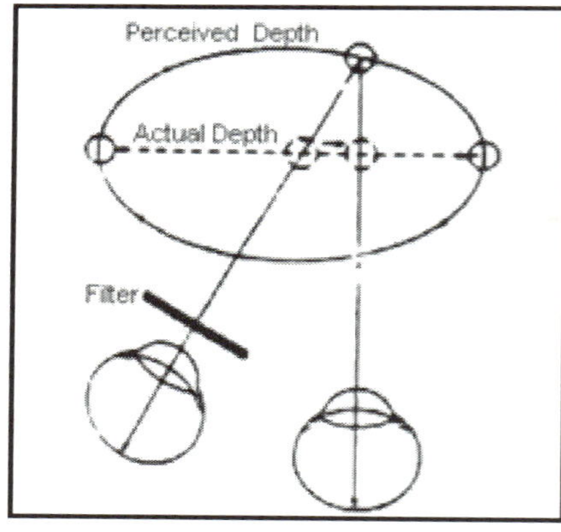

- **Real motion:** Perceived movement correlates to actual, physical movement of an object. The "image-retina" perceptual system responds to movement of an image across the retina. The "eye-head" system is responsible for following the position of a stimulus with eye and head movements. Sensitivity to motion is about 1 second of arc, and the best motion threshold is at fovea.
- **Apparent motion (illusory movement):** Perception of movement of a stationary object, in contrast to real movement where the object actually is moving in space.
  - Examples of apparent motion:
    - **Autokinetic effect:** Apparent random motion of a small stationary stimulus in a large blank field.
    - **Pulfrich effect:** Apparent motion with depth of a moving object when viewed with a filter over one eye. The filtered eye receives less light from the stimulus, causing it to respond more slowly and resulting in a delay in the transmission of signals from that eye. Therefore, at a given point in time, the position of a swinging pendulum, as seen by the filtered eye, lags behind the position seen by the other eye. As a result, a binocular disparity occurs that is consistent with a stimulus moving in an elliptical path.
  - Factors involved in the detection of apparent motion:
    - Time required to perceive apparent motion is around a 50-60 millisecond pause between the two ranges.

- **Korte's "law"** (space-time relationship for visual apparent motion) summarizes the optimum stimulus parameters for apparent motion including luminance, stimulus duration, linear separation, and duration of pause. As the distance between lights increases, the onset interval must be simultaneously increased to maintain the perception of smooth apparent movement.
- Types of apparent motion:
    - **Alpha motion**: Apparent expansion or contraction; the second target is presented in the same position as the first but is larger.
    - **Gamma motion**: Same perception as alpha motion but stimuli are different; same size but second is brighter.
    - **Beta motion**: Linear; similar to lights on a roller coaster.
    - **Sigma motion**: The motion perceived when a target is projected constantly on the fovea as the eye moves. Motion is perceived even though it always stimulates the same retinal position.

- **Stroboscopic movement** (Phi phenomena or pure movement): Apparent motion produced by successive presentation of stationary stimuli. A moving target is not actually seen, but there is a sense of motion. Various sensations of movement are produced by different intervals between flashes of light. An interval of 60 msec produces realistic movement (optimum or beta movement). An interval of less than 30 msec produces no sensation of movement. Durations of 60-200 msec produce a partial illusion of movement (pure or phi movement).

2. Motion After-Effects

- The apparent movement of an object in a direction opposite to that of the actual movement of the object just previously seen. Evidence suggests that the presence of direction-specific movement detectors in the visual system may be responsible for motion after effects.
- Examples:
    - **Waterfall illusion**: After staring at a waterfall for a couple of minutes, then looking away at a stationary object, it will appear as if that object is floating upwards. This phenomenon is due to the adaptation of motion-specific detectors that are tuned to downward movement, becoming less sensitive to downward movement. When shifting gaze to other objects, movement detectors in the other directions will be more active than the downward motion detectors, resulting in an illusion of the scene moving upwards. Since presenting the stimulus to one eye produces the same effect in the other eye, the detectors being adapted must be in the visual cortex. People with no binocularity fail to show the transfer from one eye to the other.
    - **Plateau spiral illusion**: A moving spiral, when viewed for a period of time, will produce a spiral motion after-effect in the opposite direction when another object is viewed.

3. Dynamic Visual Acuity, Visual Performances with a Moving Object, and Visual Performances with a Moving Observer

- **Dynamic visual acuity:** Visual acuity of a moving test target.
- Visual performance with a moving object and with the moving observer—there is a decrement in certain visual functions during saccades and also generally when there is significant movement of the retinal image. Small movements of the image do not detract from acuity. Strict stability of the retinal image is not required for optimal resolution. As stimulus velocity increases, resolution acuity remains relatively constant until the stimulus velocity reaches about 60 to 80 degrees/second. Beyond this velocity, the ability to resolve a moving stimulus (the dynamic visual acuity) deteriorates. The reduction in dynamic visual acuity at increasing target velocities is apparently due to the inability to accurately follow the stimulus with tracking eye movements (smooth pursuits).

TEMPORAL PERCEPTION

1. Critical Flicker Fusion Frequency, Including factors Influencing Test Object

- **Critical Flicker Fusion Frequency (CFF)** is the rate of presentation of intermittent, alternate, or discontinuous photic stimuli for which the flicker can no longer be detected. The critical flicker fusion frequency is the rate at which a flickering light appears steady. The effective light coming from such a flickering light is the average amount of light in a cycle.
- When a light flickering at ~10 cycles/sec is compared to a steady light of the same average luminance, the flickering light appears brighter. This is known as the **Brucke-Bartley Effect**. The subject can tell the light is flickering but can't accurately compensate and judge its brightness. This phenomenon can be explained by recalling that the Y-type cells respond minimally in steady light.
- A flickering light continually re-excites the peak response; therefore, the flickering light appears brighter. Recall that 10 Hz is the peak of the temporal contrast sensitivity function. The changeover from flicker to fusion is not abrupt but takes place over a transitional range of frequencies.
- Within this range, a frequency may be found by experimental methods that may be taken as the boundary between the two modes or appearance. This frequency is the critical flicker fusion frequency (CFF). The CFF is a measure of the temporal resolving power of the visual system under the particular conditions of stimulation.
- **Determinants of CFF:** Many variables of the stimulus and observer interact to determine the value of the CFF.
    - Test stimulus size: As the size of the stimulus is increased, the CFF becomes higher due to the fact that more photoreceptors are being stimulated. This is the **Granit-Harper Law**.
    - Retinal location: Since the CFF is lower for rods (20 flashes/sec) than for cones (60 flashes/sec), the CFF for a test stimulus is confined to a limited area of the retina and depends on the relative number of rods and cones stimulated in that area. If the test light is confined to the fovea, it activates only cones and the CFF function rises according to the **Ferry-Porter Law** (the CFF is directly proportional to the logarithm of the stimulus intensity). The CFF for small targets is greater in the fovea at any given photopic level of retinal luminance.
    - For spectral composition at low levels of luminance there is a difference in the CFF with various wavelengths that is due to the fact that the ability of rods and cones to detect light varies for different wavelengths.
    - Other test stimulus factors include: Temporal wave form, duty cycle, duration of flashes, number of flashes in the series, monocular vs. binocular presentation, and shape of the stimulus.
    - Test background luminance: The highest CFF is obtained when there is the condition of minimal border contrast.
    - Test background size: CFF varies with the area of surround; CFF generally rises as this area is increased.
    - Observer adaptation level: Adaptation determines CFF largely because it governs the relative sensitivity of rod and cone mechanisms. Also, light adaptation reduces the size and changes the organization of retinal receptive fields in a way that enhances the likelihood of inhibitory interactions. In general, the higher the level of light adaptation, the higher the CFF for a given test stimulus.
    - Pupil size
    - Presence of pathology
    - Non-visual properties: This includes age (CFF declines with increasing age), fatigue, hunger, drugs, body state, general health, personality, and brain damage

2. Subfusional Flicker phenomena (Bartley Brightness Enhancement)

- **Sub-fusional flicker phenomena:** The increase in brightness resulting from making a stimulus intermittent. The rate of intermittence must lie materially below the critical flicker frequency, and the photic pulses must not be feeble or enhancement will not occur.
    - The apparent increase of brightness of a surface when surrounded by a dark area as compared to when it is surrounded by a light area.
- **Brucke-Bartley effect**: The increased brightness of intermittent stimulation (compared to continuous illumination of the same intensity).
    - The Brucke effect proper is the effect gained by using a revolving disk with dark and light sectors and comparing it to a solid surface similar to the light sector. The Bartley effect proper is produced by using a motionless surface intermittently illuminated and comparing it to a continuously illuminated one. There is an increase in brightness as the repetition rate of flashes approaches a value near 10 cps, and a decline of brightness at higher frequencies. The Brucke-Bartley effect deals with the response of cells to a flickering stimulus that is administered against a background. For example, if 200 msec flashes of constant intensity are presented in series upon a background light, the response of a cell shows a decrease in the steady level of action potentials. This effect is due to **lateral inhibition**. It takes 200 msec for lateral inhibition to build up, and another 200 msec to decay. If a second flash is presented while the lateral inhibition is still present, the potentials will be decreased.
    - If the stimulus is delayed until the effects of lateral inhibition are over (say 500 msec), then the peak response of action will be unchanged. If the second stimulus is delivered at exactly the time lateral inhibition stops then the two responses will reach the same peak of action potentials, but the change in frequency of firing is greater for the second stimulus than for the first. We see the maximum change in firing frequency when the second stimulus is delivered right at the very end of the inhibitory period of the previous stimulus. The brightness of the second stimulus will be apparently greater because the darkness between the stimuli will look darker due to lateral inhibition.

3. Successive Contrast and Masking

- **Successive contrast:** Exposure to one stimulus affects the perception of a later stimulus to the same retinal areas when two stimuli are given in rapid succession.
- **Masking:** Refers to using one stimulus to hide another in masking experiments. The test stimulus is exposed briefly, and its presence must be detected against the masking effects of a second briefly exposed stimulus. The effect of the masking stimulus is to raise the threshold for the test stimulus. The magnitude of the effect depends mainly upon the luminance of the masking stimulus and the temporal relationship between the two stimuli. Masking effects are stronger in areas away from the fovea. Masking can be simultaneous, backward, or forward.
    - In simultaneous masking, both the test and the mask are presented at once (i.e. one may be printed on top of the other on the same piece of paper). This is the principle of camouflage.
    - Backward masking occurs when the mask stimulus is presented immediately after the test stimulus. **Metacontrast** is the special name that has been given to backward masking in which the test figure and the mask fall on different areas of the retina.
    - When the test contour and masking contour are of approximately the same intensity, the distance between the two flashes is not too great, and the timing is within 50-100 msec, the second flash inhibits the ability to detect to first flash. Metacontrast may be explained as a form of lateral inhibition, if we assume that the inhibitory effect (from the mask) develops more slowly than the excitatory effect (from the test).
    - Metacontrast is not just a simple retinal interaction. For example, the mechanism of metacontrast is different for short delays between mask and test than the mechanism for long delays. Also, if the brightness of the second flash, the mask, is greater than the first flash, then the first flash is perceived as not being as bright as it actually is by itself. The mask prevents detection of the test even though it occurs after the test.

- Forward masking, also known as **paracontrast**, occurs when the mask precedes the test stimulus. The effect on visibility of the second flash by the first flash depends on the brightness of the masking flash as well as the spatial and temporal separation of the two flashes.

4. Temporal Contrast Sensitivity Function

- Contrast is defined as: $C = (I_{max} - I_{min})/(I_{max} + I_{min})$. Sensitivity is 1/(contrast threshold). "Function" refers to the fact that the sensitivity depends on the flicker rate used. Temporal CSF has the same shape as spatial CSF, and is analogous to the spatial CSF except that temporal CSF is modulated over time versus over space.
- The temporal CSF measures the visual system's sensitivity to different temporal frequencies or flicker rates. The visual system is maximally sensitive to frequencies between about 10 and 30 Hz. Kelly (1961) presented subjects with a large uniformly illuminated disk (blurred at the edges) whose intensity could be varied sinusoidally in time over a range of frequencies and amplitudes.
- The subject looked at the disk while its intensity was being varied sinusoidally at some particular frequency. The amplitude was adjusted until the variation was just barely visible (the subject barely saw flicker rather than steady brightness). It was found that sensitivity falls off at the low and the high temporal frequencies.
- At the low end, the fall off is due to the visual system not noting the flicker. It seems that humans lack receptors that operate on such a low frequency. At the high frequency, the flicker is too fast to keep up with. Above 60 Hz, flicker is no longer detected, which is why we don't notice fluorescent lights flickering (they flicker at a rate slightly greater than 60 Hz).

5. Stabilized Retinal Images and Monocular Suppression

- **Troxler Effect:** The temporary and irregular fading or disappearance of a small object in the visual field during steady fixation of another object.
- As flash duration increases, visual efficiency declines. This is illustrated by Troxler's phenomena, or local adaptation. If an observer fixates carefully on a small stationary object but pays attention to a steady light presented to the peripheral retina, he will notice that the peripheral stimulus fades away within several seconds while the fixated object remains visible. The dimmer the target, the sooner it disappears.
- Both the lengthening of visibility despite increased rates of bleaching and the continued availability of unbleached pigment at the time of disappearance show that Troxler's phenomenon is neurally dependent as opposed to photochemical in nature. Disappearance is longer with increasing target size.
- Receptive field sizes at the center of the fovea are smaller than in the periphery. Small receptive fields with fine eye movements will keep the object refreshed even if it is stationary. In the periphery, receptive fields are larger so the eyes must move more to keep the object from fading.

6. Saccadic Suppression

- **Saccadic suppression:** A brief suppression of vision before, during, and after a saccadic eye movement.
- Saccades are accompanied by reduced visual efficiency. For example, test flashes presented during saccades are less likely to be seen (regardless of their position in the visual field) than similar flashes in similar positions presented while the eye is stationary. Saccadic suppression affects foveal as well as peripheral vision. The critical period of time in which there is a decrease in the ability of the visual system to perceive an object is 100 msec before the initiation of an eye movement or 150 msec after the eye movement. The ability of short flashes to evoke a pupillary response is also reduced greatly if the flashes precede or accompany a saccadic eye movement.

COLOR PERCEPTION

- Component or trichromatic theory (Young and Helmholtz): States that there are 3 principal mechanisms with different spectral sensitivity; when the visual system is activated, these mechanisms are activated – one more than the others – and this determines color; derived from the fact that color normals could match any color seen by adjusting the intensities of 3 primary colors at receptor level. This is good evidence for this theory since there are 3 cone photopigments – as evidenced by microspectroscopy.
- Hering's opponent color theory (antagonism): States there are six primary sensations which include red, green, yellow, blue, white, and black.
  - There are three receptors, each containing an antagonistic or opponent pair of colors: red-green, blue-yellow, and black-white.
  - Opponent theory is a post-receptor property. This is evidence of opponent spectral processing, which involves spectrally non-opponent cells and spectrally opponent cells.
    - Brightness: quantitatively predicted from activity of non-opponent cells
    - Hue: predicted from opponent cell activity
    - Saturation: predicted by ratio of opponent to non-opponent.

1. Chromatic Discrimination for Normal and Defective Color Vision

- Chromatic discrimination (hue and saturation) for normal and defective color vision: Be able to distinguish between the chromatic entities of hue and saturation and the achromatic entity of brightness. Color attributes are trivariant. To describe a color response, 3 variables are necessary: (1) **hue** (2) **saturation** (3) **brightness**.
- **Hue** is a color sensation usually correlated with wavelength or a combination of wavelengths. Hue discrimination is wavelength discrimination or *color acuity* – the ability to distinguish a color from a neighboring color. Hue discrimination is best at blue-green (490nm) and yellow-red (590). The *photometric equivalent* is ***dominant wavelength***.
- **Saturation** is the pureness of a color or degree to which the color is not mixed with white. Saturation discrimination is the ability to distinguish a color from white (standard illuminant C). Saturated colors appear to be full of color, whereas a desaturated color appears to have been mixed with white. The *photometric equivalent* is ***purity***.
- **Brightness** is the luminosity of color, that is, how dark or light/bright the color is. Brightness is the sensation giving rise to the perception of *luminous intensity*. The *photometric equivalent* of brightness is ***luminance***. 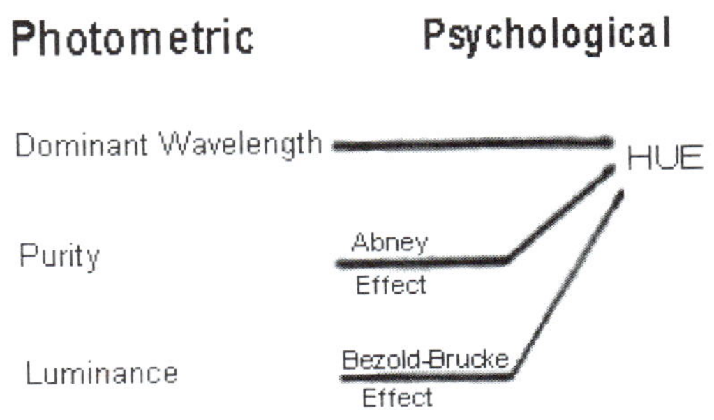
- There is not a 1-to-1 relationship between photometric quantities and psychological perception. One can experience a change in hue by changing the dominant wavelength, purity, or luminance.
  - Abney Effect: The change in hue associated with a change in purity (saturation).
  - Bezold-Brücke Effect: The change in hue associated with a change in luminance. Simple Rule of Thumb: stimuli below 500nm (blue-green) appear more blue as intensity increases. Stimuli above 500nm appear more yellow when intensity increases.
  - Purdy Effect: The change in saturation with a change in luminance.

Photometric | Psychological

Dominant Wavelength — HUE

Purity — Abney Effect

Luminance — Bezold-Brucke Effect

- Chromatic discrimination:
  - Normal trichromat: Hue discrimination is best at 490nm and 590nm.
  - **Protanope**: Does not discriminate differences in hue at long wavelengths (above 520nm provided the wavelengths are equal in brightness). Minimum saturation is 494nm – which is the

neutral point, or the point that cannot be distinguished from white. Near the neutral point, there is very sharp discrimination.
  - **Deuteranope**: The neutral point is 499nm.
  - **Tritanope**: can easily distinguish red and green; their neutral point is at 570nm.
  - *Anomalous trichromats do not have a neutral point*.
  - **Chromaticity confusion locus**: The locus of chromaticity coordinates that represent colors that will have the same appearance for the dichromat. Confusion lines delineate sections of the CIE diagram that color defectives perceive as being the same color. Each color deficiency has its characteristic pattern where the confusion lines appear to radiate from a specific co-punctal point.
  - The co-punctal point is the point of intersection of the chromaticity confusion loci.
  - The neutral point is the wavelength on the spectral locus that corresponds with a line drawn through the standard illuminant from the co-punctal point. This color is confused with white.

2. Color Mixture and Appearance

- **Primary colors:** A primary color is one color in a set of three wavelengths that cannot be matched by a mixture of the other two wavelengths. The additive primary colors are red, green, and blue. When red and green are mixed, the result is yellow. No shades of red or green are seen in yellow; therefore, *yellow is sometimes called a psychological primary*.
- **Complementary colors:** A complementary color is one of two colors which, when mixed additively, produce white or gray.
  - R + B + G = WHITE.
  - R + B = MAGENTA.
  - B + G = CYAN, complement of red.
  - G + R = YELLOW, complement of blue.
- **Additive color mixtures**: The superposition of two or more lights (of either single or multiple wavelengths) to produce a color composed of the algebraic sum of all the wavelengths involved. Examples: Color TV uses mixture of red, green, and blue dots at a given point on the screen to produce the desired color when viewed from a distance. Impressionist paintings are also an example of additive color mixtures.
- **Subtractive color mixtures**: Removal of certain wavelengths of light via filters yield subtractive color mixtures. Yellow filters cut out blue wavelengths. Red filters cut out green wavelengths. Example: with regular paintings, the particles in the paint act like small filters which reflect only the wavelengths that are not absorbed.
- **Metameric colors:** Two colors that match exactly in color appearance, but whose physical components are different, i.e. the wavelength mixtures are different.
- A color stimulus produced by a mixture of wavelengths is identical in appearance to the single wavelengths that describe that color.

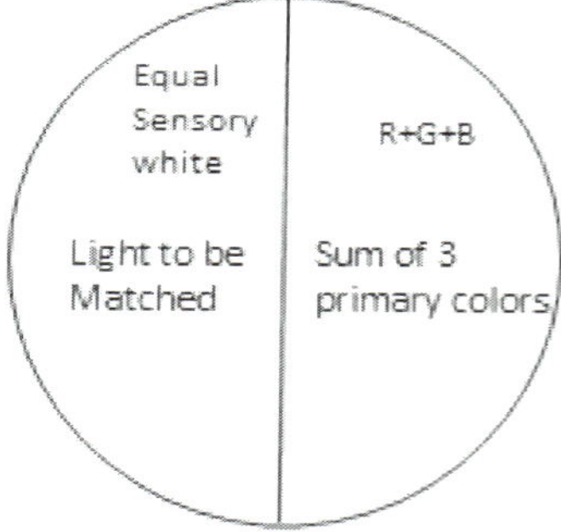

Metameric Match Design

3. Color Contrast, Constancy, and Adaptation

- **Simultaneous color contrast:** The color of an isolated object changes when it is surrounded by different colors. Chromatic areas surrounding achromatic areas will induce the perception of the hue complementary to the surrounding within the achromatic area. A form of spatial induction is demonstrated by observing the perceived color of a gray spot with a colored surround. Example: a gray spot in a red surround appears cyan (B + G = cyan, complement of red) at its edges.
- **Successive color contrast:** The negative afterimage of a colored stimulus is seen as the complement of the primary colored stimulus (AKA colored afterimages). Examples: The negative afterimage of red is seen as cyan; that of green is seen as magenta; and that of blue is seen as yellow.
- **Color contingent after-effects:** This is due to fatigue/adaptation effect. Several aftereffects have been described which involve orientation, motion, and spatial frequency. The McCollough effect is

associated with orientation. It is formed by looking at a horizontal red-black grating alternating with vertical green-black grating every few seconds for a period of several minutes. Afterwards, vertical white-black gratings appear reddish and horizontal white-black gratings appear greenish. This phenomenon can have a long-lasting effect.

- **Color constancy:** The color of an object does not appear to change much when illumination is altered over a wide range. Color depends primarily on relative brightness of an object at various wavelengths, compared to other objects in the fields of view, and that these relative values do not change when illumination is altered – even though absolute values do.

4. Color Specification and Colorimetry (CIE)

- The CIE utilized human observers and had them view a bipartite field on a white screen. On one-half was one wavelength – the test lamp; on the other half of the screen, three different colors were projected. For each test wavelength, the intensities of the three projectors could be changed to match its color. The values for the visible spectrum (from 380 to 760 nm) were found, and these were termed tristimulus values.

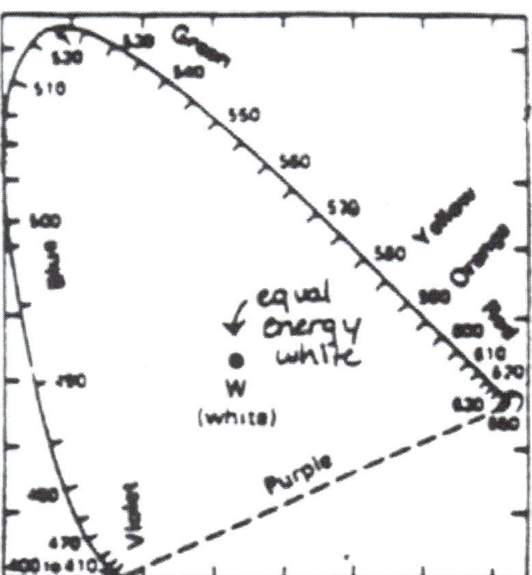

CIE Color Diagram

Source: Schwartz, 1994

The CIE color diagram

- Purpose: International system used to describe colors and summarize rules of color mixture.
- Properties: Within the diagram, a specific color sample can be identified X, Y, Z.
- **Primary colors:** Any set of three colors from which all other colors can be produced via additive mixing. X, Y, and Z are imaginary colors.
- **Tristimulus values:** The amounts of each of the primary colors that additively give the color or light desired.
- **Chromaticity coordinates** of a color are the ratios of each tristimulus value of the color to their sum.
- Features:
    - **Spectral locus:** Curve that locates all the monochromatic wavelengths (400-700nm); the coordinates of the spectrum.
    - **Dominant wavelength**: The wavelength to which you would add white to match the color in question. This is determined by drawing a line on the diagram from the chromaticity point of a reference source (white) to the chromaticity point of the sample and extending it until it intersects the spectrum locus.
    - If you take any two colors on the chromaticity diagram, the mixture of these will always be a point on a line between the two colors.
    - If you mix three colors, the resulting color will fall within their triangular boundary.
    - **Complementary wavelengths:** Two spectral wavelengths that can be mixed to match white. For purple samples, there is no dominant wavelength. Instead, extend the line going back in the other direction which is the complement of spectrum purple. The dominant wavelength for purple is specified in terms of its complementary dominant wavelength.

Munsell Color System

- This is a system of color-stimulus notation in which an attempt has been made to have the notation correspond to the sensory experience given.

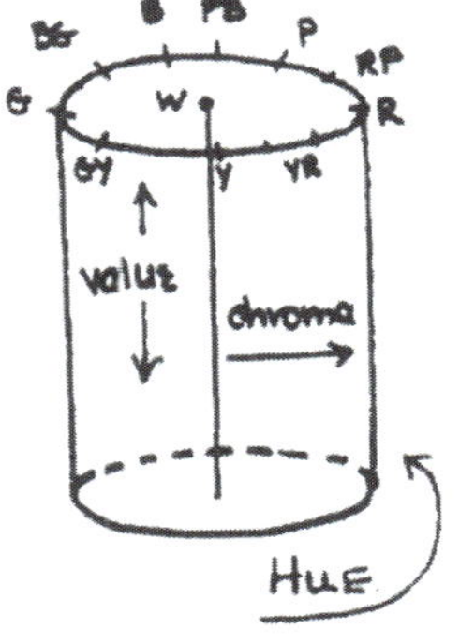

Munsell Color System Diagram

- Method of describing a color in terms of its three subjective attributes:
    - **Hue:** the characteristic or attribute of visual sensation. There are 100 Munsell Hues arranged in a hue circle and uniformly spaced around the circumference of the circle; each is symbolized by a number from 1 to 10 and a letter-symbol for the segment of the hue circle concerned. There are ten major colors, with ten steps each resulting in 100 total hues.
    - **Value** (lightness): The color solid is divided along its vertical axis into equally perceptible value units; specified on a numerical scale from 1 (black) to 10 (white).
    - **Chroma** (whiteness): Indicated numerically on a scale from 0 to various maxima; dependent on the saturation attainable with available pigments that give the desired hue and value.
- Munsell notation: the hue is cited first, then the value, followed by the chroma in the form of a pseudo-fraction: H/V/C.
- **MacAdam Ellipses:** Represent perceptual areas within the CIE diagram; all colors will perceptually appear the same even if they are physically different.

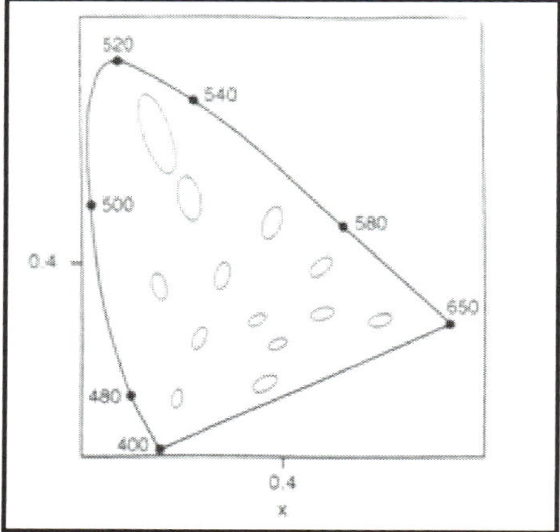

5. Spectral Sensitivity of Normal and Defective Color Vision

- Relative spectral sensitivities of the light-adapted (photopic) eye and the dark-adapted (scotopic) eye are shown in the **Spectral Sensitivity Diagram**. Note that: in the dark adapted state, the rods are always more sensitive than the cones throughout the spectrum; although in the red region, both rod and cones are equally sensitive.
- Absorption spectrum for cones:
    - S cones (short wavelength) - B cone 420 to 430nm.
    - M cones (middle wavelength) - G cones 535nm.
    - L cones (long wavelength) - R cones 565nm.
- Cones have greatest sensitivity at green-yellow (555nm).
- Rods have greatest sensitivity at blue-green (505nm)

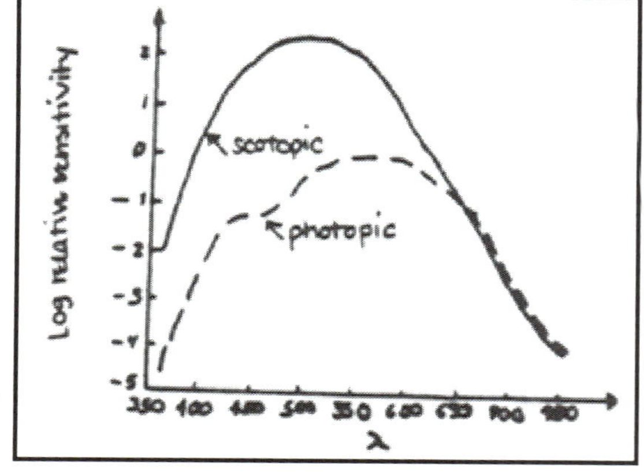

6. Mechanisms of Color Deficiencies

- These deficiencies can result either due to an inability produce certain photopigments in the case of inherited defects, or to a targeted loss of retinal cells or nerve fibers, or by damage to the ventromedial occipital cortex, posterior lingual, and fusiform gyri, in the case of acquired deficiencies. See Section on Anomalies of Color Vision; Inherited, Acquired for more on inheritance patterns and etiology information.

7. Inherited Anomalies of Color Vision

Classification:

- **Trichromats:** Trichromats have normal color vision. Three primary colors are required to match any other color. Most trichromats use the same ratio of red and green to match yellow on an anomaloscope.
- **Anomalous trichromats**: Anomalous trichromats have abnormal color vision. Three primary colors are required to match any other color, but in different proportions than the normal population.

- Deuteranomaly is the most common of all deficiencies and requires more green in color mixtures than normals require. The M-cones are mutated.
- Protanomaly requires more red in color mixtures than normals require. They have a different type of L-cone.
- Tritanomaly requires more blue in the color mixture than normals require. They have a different S-cone.

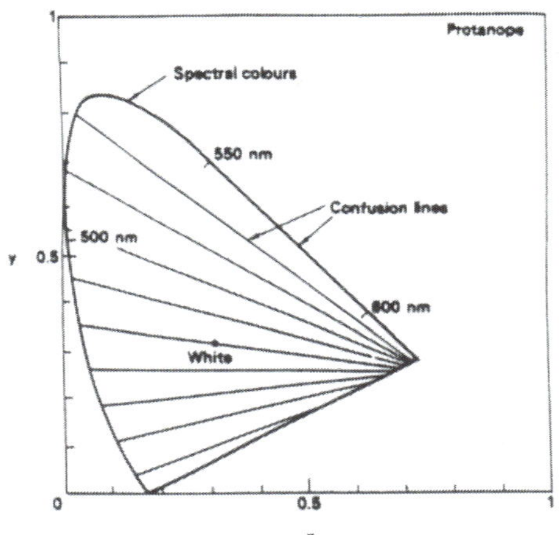

Colour confusion loci for protanopes plotted on the CIE (xy) chromaticity diagram.

- **Dichromats:** Dichromatic people only require two primary colors to perceptually match any other color.
  - Protanopes are missing the red cone pigment, erythrolabe. These people confuse red with any color and B-G with white. Protanopes have the best color discrimination for 492 (blue-green).
  - Deuteranopes are missing the green cone pigment, chlorolabe, and confuse green with white. Deuteranopes have the best color discrimination for 498nm (greener blue-green) and have nearly normal photopic spectral sensitivity.
  - Tritanopes are missing the blue cone pigment, cyanolabe and confuse yellow with white. Tritanopes have their best color discrimination for 570nm (yellow-green) and have normal photopic spectral sensitivity.
- **Monochromats**: all portions of the visible spectrum are seen as a single hue of differing brightness.
  - Rod monochromats - rod monochromats are missing all three cone pigments and are characterized by poor VA (20/200), photophobia, and jerk nystagmus.
  - Cone monochromat - atypical achromatopsia which includes rods and one cone (lacking 2 cone pigments).

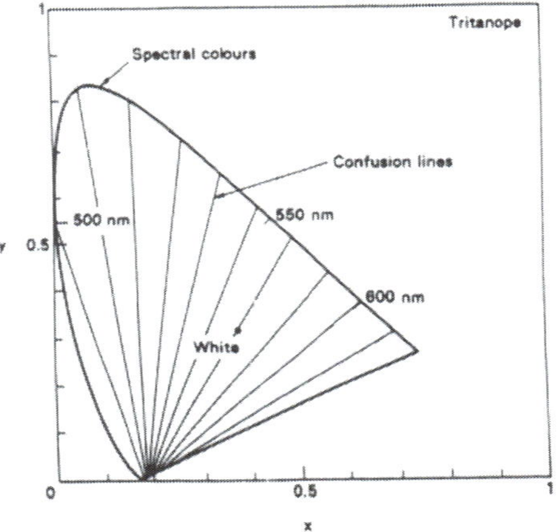

Colour confusion loci for tritanopes plotted on the CIE (xy) chromaticity diagram (data not well authenticated).

Inheritance Patterns:

- Red-green defects are most often inherited in an X-linked recessive manner; therefore, they are more common in males than females. The prevalence of red-green defects in males and females is 8.0% and 0.4%, respectively.
- Tritan defects are extremely rare (0.005%), and transmitted as autosomal dominant anomalies.

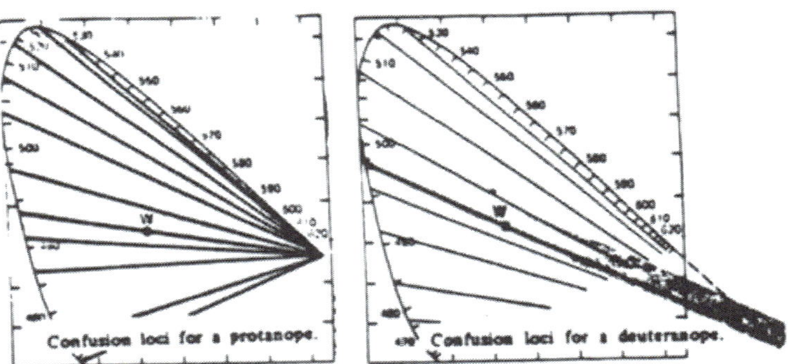

Confusion Line Diagrams for Color Deficients

Color Vision Tests:

- Pseudoisochromatic Plate Tests are the most often used. These include the Ishihara, SPP2 and HRR. Each work off the same basic principle: having a vanishing figure within a background based on chromatic differences. These differences cannot be perceived by patients with color vision anomalies because they lie on their dichromatic confusion lines. SPP2 and HRR tests are designed to detect blue-yellow defects in addition to red-green, whereas Ishihara is restricted to red-green.
- Arrangement tests include:

- The Farnsworth dichotomous tests (Panel D-15): Allows the detection of protan, deutan, and tritan defect, but does not differentiate dichromats from anomalous trichromats
- Desaturated D-15: detects subtle acquired defects, as it is extra sensitive
- The Farnsworth-Munsell 100-Hue Test: May be used in industry for screening employees, but has little application otherwise.

- **Nagel Anomaloscope**: the *Rayleigh equation* is the ratio of red to green required by an observer to match spectral yellow; as measured by an anomaloscope.
- Trichromats:
    - Normal will accept one R/G ratio to match yellow
    - Protanomalous will accept one R/G ratio to match yellow, but compared to the normal will require more red.
    - Deuteranomalous will accept one R/G ratio to match yellow, but will require more green compared to a normal.
- Dichromats:
    - Protanopia compared to the normal will require less luminance of the yellow to match the brightness of pure red.
    - Deuteranopia compared to the normal will require about equal luminance of yellow to match the brightness of either pure red or pure green.

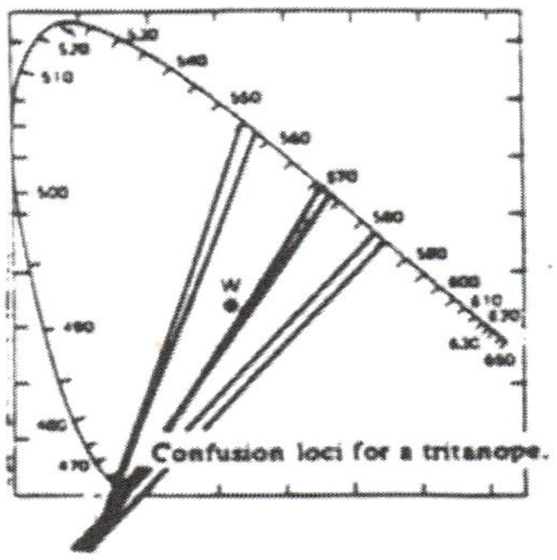

Confusion loci for a tritanope.

Confusion Line Diagram for Color Deficients

8. Acquired Anomalies of Color Vision

Classification

- Acquired defects are classified as being either a red-green or blue-yellow.
- **Kollner's Rule**: Applies only to acquired color vision deficiencies; diseases of the retina and changes of the ocular media are associated with blue-yellow defects, while diseases of the optic nerve and visual pathway are associated with red-green deficiencies (e.g., nuclear sclerosis yields a blue-yellow defect; ARMD yields a blue-yellow defect; Leber's optic atrophy yields a red-green defect); there are a few well-known exceptions to this rule however (e.g., primary open-angle glaucoma typically yields a blue-yellow defect). Note: most hereditary color defects are red-green.
- Because the etiology of acquired color vision defects is due to disease or toxicity, the pattern of the defect can change over time.

Color vision tests

- It is best to screen adults for tests that will detect blue-yellow defects, as many acquired defects result in this pattern of color deficiency. Of special consideration is Short Wavelength Automated Perimetry (SWAP), which targets the S-Cone system (which is often the earliest system affected in glaucoma).

9. Conditions for Color Vision Testing

- Most color vision tests require standard Illuminant C lighting in order to be administered properly. A MacBeth Lamp provides the proper illumination similar to Illuminant C. Indirect sunlight has also been suggested as an alternative light source. Each eye should be tested independently in order to better differentiate acquired and inherited defects. Inherited defects should affect each eye similarly. When an acquired defect is suspected, the eye likely to be most affected should be tested first.

10. Societal Implications of Color Vision Anomalies

- Schools often use color-coded visual aids to teach lessons. Special consideration should be taken to test preschool-aged children to prevent children from falling behind due to color vision anomalies.
- Vocational requirements, especially in areas of public safety (firefighters, police, and emergency response, for example) often include good color discrimination.

- Patient interest, even in non-academic or vocational consideration, stems from reliance on color vision with everyday tasks. Protan defects, for example, are correlated with higher numbers of automobile accidents because of their reduced ability to see brake lights.

11. Patient Management Strategies

- Counseling: Patients, and parents of patients, with color anomalies should be assured that color vision anomalies are stable, common, and do not pose any threat to vision.
- Special aids: Dichromatous and anomalous trichromats may benefit from wearing a red contact lens (X-chrom) lens, or other special filters that have a long-pass filter (blocking short wavelengths). When a stimulus is viewed by the eye with the contact lens, more photopigments will be bleached by higher wavelength light as compared to in the eye without the contact lens. By comparing the stimulus presented to each eye, wavelength (and, therefore, color) discrimination is improved.

BASIC PSYCHOPHYSICAL METHODS AND THEORY

1. Measurement of Absolute and Difference Thresholds

- Absolute threshold = least stimulus value that will produce a response or cause a transition from no sensation to sensation. aka: stimulus threshold
- Difference threshold = the smallest difference between two stimuli that for a given individual gives rise to a perceived difference in sensation. aka: just noticeable difference (JND).
- Both of these threshold types are measured through variations of the methods of limits, adjustment, and constant stimuli.

2. Threshold Determination

- **Method of Limits** = experimenter manipulates stimulus. Most commonly used in a clinical situation.
  - Ascending method of limits = raising intensity until a stimulus is seen.
  - Descending method of limits = lowering intensity until stimulus disappears
  - The sets of ascending trials and descending trials are averaged separately and then averaged together.
  - Advantages:
    - Fast
    - Response-dependent
  - Disadvantages:
    - At any point the subject knows how intense a stimulus to expect.
    - The initial intensity at which the series begins with can influence the point at which the subject reports the threshold. In addition, the number of stimuli that are presented is dependent on the subject's response (i.e. Snellen chart).
- **Method of Adjustment** (aka Method of Average Error) = subject manipulates stimulus to match a standard. After a determined number of trials, the readings are averaged. The stimulus must be continuously varied.
  - Advantages:
    - Rapid way to obtain threshold measurements
    - Good for dark adaptation.
  - Disadvantages
    - Subject has tendency to place threshold according to how far down she/he thinks it should go.
- **Method of Constant Stimuli** (aka "Yes/No Procedure") = stimulus is presented varied and randomly; the stimulus is NOT presented constantly but the observer is made to think so.
  - Blank trial is when no stimulus is presented, but the response is still recorded to validate the reliability of the data.
    - Hit = when the stimulus is present, and observer reports seeing stimulus
    - Miss = when stimulus is present, and observer reports not seeing stimulus

- False positive = when stimulus is not present, and observer reports seeing stimulus
- Correct reject = when stimulus is not present, and observer accurately reports not seeing stimulus

- Advantages:
  - Subject is always alert
- Disadvantage
  - Subject may become bored
  - Time consuming

- **Forced Choice** = observer must choose between two or more choices, thereby minimizing the effects of the observer's criteria (that is, their uncertainty)
  - Advantages:
    - Quick
    - Removed observer's criteria
    - Results in lower thresholds (observers do well even when guessing)
  - Disadvantages
    - If multiple alternatives are presented, observer may get overwhelmed and experiment may be time consuming

PSYCHOPHYSICAL SCALING METHODS AND THEORY

- Scaling methods = psychological measurements used to establish the intensity of the sensation experienced by the subject. Magnitude estimation is a direct method of measurement useful for determining supra-threshold events.
  - Direct scaling = The subject assigns appropriate numbers to a series of stimuli in accordance with subjective impressions. Most variance can be accounted for by a power function relationship between the stimulus magnitude and assigned numerals.
    - Other direct scaling methods: methods involving judgments of assigned equal appearing intervals between two stimuli, fractionation methods, methods of multiple judgment, and the constant sum or ratio partition method.
    - These are similar with respect to a comparison made by the subject between the subject's estimate of how much stronger or weaker a given sensation to be measured is, as compared with a standard sensation unit. For example, if light A is 3x as bright as B, assign a number to the brightness of A that is 3x larger than the brightness of B.
  - Indirect scaling = in this technique, measurements are derived from data on how well observers can tell one stimulus from another, rather than from their direct judgments of the sensation magnitudes.
    - Indirect or Fechnerian methods = require considerable statistical manipulation to construct a measurement scale. Based on Weber's Law and Fechnerian statement: $S = K \log R$. (R = stimulus intensity)
    - There are two indirect scaling methods: Law of Comparative judgment and Law of Categorical judgment.
      - Comparative judgment occurs when a stimulus gives rise to a hypothetical discriminative process which the subject varies from presentation to presentation of the same stimulus.
      - Categorical judgment occurs when a point scale is used by the subject to place the stimuli in appropriate piles or categories, i.e. like very much, like a little, neither like nor dislike, dislike little and dislike very much.
- Four basic types of measurement scales:
  - Nominal, ordinal, interval, and ratio.

SIGNAL DETECTION METHODS AND THEORY

- Signal Detection Theory is a statistical model that represents how people actually behave in detection situations. It is a psychophysical theory in which detectability of a stimulus replaces classical "threshold" value. Designed to overcome shortcoming of whether or not the subject sees a stimulus when it is actually there and when the subject could be right or wrong depending on a guess.

- Signals must be detected from a background of activity, called noise, which is usually random and may be of an internal or external source.
- In the process of detection, the observer must decide whether an observation is added to the noise or it is simply noise.
- There are two probability distributions: random variation of noise (N); and signal plus noise (SN). Detectability measures the distance between the "noise" and the "noise + signal" distribution.
- As the signal strength is decreased, the two distributions overlap which makes decision making difficult.
- Given a sensory observation, the observer decides whether it was sampled from N or SN distribution; ordinate of N gives likelihood of the observation occurring when it is only noise and the ordinate of SN gives likelihood of it actually being present.
- For each observation there is a likelihood ratio:

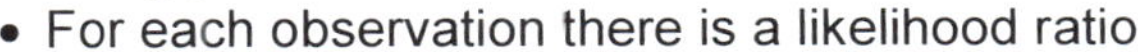

  - $L(x)$ = ordinate of SN/ordinate of N
    - If $L(x) = 1.00$, then the observation is equally likely to result from noise as it is from noise plus signal.

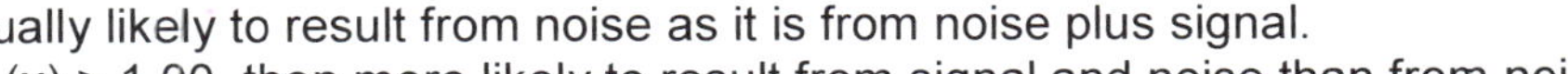

    - If $L(x) > 1.00$, then more likely to result from signal and noise than from noise alone.
    - If $L(x) < 1.00$, then the sensory observation probably resulted from noise. The observer's final decision is based on this ratio.

- Based on the fact that the stimulus was either presented or not and the subject said it was or was not presented, there are four categories that must be defined.

	Stimulus Detected	Stimulus Not Detected
Stimulus Present	Hit (a)	Miss (b)
No Stimulus	False Alarm (c)	Correct Rejection (d)

  - Hit = reports yes when the signal is presented (true positive).
  - Miss = reports yes when only noise is present (false negative).
  - False alarm = reports yes when only noise is present (false positive).
  - Correct rejection = reports no when only noise is present (true negative).
  - Hit rate = a/(a+b)
  - False alarm rate = c/(c+d).

- ROC curves = one of main sources of evidence supporting signal detection.
  - Each point on an ROC curve is determined by the location of the observer's criterion on the x dimension. As criterion is changed from strict to lax, false alarm rate and hit rate increase, and when plotted, form the ROC curve.
  - The shape of the curve determined by the way the areas under N and SN distributions above the criterion change when the location of the criterion is changed.
    - d' is a measure of detectability and is equal to the difference between the measure of the SN and N distributions divided by the standard deviation of N distribution.
  - Three basic psychophysical procedures of the Theory of Signal Detection
    - Yes/No procedure: must judge presence or absence of a signal in a long series of trials
    - Forced choice procedure: a trial consists of the presentation of 2 or more observation intervals and the task is to report which observation interval contained a signal.
    - Confidence rating procedure: involves the observer making a confidence rating for yes-no judgment.

Chapter 10 – Visual and Human Development

VISION DEVELOPMENT IN THE INFANT AND CHILD

1. Spatial Vision

- **Visual Acuity:** Acuity is a measure of sensitivity of spatial discrimination.
    - Acuity increases at approximately one cycle per degree (cpd) per month until 20 months.
    - There is a critical period in normal visual development for humans probably before 6-8 months in age. It appears that the primary limitation to early acuity is not quality of the retinal image but rather the nervous system's ability to process the image.
    - Different test methods yield different acuity results:
        - **Optokinetic nystagmus (OKN)** works well with infants
        - **Forced preferential looking (FPL)** acuities are similar to those attained with OKN
        - **Visual Evoked Potential (VEP)** measurements show that VA increases from birth.
            - By 6-8 months the VAs attained by VEP are similar to adults.
- **Contrast Sensitivity:**
    - Sensitivity shows a similar developmental trend to that for acuity. Such tests involve stimulus manipulation in the domain of contrast rather than of space and they are not, strictly speaking, visual acuity tests.
        - An infant is sensitive to a much lower and more restricted range of spatial frequencies than the adult visual system.
    - The relative loss of sensitivity at **low spatial frequencies** generally indicates the working of **lateral inhibition**. However, this is not noticed in infants before 2 months of age. Thus contour enhancement may not be present until 2 months after birth. Low frequency fall off increases notably with age.
        - **The high frequency cut off increases from 2 cpd at 2 months to 20 cpd by 10 months** and the peak contrast sensitivity improved from **4 to 40** over the same age range base **on FPL**.
    - Contrast sensitivity **peaks** at all spatial frequencies by **age 18** and remain at this level until 39 years of age.
        - Ages **8 through 15 show the lowest sensitivity to low spatial frequencies**, but the sensitivity increases by age 18.
        - Those from 45 through 66 years of age begin to lose sensitivity to high spatial frequencies

2. Refractive Error

- Spherical Error
    - **Premature infants** at birth have an average refractive error of **-0.50 D** with a standard deviation of 2.80 D.
    - **Full-term** infants at birth have an average refractive error of **+2.00 D** with a standard deviation of 2.00 D. This age range had almost a normal distribution (bell-shaped curve centered around the mean) versus adult's leptokurtotic (steeper curve in the middle) distribution.
    - **One-year olds** have an average refractive error of **+1.00 D** with a standard deviation of 1.10 D.
    - **Three-year** olds have an average refractive error of **+0.95 D** with a standard deviation of 1.00 D.
    - School children: There is a common increase in myopia with increasing age during the school years or a decrease in hyperopia (Hirsch's data, 1952).
    - During the preschool years, the curve (freq. distrib. of refraction) is leptokurtotic (steeper curve) towards hyperopia, symmetrical at the age of 10-11 and skewed towards myopia after that.

- Astigmatic error:
  - Prevalence of **infants with >1.00DC** of astigmatism is **17%;** prevalence **decreases rapidly by age 18-24 mos**:
  - Magnitude of overall astigmatism decreases after birth, becomes **adult level by 5 years old.**
  - The following graph shows the incidence of astigmatism with age.

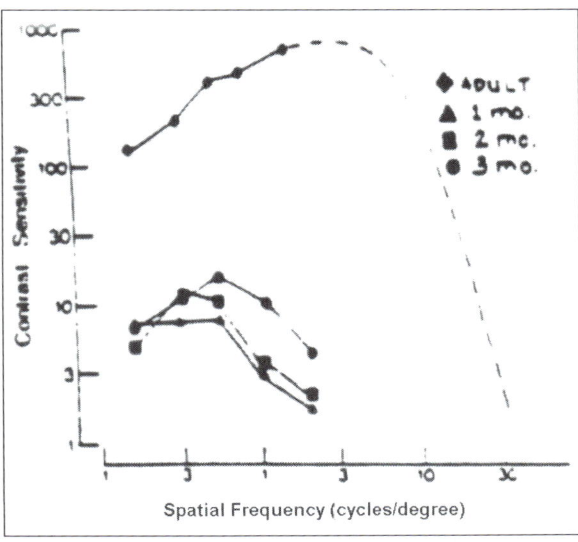

3. Color Vision

- **Color Vision**: Modern studies that measure spectral sensitivity in infants for both photopic and scotopic conditions show that the general shapes of sensitivity functions are similar to adult functions for much of the visible spectrum, although the infants were less sensitive on the whole than adults:
- **One month old infants** showed elevation in relative threshold as compared to adults for wavelengths below 450 nm. (Visual spectrum is roughly 400-700nm) In other words, infants have one log unit less sensitivity in the short wavelengths (they need more light than adults at these wavelengths to discriminate).
- **Three month old infants** did not exhibit this threshold elevation. This may be due to a less dense lens and macular pigmentation early in life. Possibly, the processing or neural pathways are not developed yet for that system.
- **By five months**, infant sensitivity curves closely agree with adult curves. This suggests normal rod and cone functioning possibly at levels of adult chromatic vision by as early as 3 months of age. It has not been proven that the existence of these functioning photoreceptors can be used by the infant to distinguish hues.

4. Spectral Transmission of the Ocular Media

- **Spectral transmission of the ocular media**: Theoretically, spectral transmission of ocular media is at its **highest point at birth** and infancy. Changes in the spectral transmission may occur and be due to ocular pathologies, but changes in transmission that occur naturally do not occur until later in life. **Brunescence** (yellowing of the lens, thus absorbing shorter wavelengths) increases as one increases in age.

UVC: 100-290
UVB: 290-320
UCA: 320-400

	Absorption	Transmission
Cornea	>3000 nm <290 nm	315 - 3000 nm (with some absorption bands)
Aqueous	very little	
Lens	>2500 nm <320-400 nm depending on age	1000 nm 2500 nm (with some absorption bands)
Vitreous	400-1000 (100%) >1600 nm 270-320 nm	270-1600 nm

table 2.1 Spectral transmission of the ocular components of the eye

Wavelength (nm)	% T to retina
>1500	0
900	90
770	94
770-400	100
400-320	age
<290	0

table 2.2 Transmission of the eye as a whole

5. Accommodation and Convergence

- Birth: Accommodation present, but not accurate. The relatively poor accommodation of newborns and 1 month olds is due to the inability to detect the consequences of focusing errors because of their inherently large depth of focus. As the infant ages, depth of focus decreases while visual acuity and pupil diameter increase, allowing greater sensitivity to accommodative error and improving focusing accuracy

- Considerable amounts of improvement in ability to accommodate to distant targets occur between birth and 3 months.
- At 4 months, accommodation is well developed.

6. Light Sensitivity

- **30 weeks gestation**: lid closure in response to bright light.
- **2-5 months**: blink response to visual threat.

7. Binocular Vision and Stereopsis

- Binocular fusion is present at a mean age of 12.8 weeks
- Disparity is detected by 3-4 months
- Stereopsis:
    - At 16 weeks with Preferential Learning: 5-6 months achieve <1 arcmin
    - At 3-4 months with VEP: youngest age of stereopsis 7-8 weeks
    - Between **3 and 6 months**: begins to develop and has rapid onset.
- Based on a number of studies, patients 5 years or older with **normal binocular vision** have **50 seconds or better at near and 120 seconds or better at distance**
- Logical order for BV development:
    - **At birth:**
        - Fovea immature, poor grating acuity
        - Eyes look in roughly the same direction
        - Some binocular coordination
    - **Birth to 3 months:**
        - Fovea matures, grating acuity improves
        - Eyes more able to fixate together on an object
        - Cells in Layer IV of cortex acquiring characteristics to enable them to act as an appropriate input to near and far cells after stereopsis occurs
    - **3-6 months:**
        - Dramatic alterations in visual cortex and ability of eyes to work together
        - Stereopsis becomes detectable, rapid increase in stereoscopic acuity
        - Full convergence EM: orthotropia
        - Binocular summation and rivalry occur
    - **After 6 months:**
        - Grating acuity improves
        - Stereoscopic acuity reaches 1 arc min

8. Form Reproduction and Perception

- **6 months** can discriminate faces
- However, infants can only identify objects if they have been familiarized with the full visible form first. If presented with parts of an object (such as a figure sitting behind a slit), even 4 year olds cannot perceive the full form

9. Temporal Vision

- **CFF** reaches adult levels by **2-4 months** of age

10. Visual Fields

- Testing visual fields in infants is difficult due to inattention
- Visual fields show little development between birth and 2 mos, then expands rapidly until 8 mos before slowing down again.
- ***Binocular*** upper VF reaches adult levels **by 12 mos**; Horizontal and Inferior fields **by 15 mos**.
- ***Monocular*** fields reach adult levels at **17 mos**.

11. Motion Perception

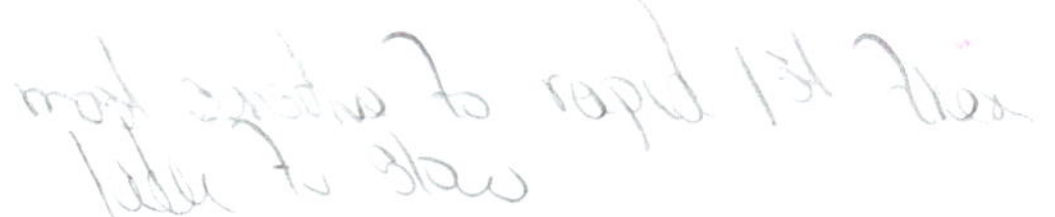

- Sensitivity to **rapid motion** is adult level **soon after birth**.
- Sensitivity to slow motion improves gradually with age.

EFFECTS OF EARLY ENVIRONMENTAL RESTRICTIONS

---

1. Plasticity of the System

- There is a critical period in the normal development of the ocular dominance columns in the visual cortex. It is during this period that the neural system is plastic and development can be altered. Once the critical period has passed the state of the neural system cannot be altered.
- The **critical period** for **humans** is somewhere between **6-8 months to as late as 2.5 years**
- The critical period for **monkeys** is during the first **6 weeks** of life and for **kittens** is between **1 to 3 months**.

2. Animal Models

- Monkeys and kittens are used to determine the effects of environment on ocular dominance columns:
- **Monkeys:** Make good comparison models; recently a lot has been done with the study of this area. These animals do have a fovea. The development of monkey visual system is very mature at birth compared to humans. It is comparable to a 3 week old human infant. A monkey's acuity develops 3 times faster than humans and has a contrast sinusoidal grating frequency of 40-50 cpd.
- **Cats**: They have an area centralis, but it's not a high acuity area like the fovea. The visual system of kittens is immature at birth. The lids are fused for 8 days postnatally. When the eyes do open, visual performance is poor because of cloudy media caused by the tunica vasculosa (remnants of the hyaloid vasculature). The quality of the image approaches adult levels at 6 wks.
- **Deprivation experiments** on both monkeys and kittens show that the retina is not affected and thus the retina must be hardwired at birth. The LGN is not as hardwired as the retina because deprivation experiments cause some cell shrinkage in all layers of the LGN. The visual cortex, on the other hand, is severely affected and alteration of ocular dominance columns occurs. Ocular dominance columns don't form until a few weeks after birth in cat and monkey.
- **Rabbits**: Not a good model to compare to humans because they don't have a fovea.

3. Light and Pattern Deprivation

- Light deprivation: Preventing all light from coming in.
- Pattern deprivation: Preventing patterns from being formed. There is more extensive alteration of normal development of binocularity from pattern deprivation than from light deprivation. This is mostly due to the absence of contoured visual patterns because it causes unequal uncoordinated input through the eyes and this can't be matched up in the visual cortex.
- **Amblyopia** can be caused by a deficient input of light and form (**pattern deprivation) or** no input at all (**light deprivation**). It can occur in one or both eyes. Unilateral or bilateral **cataracts** are the most common cause of deprivation amblyopia. **Corneal scarring, ptosis**, and **bilateral ametropia** can also lead to deprivation amblyopia.
- Unilateral cataracts or unilateral media opacities produce a dual amblyogenic mechanism. **Unilateral vision deprivation** occurs, and suppression of this blurred image by the fixating eye contributes to abnormal binocular interaction, or **strabismus, as well as form deprivation, amblyopia**.

4. Monocular and Binocular Deprivation

- **Monocular deprivation** causes the non-deprived eye to drive more cells in the visual cortex than the deprived eye.
- **Binocular deprivation** causes symmetrically reduced acuity in both eyes which can be recovered if the deprivation is ceased early enough in the critical period.

mono dep worse than bino

- Monocular deprivation effects are more severe than binocular deprivation since binocular competition and shifting in cortical cells occur.

5. Refractive Error

- When considering the effects of early environmental restrictions, one should always consider the possibility of refractive amblyopia. The key indicators of refractive amblyopia are significant hyperopia and/or astigmatism combined with a history of delayed initial lens application. A child born with some impediment to clear eyesight faces the possibility of permanently reduced eyesight unless the impediment is removed, or in some way neutralized, during the early stages of his life.
- Anisometropic amblyopia also results from a dual amblyogenic mechanism. The fixating eye has a clear image, and the anisometropic eye has a blurred image which causes unequal binocular input and leads to suppression of the anisometropic eye. In addition, the suppressed eye (usually the more ametropic eye) invariably becomes strabismic either with a microtropia or small-angle deviation.
- Also, high aniso-astigmatic infants have distortion in form or pattern detection and this can lead to other visual acuity problems such as amblyopia.
- In general, the younger the patient, the more rapidly amblyopia will develop from any cause, and the more rapid will be successful treatment by appropriate methods such as patching.

Anisometropic amblyopes:

- Caused by both anomalous binocular interactions and form deprivation. **One eye has been out of focus, which causes form deprivation, but there is also abnormal binocular interaction**. Both cause reduced visual acuity.
- Peripheral visual acuity: There is a symmetrical loss of visual acuity temporally and nasally as compared to the normal except for a small region in the nasal retina where visual acuity is about the same.
- Spatial distortion and uncertainty: No distortion, and range of uncertainty about 1 minute on either side.
- Fixations: Do not show as large of drifts as seen in strabismics and they are symmetrical, but they are larger than normal. Also, the tremors are 60 Hz.
- Pursuits: Anisometropes don't show the asymmetry in pursuits like strabismics, but they may not be as good as normals.

6. Strabismus

- Amblyopia caused by anomalous binocular interactions. The normally fixating eye tends to suppress the deviating eye causing a reduction in visual acuity.
- Peripheral visual acuity: There is an asymmetric **loss of VA where the greater loss is seen nasally.**
- **Spatial distortion** and uncertainty: Distortion up to 25 minutes, and range of uncertainty from 25 to 30 minutes.
- Fixations
  - **Normal:** High frequency tremors of about 60 Hz with 1 drift per second and magnitudes of about 1 to 2 minutes.
  - **Strabismic:** Fixation is usually eccentric (nasal) and unsteady. They have 60 Hz tremors, but drifts are large, as much as 5 degrees.
- **Pursuits**: Objects in their nasal field can be tracked pretty well, but tracking objects in the temporal field is difficult.
- The # of binocular cells decreases from 80% to 20% in the strabismic animal.
- The ocular dominance columns become well defined reflecting the separation of inputs from the 2 eyes. The asynchrony of signals sometimes leads to amblyopia

7. Cataract

- The presence of cataracts is comparable to unilateral or binocular eyelid suturing in the monocular and binocular deprivation experiments done on animal models.
- Congenital cataracts, if not surgically removed **by 3 months**, will cause abnormal development of the visual system. Visual acuity will most likely not be better than 20/200 corrected. If however, the cataract was treated by age 3 months, visual acuity of 20/60 corrected or better can be attained. If bilateral the result is almost the same as normal. If a unilateral cataract is present, normal development is not promoted due to inadequate stimulus. Also, the deprived eye gets worse due to binocular competition between the two eyes.
- If the onset of cataracts occurred after birth, i.e. traumatic cataracts, the amount of vision loss is dependent upon the age of onset; if afflicted at a later age, there is less visual loss. However, if a traumatic cataract occurs in the first 3 years of life, only rudimentary vision will result.
- In children with either unilateral or bilateral cataracts, both binocularity and stereopsis can be severely reduced or eliminated

---

CHANGES IN VISION WITH AGING

---

1. Spatial Vision

- Visual acuity:
  - Prior to 10 weeks of age, there is no measurable vernier acuity
  - By 10-12 weeks of age there is a rapid emergence of vernier acuity. Grating acuity takes longer to develop
  - Is not a significant factor with changing age post-infancy. There may be some change in central acuity, but usually as a summation of other changes or disease. Commonly up until age 80, we can get at least one eye corrected to at least 20/40. Larger losses are seen for low contrast charts and when testing under conditions of reduced illumination (pupil size, lens changes, retinal changes are causes).
- Contrast sensitivity
  - The infant CSF is shifter down and to the left compared to adults. CSF improves in sensitivity and scale from infancy and is mature by 2-3 months
    - Sensitivity to high spatial frequencies continues to develop beyond 6 months, improvement may be due to photoreceptor maturation and cone packing
  - Decreases with age (important for contact lens wearers)
  - Glaucoma, cataracts, macular pathologies and other abnormalities may result in decreased contrast sensitivity.
- Different eye diseases impact these parts of spatial vision differently, including neurological problems, medial opacities, and optical blur

2. Refractive Error

- Refractive error development is more complex and dynamic change over the first 5 years of life than at any other period of human development
- Refractive error can significantly impact visual development (amblyopia, binocularity) as well as general development (fine motor skills, learning, associated with developmental disabilities)
- 15-30% of preschoolers have refractive error
- The distribution (variability) of refractive error decreases with age
- **Emmetropization:** The eye senses the sign and magnitude of the refractive error than modulates its rate of growth through an active visual feedback mechanism in order to reduce that error.
  - The highest rates of emmetropization occur during months 12-17.
  - After 17 months, refractive error probably won't go away
- Astigmatism
  - Prevalence of astigmatism in infants >1DC
    - Noncycloplegic 53%, cycloplegic 17%, adults 10%
    - Decreases rapidly by 18m-24m

- Magnitude of astigmatism decreases during the first year and reaches adult level by 2.5 to 5 years
- Type of astigmatism:
  - Higher prevalence of ATR from birth to 3 years than adults
  - By 5 years, higher prevalence of WTR
  - Most changes in ATR astigmatism shift to WTR, oblique shows most stability (prescribe for oblique)

- Anisometropia
  - Prevalence of anisometropia >1D is negatively correlated with age. A child with little anisometropia at year 1 if found to have significant anisometropia at age 4
  - Anisometropia decreases with time
- Myopia
  - Greater magnitude and prevalence in premature than full term infants
  - Myopic babies are likely to be myopic at age 1
    - Most infants are born hyperopic at birth and become emmetropic by year 1
- Ametropias that may result in amblyopia
  - Hyperopia >2D
  - Myopia >8D
  - Astigmatism >1.50 DC

3. Color Vision

- Rods and at least 1 cone type are functional by 1 month
- Infants show dichromic (tritanopic) color vision by 8-10 weeks.
- Trichromatic vision is present by 3 months
- There is a loss of discrimination of the **blue** end of the spectrum, caused by **macular degeneration** and **nuclear sclerosis** in old age. Results in **tritanopia**

4. Spectral Transmission of the Ocular Media

- Transmission of light decreases with age (relatively small effect).
- The lens becomes more yellow with age and absorbs more light, significantly changing the amount and quality of light reaching the retina; the yellowing of the lens may accelerate after the age of 60.
- Cataracts in the lens causes decreased vision and changes in refractive error
- The vitreous liquefies (syneresis) causing reflections of light that patients notice as “floaters”

5. Accommodation and Convergence

- The amplitude of **accommodation decreases linearly with age**. This normal decrease in the elasticity of the lens if classified as presbyopia.
- **Convergence ability stays the same or better** because of the unlimited use of accommodative convergence (which is due to the fact that the innervation to accommodation is still there).

6. Light Sensitivity

- The retinal illuminance for an 80 year old is at least 10 times lower than that of a 25 year old; therefore the sensitivity decreases with age. Patients will need additional light to see targets with age

7. Glare (Disability and Discomfort)

- **Light scatter by the lens** causes more glare problems with increasing age.
- **Disability glare recovery** (time it takes for visual acuity to recover following exposure to bright light) **increases** with age

8. Dark Adaptation, Glare Recovery

- The ability to adapt to darkness is significantly slowed with age. This is caused by inadequate regeneration of rhodopsin and decreased ability to metabolize vitamin A

- Each decade brings a 2 to 3 log unit higher threshold of the rods and cones, but the time to the rod-cone break remains constant; the ability to recover visual sensitivity from bright lights worsens after age 40.

9. Visual Fields

- The peripheral fields decrease somewhat primarily due to senile miosis and nuclear lens sclerosis. Retinal sensitivity is decreased, as is retinal illumination, both causing a decrease in peripheral visual acuity.

10. Temporal Vision

- CFF decreases about 7 cycles/sec by age 40.
- 70% of the loss is attributed to senile miosis, which reduces light by a factor of approximately two.

11. Oculomotor System

- Under **scotopic conditions**, aging patients had **difficulty with fixation**.
- The older patients showed a decreased gain (increased lag) and consequently an increased number of saccades in order to maintain fixation.
- The range of voluntary eye movements becomes limited with advancing age.
- Tonic vergence appears to increase somewhat with increasing years, as evidenced by increasing esophoria for distance fixation.
- The positive fusional vergence decreases with age, but the negative fusional vergence does not.
- The total vergence as determined from the far point to the near point of convergence does not appear to change significantly with age.

Normal Motor Development in the Infant Child

- Oculomotor system:
  - Looking is an active response controlled by the 12 extraocular muscles. Newborn eyes roam around both in the presence and absence of visual stimulus. They can make coordinated and directionally correct oculomotor responses to auditory stimuli. Early fixation is monocular. They can fixate an object a few inches from the eyes. They can maintain conjugate fixation and conjugate eye movements.
  - Pupillary light reaction
    - 31 weeks after gestation: pupillary light reaction present.
  - Milestones
    - Looking at patterns: several weeks after birth
    - Following moving objects: several weeks
    - Reaching for objects: 4 mos

12. Motion Perception

- **Visual perceptual-motor abilities:** Visuomotor-sensory-motor control or coordination. Our visual field contains sharp details only in its central region and as we move toward the periphery, these details are lost. In order for our visuomotor system to expand our effective visual fields, our eyes make several types of movements: saccades, smooth pursuit, vestibular controlled and optokinetic movements.
- **Saccades** rapidly change our fixation from one stimulus to another. At birth a functional saccadic movement exists but is not adult-like. Instead of one distinct saccadic movement as performed by an adult, the infant performs smaller multiple saccades to get to its fixation. At 4-5 months, the step saccades are no longer present. Also, the infant's saccades have longer latency periods.
- **Smooth pursuit** movements hold fixation on a moving target. It is present at birth but is only seen in OKN. At 5-6 weeks of age all tracking is completed by saccadic movements and not by smooth pursuits. By 2 months, infants can use smooth pursuits for low velocities.
- **Vestibular-controlled** eye movements compensate for motion of the head and help maintain fixation on a constant point in space. It is generally present at birth, but is not well coordinated with other forms of eye movements until 3 months.

- **OKN** are smooth pursuits with saccadic refixations in the opposite direction. Elicited in newborns and infants of all ages under binocular stimulus, but not under monocular conditions until 3 months. Asymmetric OKN exists under monocular conditions for infants younger than 3 months. The asymmetry is for temporal to nasal movements of the stimulus.
- Binocular convergence appears first accompanied by marked jerks and later smaller ones, until convergence becomes smooth. The infant's ability to stand upright unattended is accomplished through vision, since vestibular sense is not fully developed until 4-5 years of age. Motor and sensory capacity for fusion may be present soon after birth, because it can be stimulated by an optokinetic response.
- Development of conjugate gaze
  - **Birth:** conjugate horizontal gaze well developed.
  - **2 months:** conjugate vertical gaze well developed.

Normal Motor Development in the Infant and Child

- Development of motor control parallels CNS development
  - goes in a cephalocaudal direction (head before toes)
  - goes in a proximal-distance direction (trunk before extremities)
- Gross motor/language development milestones:
  - Primitive reflexes present at birth include finger gripping
  - Control of neck and head: 6 mos
  - Sitting alone: 7 mos
  - Crawling : 7 mos
  - Pulling themselves up: 8 mos
  - Pointing: 9 mos
  - Standing: 11 mos
  - Walking: 12 mos
  - Running/jumping: 2 years

13. Visual Attention

Normal Cognitive and Social Development in the Infant and Child

- Infants progress from reflex activities, to a more systemic and organized behavior learned through imitation
- Some milestones:
  - Able to discriminate mom's voice: 12 hrs
  - Looking at faces with interest: at birth
  - Smiling: 2 months
  - Crying when mom is absent: 8 months
  - Stranger anxiety: 8-12 mos
  - One clear word: 9 mos
  - Combination of words: 21 mos
- Effects on visual impairment on cognitive and social development:
  - The inability to see things will greatly affect the way an infant learns about things that cannot be felt with their hands, such as large distant objects (cars, trees). Concept of distance will be difficult to form.
  - Without eye contact or the ability to see facial expressions clearly, it will be difficult for the child to learn facial signals, flow of conversations, social mannerisms, etc.

Normal Development in Infancy and Childhood				
Age (months)	Motor	Social	Hear/Speech	Eye/Hand
1	Head erect for a few seconds	Quieted when picked up	Startled by sounds	Follows light with eyes
2	Head up when prone		Listens to bell or rattle	Follows toy up, down, sideways
3	Kicks well	Follows person with eyes	Searches for sound with eyes	Glances from one object to another
4	Lifts head and chest prone	Returns examiner's smile	Laughs	Clasps and retains toy
6	Rises onto wrists	Turns head to person talking	Babbles or coos to voice, music	Takes toy from table
8	Sits without support	Looks at mirror image	Understands "no" and "bye-bye"	Passes toy from hand to hand
10	Stands when held up	Smiles at mirror image	Says "mama" "dada"	Manipulates two objects together
12	Walks or side steps around pen	Plays pat-a-cake	Three words with meaning	Finds a toy hidden under cup
14	Walks alone	Uses spoon	Recognizes own name	Makes marks with pencil
16	Push chairs, toy horse, etc	Shows shoes	6-7 clear words	Scribbles freely
18	Climbs onto chair	Takes off shoes, socks	Enjoys rhymes, joins in	Constructive play with toys
20	Jumps	Bowel control	12 words	Tower of 4 bricks
22	Walks up stairs	Tries to tell experiences	Listens to stories	Tower of 5+ bricks
24	Walks up and down stairs	Knows 4 body parts	Names 4 toys	Tries to copy line drawings

VISUAL PERCEPTUAL-MOTOR SKILLS

- Visual processing requires perception (the ability to break down a form, code it, identify it) then motor integration (the ability to reproduce the form.)
- Visual perceptual-motor skills require four main processes:
  - Stimulus reception and processing – looking at the letter or figure
  - Sensory integration – comparing the stimulus to information stored in long-term memory
  - Effector activity – making a decision to draw and then implementing the decision
  - Information feedback – proprioceptive, kinesthetic, visual, verbal
- During assessment, focus on the process and product of a visual-motor task:
  - Handedness
  - Presence of motor overflow (mirroring of the other hand, tongue protrusion)
  - Degree of impulsivity
  - Rotation of paper or stimulus materials
  - Difficulty with certain functions
  - Pencil pressure
  - Awareness of errors
  - Placement, erasures
- Visual Perception Tests:
  - **Gardner Test of Visual Perception Skills (TVPS):** Ages 4 – 12. Composed of seven parts to determine visual discrimination, visual memory, visual spatial relations, visual

Development Timeline	
Birth - 1 month	- Rapid motion perception soon after birth (slow motion improves gradually with age) - Vestibular-controlled eye movements - OKN under binocular conditions - conjugate horizontal gaze
2 months	- CFF reaches adult level (temporal vision) - Smooth pursuits - Conjugate vertical gaze
3 months	- CFF reaches adult level (temporal vision) - Normal rod and cone functioning. No longer have increased threshold for wavelengths below 450nm. - Vestibular eye movements well coordinated with other eye movements - OKN under monocular conditions
4 months	- CFF reaches adult level (temporal vision) - Accommodation is well developed - Saccades
5 months	- Pretty close to normal stereo - Saccades
6 months	- Critical period - VEP VA similar to adults - Can discriminate faces
7 months	- Critical period - VEP VA similar to adults
8 months	- Critical period - VEP VA similar to adults
9 months	- Average ametropia changes to myopia
12 months	- Binocular upper VF
15 months	- Binocular horizontal and inferior VFs
17 months	- Monocular VF
4 years	- Convergence
5 years	- Convergence - Adult level of astigmatism
18 years	- Contrast sensitivity

form constancy, visual sequential memory, visual figure ground, visual closure. Most widely used test.
    - Primary Mental Abilities (PMA): evaluates speed and spatial relations
    - Motor Free Visual Perception Test (MVPT-3)
    - Motor-Free Visual Perception Test Vertical (MVPT-V): **ages 55-80**, uses stimuli at the **vertical midline** to tests pts who may have a **hemifield visual neglect.**
- Visual Motor Integration
    - Visual motor integration is closely associated with fine motor skills. A patient with normal visual motor integration skills may not have normal fine motor skills. Most patients who have poor fine motor skills will perform poorly on visual motor **integration tests**.
    - Tests that assess visual motor integration
        - Beery-Butenica Developmental Test of Visual-Motor Integration (VMI)
        - Rosner Test of Visual Analysis Skills (TVAS)
        - Wold Copy Sentence Test
    - Tests that assess fine motor skills:
        - Beery Developmental Test of Motor Coordination
        - Frostig Test, Part 1
        - Grooved Pegboard

ANOMALIES OF CHILD DEVELOPMENT

1. Epidemiology, History, and Signs/Symptoms Manifest by Infants, Toddlers, Pre-Schoolers, and School-Age Children

History

- Parents of infants (birth to 18 months) want to know what/if the child can see
- The following are good questions to ask the parents
    - Are you concerned about any aspect of the child's health or development?
        - Motor and social development is visually dependent
        - A child with poor growth/development may have abnormal optic nerve and visual pathways
        - Hearing problems could be associated with **Retinitis Pigmentosa, Waardenburg,** and **Alport Syndromes**
    - Was the child exposed to toxic or infectious agents during pregnancy?
        - **TORCH**
    - Was the baby premature or hospitalized?
    - What medications was the mother on during pregnancy and breast feeding

Signs/Symptoms of Visual Anomalies

- Physical
    - Nystagmus
    - Constantly watering
    - Flickering eyelid movements
    - Cloudy pupil
    - Redness
    - Crustiness
    - Strabismus
    - Proptosis
    - Ptosis
- Behavioral
    - Sensitive to light – photophobic
    - Stares at bright lights
    - Eye poking
    - Waving hand in front of their eyes
    - Child does not smile or seems disinterested in environment

Epidemiology	
Common Disorder	Prevalence
Autism	1-2 per 1000 births
Cerebral Palsy	1.5-2 cases per 1000 births
Down Syndrome	1 per 1000 births

        - Does not make eye contact by 3 months of age
        - Does not reach for object by 6 months of age
    - Is not interested in activity or TV
    - The child holds a toy extremely close to view it
- Infantile ocular abnormalities rarely present in older children and are closely associated with embryological malformation, a problem during the birth process or disruption in the early postnatal visual development

Pre-Schooler (3-5 years) and School-Age Child

Conjunctivitis

- **Acute Bacterial Conjunctivitis**
    - Common in young children
    - Bilateral, mucopurulent with papillary conjunctivitis
    - Transmission by hand or spread from nasopharynx
    - 25% of children with conjunctivitis have otitis media
- **Hyperpurulent Bacterial Conjunctivitis**
    - A severe, rapid onset of lid swelling, excessive discharge, tenderness, conjunctival swelling and preauricular adenopathy
    - Important because of its morbidity
- **Acute Follicular Conjunctivitis**
    - Common in children
    - Associated with an acute upper respiratory tract infection

Trauma

- The majority of pediatric lid and adnexal injuries are accidental

2. Clinical techniques and Tests to Assess the Development of an Infant, Toddler Pre-schooler, and School Age Child

Landmark	Normal
Creeping-pulling	5 months
Hands and knees crawling	7 months
Walking/unsupported	12-14 months
Speaks clearly	1 year
Speaks in short sentences	2 years

- Talk directly to the child not the parents
- Don't wear a white coat
- Start by observing the child – are they interested in their surroundings? Do they notice small objects in the room? Are they coordinated? Make note of facial features (abnormalities of ears, ocular adnexa, eyelids, and facial asymmetry) and head posture
    - Fine and gross motor development – eye/hand coordination
    - Personal – social development
    - Speech – language development
- **Retinoscopy** – media opacities, refractive error, astigmatism, anisometropia
- **Slit Lamp** Examination – corneal abnormalities, congenital glaucoma, anterior segment dysgenesis, iris abnormalities (transillumination defects in albinism, Lisch nodules in neurofibromatosis) and children at risk for juvenile uveitis (juvenile rheumatoid arthritis)
    - Infants – parents may need to support the baby in the prone position
    - Young children – supported in parent's lap or place knees on exam chair
    - Older children- have them stand
- **Funduscopy**
    - Children >6 months can have pupils dilated with either 1% cyclopentolate or 1% tropicamide
    - Children<6 months can be dilated using 0.5% cyclopentolate
    - Do not use 10% phenylephrine in children because may precipitate life-threatening cardiovascular consequences
- **B-Scan** ultrasound – if media opacities preclude examination of the posterior pole
- Examination of a premature baby
    - Major concern is **retinopathy of prematurity**
    - Retinoscopy – assess clarity of media, refractive symmetry

- Hand-held slit lamp
- Indirect ophthalmoscope
- Sclera depressor
- Pediatric size speculum
- Portable tonometer

- Fixation Assessment – Cover test
  - Look for a manifest deviation, alternation of fixation and abnormal movements (unsteady fixation, nystagmus, searching)
  - **Central** or foveal fixation- assess corneal light reflex
  - **Steady** fixation
  - **Maintained** fixation- ability to maintain fixation with the same eye when the other is uncovered
- **Pupils**
  - Abnormalities to pupillary response to light are generally due to disease of the anterior visual pathway
  - RAPD – amblyopia
  - Anisocoria
  - Older children will accommodate to light source, make sure they look into the distance
- Estimating acuity in preverbal child (less than 3)
  - Optokinetic nystagmus (OKN)
    - Acuity is finest grating on a rotating drum that elicits a visible nystagmus response
  - Preferential looking (PL)
    - Infants have a greater tendency to look at a patterned stimulus than a plane field
    - If infant can see stripes (in a two-alternative, forced choice, preferential learning test) they will look at them
    - PL is a resolution acuity, which is usually better than recognition acuity, especially in amblyopes
  - Visually evoked potentials (VEPs)
    - A transient electroencephalogram that subtracts the background cerebral "noise"
    - The finest grating that elicits a waveform detectibly different from a blank screen is the threshold acuity
    - Particularly useful in children with motor developmental disabilities, ocular motor apraxia, and cortical visual impairment
- Optotype Testing (in children older than 3)
  - Even though some children can read letters at age 4, it is better to use pictures to keep children in their comfort zone.
  - Be aware of the **crowding phenomenon** where performance is better with single optotype than a line of letters which can be a sign of amblyopia
- **Color Vision**
  - Pseudoisochromatic plates – Ishihara screen for moderate-severe congenital red-green deficiencies (not BY)
    - Blue-yellow defects are common in acquired diseases (optic neuritis, retinitis pigmentosa, chorioretinitis, and diabetic retinopathy)
- **Contrast Sensitivity**
  - May not reach adult levels until 8 years old
  - May be useful in detecting previous optic neuritis
  - Use "Mr. Happy" or Pelli-Robson charts
- **Visual Fields**
  - Confrontation using toys or lights- child will make a quick eye or head movement to approaching stimulus
  - Can use finger counting or "wiggling" for older children, or even Goldmann perimetry
- **Fusion Testing**
  - **Stereopsis** implies good visual acuity in both eyes. Is a function of retinal image disparity
  - **Sensory fusion** infers that corresponding retinal points are present in each eye and project to similar areas of the cortical visual map
  - **Motor fusion** allows for vergence movements

- DDST – Denver Developmental Screening Test
  - Designed to assess the development of the 3 areas above during the first 6 years of life
  - Compares a child's physical and mental development to age norms
  - Consists of 105 tests slowly increasing in difficulty
- **Mental Abilities**
  - **Cognitive Development** – the ability to think about or reflect upon the past, present or future experiences or thoughts in order to analyze complex and abstract issues. To solve complex problems and to achieve new synthesis and understandings about oneself and one's milieu
  - **Mental Retardation** – A condition which refers to significantly sub-average intellectual functioning existing concurrently with deficits in adaptive behavior. Manifests during the developmental period. Clinical tests for mental retardation would include IQ testing and adaptive behavior testing
  - **Developmentally disabled** – those who have intellectual deficits in specific areas but their cognitive/intellectual functioning doesn't class them with the mentally impaired
  - **Idiot-Savants** – Generally classed as mentally retarded but they have a specific intelligence related function which it developed to a high degree
- **Sensory Abilities**
  - For the evaluation of hearing, the test results and interpretation will fall into 4 categories
    - Conductive hearing loss
    - Sensorineural hearing loss
    - Mixed hearing loss
    - Central hearing loss

Age (Months)	Response to Sound
Birth	Reflex response to sound
1	Reflex may be inhibited
3	Eye or head movement toward sound source
6	Localization of sound observable
9	Accurate localization
12	Recognizes own name
18	Shows awareness of body parts when named
20	Identifies familiar objects when named
24	Points to familiar pictures when named

- **Neuromuscular and Physical Abilities**
  - Motor development can be defined as the process of gradual acquisition of skills that incorporate movement. Mainly deficiencies in the nervous system lead to problems with motor development. There are 3 categories of developmental failure
    - Rate – develop through normal sequences of motor development but at a slow rate
    - Defective patterns – normal rate of motor maturation, but there is a delay in developmental progress
    - Rate and Defect- slow maturational rate and a specific defect in tone, strength, and or control
- **Personal-Social Behaviors**
  - Endogenous (constitutional) and exogenous (environmental) factors lead to disturbances in normal personal-social behaviors. Mentally retarded children have slower emotional maturity. When evaluating their personal-social level, a set of norms for the mentally retarded should be used.
- **Speech and Language Abilities**
  - Children with a specific speech and language disorder are deficient in some aspect of verbal functioning, but have average performance on non-verbal tasks. Mentally retarded children are deficient in more areas than just a specific speech and language disorder

3. Vision Problems which may be Associated with Deviations from Normal Patterns of Development

- Teratogenic factors
  - Teratogen is a drug or other agent that causes abnormal fetal development
  - Drug abuse, infection, medications (anticonvulsants, anticoagulants)
  - Factors occurring in the 1st trimester of pregnancy often result in eye defects
- **Fetal Alcohol Syndrome (FAS)**
  - Need 3/7 of the following categories to diagnose
    - Low birth weight
    - Growth retardation

- CNS dysfunction
- Microcephaly
- Midface hypoplasia
- Missing fulcrum under nose
- Ocular findings (Short palpebral fissures, epicanthal folds, ptosis, strabismus)

Intrauterine Infections

- Neonates infected by hematogenous spread or ascending infection from maternal genitourinary tract
- May injure the fetus by disturbing embryogenesis, damaging vital organs or as an ongoing infection that extends into postnatal life
- **TORCH infections** (Toxoplasmosis, Rubella, Syphilis, CMV, Herpes Simplex)
  - **Toxoplasmosis**
    - 1st trimester infection causes the most severe manifestations of the disease
    - Acquired from eating undercooked meat or exposure to cat feces
    - Ocular findings
      - Chorioretinitis – scarring that is heavily pigmented with areas of atrophy, usually bilateral and involves the macula, and is progressive with age
        - Toxoplasmosis acquired post-natally rarely has chorioretinitis
      - Microphthalmos
      - Cataracts
      - Panuveitis
      - Optic atrophy
    - Systemic findings
      - Intracranial calcification
      - Seizures
      - Hydrocephalus
      - Microcephaly, hepatosplenomegaly, jaundice, anemia, fever
  - **Syphilis**
    - Occurs in fetuses exposed to *Treponema pallidum* after the 16th gestational week
    - Can damage neonates postnatally as ongoing infections
    - Ocular findings
      - Chorioretinitis – peripheral areas of pigment mottling, can resemble retinitis pigmentosa
      - Interstitial keratitis (10-40%) – sectorial or diffuse corneal edema
      - Anterior uveitis
      - Iridoschisis
      - Optic atrophy
    - Early systemic findings
      - Skeletal abnormalities, rhinitis, maculopapular rash, fissures around the lips, nares, anus, hepatosplenomegaly, anemia, and uveitis
    - Late systemic findings
      - Sensorineural hearing loss, bone changes, dental abnormalities, interstitial keratitis
    - **Hutchinson's triad= keratitis + deafness + malformed incisors**
  - **Rubella**
    - Interfere with embryogenesis, rarely result in malformation after 1st trimester
    - Ocular findings:
      - Cataracts (20-30%)- bilateral
      - Microphthalmos
      - Glaucoma (10%)- common in eyes with iris hypoplasia and microphthalmos
      - Keratitis
      - Pigmentary Retinopathy (40%) – bilateral, mottled changes in posterior pole
      - Mottled iris atrophy
    - Systemic findings
      - Growth retardation, mental retardation, hearing loss, congenital heart defects, thrombocytopenic purpura, microcephaly, osteopathy, lymphadenopathy, diabetes

- **Cytomegalovirus (CMV)**
    - The most common intrauterine infection – occurs in 1% of newborns in US, but only 10% of children with congenital CMV are symptomatic as newborns
    - Causes necrosis of vital organs, result in severe abnormalities
    - Ocular findings
        - Keratitis
        - Optic atrophy
        - Chorioretinitis – scars in 6%, are less heavily pigmented than toxoplasmosis
        - Microophthalmos
        - cataracts
    - Systemic findings
        - Jaundice, hepatosplenomegaly, microcephaly, sensorineural hearing ion, psychomotor retardation, cerebral calcifications, malformations of cortical development, petechial rash
- **Herpes Simplex**
    - Most commonly occur in newborns delivered to mothers with active genital herpes
    - Neonatal herpes simplex infections begins as a cutaneous vesicular eruption that progresses to systemic infection in 50% of newborns
    - Ocular findings
        - Blepharoconjunctivitis with vesicles on eyelids
        - Keratitis with epithelial dendrites
        - Chorioretinitis with vitritis and optic atrophy
            - Well circumscribed hyperpigmented scars in peripheral retina
        - Cataracts secondary to uveitis
        - Cortical visual impairment due to herpes simplex encephalitis
    - Systemic findings
        - Hepatitis, pneumonia, intravascular coagulation, or encephalitis

- **Varicella**
    - Occurs after the 2nd or 3rd trimester
    - Ocular findings
        - Chorioretinitis – single or multiple deeply pigmented scars and atrophy, resembles toxoplasmosis, can be uni/bilateral, can result in tractional retinal detachments
        - Cataracts
        - Microphthalmos
        - Horner syndrome- unilateral
    - Systemic findings
        - Low birth weight, seizures, cortical atrophy, cicatricial skin lesions, and neuropathic bladder

Ophthalmia Neonatorum (Conjunctivitis of the Newborn)

- Conjunctivitis that occurs during the neonatal period and during the first month of life
- **Gonococcal conjunctivitis**
    - Usually develops 1-3 days after birth
    - Common in developing countries
    - Propensity to produce severe keratitis
    - Treat with 3rd generation cephalosporins
- **Chlamydial conjunctivitis**
    - Usually develops 5-25 days after birth
    - Most commonly isolated pathogens in industrial countries
    - Can be associated with neonatal pneumonitis
    - Treat with oral erythromycin
- **Congenital dacryostenosis**
    - Congenital nasolacrimal duct obstruction frequently associated with neonatal conjunctivitis
    - Expected in unilateral conjunctivitis with epiphora and reflux of mucopurulent material from Lacrimal puncta after Lacrimal sac massage
- **Viral conjunctivitis**

- Occurs infrequently in neonates
- Herpes simplex conjunctivitis can develop
- Vesicles on eyelids and herpetic keratitis may be seen

Globe and Anterior Segment Anomalies

- **Anophthalmos**
  - Eye is nonexistent or tiny cystic remnant of the eye is present
  - Represents complete failure of budding of the optic vesicle or early arrest of its development
- **Microphthalmos**
  - Abnormally small eye- axial length <21mm in an adult or <19mm in a 1 year old infant
  - Can be simple (without other disease) or complex (associated with cataract, retinal vitreous disease, or more complex malformations)
  - Etiology
    - Isolated idiopathic
    - Isolated inherited
      - Autosomal dominant
      - Autosomal recessive
      - X-linked
    - With ocular and systemic diseases
  - Can present with ocular abnormalities
    - Anterior segment malformations- Peters Anomaly, Reiger Anomaly
    - Cataract
    - Persistent hyperplastic vitreous – autosomal dominant oculodentodigital system
    - Retinal diseases – ROP, dysplasia, folds, degeneration, glaucoma
    - Aniridia
    - Coloboma
- **Congenital Ptosis**
  - Most common type of ptosis in childhood
  - Due to a dystrophy or dysgenesis of the levator
  - Resulting obstruction of vision can cause deprivation amblyopia
- **Congenital Glaucoma**
  - Rare in infants (1 in 10,000) with heterogenous causes. 75% of cases are bilateral, occurs more in boys than girls
  - High pressure in the eye in combination with a large cornea can cause nerve damage in newborns and infants
  - Common etiology is malformation of some parts of the eye, often an anterior segment developmental anomaly (trabecular meshwork) of neural crest cell origin, can be autosomal recessive
  - Symptoms/signs include excessive tearing, photophobia, blepharospasm
  - The pressure can damage Descemet's membrane
  - The age of onset is in utero (first few months of age)
- **Congenital Cataracts**
  - Can cause pattern deprivation vision until the lens is surgically removed
  - Symptoms/signs of cloudiness of the lens, failure of the infant to show visual awareness and nystagmus
  - May be associated with
    - Intrauterine infection (German measles)
    - Metabolic diseases
    - Congenital glaucoma
    - Trisomy 13
    - Aniridia
    - Microphthalmia
    - Coloboma
    - PHPV

Uveal Anomalies

- **Aniridia**
  - A congenital, hereditary, bilateral absence of the iris (presence of iris root upon gonioscopy)
  - Caused by an autosomal dominant deletion of chromosome 11 caused by a mutation in the *PAX6* gene
  - Associated ocular defects
    - Lack of foveal reflex (poor macular development)
    - Optic nerve aplasia/hypoplasia (75%)
    - Cataract (50-85%)
    - Glaucoma (30-50%)
    - Keratoconus
    - Arcus juvenilis
    - Albinism
    - Ectopia lentis (50%)
    - Poor visual acuity
    - Nystagmus
    - Strabismus
  - Increased incidence of Wilm's Tumor
- **Coloboma**
  - An imperfect closure of a cleft that occurs during the development of ocular structures during pregnancy. Can occur in the eyelid, iris, lens, choroid, or optic disc. Retinal and iris colobomas are the most common
  - Systemically associated with CHARGE Syndrome, Joubert Syndrome, Lenz Microphthalmia Syndrome
  - Symptoms depend on the location and size of the coloboma.
    - Iris – vision not usually affected, a keyhole shaped pupil can cause some light sensitivity
    - Retina – causes blind spots, central vision loss if macular
    - Optic nerve- greatest impairment
  - **Optic Disc**
    - A defective closure of the fetal fissure, usually affects the inferior part of the retina and choroid
    - Bilateral in50% of cases, may be inherited in autosomal dominant or sporadic mode
    - Associated with
      - Microphthalmos with or without cyst
      - Serous retinal detachments with high spontaneous reattachment rates
      - Multisystem genetic disorders
        - **CHARGE** (coloboma, heart defects, atresia, mental retardation, genitor-urinary abnormalities, ear defects)
        - **Goltz Syndrome** (X-linked dominant, focal dermal hypoplasia)
        - **Lens Microphthalmia Syndrome** (X-linked, microphthalmos w/ or w/o coloboma, mild mental retardation, large ears)
        - **Meckel-Gruber Syndrome** (Autosomal recessive, coloboma, renal abnormalities, occipital encephalocoele)
        - **Walker-Warburg Syndrome** (autosomal recessive, hydrocephalis, encephalocoele, retinal dysplasia)
        - **Goldenhar Syndrome** (lid coloboma, epibulbar dermoid, ear abnormalities)

Retinal/Optic Nerve Anomalies

- **Retinopathy of Prematurity (ROP)**
  - Disease of the developing retina and its vasculature
  - Main risk factor is extreme prematurity and incomplete development of (temporal) retinal vessels at birth
  - Excessive oxygenation of arterial blood increases ROP
    - When taken out of environment, blood vessels proliferate, but don't grow properly because they are weak and leak which pulls the retina and leads to a retinal detachment
  - Stages or ROP

        - Stage 1: demarcation line: thin, flat, white circumferential border separating vascularized posterior retina from gray avascular peripheral retina
        - Stage 2: ridge: thickening, elevation of the retina at the border
        - Stage 3: ridge with extraretinal fibrovascular proliferation
        - Stage 4: fibrotic tissue pulls retina and leads to a partial retinal detachment
        - Stage 5: complete retinal detachment
    - The lower the birth weight, the more likely the development of severe ROP
    - There is no treatment for stage 1, 2, or low grade stage 3 ROP
    - Treatment of stage 4,5 includes ablation of the entire avascular peripheral retina using cryotherapy or laser photocoagulation
- **Albinism**
    - A genetic defect of melanin production that results in little or no color in the skin, hair, and/or eyes. The genetic defect can be one of several and may be familiar
    - Ocular albinism only affects the eyes, whereas oculocutaneous albinism (most severe form) causes white hair, skin, and iris color.
    - Ocular symptoms
        - Strabismus
        - Photophobia
        - Nystagmus
        - Blond iris/fundus
        - Functional blindness
    - Systemic symptoms
        - Absence of pigment in the hair, skin or iris
        - Patchy or missing skin
- **Retinoblastoma**
    - A rare, cancerous tumor of the retina caused by a mutation in a cell division gene
    - 50% of cases the mutation develops sporadically, 50% is a familial mutation
    - Cancer generally affects children under the age of 6
    - Symptoms/signs
        - Eye pain and redness
        - Strabismus
        - Diplopia
        - Poor vision
        - Leukocoria
        - Differing iris colors
- **Retinal Dystrophies**
    - Degeneration of photoreceptors of retina
    - Generally a result of an inherited photoreceptor degeneration (IPD)
    - Not common (6-9 per 10,000 births), but a major fraction of childhood blindness
    - **Leber's Congenital Amaurosis**
        - A rare autosomal recessive disorder that causes a progressive, severe retinal dystrophy that affects both rods and cones and leads to blindness or near-blindness in children
        - Amaurosis refers to a loss of vision not associated with a lesion
        - Signs/Symptoms
            - Poor visual function <20/400
            - Franceschetti's oculo-digital sign (eye poking, pressing, rubbing)
            - Nystagmus
            - Fundus appearance is variable, may appear normal and develop pigmentary retinopathy similar to RP later in childhood
            - Lack of electrical response from the retina (ERG) is common
    - **Congenital achromatopsia** – complete loss of cone function
        - No color vision, poor acuity, nystagmus, often photophobic
    - **Congenital stationary night blindness** - failure of rod vision from birth
        - Normal acuity, color vision at high light levels, poor vision at low levels
- **Optic Nerve Hypoplasia**

- Developmental defect of the optic nerve fibers of one or both eyes, which causes a decreased number of axons
- Vision is highly variable, depending on number of intact neurons, VA can range from 20/20 to NLP, may be generalized or segmental visual field loss. If bilateral and severe, leads to complete blindness
- Caused by gestational CNS injury that results in transsynaptic degeneration and neuronal migration defects
  - Maternal ingestion of drugs (neuroleptics, alcohol, cocaine, LSD) during 1st trimester, maternal diabetes, young maternal age
- Associated with midline neurological defects (quadriplegia and hemiplegia)

- **Morning Glory Disc**
  - Unilateral large, funnel-shaped optic nerve with multiple peripheral radial retinal vessels and central glial tuft
  - Commonly have low vision, but can vary from 20/20 to no light perception
  - Associated with
    - Peripapillary RPE mottling
    - Serous retinal detachments
    - Transsphenoidal encephalocele
    - Midfacial anomalies (hypertelorism, clefting syndromes)
- **Persistent Hyperplastic Primary Vitreous (PHPV)**
  - Remnant of the hyaloids vascular system seen in 95% of premature infants, 3% of term infants
  - Premies (<34 weeks)- the hyaloids has reached from the optic nerve head to the posterior capsule of the lens. It courses from the optic nerve and appears as a "ghost vessel" going to the lens, which could be blocking vision
  - If severe, necessitates a vitrectomy
- **Retinitis pigmentosa**
  - Generally progressive inherited disease, that leads to photoreceptor dysfunction and death. It is a clinical degeneration of the outer retina
  - Children become unable to see at night (night blindness) and then lose their side (peripheral) vision. Tunnel vision develops followed by complete blindness
  - Signs
    - Intraneural retinal "bone-spicule" pigment in fundus
    - Loss of rod and cone ERG responses
    - Thinning and atrophy of the RPE in the mid and far periphery
    - Relative preservation of the RPE in the macula
    - Gliotic "waxy pallor" of the optic nerve head
    - Attenuated retinal arterioles
  - Typically bilateral
  - Severity of the features increase with age

Cerebral/Visual Pathway Anomalies

- **Cortical Visual Impairment**
  - Damage to the geniculostriate pathway
  - Etiology
    - Hydrocephalus
    - Perinatal/postnatal hypoxia-ischemia (Most common cause)
    - Hemorrhages
    - Cerebral malformations
    - Head trauma
    - Infections
  - Ocular anomalies
    - Loss of vision and OKN
    - Normal pupil responses
    - Eyes appear healthy
    - Vision loss is transient or permanent
      - Patients appear visually inattentive, with overlooking-eccentric viewing, light gazing.

        - Motion vision maintained
    - Associated neurological deficits
        - Cerebral palsy
        - Seizures
        - Hydrocephalus
        - Mental retardation
        - Microcephaly
- **Cerebral Palsy**
    - Most common developmental disability, effects 2:1000 births
    - Characterized by a general non-progressive locomotor dysfunction of varying severity due to a defect or lesion in the immature brain
    - Risk factors
        - **Pregnancy** (maternal diabetes, hyperthyroidism, high blood pressure, seizures, poor nutrition), placenta pervia/abruption placenta
        - **Delivery risks** (prematurity <37 weeks, prolonged rupture of amniotic membranes leading to fetal injection, severely depressed fetal heart rate, breached)
        - **Neonatal risks** (asphyxia, interventricular hemorrhage, periventricular hemorrhage, meningitis infection)
    - Signs
        - Delayed motor milestones
            - Not rolling by 6 months, fisting after 5 months, not sitting with support by 8 months, not walking by 15-18 months
        - Persistent or evolving increased or decreased muscle tone
            - Head lag beyond 6 months, poor trunk control and balance, opisthotonic posturing and extensor thrusting, dystonia, early rolling or standing, toe walking/scissoring, abnormal motor or gait patterns
        - Persistence of primitive reflexes
        - Focal abnormalities of movement, posture, tone
            - Declaring handedness prior to 18 months, differences in functional ability of right/left extremities, **clonus** persisting past 12 months
        - Behavioral
            - Irritability, easily startled with exaggerated Moro reflex, excessive crying, jittery, sleeping difficulties
        - Physical
            - Decreased rate of head growth, poor suck, delayed feeding milestones, poor weight gain
    - Ocular anomalies
        - Refractive error (21-85% have significant RE, 3-4D Hyperopia)
        - Strabismus (43%, ET>XT)
        - Accommodative insufficiencies
        - Nystagmus (12%)
        - Optic atrophy
        - Visual field defect
        - CVI
        - Cataract
        - Fundus anomaly
        - Microphthalmos
        - Corneal opacity
    - Systemic anomalies
        - Language disorders (90%)
        - Visual problems (70%)
        - Mental retardation (50%)
        - Seizures (35%)
        - Hearing deficits (15%)

4. Tests Used by Optometrist to Determine a Child's Level of Visual-Perceptual Development

Visual Attention and Discrimination

- **Visual Function**
  - **Visual Acuity** – important to use age-appropriate linear and single optotype acuity charts (Snellen, HOTV, Lea) at both distance and near, monocular and both eyes open
  - **Contrast Sensitivity-** Cambridge, Mr. Happy, Hiding Heidi
  - **Color Vision** – F2 plates, HRR
  - **Visual Fields** – monster fields
  - **Fixation (Eccentricity, steadiness)** – visuscope
- **TVPS-3 (Gardner Test of Visual Perception Skills)** – Ages 4 to 19. This is the most widely used test of visual perception, has 7 subparts
  - **Visual Discrimination** – the ability to match two identical forms when mixed among similar forms. Related to perceptual speed test- looking at the automaticity of doing this task
  - **Visual Memory –** Ability to remember for immediate recall (after 4-5 secs) all of the characteristics of a given form and being able to find it among an array of similar forms
  - **Visual Spatial Relations –** Ability to determine from among five forms of identical configuration, the single form that is different from the other forms
  - **Visual Form Constancy –** Ability to see a form and being able to find a form even though it may be smaller, larger, rotated or hidden
  - **Visual Sequential Memory** – Ability to remember for immediate recall (after 4-5 seconds) a series of forms from among four separate series of forms
  - **Visual Figure Ground –** Ability to perceive a form visually and to find this form hidden in a conglomerated ground of matter
  - **Visual Closure** – Ability to determine from among four incomplete forms, the one that is the same as the stimulus form (completed form)
- **MVPT-3 (Motor Free Visual Perception Test)** – Ages 4 to 94. Similar to TVPS, evaluates visual discrimination, form constancy, figure ground, spatial orientation, visual short-term memory, and visual closure.
- **MVPT-V (Motor Free Visual Perception Test Vertical)** – Ages 55 to 80. To assess visual perceptual abilities in *adults* that may have hemifield visual neglect, this test is NOT used in children
- **PMA (Primary Mental Abilities)** – Ages 5 to 13-9.
  - **Perceptual Speed** – Evaluates the automaticity of performing visual discrimination tasks. Good perceptual speed is important for reading skills
  - **Spatial Relations** – Evaluates the ability to manipulate objects and figures to make a square. The patient is shown an incomplete square and must determine which piece can be used to complete the square. Children with spatial problems may have difficulty with learning sight words (eidetic). Slightly more difficult task than TVPS
- **Beery VMI Developmental Test of Visual Perception** – Ages 3 to 17-11. This is a supplemental test to the Beery VMI. It is similar to the visual discrimination portions of the Gardner TVPS and MVPT.

Visual-Motor Integration

- Visual motor integration involves seeing a form, processing the information (breaking the form into parts) and then reproducing the forms (reassembling the parts)
- **TVAS (Rosner Test of Visual Analysis Skills)** – Ages 4 to 8
  - Test examines a child's ability to analyze a geometric pattern in an organized fashion and copy it. This test is unique in that if you teach a child how to pass this test you train them in perceptual skills
  - Dot maps of varying numbers with geometric forms are used. The child is told to copy the map exactly on the dot map provided. Stop after two consecutive errors.
- **Wold Copy Sentence Test** – Ages 6 to 13
  - Used to evaluate the child's fine motor and visual motor integration skills when copying symbols

- The task is to copy the 110 words as quickly and neatly as possible
    - Determine the copy rate in letters/minute. Evaluate the spacing, letter formation, and speed.
- **VMI (Beery-Butenica Test of Visual-Motor Integration)** – Ages 3 to 17
    - The child copies 2D or 3D forms in a box just below the form. Stop the test after three consecutive errors, and no erasing or tracing is allowed
    - Monitor the child's performance (impulsiveness, strategy used for the analyzing of the forms) and body posture

Intersensory Integration

- **AVIT (Auditory-Visual Integration Test) aka Birch Belmont** – Ages 5 to 12
    - The examiner taps out a series of long and short taps which the child must match to a visual representation of the taps using dots and spaces
    - Poor performance can be caused by auditory-visual integration deficit or poor sequential memory
- **VADS (Visual-Aural Digit Span Test)** – Ages 5 to 11
    - Tests crossed-channel/intersensory reception, processing, and expression of spoken and written information (a series of digits)
    - Child must repeat a series of digits (numbers) presented by the examiner in four subparts: Aural-oral, Visual-oral, Aural-written, Visual-written
- **REO (Melvin-Smith Receptive-Expressive Observation)** – Ages 7 to 8
    - Very similar to VADS except that letters and words are also presented
    - Four subparts are auditory-vocal, visual-vocal, auditory-motor, and visual-motor

Bilateral Integration and Laterality

- Laterality is the ability to know one's own right from left
- Directionality is the ability to differentiate another person's or thing's right from left
- These skills are important for the development of writing, reading, and math skills
- **Piaget Test of Left-Right Concepts** – Ages 5 to 11
    - Evaluates laterality and directionality skills
    - Examiner asks series of questions testing child's ability to differentiate left from right on his own body and on another person's body, and to determine the relative left-right positions of objects placed in front of him
- **Gardner Reversal Frequency Test** – Ages 5 to 15
    - Evaluates different aspects of directionality with three different subtests
    - Execution – writing numbers and lower case letters
    - Recognition – identifying the reversed letter in a pair of mirror images or in isolation
    - Matching- identifying the correct orientation of numbers or lower case letters from a choice of four alternative presentations
- **Jordan Left-Right Discrimination Test** – Ages 5 to 13
    - Evaluates different aspects of directionality with three different subtests
    - Level 1 – identification of letters and numbers that are reversed
    - Level 2A – identification of words containing a reversed letter
    - Level 2B – identification of reversed word in a complete sentence

Chapter 11 – Lids/Lashes/Lacrimal System/Ocular Adnexa/Orbit

EYEBROW (GROSS ANATOMY)

1. Function
   - Diverts sweat, dirt, lice, dandruff, and other creepy crawly things from dripping into eyes.
   - Shades eyes
   - Conveys emotions (e.g. hate, frustration, anger – all the things you feel while studying for board exams).

2. Structure
   - Lies on the supracilliary ridge of the frontal bone. It consists of thick skin covered by characteristic short cilia
   - There are three parts to the "comma" shape which are the head, the body, and the tail
   - Eyebrow layers:
     - Skin
     - Muscle
     - Fat
     - Aponeurosis

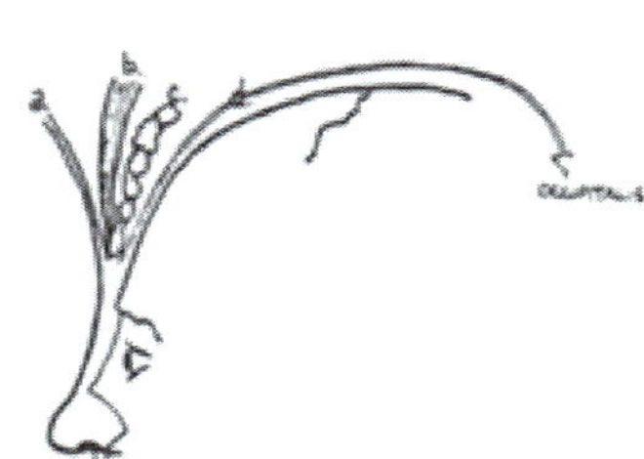

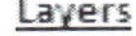

Layers
A. Skin
B. Muscular
C. Fat (Cellulo-Adipose)
D. Aponeurosis

   - **Skin layer:**
     - Outermost layer
     - Contains cilia (extra long hair) which keep sweat/rain from dripping into your eyes and numerous amounts of sweat and sebaceous glands. The sebum helps keep the hair soft and repel water.
     - **superficial fascia** beneath the skin layers. This layer has no fat. It is all loose connective tissue. "Cements" the skin to muscle.
   - **Muscular Layer** (Controlled by **CN VII**)
     - Produces eyebrow movements, critical for facial expression
     - **Frontalis muscle** elevates the eyebrows and pulls the scalp forward. Originates high on the scalp (epicranial aponeurosis) and inserts into connective tissue near the superior orbital rim.
       - Squinting also stretches the occipitalis. Tension headaches at the back of the head can be experienced along with eyestrain.
     - **Orbicularis oculi muscle**: depresses the eyebrows.
     - **Corrugator (supracilii) muscle**: pulls the head of the eyebrows medially and downward during frowning. Originates on the frontal bone and inserts into the skin superior to the medial eyebrow.
     - **Procerus (pyrimidalis) muscle**: depresses the head of the eyebrow down and medially. Forms concentration furrows on the nose. Originates on the nasal bone and inserts into the medial side of the frontalis.

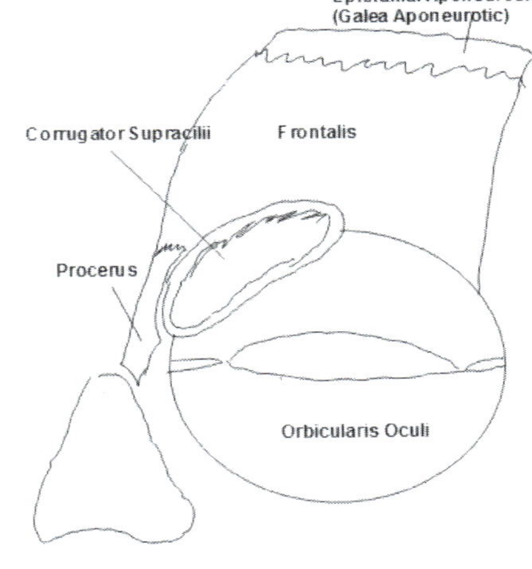

- **Celluloadipose layer:**
    - Merges with the fatty tissue in the eyelid below the muscles. Insulates and allows the muscles to slide over the bone. Because it is porous, fluid can penetrate the layer → with a black eye, blood seeps down in the fat in front of the septum orbital.
- **Aponeurosis layer:**
    - **Galea-aponeurotica** (aka aponeurosis): Connects the occipitalis muscle and frontalis muscle. Inserts in the region of the supra-ciliary ridges and occipital bone. Prevents sub-aponeurotic fluid from draining to the eyelids.

ORBIT (GROSS ANATOMY)

---

1. Contents

Extraocular muscles

- **4 recti**: medial, lateral, superior and inferior.
- **2 obliques**: superior and inferior
- **1 levator**

Cranial Nerves:

- **II - Optic nerve** is sensory from the retina.
- **III- Oculomotor nerve** is sensory (proprioception) and motor for the extrinsic ocular muscles
    - Origin: Nucleus is in the midbrain at the medial margin of the cerebral peduncle, emerges at anterior midbrain at the oculomotor sulcus in 2 to 10 or 15 strands.
        - Large, myelinated fibers – motor axons.
        - Small myelinated fibers – parasymp fibers to smooth muscles.
        - Small unmyelinated fibers – sympathetic.
    - Course: runs forward in the interpeduncular cistern between the post. cerebral A. and sup. cerebral A. It crosses the tentorial gap which is post. to the dorsum sellae. It runs lateral to the post. clinoid process of the sphenoid (below the optic tract). Then it pierces the dura and enters the cavernous sinus. Then it divides into sup. and inf. divisions within the sinus. It enters the orbit via oculomotor foramen. **Within the sinus, III can communicate with the ophthalmic division of CNV**. Also, it can receive sympathetic fibers from the carotid artery.
        - Superior division has 2 branches to the SR and to the Levator.
        - Inferior division has 3 branches: IR, MR, IO to the bulbar side of the muscle. Sends branches to the ciliary ganglion, a relay center of the autonomic nervous system to the intrinsic eyeball muscles (the iris sphincter and ciliary muscle are both smooth) motor root.
    - **Effects of lesions on III**:
        - Impaired sup div causes ptosis due to levator and SR paralysis.
        - Impaired both divs. Causes ptosis and pupil dilation, no accom, eye drifts down and out since LR and SO are intact.
- **IV- Trochlear nerve,** mixed nerve
    - Origin: In brain stem, fibers from the right nucleus cross to the left (**dorsal origin & crossed nerve**). It is the most **slender** and has the **longest** intracranial course of CN's. It passes through the **sup. orb. fissure** to **innervate the SO on the orbital side which is unique** since all other muscles are innerv. on the bulbar side. It is the only CN with an origin on the dorsal surface of the brainstem. It has both myelinated (mostly) and unmyelinated fibers.
        - If sever nerve, the same side of the injury is affected. If you sever the nucleus, the opposite side is affected.
        - It's position and length makes CH IV susceptible to damage due to **whiplash**
    - **Lesions**: SO paralysis and result in eyeball moving up, in, and extorting. **Head tilt away from side of the lesion will result.**
        - **A head tilt** can also be an indication of a **vertical phoria**
- **V- Trigeminal nerve, mainly sensory with motor to the muscles of mastication,** 3 branches: ophthalmic, maxillary, and mandibular

- Origin: From the ventrolateral surface of the **pons**. Sensory ophthalmic branch enters the orbit via the SOF. It is responsible for sensory from the conjunctiva, lacrimal gland, mucous membrane of nose and sinus, skin of the superior lids, nose and forehead. This is the **largest CN**. It innervates the masseter (muscle for mastication).
    - **Prevented from communicating with the cavernous sinus** by a pocket of dura called Meckel's cave
    - **Trigeminal ganglion also called Gasserian or semilunar ganglion**
- **VI- Abducens nerve,** mixed
  - Origin: in the pons, innervates the LR via the SOF for motor and proprioception (sensory).
    - Runs over the sharp part of the petrous bone – injury prone
    - Fibers from VII surround – so likely both will be damaged
- **VII- Facial nerve** mixed
  - Origin: from the pons and distributed via the motor root to facial and scalp muscles; and via parasymp. root to the lacrimal gland; and via sensory root to the back of the throat and external auditory meatus.
- **I- Olfactory nerve,** entirely sensory, arises from the olfactory mucosa of the nasal cavity. The axons pass through the cribriform plate of the ethmoid bone to synapse with neurons in the olfactory bulb, which lies above the cribriform plate. The axons from the olfactory tract terminate in the primary olfactory area in the cerebral cortex.

Nerve	Fiber Type	Origin	Enters Orbit Via	Targets
Oculomotor (III)	-Motor -Proprioceptive -Symp/Parasymp	III Nucleus in midbrain between pons and peduncle	Oculomotor foramen, through Annulus of Zinn	SR, Levator, MR, IR, IO
Trochlear (IV)	-Motor -Proprioceptive	IV Nucleus in midbrain	Superior Orbital Fissure (SOF), above Annulus of Zinn	SO
Abducens (VI)	-Motor -Proprioceptive	Pons	Oculomotor Foramen, through Annulus of Zinn	LR
Trigeminal (V)	-Sensory	Sensory root of Pons	*Frontal* and *Lacrimal* branches→SOF, above Annulus of Zinn. *Nasociliary* branch →oculomotor foramen.	Multiple, see below

Branches of Trigeminal Nerve (V) – Ophthalmic Division		
Branch	**Division**	**Target**
Frontal	Supratrochlear	Medial portion of upper eyelid skin Conjunctiva Forehead skin
	Supraorbital (Nerve of Kobelt)	Skin of scalp Mucosa of frontal sinus
Lacrimal	Superior Division (Lateral Palpebral)	Lacrimal Gland
	Inferior Division	Carries parasympathetic fibers from phenopalatine ganglion
Nasociliary	Posterior ethmoidal (Nerve of Lushka/Krause)	Mucous membranes of sphenoid sinus Posterior ethmoidal air cells
	Anterior ethmoidal	Anterior ethmoidal air cells Frontal sinus Nasal mucosa Skin of nose
	Infratrachlear	Skin of nose, lids Conjunctiva Lacrimal sac Caruncle Plica semilunaris
	Sensory root (emerges as short posterior ciliary nerves)	Eyeball around optic nerve
	Long posterior ciliary nerve	Iris Cornea Ciliary muscle Symp. Innervations to iris dilator muscle

Diagram of trigeminal

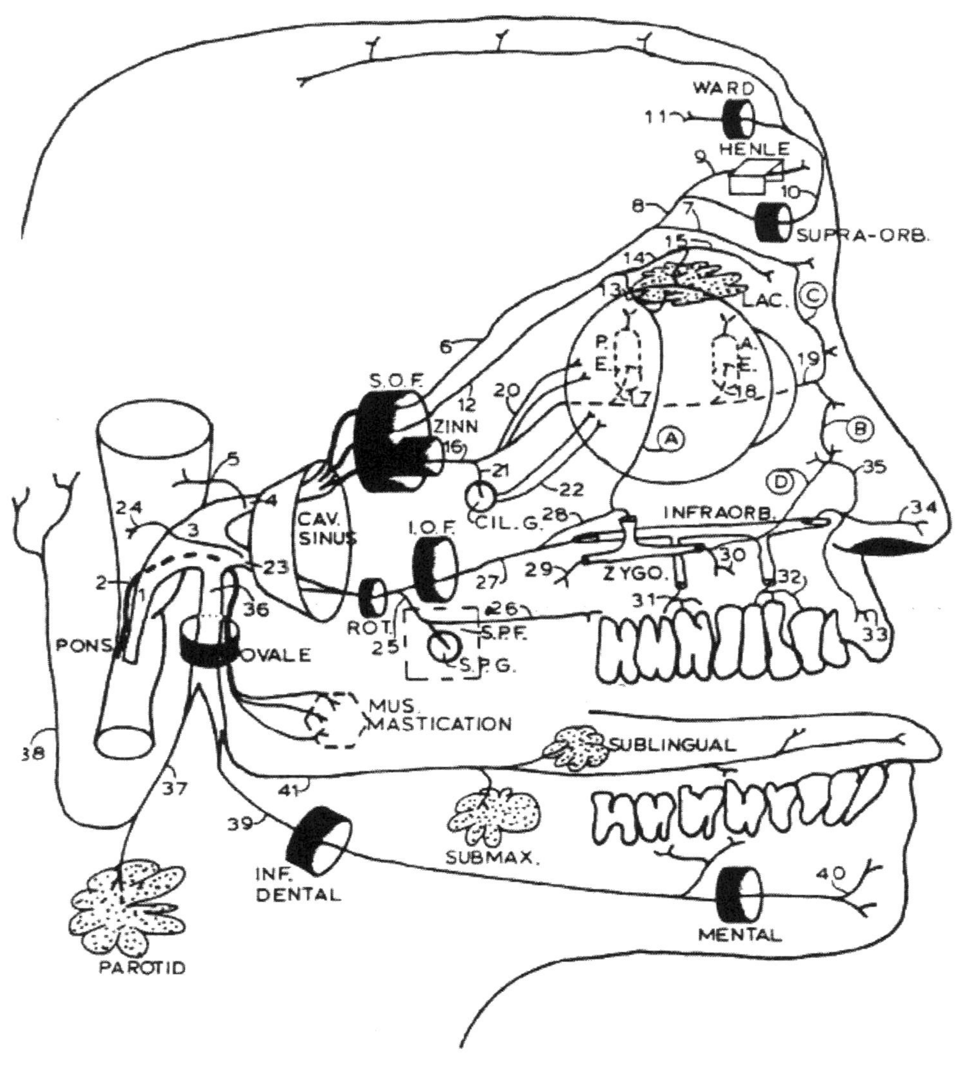

1) Sensory Root
2) Motor Root
3) Semilunar Ganglion
4) Ophthalmic Division
5) Recurrent Nerve of Arnold
6) Frontal
7) Supratrochlear
8) Supraorbital
9) Medial Frontal
10) Lateral Frontal
11) Nerve of Kobelt
12) Lacrimal
13) Inferior Division
14) Superior Division
15) Lateral Palpebral
16) Nasociliary
17) Posterior Ethmoid
18) Anterior Ethmoid
19) Infratrochlear
20) Long Posterior Ciliary
21) Sensory Root
22) Short Posterior Ciliary
23) Maxillary Division
24) Middle Meningeal
25) Sphenopalatine
26) Posterior Superior Alveolar
27) Infraorbital
28) Zygomatic
29) Zygomatico-temporal
30) Zygomatico-facial
31) Middle Superior Alveolar
32) Anterior Superior Alveolar
33) Labial
34) Nasal
35) Inferior Palpebral
36) Mandibular Division
37) Auriculo-temporal
38) Superficial Temporal
39) Inferior Alveolar
40) Mental
41) Lingual

Anastomosis

A) Inferior division of the Lacrimal – zygomatic
B) Infratrochlear- inferior palpebral
C) Supratrochlear – Infratrochlear
D) Inferior Palpebral – Zygomatico-facial

Parasympathetic nerves:

- 2 divisions: Tectal and Bulbar.
- The **preganglionic cell bodies of the parasympathetic div.** are found in nuclei in the brainstem and the lateral gray horn of the 2nd through the 4th sacral segment of the spinal cord. The ones of importance for the eye emerge as part of a CN.
    - **Tectal outflow** is with the CN III to ciliary ganglion which is the intermediate destination for parasympathetic nerves to the eye for pupillary constriction and accommodation. "Accessory ganglia of Axenfeld" = displaced cells in the episclera of the eye.
- **Ciliary ganglion roots:**
    - **Sensory root (long root)**: sensory from iris and cornea
    - **Motor root (short root)**: are parasympathetic fibers from the CN III inferior division, postganglionic parasympathetic fibers travel in short posterior cil. nerve and go to iris sphincter muscle and ciliary muscle.
    - **Sympathetic roots are postganglionic symp. fibers** from the sup cervical ganglion, make no synapses in the ganglion, supply the iris dilator muscle and ocular blood vessels. Travel to the eye via short posterior ciliary nerves.
- **Ciliary ganglion branches:**
    - **Short poster. ciliary nerves** come out of the ganglion anteriorly and are the only postganglionic pons fibers that are myelinated. They are mixed nerves containing sensory, symp., and parasym. fibers. There are 6-10 nerves which go to the area around the optic nerve
    - **Bulbar outflow** leaves the brain via CN VII, specifically nervous intermedius, and goes to the sphenopalatine ganglion. Although it leaves with VII, it also uses V as a passive carrier. The sphenopalatine ganglion supplies pons input to the orbit for lacrimation and possibly vasodilation. Projections to orbital, cranial, and ocular BV's means that pons stimulation can cause dilation of the BV's and increase the pressure. It is located on top of the sphenopalatine fossa and lateral to the pterygoid foramen. It has many branches and roots.

Pupillary constriction

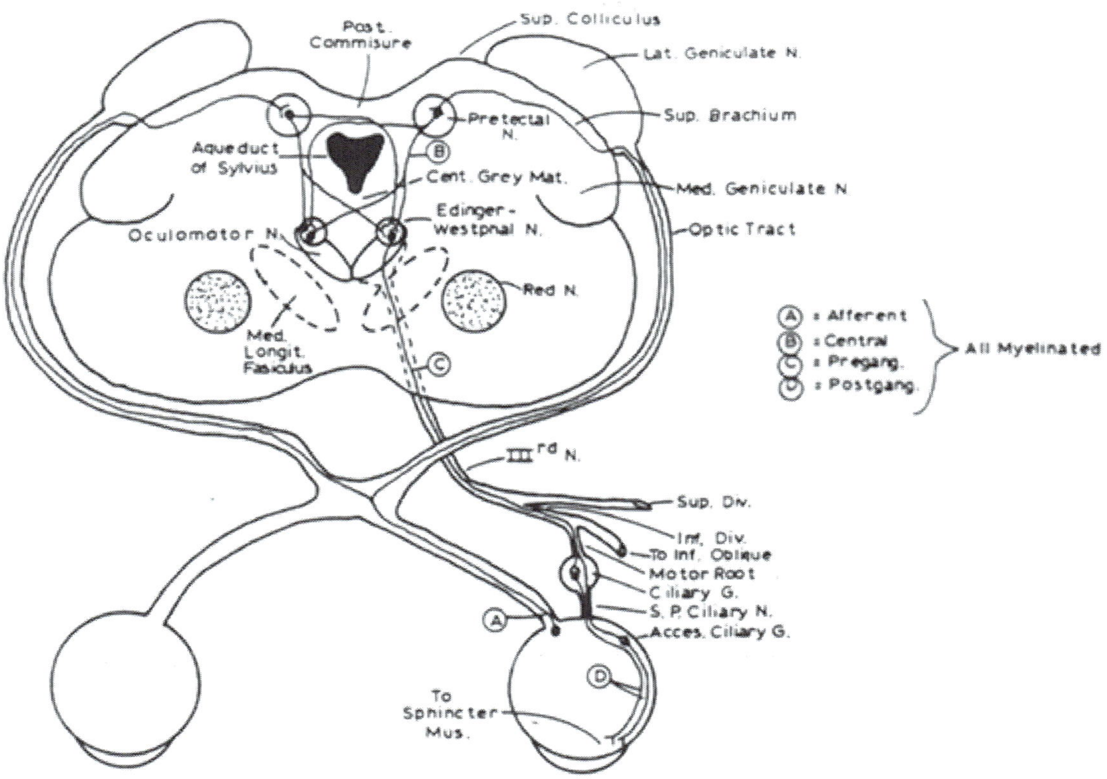

Sympathetic nerves:

- The preganglionic fibers of the sympathetic division have their **cell bodies** located in the **lateral gray horn** of the spinal cord in the thoracic and first two lumbar segments.
- The **preganglionic fibers** leave the spinal cord through the **ventral root** of a spinal nerve.
- After exiting through the intervertebral foramina, the preganglionic sympathetic fibers enter a white ramus of the spinal n. with ganglia of the sympathetic trunk.
- Generally, autonomic innervation destined for a particular level of the body comes off the symp spinal chain at the ganglion nearest that level. So for the orbit, the ganglion is the superior cervical ganglion and is located behind the internal carotid artery. Postganglionic fibers leaving here serve the head, where they are distributed to the sweat glands, smooth muscle of the eye, and facial blood vessels.
- **Internal carotid nerve:**
    - Carries the fibers of axons leaving the ganglion and project cephalically toward the head. It **bifurcates into a lateral and medial branch and gives rise to two major sympathetic plexi**, which provide autonomics to the orbit.
        - **Sympathetic carotid plexus** arises from the **lateral branch** of the internal carotid N. and breaks down into many smaller fibers and attaches to arteries or nerves that pass near by V, VI, deep petrosal N., or ophthalmic A.
        - **Sympathetic cavernous plexus** arises from the **medial branch** of the internal carotid N. is located in the cavernous sinus. III, IV, V (ophthalmic div), and ophthalmic A all get covered with autonomic innervation.
- Functions of autonomic innervation:
    - For **vasoconstriction at iris ciliary body** (CB gets dual autonomic innervation, **sympathetic to blood vessels and parasympathetic to muscle**).
    - To extraocular muscle blood vessels, smooth muscles of Muller in the orbit, lacrimal gland, choroid, RPE, and to the iris dilator muscle.

Pupillary dilation

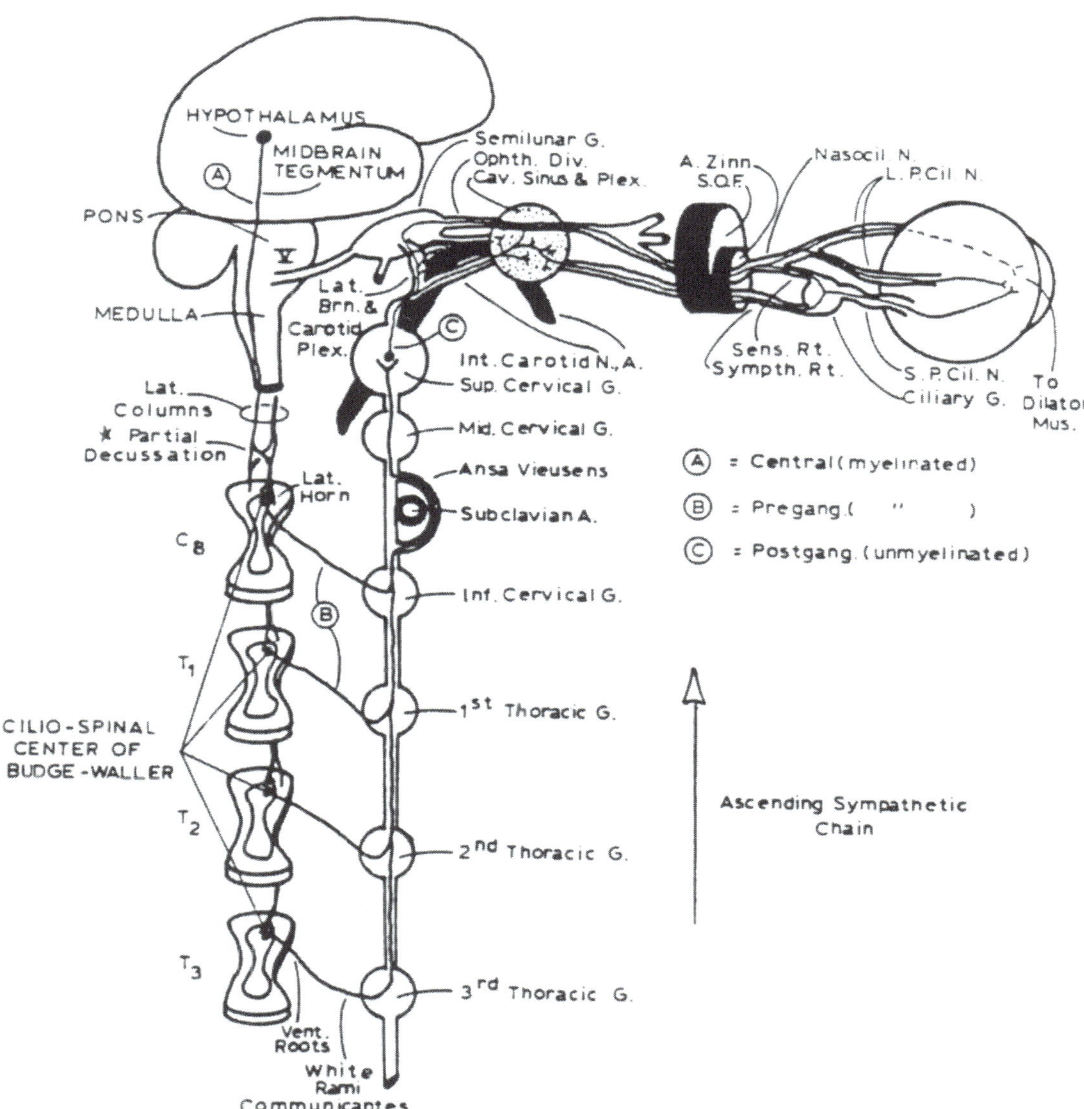

- Blood vessels
  - The **internal carotid artery** gives rise to the **ophthalmic artery**, the main supply to the orbit
  - The **external carotid** gives rise to the:
    - **Facial artery**
    - **Superficial temporal artery**
    - **Internal maxillary artery**, which gives rise to:
      - **Infraorbital** artery
      - Orbital branch of middle meningeal artery – alternative supply to orbit and eye; insufficient to maintain structures alone
  - Superior and infra-orbital branches

Arteries of the Orbit	
Ophthalmic Artery (Branches #1-12)	**Serves:**
1. Central Retinal Artery (Originates in the **Circle of Willis** after the **cavernous sinus**)	-Inner Retina (arcades seen in posterior pole)
2. Lacrimal Artery -Recurrent Meningeal -Muscular (2 branches) -Zygomatic -Superior and Inferior Lateral Palpebral	 -Lacrimal gland -One branch to SR, one to LR -Skin of the face -Join with palpebral arcades to serve eyelids
3. Muscular Artery -Superior -Inferior -Anterior ciliary arteries	 -SR, SO, Levator -IR, IO, MR -Come off both superior and inferior muscular to server their respective muscle targets
4. Posterior Ciliary Arteries -Long -Short	 -Layers of the eyeball -Come off the long posterior ciliaries to serve eyeball
5. Pial Artery	-Pia mater of optic nerve
6. Supraorbital Artery	-Anything on orbital roof, upper eyelids, brows, forehead region
7. Posterior Ethmoidal Artery	-Mucous membrane of ethmoidal air cells and the ethmoidal region in general
8. Anterior Ethmoidal Artery	-Meninges in anterior cranial fossa (serves along with anterior meningeal artery)
9. Medial Palpebral Artery -Superior -Inferior	 -Superior palpebral arcade -Inferior palpebral arcade
10. Dorsal Nasal Artery	-Terminal branch of ophthalmic artery, anastomoses with the Angular Artery
11. Frontal Artery (aka Supratrochlear)	-Terminal branch of ophthalmic artery
12. Infraorbital Artery	-Alternate route to the internal carotid path -Is the terminal branch of the internal maxillary artery which is the terminal branch of the external carotid -Serves IO, IR, lacrimal sac and structures at the bottom of the orbit

- Fat compartments
  - Serve to lubricate, insulate & cushion orbital contents
  - **Two portions**:
    - Central "fat" - loose lobulated fat located within the extraocular muscle cone (around the optic nerve) which allows for globe movement.
      - Septa of lobules insert into Tenon's capsule at the back of the globe.
      - The surface of optic nerve contains a limiting membrane separating the fat from the dural covering of the nerve.
      - Supravaginal space of Schwalbe is the space between limiting membrane and dura.
    - Peripheral fat - located outside of muscle cone between the periorbita & the recti muscle.
      - Thickest at insertion
      - Covered by thin membrane that is connected to the periorbita by thin processes.
      - Located in the intermuscular spaces.
      - Consists of 4 lobes:
        - The posterior portions of the lobes are continuous with the central fat.
        - The anterior lobes are connected to the intermuscular membrane & Tenon's capsule.
- **Fascia**
  - Connective tissue that binds and separates orbital compartments.
  - **Periorbita (periosteum of the orbit)**: derived from dura mater and separates to line the bony cavity of the orbit.

- Bulba fascia (Tenon's capsule): wraps the globe from edge of optic nerve to corneal margin.
- **Muscular fascia**: tissue that surrounds each extraocular muscle

2. Anatomical Relationships Among Orbital Structures

- The **bony orbit** can be depicted as a quadrilateral pyramid with dimensions.
- The average volume of the fossa orbitalis (orbital cavity) is 29 ml.
- Brocha's orbital index:
  - **Height** (mm) x 100 = Brocha's orbital index for the aditus orbitae.
  - **Width** (mm) (orbital opening)
  - If > 89, is **mega-seme**; Asian
  - If 84-89, **meso-seme**; White
  - If < 84, is **micro-seme**; Black
- Medial walls of two orbits are almost parallel
  - The walls are 3mm farther apart posteriorly than at the orbital margin
  - The globe is held in position by fascia and the check ligaments associated with extraocular muscles

3. Bones of the Orbit

- Single orbit consists of 7 bones.
- **Facial bones** (4 bones – **2 of each** facial bones)
  - Maxillary
  - Zygomatic
  - Palatine
  - Lacrimal
  - **Cranial bones** (3 bones **shared by both** orbits)
    - Frontal
    - Sphenoid
    - Ethmoid
  - Both orbits together consist of 11 bones total.

Bone	Facial/Cranial	Topographical Features
Maxillary	F	Maxillary sinus (aka Antrum of Highmore)
Zygomatic	F	
Palatine	F	Part of orbital, nasal, and oral cavities
Lacrimal	F	Fossa for the lacrimal sac. Opening to the nasolacrimal duct
Frontal	C	Diploe and frontal sinus, supra-ciliary ridges with glabella in between
Sphenoid	C	Sellae turcica (pituitary fossa) consisting of the tuberculum sellae (front part) and dorsum sellae (back portion)
Ethmoid	C	Air cells (sinus), crista galli, cribiform plate, lamina papyracea, superior and inferior nasal conchae

Margins

- **Supra-orbital margin:**
  - Formed by: **frontal bone**
  - Topographical features:
    - Supra-orbital notch or foramen
    - Supra-ciliary foramen and canal of Ward
    - Frontal notch of Henle
    - Supra-orbital ridges
- **Lateral orbital margin:**
  - Formed by: **zygomatic bone** (mostly)**, frontal bone.**
  - Topographical features:
    - Lateral orbital tuberculae (aka zygomatic tubercle or Whitnall's tubercle.)
- **Infra-orbital margin:**
  - Formed by **zygomatic and maxillary bones**.
  - Topographical features:
    - Infra-orbital suture
    - Infra-orbital foramina and canal
- **Medial orbital margin:**
  - Formed by **maxillary, frontal, and lacrimal bones.**

- Topographical features:
    - Dacryon
    - Fossa for the lacrimal sac
    - Anterior lacrimal crest
    - Posterior lacrimal crest
    - Sutura notha

Orbital Walls

- **Roof:**
  - Formed by: **frontal and part of sphenoid bone**
  - Topographical features:
    - Fossa for the lacrimal gland
    - Trochlear fossa
- **Lateral wall:**
  - Formed by: **great wing of sphenoid** (mostly) and **zygomatic**.
  - Topographical features:
    - Spinae recti lateralis – small bony spur that servers as a attachment point for part of the lateral rectus muscle.
- **Floor:** Formed by **maxillary, zygomatic, palatine, and sphenoid**.
- **Medial wall:** Formed by: **maxillary, lacrimal, sphenoid, and ethmoid** (lamina papyracea mostly).

4. Foramina and Openings of the Orbit

Foramen	**Contents**
Supra-Ciliary Foramen and Canal of Ward	-Nerve of Kobelt (Branch of Trigeminal V) -Branch of Supra-Orbital Artery -Diploic vein
Frontal Notch of Henle	-Medial frontal nerve (medial branch)
Optic Foramen and Canal	-Optic Nerve -Ophthalmic Artery -Meninges -Autonomic Nerves
Zygomatico-Orbital Foramen	Zygomatic Artery, Vein, Nerve
Zygomatic-Facial Foramen	Zygomatico-Facial Artery, Vein, Nerve
Zygomatico-Temporal Foramen	Zygomatico-Temporal Artery, Vein, Nerve
Meningeal Foramen	Medial Meningeal Artery and vein
Superior Orbital Fissure (SOF) – above the Annulus of Zinn	-Trochlear Nerve (IV) -Lacrimal and frontal branches of the Trigeminal Nerve (V) – Ophthalmic division of V)
Oculomotor Foramen – portion of SOF within the Annulus of Zinn	-Superior and Inferior division of the Oculomotor Nerve (III) -Nasociliary Branch of Trigeminal (V) Ophthalmic Branch -Abducens Nerve (VI) -Autonomic Nerves -Maybe Superior and Inferior Ophthalmic Veins
SOF – Below the Annulus of Zinn	-Maybe Inferior Ophthalmic Vein
Inferior Orbital Fissure (IOF)	-Zygomatic and Infra-Orbital branches of Trigeminal Nerve -Infra-orbital Artery, Vein, and Nerve -Branch of Inferior Ophthalmic Vein -Autonomic Nerves

Note: With any of the orbital openings, the name usually specifies the contents, and in some cases, the location of the opening also.

ORBIT (DEVELOPMENTAL ANATOMY)

1. Development of Bones of Orbit (Closure of Sutures)

- The bony walls of the orbit are formed from **mesoderm** surrounding the eye, which include the following:
  - The floor and lateral wall from visceral mesoderm of the maxillary process.
  - The roof from the mesoderm capsule of the forebrain.
  - Medial wall from the lateral nasal process.
  - Sphenoid bone from the base of the skull (sphenoid mesoderm forms the greater wing while the anterior mesoderm process forms the lesser wing).
- At 6-7 weeks the centers of the orbital bone appear (ossicles).
- By 4 months the **orbital walls are well developed.**
- Up until the 6th month, the orbit boundaries are shaped by the developing optic cup.
- Between the 6th and 7th months, the lacrimal apparatus and the oblique muscles play an important role in shaping the orbit.
- At 6-7 months the **sutures close**, **with the exception of the sphenoid bone** which closes at the end of the first year.
- The sutures are united by a sheet of periosteum.
- As the development continues, the orbital axis swings forward. At the end of the second month of development, the orbital axis is 180 degrees while at birth the axis is at 71 degrees. The adult axis is 68 degrees.

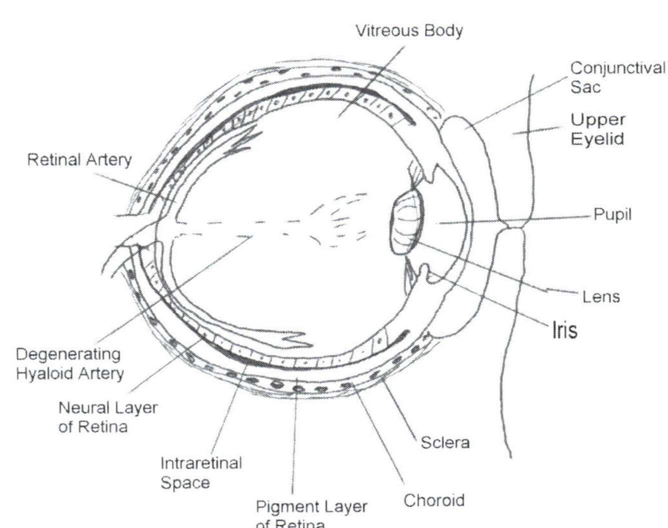

Cross Section of Eye Near Completion

2. Abnormalities (Faulty Development of Facial Bones)

- Anomalies of ossification result in accessory sutures and a large number of ossicles (a.k.a. supernumery ossicles).
- Variation in orbital notches and canals are relatively minor and common in the trochlear spine, supraorbital notch, zygomatico-facial foramen.
- Defects in orbital walls are congenital and rare. When they occur, the orbital, maxillary or frontal bones are absent.
- Generalized orbital deformities can be caused by abnormal posture of the fetus in the uterus (intra-uterine molding).
- Orbital **meningoceles and cephaloceles** are rare but occur when cranial components bulge into the orbit.

ORBIT (PATHOLOGY)

1. General Signs of Orbital Disease

- Soft Tissue Involvement (See Pathology of the Eyelids Below)
  - Lid and periorbital edema
  - Ptosis
  - Chemosis
  - Epibulbar injection
- Proptosis
- Enophthalmos
- Dystopia
- Ophthalmoplegia

2. Proptosis

- **Proptosis-** an abnormal protrusion of the globe which may be caused by retrobulbar lesions or a shallow orbit (less frequent)
  - **Axial proptosis** (symmetrical widening of the palpebral fissure) indicates lesions within the muscle cone, such as cavernous hemangioma and optic nerve tumors.
  - **Eccentric proptosis** indicates masses in the anterior orbit which displace the globe away from the site of the lesion.
- **Assessment of Asymmetrical Fissures**
  - One should always stand back from the patient and examine the faces.
  - Facial asymmetry or malposition of the lids may cause a mistaken impression of protrusion of the eyes (proptosis)
  - **Unilateral high myopia** will give the impression of a projecting eyeball; in fact, any condition that bares a portion of the inferior or superior sclera can provide a visual cue that invites the mistaken diagnosis of proptosis
- **Exophthalmometry**
  - Measure the degree of proptosis with an exophthalmometer. (Hertel or Luedde)
  - The feet of the instrument are placed on each bony lateral orbital margin and the distance between each lateral orbital rim is recorded to make future comparisons valid.
  - Correct for parallax and measure apex of the cornea.
  - **A difference of 2 mm** or more of proptosis between the two eyes is taken as significant.
  - Differentiate proptosis from pseudoproptosis (ie; congenital bony deformity, enophthalmos of the fellow eye, or lid disease).
  - Occasionally a Horner's syndrome will present as proptosis of the contralateral eye.
  - Direction of proptosis may give clues to possible pathology (eccentric of axial proptosis).
- **Valsalva Maneuver in Proptosis**
  - Forced opening of closed passage way; ex: blowing with mouth and nose shut. This increases venous pressure and can exacerbate the proptosis in patients with venous abnormalities.

3. Enophthalmos

- **Enophthalmos-** a recession of the globe within the orbit. Often subtle. Possible causes:
  - Post-traumatic (blow-out fracture of the orbital floor) or congenital structural abnormalities of the orbital walls
  - Orbital content atrophy caused by radiotherapy, scleroderma, or eye poking in blind infants
  - Sclerosing orbital lesions (metastatic schirrous carcinoma, chronic inflammatory orbital disease)
- **Workup for Suspected Blow Out Fracture**
  - Usually caused by a direct blow to the eye through closed lids. This wave of pressure results in a **blowout into ethmoidal or maxillary sinuses**.
  - A portion of orbital **tissue may become trapped** (ie: if in maxillary sinus known as **tear drop sign**) and thus **restricts rotation of the globe**. This trapped tissue can be confirmed with a **skull x ray and orbital tomography**.

- Symptoms
  - **Vertical diplopia** on up and down gaze
  - Restriction of rotation of eye
  - E**nophthalmos**
  - Decreased single binocular visual field.
- Prolapse of the orbital fat with these septa is often responsible for the limitations of ocular motility seen.
- Take a careful case history including onset, duration, pain, diplopia, visual failure.
- Survey old photographs if possible.
- Progressive symptoms may indicate an expanding lesion.
- Since many orbital diseases are associated with systemic disease, a neuro-ophthalmic exam is obligatory.

- **Palpation of Orbital Rim and Anterior Orbit**
  - Generally, one is able to use the index finger to probe between the globe and orbital bone anteriorly.
  - Encountering any fullness or firmness is almost always pathologic because not even the lacrimal gland is normally palpable.
  - **Lymphoid tumors** of the orbit are frequently situated immediately **behind the superior orbital septum** and in the **lacrimal gland**; they have a **firm and rubbery consistency** rather than a rock hard texture.
  - Malignancies and sclerosing inflammatory processes of the orbit can feel rock hard, but this finding is not necessarily an indication of malignancy.
  - One of the most woody feeling orbital conditions is **sarcoidosis**, caused by the abundant fibrous tissue that accompanies the granulomas
- **General workup for Periorbital Ache/Pain of Unknown Cause**
  - Visual Acuity, Color vision, Retinoscopy, Pupil Reflexes, Versions, Visual fields, Fundoscopy, and Evaluation of Diplopia (if any)

4. Dystopia

- **Dystopia** is a displacement of the globe in the coronal plane, usually due to an extraconal orbital mass (Lacrimal gland tumor). Can be associated with proptosis or enophthalmos

5. Recongition of Dysplastic Cranio-Facial Appearance

- **Craniostenosis** is the premature closure of the bones in the head. It results in flat orbits, exophthalmos, and hypertelorism.
- **Craniofacial dysostosis (crouzon's disease)** is a specific type of craniostenosis. Premature closure of all sutures, and in addition, the bones of the lower face grow in peculiar positions. It results in shallow orbits, exophthalmos, and hypertelorism.
- **Orbital cellulitis** is a common infection of the orbit. It results from something as simple as a chalazion or most often from the sinuses.
- **Pseudotumor** is a chronic presence of inflammatory cells in the orbit. Patient presents with pain, limitation of movement, and exophthalmos. This is treated with oral steroids, and the etiology is unknown.
- **Pseudotumor cerebri** presents with papilledema and no pathology. It has nothing to do with an inflamed orbit (don't confuse with pseudotumor described above).
- **Hyperthyroidism** in Grave's disease is the most common cause of unilateral and bilateral exophthalmos.

6. Diagnostic Testing (Applications and Interpretations)

- Special tests (including tomograms, ultrasound, CAT scan, venograms, and X-Ray)
  - Electromagnetic energy is transmitted from a source through a patient. The patient absorbs some of this energy depending upon the type of tissue within the x ray beam. Subsequently, the resultant energy that is transmitted through the patient is used to form an image on photographic film. Higher atomic numbers (and density) of the tissue give a "whiter "image. Air,

O2 and nitrogen low atomic members show up as black. Order for acute boney trauma.

- CRT computerized tomography
  - An **x-ray tube** passes around the patient in a circle. The amount of x ray absorbed by the patient is measured by multiple detectors within the circle. This information is then fed to a computer that reconstructs an image of the patient being examined in an axial plane. CAT scan is used for; acute cranial trauma, orbits, tumors, optic atrophy, and unexplained loss of vision.
- MRI
  - A patient is placed in a large **magnetic field**. This **aligns all the protons** (usually Hydrogen). A **radio signal** is transmitted through the subject which changes the magnetic alignment depending upon the tissue being examined.
  - A radio receiver is utilized to listen as the molecules then realign themselves within the magnetic field.
  - The computer then creates an image of the part being examined in multiple planes. It measures H2. It does NOT image bone. Bone appears BLACK.
  - In MRI, **type 1** fat appears white, and spatial resolution is good. In general, type 1 is used more
  - In **type 2,** fat appears dark. Type 2 is used when one wants to get a specific idea of the water content.
  - You can see a **retinal detachment** in an MRI.
  - MRI is used for demyelinating diseases, posterior fossa tumors, orbits and tumors, optic atrophy, unexplained loss of vision, and cranial nerve palsy.

BLOOD SUPPLY (GROSS ANATOMY)

1. Relevant Branches of the Internal and External Carotid Arteries

- Branches of the **Internal and External Carotid Arteries** supply the orbit, eyelid, and upper face.
- The pathway from the heart to the right eye and face: arch of aorta → brachiocephalic artery. → right common carotid → splits into right internal & external carotid artery at the level of the larynx.
- The pathway from the heart to the left eye and face: arch of aorta → left common carotid → splits into left internal & external carotid artery at the level of the larynx.
- The **External Carotid Artery**'s branches supply the face and dura mater.
  - **Facial Artery**: A medial branch of the external carotid artery. It branches to the angular artery which supplies eyelids and side of nose.
  - **Superficial Temporal Artery**: The most lateral branch of the external carotid artery. It supplies side of the face and the eyelids.
  - **Internal Maxillary Artery:** Is a back-up supply to the orbit via the infraorbital artery. and orbital branch of the middle meningeal artery. This is also called "collateral circulation."
- The **Internal Carotid Artery** supplies the orbit via the ophthalmic artery. It emerges from the mid-cranial fossa on either side of the body of the sphenoid. It ascends through the side of the body of the sphenoid. It ascends through the cavernous sinus which is located on both sides of the sphenoid, before giving off the ophthalmic artery.
  - **Ophthalmic Artery:** the 7th branch of the internal carotid. It supplies 90% of orbital blood.
  - Ophthalmic artery's pathway:
    - The artery moves vertically and medially from the inferior side of the optic nerve.
    - Then, it moves laterally to circle above the nerve.
    - It enters the orbit through the lateral portion of the optic foramen.
    - Inside the orbit the artery crosses over the top of the optic nerve to hug the medial wall as it enters the orbit.

Branches of Ophthalmic Artery

- **1. Central Retinal Artery**: 1st branch. of ophthalmic A. It starts infero-lateral in the orbit and supplies most of the blood to the retina. It runs in the dura and under the optic nerve until 12-13 mm posterior to the eye where it runs into the center of the optic nerve.

- **2. Lacrimal Artery**: Usually the 2nd branch but can be the 1st. It runs anteriorly along the lateral orbital wall to the lateral surface of the LR muscle then terminates anteriorly at the lacrimal gland. It has 4 branches:
  - **Recurrent Meningeal Artery**: Also called recurrent lacrimal artery. It passes out of the orbit through the meningeal foramen or superior orbital fissure's lateral limb, and can anastomose with the orbital branch of the middle meningeal artery (which is from the internal maxillary artery branch from the external carotid.
  - **Muscular Artery** to the LR & SR muscles, can be variable
  - **Zygomatic Artery** splits into 2 branches: - zygomatico-facial & zygomatico-temporal (via a T-shaped canal in the zygomatic foramen) which both follow the zygomatic nerve, pierces the septum orbitali and emerges in the eyelids near the lateral canthus, splitting into the superior and inferior palpebral branches to join the arcade in the eyelid and **anastomose** with medial palpebral arteries
  - **Superior and Inferior Lateral Palpebral Artery** the terminal branches of the lacrimal artery. They join the arteriole arcades of the eyelids.
  - **Note:** Sometimes the posterior ciliary arteries are a branch of the lacrimal instead of the ophthalmic.
- **3. Muscular Artery**: Direct branches of the ophthalmic artery. It has 2 groups:
  - Superior muscular artery → supply SR, SO, Levator
  - Inferior muscular artery → supply IR, IO, MR.
  - The recti arteries branch to **anterior ciliary artery** which run down the orbital, bony side of the muscle and pierce the globe where the muscle inserts anteriorly, emerges on the sclera and heads toward the cornea (where neovascularization would occur)
    - Two **anterior ciliary arteries** per muscle (except LR that has 1) - also feeds the iris and ciliary body
- **4. Posterior Ciliary Artery**: Two long branches *lateral and medial* between sclera and choroid give rise to many short post. ciliary arteries which pierce the back of the globe forming the **Circle of Haller-Zinn** around the optic nerve which is decentered nasally (blood vessels are centered on the posterior pole).
  - Could be a branch of the lacrimal instead of the ophthalmic
- **5. Pial Artery:** Vascularizes the pia mater of the optic nerve.
- **6. Supra-Orbital Artery** runs along the roof medially and exits by the supra-orbital notch. If the artery splits into 2 branches inside the orbit, each follows the medial and lateral frontal nerves. This causes the supratrochlear artery to not exit by the frontal notch of Henle.
  - It supplies blood to the frontal sinuses, the SR, levator, periosteum and bone of the roof of the orbit, upper lids (another contributor to the arcades in the eyelid), scalp, and eyebrows.
- **7. Posterior Ethmoid Artery:** Goes through the posterior ethmoid foramen to the nasal and ethmoidal air cells and parts of the nasal cavity, dura mater, anterior cranial fossa
- **8. Anterior Ethmoid Artery:** (larger than posterior) Exits through the anterior foramen to supply the mucosa of the ethmoidal air cells and frontal sinus and skin of the nose. Branches to the anterior meningeal artery in the anterior cranial fossa meninges.
- **9. Medial Palpebral Artery:** Branches off the ophthalmic artery near the trochlea and it bifurcates to make the inferior and superior medial palpebral artery. It supplies blood to marginal and peripheral arcades of the lids.
- **10. Dorsal Nasal Artery** is one of 2 terminal branches of the ophthalmic artery. It runs with the infra-trochlear nerve above the medial palpebral ligament and anastamoses the external carotid artery via the angular branch (in the cheeks) of the facial artery. It supplies blood to the lacrimal sac and skin of the nose.
- **11. Frontal (Supratrochlear) Artery** passes through the frontal notch of Henle or pierces the septum orbitale to vascularize the forehead and scalp, medial eyebrow.
  - The notch of Henle can have one of two arteries – if the **supraorbital artery** branches within the orbit, it will pass through the notch instead of the **frontal artery**

- **12. Infra-Orbital Artery** (branch of internal maxillary): A source of orbital blood supply (collateral) as an alternative to the internal carotid source since this is from the external carotid.
    - Inside the orbit, it supplies blood to the IR, IO and lacrimal sac. Other branches supply the lower eyelids and upper mouth, lips, cheeks, meninges.
    - Goes through the **IOF** and emerges through the **infraorbital foramen** just under the orbit.
- **Orbital branch of the Middle Meningeal artery**: Provides a minor blood supply to the orbit. It is a branch of the internal maxillary artery, and it anastomoses with the recurrent lacrimal artery. (also called the recurrent meningeal artery). It may also enter the orbit by itself through the superior orbital fissure or meningeal foramen

2. Relevant Branches of the Internal and External Jugular Veins

- The internal and external jugular veins drain the orbit:
    - **Posteriorly** through the inferior or superior. Ophthalmic vein
    - **Anteriorly** to the angular vein, or **Inferiorly** through the infra-orbital vein
- Veins do not have valves and allow bidirectional flow, which is a disadvantage since infections may spread more easily. Also, veins have a much more variable pathway than arteries.
- **Superior Ophthalmic Vein (SOV)**: D**drains to internal jugular**; the largest orbital vein lies at the superior medial margin of the orbit (except for the lacrimal branch) anastomoses with the angular vein at the front of the orbit via the orbital vein. This is one of the two drainage routes: frontal.
- Drainage through the back of the orbit is the major route
    - The superior ophthalmic vein goes through the superior orbital fissure to get out of the orbit, then goes to the cavernous sinus, to the inferior petrosal sinus, and finally to the internal jugular vein, which drains to the brachiocephalic, then the superior vena cava and finally the right atrium
- Branches of the superior ophthalmic vein corresponding to arteries:
    - **Anterior and posterior ethmoidal, muscular, and lacrimal veins** all travel with the corresponding A. However, the lacrimal vein may pass out of the orbit without the artery through the superior orbital fissure to the cavernous sinus.
    - **Central retinal vein** travels within the optic nerve to the posterior part of the orbit where it connects with the superior ophthalmic vein. Sometimes it leaves the orbit independent of the SOV. It drains the blood from the retina.
    - **Anterior ciliary vein:** drains the front part of the eyeball to which the anterior ciliary A. serves.
    - **Palisades of Vogt –** spokes near limbus where blood vessels go, near the canal of Schlemm
    - **Vortex veins:** aka **venae vorticosa**. There are four-- each drains a quadrant of the posterior eye to the SOV.

  Note: There are no vortex arteries, no posterior cililary veins, and the upper temporal vortex vein may drain into the lacrimal SOV.
- **Inferior Ophthalmic Vein (IOV)**: Passes out of the orbit independently of the SOV, through the **inferior orbital fissure** to the **pterygoid venous plexus** in the **infra-temporal fossa** where it is connected to the **cavernous sinus** (below the orbit and under the arch of the zygomatic bone).
    - It continues to the internal maxillary vein, then to the retro-mandibular vein, to the **external jugular vein**, then to the subclavian, innominate, superior vena cava, and finally to the right atrium.
    - It drains the bottom of the orbit.
    - Joins up with SOV or leaves orbit by itself
- **Pterygoid venous plexus**: In the medial part of the infratemp. fossa
    - Venous plexus is not the same as a venous sinus.
    - Venous sinus is in the cranium and lined with dura mater.
    - Venous plexus is outside the cranium, not lined with dura mater, and is a mass of very small veins. It lies below the cavernous sinuses and connects to them by emissary veins which go through the sphenoid foramen ovale, lacerum, rotundum, and vesalius. Drainage may be to the internal maxillary to the retro-mandibular vein to the external jugular vein, or to the anterior facial vein through the deep facial vein. It communicates with the IOV through the inferior orbital fissure.

3. Sinuses

- **Cavernous sinuses**: In the middle cranial cavities on either side of the body of the **sphenoid bone** and **sella tursica** made up of spongy vascular tissue in a pocket that the **dura mater** makes. The two are connected by two little branches in the front.
  - It is formed anteriorly by the SOV and posteriorly communicates with the inf and sup. petrosal sinus.
  - It is located directly behind the SOF.
  - The two cavernous sinuses communicate by the anter. and poster. intercavernous sinuses creating the circular sinus.
  - All inter-cranial sinuses are lined with dura mater.
  - It communicates with the IOV, and drains via the pterygoid plexus. Blood in the cavernous sinuses can flow in any direction.
  - **Carotid cavernous fistula**: If internal carotid ruptures within the cavernous sinus
  - **Ophthalmoplegia**: Pituitary gland tumor can compress the cavernous sinus compromising the function of CN III, IV, and VI which travel through the sinus
- **Lymphatics**: No nodes or vessels are in the orbit.
- **Dural Sinuses**: Also known as the dural venous sinuses, cerebral sinuses, or cranial sinuses
  - Receive blood from internal and external veins of the brain, receive cerebrospinal fluid (CSF) from the **subarachnoid space**, and ultimately empty into the internal jugular vein.
  - The walls of the dural venous sinuses are composed of dura mater lined with endothelium, a specialized layer of flattened cells found in blood vessels. They differ from other blood vessels in that they lack a full set of vessel layers (e.g. tunica media) characteristic of arteries and veins.

EYELID (GROSS ANATOMY)

---

1. Anatomic Boundaries

- The upper eyelid extends to the eyebrow and is divided into two portions:
  - **Tarsal Portion** which lies closest to the lid margin, rests on the globe, and contains the **tarsal plate** (a dense connective tissue made of collagen that has Meibomian glands embedded in it)
  - **Orbital (Preseptal) Portion)** which extends from the tarsus to the eyebrow
  - **Superior Palpebral Furrow (Sulcus)** separates the tarsal portion from the orbital portion. It can be absent in East Asians.
- The lower eyelid also has a tarsal and orbital part, but these parts are not as pronounced as the upper lid.
  - **Inferior Palpebral Furrow (Sulcus)** separates the tarsal and orbital parts, it becomes more visible with age
  - **Naso-jugal Furrow (Sulcus)** attaches the skin to the underlying connective tissue in the nasal area, extending past the inferior orbital margin
  - **Malar Furrow (Sulcus)** defines the lower boundary of the eyelid on the lateral side

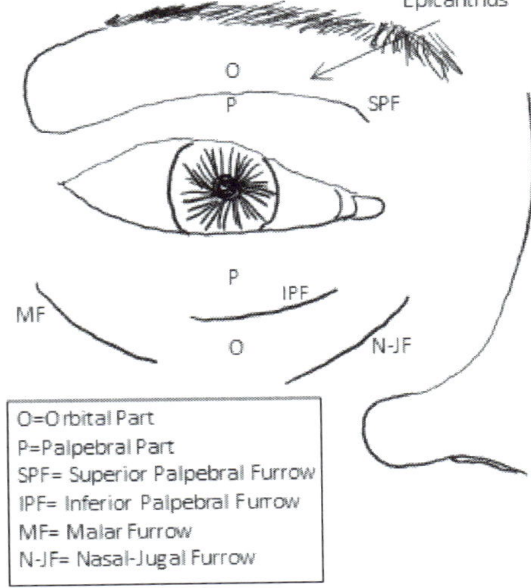

- The **Palpebral Fissure (Medial Margin)** is the slit or opening that the eyelids form, it is the entrance into the conjunctival sac. It is lower medially than laterally (by 2-4mm) sloping toward the medial canthus allowing for tear drainage. The shape and size of the palpebral fissure may vary:

- **Plica Semilunaris**: Moon shaped fold of conjunctiva
- **Lacrimal Caruncle**: Small tissue bulge
- **Epicanthal Fold/Epicanthus (Mongolian Fold)**: Vertical fold of skin at the nasal canthus that covers the caruncle and plica semilunaris. In Asians, epicanthus covers the medial canthus and orbital septum fuses with the levator tendon much closer to the tarsal plate, eliminating the superior palpebral furrow. In Asians and infants, this can be misperceived as a "pseudo-tropia"

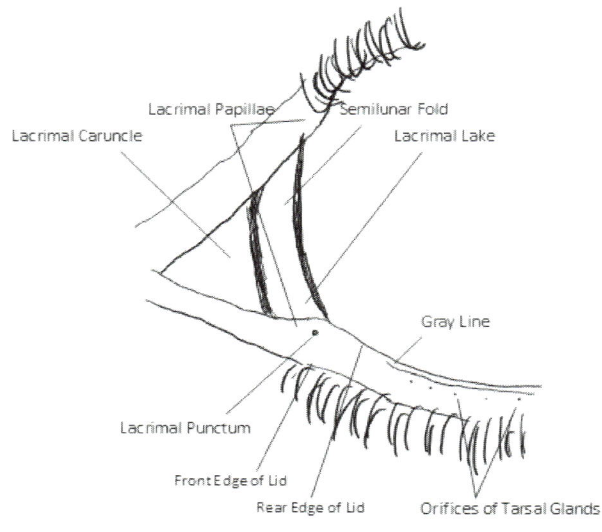

- **Eyelid Margin** rests against the globe (conjunctiva). Two margins of the eyelid come together when we close our eyes. Each margin is divided into two portions:
  - **Ciliary portion** is where the lashes are, it is the lateral 5/6.
    - **Palpebral Cilia** (eyelashes) are arranged in 2-3 rows on each lid, with an average of 100 to 150 lashes on the upper and 50-80 on the lower lid. They grow in 10 weeks and have a life span of 3-5 months
  - **Lacrimal portion** is the medial 1/6 of the margin. The two portions are divided at the **lacrimal papilla,** a small division that contains the lacrimal punctum.
  - The lid margins contain the glands of Zeis and Moll.
- **Gray Line**: a groove that runs along ht eyelid margin between the cilia insertions and pores of the Meibomian glands, it is the boundary between skin and conjunctiva
- **Mucocutaneous Junction** is the transition from the skin of the eyelids to the conjunctiva.

2. Layers of the Eyelid

- Four layers (from the front to the back):
  - Cutaneous
  - Muscular
  - Fibrous
  - Conjunctival.

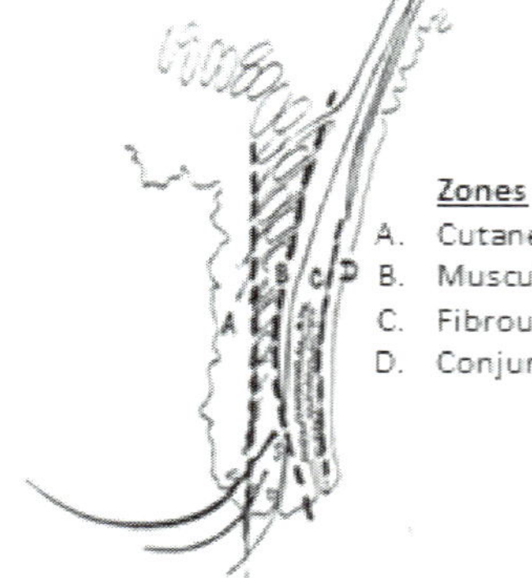

- **Cutaneous Zone:**
  - 1 mm thick (thinnest skin layer in the body)
  - Sublayers:
    - **Stratified squamous epithelium**
    - **Dermis-connective tissue** layer (deeper) with nerves, blood vessels and lymphatics.
    - **Sub-cutaneous areolar zone**
      - Does not have any fat
      - Moves freely over the underlying muscles, but is attached tightly at the margins.
- **Muscular Zone:**
  - Smooth muscle, sympathetically innervated
  - Three sets of muscles associated:
    - Orbicularis oculi (the sphincter)
    - Superior and Inferior Tarsal Muscles (Mullers muscle)
    - Levator LPS
- **Fibrous Zone:**
  - Contains the **Tarsal Plate**, a dense connective tissue or collagen fibers that run both vertically and horizontally to surround the Meibomian glands. It gives the lid rigidity, structure, and shape. The orbital border of the tarsus is attached to the orbital septum.

- **Septum Orbitale** is the palpebral fascia, sometimes called the "fire curtain of the orbit". It hangs in front of the orbit and is a tough barrier to infection spreading to the eye. It is very hard to pierce. Its attachments include:
  - The arcus marginalis, which is a connection to bone all the way around the orbit. The weakest portion is medial.
  - The periorbita of the orbital bone, which is continuous with the periosteum of the bone
- **Aponeurosis** (tendon) **of the Levator Palpebra Superioris** is a fibrous structure that inserts in the palpebral part of the eyelid.
  - The aponeurosis becomes continuous with the sheath that lines the levator and the superior rectus so that the eyeball, eyelid and conjuctiva move together.
  - There are three subdivisions to the aponeurosis:
    1. Cutaneous portion
    2. Osseous or orbital portion
    3. Conjunctival portion
- There is also a check ligament that limits the range of motion of the levator muscle

o **Conjunctival Zone:**
- A thin translucent membrane that runs from the limbus over the anterior sclera and turns anteriorly to line the eyelids. It ensures the smooth movement of the eyelids over the globe. The **palpebral conjunctiva** lines the eyelids while the **bulbar conjunctiva** covers the sclera.

3. Muscles (Actions)

- **Orbicularis Oculi** (sphincter)
  - Innervated by the upper and lower zygomatic branches of the facial nerve
  - Palpebral fissure is closed by contraction of the orbicularis oculi muscles
  - Marginal Portion
    - **Muscle of Riolan: A**djacent to the lid margins on both sides of the Meibomian gland openings. They maintain the lid margins close to the globe
    - **Muscle of Horner:** Fibers that encircle the lacrimal canaliculi
  - Palpebral Portion
    - **Pretarsal:** Fibers in front of and lying on the tarsal plates
    - **Preseptal:** Fibers in front of tarsal plates to the medial orbital margin and the medial palpebral ligament to the lateral palpebral raphe

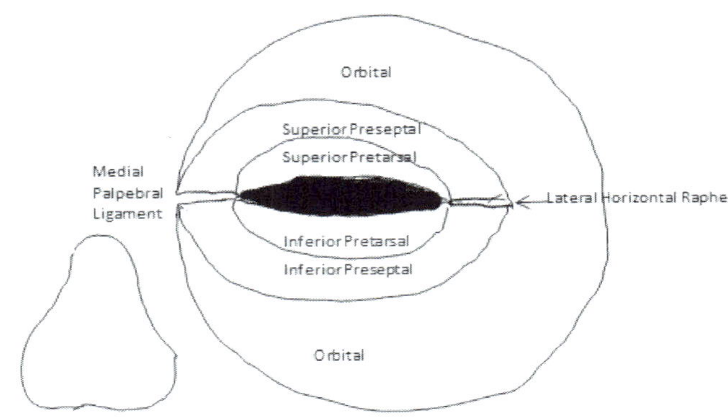

  - Orbital Portion
    - Contains the muscle that extends past the orbital rim onto the brow and cheek regions. Attached superiorly to the medial orbital margin (deep origin) and medial palpebral ligament (superficial origin), medial too the supraorbital notch.
    - **Muscularis Superciliaris:** Outer portion that lies over the supraciliary ridge, superior to the orbit, which depresses the eyebrow
    - **Muscularis Malaris:** Inferior to the orbit, which raises up the cheeks
  - Blinking
    - You use the entire orbicularis muscle during a forceful blink
    - Reflex blinks are elicited by sensory stimuli and are excursions of the upper lid and are faster and larger in amplitude than spontaneous blinks.
    - Lid movements during spontaneous blinking moves the tears across the cornea both vertically and medially towards the sites of drainage at the medial canthus
    - **Bell's Phenomenon** is an involuntary rolling up of the eyeballs during a blink.

- **Levator Palpebrae Superioris**
  - Retractor of the upper lid, it is the antagonist of the palpebral portion of the orbicularis oculi.
  - It is innervated by **cranial nerve III.**
  - Originates at the apex of the orbit on the sphenoid bone above the superior rectus.
  - Muscular portion ends within the orbit and expands into a broad flat tendon – **levator aponeurosis**, which inserts onto the anterior surface of the superior tarsal plate and the connective tissue of the pretarsal portion of the orbicularis oculi.
- **Superior and Inferior Tarsal Muscles of Muller**
  - Innervated by the sympathetic system (superior cervical ganglion). It can open the eyes wider in response to fear.
  - The superior tarsal muscle of Muller aids the levator to lift the upper lid. It arises near the origin of the levator aponeurosis, and runs behind it to the upper ridge of the superior tarsal plate.
  - The inferior tarsal muscle of Muller depresses the lower lid. It runs between the bottom edge of the inferior tarsal plate and the connective tissue of the surrounding inferior oblique and inferior rectus muscle insertions on the eye.
- Palpebral ligaments suspend the tarsal plate in front of the eye.
  - **Medial palpebral ligament:**
    - Well-developed
    - Attaches to bone
    - Bridges over fossa for the lacrimal sac
  - **Lateral palpebral ligament:**
    - Small and not well-developed
    - Not a true ligament at all made of connective tissue

4. Glands

- **Meibomian (Tarsal) glands:**
  - Located in the tarsal plate. The conjunctiva and skin end at duct of the Meibomian gland
  - Sebaceous (fatty) –secretes sebum (combination of cholesterol and fatty acids) to help seal the palpebral fissure The sebum forms the top layer of the tears, which decreases surface tension and prevents evaporation.
  - A chronic inflamed Meibomian gland is called a **chalazion** (aka **internal hordeolum**, hailstone or pimple).
- **Zeiss glands:**
  - Located at the eyelid margin
  - Sebaceous (fatty) glands associated with hair follicles. Secretions released directly onto hair follicle to prevent cilia from becoming dry and brittle
  - An infected Zeis (or Moll) gland is called a **stye** (aka **external hordeolum**). Zeis glands are more easily infected because the ducts are close to the skin
    - To determine if external or internal hordeolum: place a cue tip on the bump and move the skin. If skin slides over the bump it is an internal hordeolum (Meibomian), if the bump goes with the skin it is an external hordeolum (Zeiss/Moll)
- **Moll glands:**
  - Located near the hair follicles.
  - Modified sweat (sudoriforous) glands. It is an apocrine gland that empties into the hair follicles and skin (not onto the conjunctiva)

5. Blood Supply and Drainage/Lymphatic Drainage

Eyelid Arteries

- There are two main systems that supply blood to the eyelids: the **facial** system and the **orbital** system. These two sources branch out into the superior and inferior **peripheral arteriolar arcades**
- Facial system:
    - Derived from the **external carotid** artery

        - The **facial artery** ascends the face and becomes the angular artery, a terminal branch that goes to the medial canthus. The **angular artery** supplies the lacrimal sac, medial part of the lid, and skin of the cheek.
        - The **superficial temporal artery** (another terminal branch of the external carotid) gives three branches that supplies areas near the orbit.
            - **Transverse facial artery** supplies the skin of the cheek and anastomoses with the infraorbital artery.
            - **Anterior temporal artery** supplies the skin and muscles of the forehead and anastamose with the suprorbital and supratrochlear arteries.
            - **Zygomatic artery** supplies the orbicularis muscle.
        - **Infraorbital** artery is a branch of the internal maxillary. The **internal maxillary** artery branches off the external carotid, then runs the floor of the orbit and comes out on the face via the facial infra-orbital foramen. The infraorbital artery supplies the lower eyelid and lacrimal sac.
- Orbital system:
    - Originates from the **ophthalmic branch** of the **internal carotid artery**. The ophthalmic artery has many branches which spill out to the front of the orbit to the eyelid.
        - One branch, the **lacrimal artery** runs forward along the upper border of the lateral rectus muscle. Aside from supplying blood to the lacrimal gland, it also branches, and the **lateral palpebral arteries (superior and inferior)** pierce the orbital septum, anastomose with the **medial palpebral arteries** and form the **palpebral arcades.**

Eyelid Veins

- There are two main systems that drain blood from the eyelids, the **facial** and **orbital systems.**
- Facial system:
    - Drains to the **external jugular** vein via:
        - **Anterior Facial** vein, which gets its blood from the **angular** vein and drains to the posterior facial and into the external jugular.
        - **Superficial Temporal** vein drains down the side of the face into the **retro-mandibular** vein, which becomes the external jugular.
        - **Infraorbital** vein, which may or may not be present at all. If it is, it drains to the pterygoid venous plexus and then into the internal maxillary and finally to the external jugular vein.
- Orbital system:
    - Drains to the **internal jugular** vein via the:
        - **Superior Ophthalmic** vein, which collects blood from the **supraorbital** vein and the **supratrochlear** vein, which drains to the cavernous sinus.
        - **Inferior Ophthalmic** vein, which drains from the **lacrimal** vein and sometimes the infraorbital vein and empties into the cavernous sinus and then into the internal jugular vein.
        - **Anterior Facial** vein can drain 2 possible ways. Under the orbital system, the anterior facial vein drains to the common facial vein and then into the internal jugular vein.

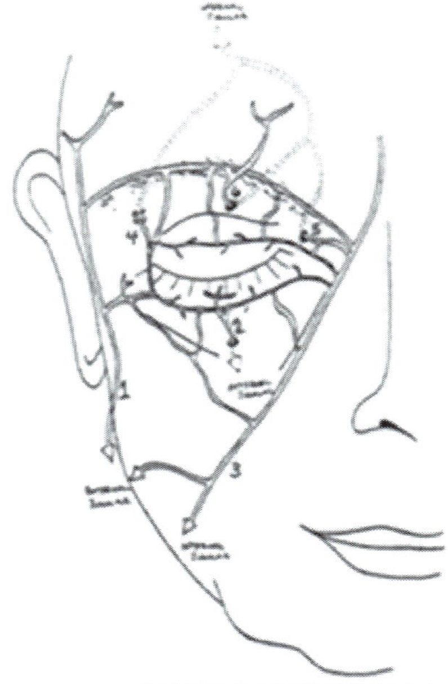

<u>Facial Venous System</u>
1. Superficial Temporal
2. Infra-Orbital
3. Anterior Facial

<u>Orbital Venous System</u>
3. Anterior Facial
4. Lacrimal
5. Supratrochlear
6. Supraorbital

Lymphatic Drainage

- The **lymph plexi** of the eyelids are found both **deep** (between the tarsal plate and the conjunctiva) and **superficial** (pre-tarsal plate).
- There are two drainage routes for lymph from eyelid skin and the orbicularis oculi:

- Lymph from the **medial** portion of the eye drains to the **submaxillary** or **submandibular** nodes.
- Lymph from the **lateral** portion of the eye drains to the **preauricular** or **parotid** nodes.

6. Innervation

- Motor innervation comes from the **oculomotor nerve** (**CN III**), which innervates the levator palpebrae superioris and the **facial nerve (CN VII)** which innervates the orbicularis oculi.
- **Sensory** innervation comes from the **trigeminal** nerve (**CN V**). There are two divisions which supply the orbital region:
  - **Ophthalmic division**: receives sensory input from the upper eyelid via the external/dorsal nasal, infratrochlear, supratrochlear, supraorbital, and lacrimal nerves.
  - **Maxillary division**: receives sensory input from the lower eyelid and cheek via the infraorbital nerve, zygomatic-facial nerve, and zygomatico-temporal nerves.

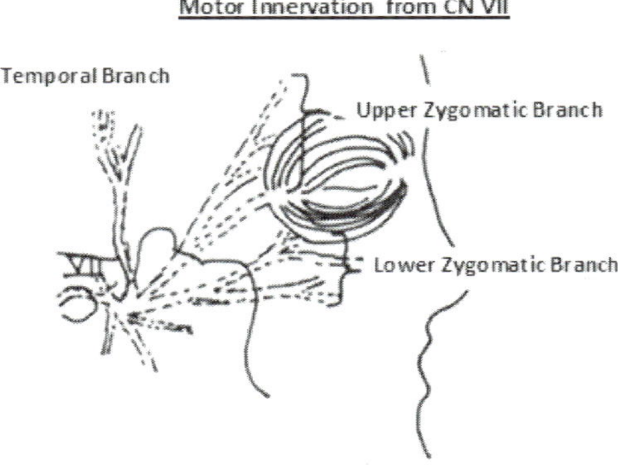

- **Autonomic** innervation: **sympathetic** innervation goes to the smooth muscle of Muller, the glands of the eyelid, and the blood vessels. The route the innervation takes is highly variable.

EYELID (DEVELOPMENTAL ANATOMY)

---

1. Tissue Origin

- The **eyelid** is derived from **mesoderm**.

2. Lid Folds

- The upper lid fold is formed from the **frontonasal processes**.
- The lower lid is formed from the upgrowth of the **maxillary process** and usually lags behind the upper lid in development.
- The folds form during the **2nd month** from mesodermal condensation curving up and over the eye.

3. Fusion of the Eyelids

- The **eyelid starts fusing** from the inner canthus during the 7th-8th week and remains fused until the eyelid glands are developed.
- By the 7th month, **the lid adhesion dissolves** as a result of secretions from sebaceous glands and cornification of lid cells.

4. Ectodermal Derivatives (Skin, Glands, Conjunctiva)

- Ectoderm surrounding mesoderm develops into skin on the outer ectodermal edge and into conjunctiva on the inner ectodermal edge.
- The conjunctiva is continuous with corneal epithelium and provides the derivation for the lid glands.

5. Mesodermal Derivatives

- Tarsus, Orbital Septum, Orbicularis Oculi, Aponeurosis of Levator, Smooth Muscle
- By the end of the 3rd month, a **primitive tarsus forms** as a connective tissue condensation. By the end of the 7th month, it is a **well-formed upper lid**.
- The **orbicularis oculi** is developed by the end of the 3rd month.
- 5th month. The **aponeurosis of the levator splits** into superficial and deep portions.
- Smooth muscle of the eyelid is also derived from mesoderm.

EYELIDS (PHYSIOLOGY)

1. Normal Closure of Eyelids (Forced, Spontaneous)

- **Forced closure** is accomplished by the orbital portion of the **orbicularis oculi** which is under voluntary control and is innervated by cranial nerve **VII**.
- **Spontaneous closure** (blinking and voluntary winking) is accomplished by the palpebral portion of the orbicularis. The lower lid remains almost stationary while the upper lid closes in a lateral to medial fashion. The average **blink rate** is **15/min**, with **0.3-0.4 sec duration per blink.**
- Blinking also serves the purpose of helping to remove irritants which have landed in the eye. Also, eyelids serve the purpose of helping to control the amount of light entering the eye (control of the iris is autonomic). Without eyelids, it would be helpless to block visual sensory overload under very bright light. Eyelids also used to block light from reaching the eyes during sleep.

2. Blink Reflexes (Spontaneous, Menace, Auditory, Touch, Dazzle)

- **Spontaneous**: Occurs without stimuli; see above description.
- **Menace**: Occurs when an unexpected or threatening object comes suddenly into the near field of vision; it's a **cortical reflex** and the **afferent pathway is via the ON.**
- **Auditory**: Loud noises can cause a blink reflex.
- **Touch**: Occurs when any object touches an anaesthetized eye; it's a corneal reflex and the **afferent pathway** is via the nerve **V** and **efferent** via nerve **VII**.
- **Dazzle**: Occurs with bright lights. Afferent pathway is via the ON.

3. Role of Eyelids in Production, Distribution, and Drainage of Tears

- **Production**: The aqueous component of the normal tear flow is produced by continuous secretion from the accessory lacrimal glands (**glands of Krause**) scattered throughout the conjunctival sac. The Krause glands are located in the **conjunctival fornices** (about **30-40** of these glands are located in the lateral part of upper fornix near or attached to the main lacrimal gland). The **Wolfring / Ciaccio** glands are located along the **superior border of the upper tarsal plate conjunctiva and inferior border of the lower tarsal plate conjunctiva**. Excessive production of tears, as in crying, is due mainly to reflex stimulation of the main lacrimal gland. **Meibomian glands** produce the **oily** layer of the tear film, with input also from **Zeiss and Moll** glands to some extent. These large sebaceous glands are located in the **tarsal plate**. The mucous layer is produced by goblet cells in conjunctival fornices.
- **Distribution:** The upper lid blinks laterally to medially wiping a thin film of tears over the corneal epithelium and bulbar conjunctiva.
- **Drainage:** With each blink, the orbicularis ring moves nasally forcing tears into the puncta as it closes from the lateral to medial direction. The tears enter the puncta and go through the canaliculi into the lacrimal sac due to the blink action. The *contraction* of the orbicularis creates a *negative pressure* in the lacrimal sac. When the orbicularis relaxes, the sac collapses and drives the tears into the nasolacrimal duct.

Gland	Secretion	Location	Number of Glands
Krause	Aqueous	Conjunctiva Fornices	30-40
Wolfring/Ciaccio	Aqueous	Conjunctiva- borders of tarsal plates near lid margins	
Zeiss and Moll	Sebaceous		30-40 upper lid, 20-30 lower lid
Meibomian	Lipid	Tarsal plates	
Goblet and Crypts of Henle	Mucous	Conjunctiva Fornices	
Epithelium Cells	Glycocalyx – creates hydrophilic surface on cornea for tears to adhere	Corneal epithelium	All epithelium

4. Protective Functions of Eyelids

- **Cilia:** Sensing actions **induce a blink reflex**, which attempts to limit eye damage.

- Secretions of the conjunctival, Meibomian, and lacrimal glands have a protective function against:
    - Dehydration
    - Foreign particles.
- Movement removes debris during a blink.
- Squinting protects the eyes from intense light.

5. Purposes and Roles for Vision

- Eyelids spread the tear film over the anterior surface of the eye, maintaining a smooth uniformity of the tear film through blinking which creates a smooth refractive surface.
- Optically, the eyelids increase depth of field, reduce aberration effects when squinting, and control the entry of light into eye.

ADNEXA (PATHOLOGY)

---

1. Head

- Position and Posture:
    - **Head** may be displaced, or **unable to be held up [eg. in Tay Sachs disease**], or elevated [eg. in ptosis], or tilted to one side [e.g. paralysis or overacting of extraocular muscles IO or SO], or **rotated and tilted [eg**. **true torticollis**].
- Size and Shape: **Hypocephalus and microcephalus** may be associated with **lamellar cataracts**.
- Scars may suggest the probable cause in cases of optic atrophy or in paralysis of the extraocular muscles.
- **Palpate the head** to detect presence of sclerosis of the temporal artery, nodules or depressed fractures, arteriosclerosis characterized by tortuosity and hardening of the vessels, or of **arteritis**, which presents cordlike thickening of the temporal arteries, palpable nodules, and **painful tender areas over the temple and the scalp**.
    - Metastatic sarcomatous nodules may be present in the skull in cases of primary or **metastatic sarcoma of the choroid.**
    - Depressed fractures may be associated with asthenopia, chronic headaches, optic N. atrophy or papilledema.

2. Face

- Asymmetry may result in hypertropia or unilateral proptosis. **Unilateral hypertrophy of the face** may occur in **Recklinghausen's** disease.
- Edema, swelling, or puffiness observed in **chronic nephritis, trichiasis, whooping cough, aneurysm of the aorta, or in hyperthyroidism**.
- Distortion
    - As in facial paralysis [**Bell's palsy**], in spasm of the orbicularis muscles, in **tic douloureux (trigeminal neuralgia)**.
- Skin Lesions
    - As in **Herpes Zoster** characterized by cluster of vesicles along the course of the Trigeminal nerve, with respect to face **midline**, associated with **conjunctivitis, corneal ulceration, iridocyclitis and glaucoma**.
    - Rashes of **syphilis** may be associated with **paresis of the levator, extra or intraocular muscles.**
- Scars in lacrimal gland region (ex. old tuberculous lesions of the gland), in lacrimal sac region [eg. old dacryocystomy].
- Enlargement of gland:
    - Preauricular gland (ex. in cases of hordeolum, infected chalazions, **herpes, abscess, sarcoma of the eyelids, syphilis or tuberculosis of the conjunctiva, adeno virus conjunctivitis**).
    - Parotid gland associated with chronic inflammation of the lacrimal gland.
    - **Submaxillary gland** may occur in **epidemic keratoconjunctivitis.**

- **Glands:** The **preauricular gland** [area in front of the ear] becomes palpable as a result of acute infections. Also palpate the submaxillary and the salivary and lacrimal glands.

Testing of Facial and Lid Muscles Served by the Cranial Nerves

- **CN III**
  - Test extraocular muscles, ciliary muscles [**NPA**], size, shape, position and reactions of the **pupils**, ability to **elevate** the upper lid.
- **CN VII**
  - Note any flattening or asymmetry of one side of the face and test the sense of **taste** of the anterior two thirds of the tongue.
  - Direct patient to **frown**, to **raise his eyelids**, to **open and shut eyes**, to **show teeth**, to **smile**, to **whistle**, to **blow out cheeks**.
  - If the VII nerve of one side is involved, **direct winking is absent, but normal consensual response occurs (absent with CN V)** with both eyelids of the other eye.
- **CN V**
  - Test the motor division by palpating and noting the position of the **lower jaw**, especially with relation to the median incisors of both dentures.
  - Test the sensitivity of the three branches of the sensory division which supply the **nasal, lingual and buccal mucous membranes** and part of the **scalp to touch, pain and temperature**.
  - Test the **corneal sensitivity** to touch. **Neither direct nor consensual winking** will occur if the 5th cranial nerve is involved.

Testing for Facial Anhydrosis

- Findings are dry face, **elevated eyebrows**, prominent frontal fossa, depressed nasal root and bridge, and delayed appearance of hair, eyebrows, and eyelashes.
- Pathognomonic of this is total absence of sweat glands or nonfunctioning glands and ducts. This condition is called anhidrotic ectodermal dysplasia. **Sensory neuropathy with anhydrosis** is characterized by mental retardation, frequent unexplained fever and pain insensitivity.

Sinus Elevation

- Pain originating from the paranasal sinuses may be perceived as stemming from the eyes.
- Characteristics: follow a rhythmic pattern, being most prominent as the sinus fills with fluid and ebbing with drainage, is chronic for days to weeks and usually is **dull, pressure sensation, unilateral, and retro-orbital**, with increased discomfort on tapping of the affected sinus area.
- A history of chronic post nasal drip may be elicited. Rarely, in acute bacterial inflammation, there may be fever, erythema and swelling of the area.
- Actual involvement of the orbit with **cellulitis** and possible abscess formation may occur.
- Radiographs may show a thickened fluid level or polyp formation.

Assessment of Periorbital Edema-Testing for Orbital Bruits

- Use the **bell portion of your stethoscope** and hold the bell over the patient's eye. If you hear a loud "train" sound or bruit you may have a cavernous sinus fistula on your hands
- 80% of **carotid cavernous sinus fistula** result from trauma to the head.
  - Signs: **pulsating exophthalmos** and a very loud **bruit** when listening with a stethoscope.
  - A characteristic of carotid cavernous fistula is lessening or cessation of the bruit with gentle compression in the neck of the **ipsilateral carotid artery**

3. Eyelids

- **Eyelids:** Palpate the eyelids for swelling or irregularity. Reexamine the lids after eversion and double eversion.
  - Causes of swelling include: chalazion, localized infection, foreign body, prolonged blepharospasm, trichinosis (parasitic infection from eating undercooked meat), canaliculitis,

tuberculous nodule, hordeolum, infected Meibomian gland, dacryocystitis or neoplasmic mass, severe types of conjunctivitis, iritis or orbital cellulitis.

- **Erythema** of the lids implies an inflammatory condition and may be marked in idiopathic orbital inflammation in which the redness abruptly stops at the orbital rim where the periorbita recurves to form the orbital septurn in the lids. In all instances the orbital rims should be palpated for any evidence of bony irregularities or the discovery of a mass lesion.
- Eyelid Abnormalities:
  - **Palpebral hernia** is the protrusion of orbital fat at the lateral orbital fold. It occurs naturally with age. In its exaggerated form it is known as **lateral ptosis adiposa**.
  - **Ectropion** is the turning out of the lid margin away from the eye could be from **wound** or **scar.** The Meibomian gland ducts are moved which leads to **exposure conjunctivitis or keratitis**
  - **Entropion** is the turning in of the lid margin towards the eye.

Lid Eversion

- **Upper Tarsal Conjunctiva**
  - Whether smooth or rough, hyperemic or anemic [conjunctivitis], excessive discharge [tear, mucoid, or mucopurulent], signs like undue pallor, dryness and smoothness of the tarsal conjunctiva are characteristics of late stages of **trachoma**.
  - Any hard, flat, red or pale, discreet or grouped papillae with milky or threadlike discharge are characteristics of **vernal catarrhal conjunctivitis.**
- **Lower Tarsal Conjunctiva**
  - Note for concretions, infarcts, ulcerations, lacerations, erosions, foreign bodies, localized granuloma.

LACRIMAL SYSTEM (GROSS ANATOMY)

---

1. Lacrimal Gland (Structure, Innervation, Blood Supply)

- The gland is located in the **lacrimal fossa**
- The gland is more lateral, sac is medial. And divides into two lobes:
  - **Superior (orbital)**, which is larger, located closer to bone
  - **Inferior (palpebral)** sticks down into orbit a little
  - The two halves are separated by the aponeurosis of the levator.
- The 12 ducts empty in the superior fornix (2-5 large ducts superiorly, 6-8 small ducts inferiorly).
- Secretes a serous, water-like secretion (tears). Most of the tear fluid is supplied by the main lacrimal gland, additional secretions come from accessory lacrimal glands (Krause/Wolfring)
  - The lysozyme in tears is bacteriostatic
- Innervation of the lacrimal gland stimulates secretion and is regulated by autonomic inputs
  - **Lacrimal nerve**, a branch of the ophthalmic division of the oculomotor nerve (Trigeminal CN V). This nerve is sensory
  - **Facial nerve (CN VII)**, stimulates tear production, parasympathetic normal homeostatic lacrimation. **Parasympathetic innervations** originate from cells in the pterygopalatine ganglion
  - **Sympathetic innervation**, for excess tear production in response to pain or emotions, comes from cells in the superior cervical ganglion.
- Blood supply is via the **lacrimal artery and vein**.
  - The **superior temporal artery** sometimes provides blood as well.

2. Accessory Lacrimal Glands (Location, Function)

- Includes **Wolfring glands** (sometimes in the middle part of the lid) and **Krause glands** (along the superior and inferior fornices of the conjunctival sac).
- Located in the subconjunctival tissue from the fornix area to near the tarsal plate.
- Function:

- Secrete a small amount of tear fluid into the conjunctival sac; ectopic portions of the lacrimal gland tissue; all produce the same kind of tears, secreting onto the conjunctival surface. Henle and Baumgarten "glands" are in fact not glands at all, but mere epithelial invaginations.

3. Distribution of Tears (Role of Eyelids)

- When close eyelids in a reflex blink, eyelids meet first at the temporal canthus, and then moves toward the medial canthus where tears pool in the lacrimal lake. The last part closing is the medial part. Eyelid closing mechanically pushes tears/dirt medially and vertically towards the sites of drainage.
- Contraction of the lacrimal part of the orbicularis oculi compresses the canaliculi, forcing tears into the lacrimal sac. The contraction also pulls on the fascial sheath attached to the lacrimal sac causing lateral displacement of the lateral wall, sac expansion, and negative peruse (pulling the tears from the canaliculus).
- Relaxation of the orbicularis oculi allows the lacrimal sac to collapse and the tears are driven into the nasolacrimal duct by gravity.

4. Drainage of Tears

- **Valve of Hasner (Plica Lacrimalis)**
  - Residual nictitating membrane (fold of mucosal tissue) that prevents retrograde movement of fluid up the duct from the nasal cavity
- **Lacrimal papillae**
  - Tear drainage occurs through the superior and inferior lacrimal papillae by way of the **lacrimal puncti**.
  - **Superior punctum** is 6 mm from the medial canthus and the **inferior punctum** is 6.5 mm from the medial canthus.
- **Canaliculi**
  - Each punctum opens into a canaliculus which is 10 mm long. They join at the sinus of Maier and then empty into the lacrimal sac. The two are offset so they don't overlap when the eyes close.
  - The medial third of the canaliculi are covered in front by the two bands which connect the medial palpebral ligaments to the tarsi, while behind is the lacrimal part of orbicularis oculi, known as **Horner's muscle**
  - Horner's muscle serves to pump tear fluid down the nasolacrimal canal
- **Lacrimal sac**
  - Membranous lacrimal sac lies within a fossa formed by the lacrimal bone and frontal process of the maxilla near the anterior border of the medial orbital wall
  - The sac, closed above and open below, is continuous with the nasolacrimal duct, a mere constriction marking their junction
  - The sac is enclosed by a periorbita, which splits at the posterior lacrimal crest, encloses the sac, reuniting at the anterior crest, and thus forms the lacrimal fascia
  - Lateral to the sac are skin, part of orbicularis oculi, and lacrimal fascia, attached to which are a few fibers of the inferior oblique
  - Anterior to the sac are the medial palpebral ligament and angular vein

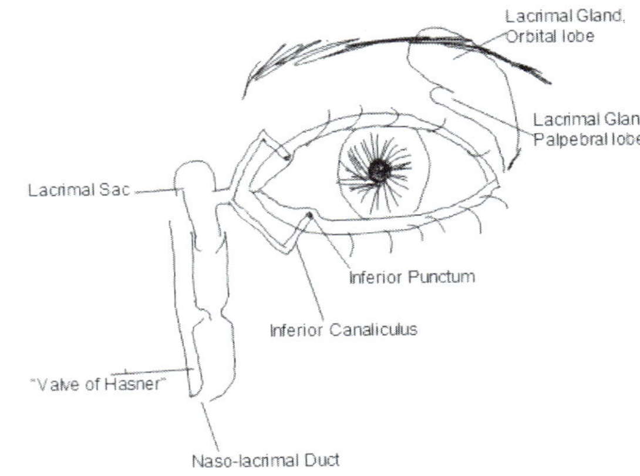

- **Naso-lacrimal duct**
  - Tears drain from the lacrimal sac to the inferior meatus of the nose. Travels through the **nasolacrimal canal**, which is formed mainly from the maxillary bone. Parts of the nasolacrimal canal are also made from the lacrimal bone and the inferior nasal conchae (turbinate bone).

- **Ostium lacrimale**
    - The opening of the nasolacrimal duct into the inferior meatus of the nose. It closes when sneezing or blowing your nose.

5. Lacrimal Fossa (Bony Structure)

- The **fossa for the lacrimal gland** is near the roof of the orbit, behind the zygomatic process of the frontal bone. It houses the lacrimal gland and also orbital fat.
    - The fossa is usually smooth, but is pitted by attachment of the suspensory ligament of the lacrimal gland when it is well developed
- The **fossa for the lacrimal sac** is in the lacrimal bone and sealed by connective tissue (the **lacrimal fascia**).

6. Nasolacrimal Canal (Bony Composition, relationship to maxillary sinus)

- The **nasolacrimal canal** is composed of the lacrimal bone and the inferior nasal conchi. It extends from the orbit into the nasal cavity.
- The **maxillary sinus** is located inferior to the orbits and borders the medial wall next to the lacrimal and maxillary bones. Trauma to the bony orbit (for example a blowout fracture) poses risk for infection of the orbital cavity leading to orbital cellulitis. If the maxillary sinus is infected, the nasolacrimal canal allows the infection passage to the anterior orbit.

LACRIMAL APPARATUS (DEVELOPMENTAL ANATOMY)

1. Tissue Origin of Lacrimal Glands (Main, Accessory)

- Main **lacrimal gland**: During the 8th week several buds of **ectoderm** appear on the superior lateral portion of the conjunctival fornix. These buds divide several times to form lobules (acini) of the main lacrimal gland.
- **Accessory (Krause, Wolfring, or Ciaccio): growths of basal cells** on the superior and inferior conjunctival fornices appear during the 6th month.

2. Tissue Origin of Lacrimal and Nasal Passages

- Originates as buried surface **ectoderm** in the nasolacrimal groove located between the paraxial and maxillary mesoderm.
- At week 7, the maxillary process grows up and over the nasolacrimal groove, fusing with the lateral nasal process and paraxial mesoderm.
- A cord of cells form from the separated epithelial cell of surface ectoderm and form the upper and lower lacrimal canaliculi.
- The canaliculi enlarge to form the lacrimal sac and the nasolacrimal duct, which empties into the inferior meatus of the nasal cavity. This process is **completed** by 3.5 months.

3. Abnormalities

- According to Pearson and Duke-Elder:
    - Newborns cry without tears.
    - Tearing may begin from 20-104 days after birth. (conflicting theories, see below)
    - The lacrimal gland does not reach its full growth until 3 or 4 years of age.
- According to Adler. Apt. and Cullen (1964):
    - Infants may cry with tears within the first 24 hours after birth.
    - Premature infants may fail to tear.

TEARS AND LACRIMAL APPARATUS (PHYSIOLOGY)

1. Function of Tears

- Optical: maintains an almost perfect **optical surface** on the cornea.
- Nutritional: Provides medium for $\mathbf{O_2}$ transport to the cornea.
- Antibacterial: **Lysozyme is bacteriocidal**.
- Lubricant: **Protection from mechanical rubbing** of blinking and protection of mucous membranes.
- Mechanical: **Flushing away of debris** from corneal surface.
- Corneal transparency: Helps maintain corneal transparency by providing the correct ***pH and *osmolarity needed to avoid cornea edema.**

2. Production of Tears

- Sources: The tears are produced mainly by the lacrimal gland (90%) and also by the accessory glands of Wolfring and Krause
- Neural control: Sensory innervations to the lacrimal gland are through the lacrimal nerve. The gland receives vasomotor sympathetic innervations.
    - Reflex tearing occurs when the branches of the ophthalmic nerve are stimulated or in response to an external stimuli.
    - Afferent pathway is through the trigeminal nerve
    - Parasympathetic pathway is through the facial nerve

3. Composition of Tears

- New Model: Tear layers are **30μm thick** (old model said 7μm thick)
- **Outermost oil layer (1%)** comprised of a mix of liquids; has a **high melting point.**
    - **Reduces rate of evaporation** of underlying aqueous layer.
    - Forms a barrier along the lid margin that retains the lid margin tear strip and **prevents epiphoria**, which is spillage of tears onto the skin.
    - Provides **good optical surface**.
- **Central aqueous phase (60-95%):** Depends on thickness percentage of the mucous layer and model; contains **98.2% water** and **1.8%** dissolved solids (inorganic salts, glucose, urea, proteins, and glycoproteins). Aqueous:
    - Volume
    - Nutrients
    - Gas exchange
    - Waste exchange
- **Innermost mucous layer (30-40%)** according to older models, newest model proposes that this is the thickest layer). It is composed of mucin and other glycoproteins, proteins and electrolytes. It aids in tear film stability, captures bacteria and debris (coats foreign bodies), and mechanical protection
- **Glycocalyx**: Very thin layer composed of glycoproteins made from the corneal/conjunctival epithelial cells. Provides hydrophilic surface for tears to adhere to cornea, repels bacteria and other debris due to negative molecules, and can aid in environmental sensing due to chemical changes in the tear film
- **Electrolytes**
    - Low molecular weight organics (**glucose, amino acids**)
    - High molecular weight organics **(proteins, lipids, glycoproteins)**
- **Cells**: Ocular surface cells of the glycocalyx allow for adhesion of the aqueous layer of the tears to the ocular surface
- **Physiological variations** (e.g. aging, open vs. closed eye, contact lens wear) in tear constituents
    - Normal aging can cause a decrease in aqueous tear production (which can lead to dry eye)
    - Contact lenses cause tear compartmentalization (order of layers is altered), change in tear production (nerves in cornea cannot detect stimulus), component modification, and can trap bugs and debris. This consequently leads to alterations in tear defenses and corneal epithelial cell defenses
    - Open eye – blinking and tear film can protect the eye, more O2

- Closed eye – inflammatory response for protection where pH decreases → sigA/Albumin/plasmin/IL-8/PMN's increase

4. Tear Film Distribution, Structure, and Stability

- In the normal eye, the tear film is complete, without holes, over the 5 second period between blinks.
- At least 10 seconds is required to evaporate away the aqueous phase of a normal tear layer. The normal **evaporation is 10% of the production rate, or 0.12μL/min**.
- The tear film thins uniformly by evaporation. **Lipid molecules** from the top surface begin to **migrate downward towards the mucous layer**. When the mucous layer covering the epithelium is **sufficiently contaminated by lipid, it becomes hydrophobic** and the **tear film ruptures**
- **Blinking** can repair the rupture by **removing the lipid contaminants** from the mucous layer and restoring a thick aqueous layer.

5. Elimination of Tears

- Some tear fluid is lost by **evaporation** and/or **absorption** through the conjunctival tissue.
  - 10% to 25% of secreted tear volume is lost to evaporation under normal conditions.
  - The remaining tears are drained through the lacrimal excretory system into the nose.
  - Some of the tear volume may be absorbed in the nasolacrimal system.
- 75% of the tear fluid passes through the **nasolacrimal drainage** apparatus.
  - Tears are swept across the ocular surface by the mechanical closing of the upper eyelid.
  - The tears pool in the lacrimal lake. The force of contraction from the orbicularis oculi causes the canaliculi to close pushing the tear fluid in them into the lacrimal sac.
  - Upon relaxation of the orbicularis oculi, the canaliculi open and pull the tears from the lacrimal lake through the punctum due to a built up force of negative pressure.
  - From the lacrimal sac, the tears flow down through the nasolacrimal duct and into the inferior meatus of the nose.

6. Physico-Chemical Properties of Tears

- Anatomic and physiologic studies have confirmed **positive pressures** pumping of the **canaliculi** during eyelid closure.
- Osmotic pressure
  - Contributed by electrolytes in tear, about **305 mOsm/kg**. A decrease to **285 mOsmo/kg has been reported following lid closure,** which is accounted for by the reduced evaporation.
- pH and buffering
  - **pH** of tear film quotes to be between 7.14 and 7.82 with a mean value similar to plasma **7.4-7.5**.
- Temperature and viscosity
  - About 46% of the heat of the eye is carried off by convection—by heat transfer directly to the surrounding air, 41% by radiation. Radiactive heat transfer is by means of transfer of heat energy in the form of electromagnetic waves in the **IR** wavelength region from the warm eye to colder surfaces in the surrounding environment.
  - A windy (**10mph**), cold (**-15 deg C**) environment can lower the tear temp to such low levels, about 5 deg C that metabolism in the epithelial cells will cease.

LACRIMAL SYSTEM (PATHOLOGY)

---

1. Epidemiology, History, and Symptom Inventory

- The lacrimal secretions are distributed over the surface of the eye by gravity, capillary action, and the eyelids. In order for fluid to enter the drainage system, the **puncta must be in anatomic apposition**

to the tear film meniscus on the surface of the eye.

- Disorders of the lacrimal system are manifested usually either by excessive tearing (epiphora) or dry eyes (keratitis sicca).
- Redness in the region of the lacrimal sac usually results from an acute **infection of the lacrimal sac (acute dacryocystitis**). Redness may also result from an inflammation anterior to the sac (prelacrimal abscess) from a cutaneous eruption or from perforation of the ethmoid cells (acute **ethmoiditis**). Redness in the region of the lacrimal gland usually indicates inflammation of the lacrimal gland (**dacryoadenitis**). Redness of the margin of the orbit suggests **periostitis**.
- Obstruction or patency of the lacrimal passages may aid in differential diagnosis. **If fluid injected into the sac does** not pass freely into the nose = **probable infection**
- If pus or mucus can be expressed from the sac the diagnosis is certain (**canaliculitis**).

2. Observation, Inspection, Recognition of Signs, and Techniques and Skills

Palpation of Sac, Canaliculi and Lacrimal Fossa

- Observation of lid dynamics, punctal position Palpation of sac, canaliculi, and lacrimal fossa used to detect discharge from sac, stenosis or laceration of canaliculus. Can detect imperforate, accessory, or everted puncta.

Biomicroscopic Appearance

- Note location of redness and swelling, tear quality and quantity.

3. Diagnostic Testing (Applications and Interpretations)

Use of Diagnostic Dyes

- **Fluorescein** is used in the tear break up time **(TBUT) test to assess the mucin layer of the tears**. One drop of fluorescein is instilled in the conjunctival sac, then the patient blinks and holds his eyes wide open. The appearance of the first dark spot, using the slit lamp with blue filter, on the cornea indicates the TBUT which is normally 15-30 seconds. A finding of **less than 10 seconds indicates deficient mucin layer**.
- **Rose bengal** stains devitalized epithelial cells and any cell not covered by tear film, mucous and keratin. Usually a very small amount is instilled into the lower conjunctival sac. A positive test will show **triangular stipple staining of nasal and bulbar conjunctiva**. Staining is graded 0-4+ with 3-4 being heavy staining. This test measures abnormalities in the oily layer of the tear film.
- **Lissamine Green** stains similarly to Rose Bengal w/o stinging.

Fluorescein Dilution Test

- Instill a tiny drop on the superior bulbar conjunctiva. Look at the tear film with the cobalt filter in the slit lamp at 5 min. intervals.
- In normal, it becomes very difficult to see any fluorescein at 10 or 15 min.
- If there is still a lot of fluorescence after 15 min., this indicates an aqueous production deficiency.

Tests of Basic and Reflex Secretion

- Basic secretion is by the **Krause and Wolfring glands**, about 0.5-1.25 ml per day.
- Reflex secretion is by the **lacrimal gland.**
- **Schirmer 1:** (*reflex and basal tears, no anesthetic*)
  - Using a **Whatman 41** filter paper, the ends are folded and placed over the lower palpebral conjunctiva. The patient keeps his eyes open, **looking upwards**, and blinking when needed. After **5 min**. the strips are removed and the wet area is measured.
  - A normal patient wets 10 30 mm in 5 min.
  - Below 5mm is considered abnormal. (5-10mm is borderline)
- **Schirmer 1a**: (*basal tears only, anesthetic used*)
  - The Schirmer I test is modified by using a topical anesthetic eliminating any reflex tearing. Less than 5 mm of wetting is considered abnormal.

- **Schirmer 2**: (*reflex secretion*)
  - Use **oph.** Anesthetic, use cotton tip applicator to irritate nasal mucosa on each side for 10-15secs. Leave strip in place for **2min**. **>15mm is abnormal**.

Fluorescein Transit Tests to Nose and Oropharynx

- Fluorescein transit tests (**Jones test I**):
  - In this test, fluorescein is instilled into the conjunctival sac and if the excretion is normal, the dye can be recovered from the nose with a cotton swab or **blowing nose within 5 min**. (Jones test 1a):
  - If after Jones 1, no staining is present, the cul de sac is irrigated with saline **(Jones 2)**. If the cotton swab is wet after irrigation, there is partial obstruction of the system. If there is no wetting even after irrigation, there is complete obstruction of the nasolacrimal passage.

Saccharin Taste Test

- If the **patient reports that he can taste the agent** instilled into the conjunctival sac this indicates **normal tear outflow**. The time interval is usually about **30 minutes**.

4. Pathophysiology and Diagnosis

Congenital and developmental lacrimal anomalies

- **Nasolacrimal duct obstruction**
  - The most common congenital abnormality of the lacrimal system.
  - **As many as 30% of newborn infants** are believed to have closure of the duct at birth.
  - The most **common site is the valve of Hasner**.
  - In most cases, this obstruction is **transient**, and patency occurs within **3 weeks of birth**.
  - Tears and mucus may accumulate in the lacrimal sac, causing distention of the sac and sometimes leading to dacryocystitis.
  - Treatment consists of sac **massage, hot compresses, and antibiotics**.
    - If the obstruction is not relieved, and the baby is at least 6 months old, nasolacrimal **duct probing** is done.
    - If the valve is not opened, even with probing, by the time the child is 3 years old, DCR (**dacryocystorhinostomy**) is performed.
- **Dacryocele**
  - Hardened mass that obstructs outflow in the nasolacrimal sac.
  - It presents as a bluish purple discoloration over the inferior medial canthus.
  - Usually resolves without treatment; however, if it becomes infected, systemic antibiotics are used. It is useful to apply hot compresses to soften the mass.
- **Punctal and canalicular abnormalities**:
  - Include absence, stenosis, duplication, and fistulization.
    - Imperforate or absent puncta can sometimes be opened by a sharply pointed dilator.
    - Fistulas can be surgically excised.
    - Absent canaliculi can be bypassed.
- **Diverticula**
  - **Cystic outpouchings** may accumulate fluid and simulate a mucocele of the **lacrimal sac**. They may become infected and mimic dacryocystitis. Treatment is **surgical excision**.
- **Neoplasia**
  - Lacrimal gland:
    - Usually occurs with patients **over age 50** and tend to be **malignant**. The gland is swollen, tender and sometimes the patients report **diplopia**. Diagnosis is by biopsy. Treatment is surgery.
  - Lacrimal sac
    - **Typically benign**. Hardened regions **cannot be softened by massage** and **when pressure is applied, blood regurgitates**. Diagnosis is by **dacryocystography** and

treatment is surgical removal.

Inflammations and Infections

- **Dacryoadenitis**:
  - Inflammation of the lacrimal gland is rare and is usually due to an injury being complicated by an acute bacterial infection.
  - There can be pain, redness, heat, swelling and possibly loss of function of the gland. There is **often epiphora** and the **preauricular lymph nodes may be enlarged** along with the lacrimal gland.
  - Treatment is systemic antibiotics.
  - **Acute viral dacryoadenitis** usually accompanies systemic illness.
    - In children's flu, in adults' mumps and measles, it is usually **mononucleosis with preauricular adenopathy**.
    - Viral infections are milder in presentation than bacterial and there is no pus present.
    - Analgesics and compresses may be used.
  - **Chronic dacryoadenitis** is the chronic enlargement of the gland secondary to systemic diseases such as collagen disease (**sarcoid), tuberculosis, lymphosarcoma, and leukemia**.
    - Chronic enlargement of the salivary, parotid, and lacrimal glands can be seen in Mikulicz Syndrome.
- **Dacryocystitis**:
  - **Acute dacryocystitis** (inflammation of the lacrimal sac) is usually unilateral, red, swollen, and painful to touch.
    - There is **diffuse pain in and around the eye** and usually accompanied by **headaches**.
    - Caused by bacterial infections by *Streptococcus pneumoniae* and *Staphylococcus.*
    - Usually leads to obstruction of the nasolacrimal duct. Occurs more often in females.
    - Treatment is with systemic antibiotics and hot compresses.
  - **Chronic dacryocystitis** presents with no pain or tenderness. It presents with **epiphora**. Usually unilateral and more often in females over 35.
- **Lacrimal sac obstructions**:
  - Uncommon and generally the result from dacryoliths.
  - Solid concretions within the sac may be caused by infection with Streptothrix.
  - Sometimes respond to irrigation with antibiotics.
  - The **sac** must frequently be opened and a **DCR** (**Dacryocystorhinostomy)** performed. An incision is made in the nose and a small piece of bone is removed. A Jones tube is inserted to facilitate the flow of tears.
- **Canaliculitis:**
  - Narrow or inflamed canaliculus caused by **Actinomyces infection (Streptothrix). Sulfur granules** indicate the presence of actinomyces infection. Treatment is with systemic antibiotics, hot compresses, and massage.

Lacrimal trauma

- **Lacerations of the canaliculi**
  - A wide variety of sutures, wires, and tubes have been described for the support of lacerated canaliculi during surgical approximation and healing. If possible, these **supports** should remain within the canaliculus until **4-6 weeks after injury.**

Dry eye syndrome

- Usually abnormality or deficiency of one of the components of the tear film. **A common symptom is photophobia**
- Differential diagnosis: **Sjogrens, lupus, rheumatoid arthritis, pemphigoid** (autoimmune blistering skin disease)**, Stevens Johnson** (life-threatening skin condition causing dermis to separate from epidermis)**, dermatitis, psoriasis**, and
- Medications like **diuretics, Accutane, antihistamines, and birth control pills.**
- Treatment includes mucomimetics, polyvinyl alcohol derivatives, lipid derivatives, ointments, soft contact lenses, and inserts

EXTRAOCULAR MUSCLES (GROSS ANATOMY)

1. Names

- Lateral rectus (LR)
  - Thinnest and weakest of the rectus muscles
- Medial rectus(MR)
  - Largest, thickest, and strongest of the rectus muscles, though similar in width and length
- Superior rectus (SR)
  - Makes 23-25° angle with visual axis
  - The levator originates from the small wing of the sphenoid and melds with the SR
- Inferior rectus (IR)
  - Makes 23-25° angle with visual axis
- Superior oblique (SO)
  - Longest and thinnest EOM. Makes 55° angle with visual axis
- Inferior oblique (IO)
  - Makes 55° angle with visual axis

2. Origins and Insertions

Muscle	Origin	Insertion (Distance from Cornea)
LR	Spinae Rectae Lateralis (Greater wing of sphenoid)	6.9mm
MR	Medial part of Annulus of Zinn	5.5mm
SR	Upper Annulus of Zinn	7.7mm
IR	Lower Annulus of Zinn	6.5mm
SO	Short narrow tendon anterior and medial to optic foramen and Trochlea, body, and small wing of the sphenoid	Inserts in posterior temporal superior quadrant 14-19mm from limbus (ventral to SR)
IO	Small narrow fodda in floor of orbit just within orbital margin, lateral to nasolacrimal canal, maxillary bone	Inserts in posterior globe just anterior to macular area (under LR)

- Annulus of Zinn: Tendon blended with that of the levator palpebrae superioris directly above.
- Physiological/Functional Insertion – where force acts on the eye (theoretical, don't actually find exact point
- Width of insertion increases counterclockwise
- Insertion distance of the rectus muscles from limbus increases clockwise from MR of right eye

3. Innervation, Blood Supply

Muscle	Cranial Nerve	Artery Supply	Venous Supply
LR	VI	Ophthalmic Artery or Lacrimal Artery	Superior or Inferior Ophthalmic Vein
MR	III	Ophthalmic Artery (Medial Musc. Branch)	Inferior Ophthalmic Vein
SR	III	Ophthalmic Artery (Lateral Musc. Branch)	Superior Ophthalmic Vein
IR	III	Ophthalmic Artery (Medial Musc. Branch)	Infraorbital Vein
SO	IV	Ophthalmic Artery (Superior Musc. Branch)	Superior Ophthalmic Vein
IO	III	Ophthalmic Artery (Infraorbital and Medial Musc. Branches)	Inferior Ophthalmic Vein

*Assume Muscular Branches of arteries and veins unless noted otherwise

4. Relationship to other Orbital Structures

- The four recti originate from the Annulus of Zinn, an oval band of connective tissue located at the apex of the orbit, anterior to the orbital fissure
- The EOMs have a layered organization. One layer, the "global" layer lies adjacent to the globe and inserts into the sclera allowing movement of the globe. The "orbital" layer lies adjacent to the orbital bone inserts into connective tissue muscle and influences rotational axis
- Dense connective sheaths between the EOMs and orbital bones allows for the supportive framework of the globe within the orbit

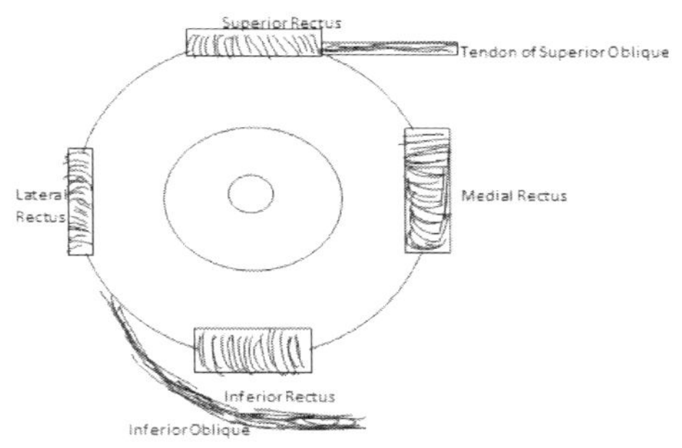

EXTRAOCULAR MUSCLES (DEVELOPMENTAL ANATOMY)

1. Condensation of Mesenchyme (bilateral condensation)

- By the 7th week, bilateral mesodermal condensations begin forming in the anterior orbit taking on the shape of a cone. This extraocular muscle development is independent of the optic vesicle development.
- Superior rectus, superior oblique, and levator palpebrae superioris develop from the superior mesoderm condensation.
- Inferior rectus and inferior oblique develop from the inferior mesoderm condensation.
- Medial and lateral recti develop from both complexes

2. Motor Innervation Development

- Oculomotor (**III**), the trochlear (**IV**), and the abducens (**VI**) evolve in the **cranial portion of the neural tube**.
- By the **4th week**, the **oculomotor nerve** reaches its respective muscle destinations from its cranial origin.
- By the **6th to 7th week**, the **trochlear nerve** is visible.
- There is a possibility that the trochlear and the abducens nerves originate as separate parts of the oculomotor nerve.
- By the **8th week**, all motor nerves are well developed.

3. Insertion of Extraocular Primordia into Anterior Sclera

- During the middle of the **second month**, some tissue strands that correspond to the undifferentiated **tendons emanate from the recti** and divide into **two portions**.
  - The **heavier portion** radiates into and interweaves with the loose **periocular connective tissue**.
  - The **thinner portion** intertwines with **scleral fibrils**.
- Near the end of the **3rd month**, the tendons of the recti muscles **fuse with the sclera** in the vicinity of the **equator**.

4. Late Development

- Defective development of the oculomotor nerves is rare though it can be observed in **hydrocephalus** (fluid accumulation in the cranium).
- If the muscle cone is in a primitive state, **defective division in the developing mesoderm** can result in **cyclopia**. In a well-developed eye, **defective division of the mesoderm** can lead to **extra muscle** tissue development leading to **strabismus**.
- Abnormal insertion of extraocular muscles can result in heterophoria or strabismus.

- Absence of an extraocular muscle (hypoplasia) can result in congenital ocular paralysis.

EXTRAOCULAR MUSCLES (PHYSIOLOGY)

1. Vestibular Control Mechanisms

- **Vestibulo-ocular reflex (VOR)**:
  - The VOR **keeps the eyes fixed on a target when the head moves**. The head motions are sensed by the vestibular labyrinth and the eye motions are monitored by the outflow mechanism.
  - When the membranous labyrinth, or **semi-circular canal,** senses a head movement, it sends a signal to the **vestibular nuclei** which then sends a signal via a **long pathway to the EOMs** (cerebellum → medial longitudinal fasicullus → ocular nuclei in EOMs)
  - The excitation of some cells, and the inhibition of others helps to speed the movement of the eye to keep the retinal image stable. The reflex can be modified by the use of prisms.
  - An example of this is when a patient receives a new spectacle prescription and looks to the side. The eyes will actually move too far (or not enough, depending on the change in Rx), causing retinal slip. Cortical outflow will then tell the muscles to make a corrective motion.
- **Nystagmus**: Nystagmus by definition is a regularly repetitive, usually rapid and generally involuntary movement of the eye.
  - **Jerk nystagmus** is often slow in one direction and fast in the other direction
  - **Vestibular nystagmus** is the ocular response to vestibular stimulation. Vestibular nystagmus is nystagmus induced by the caloric stimulation of the endolymph. **COWS** stands for cold opposite, warm same. Cold water in the ear causes a fast phase to the contralateral side.
  - **Optokinetic nystagmus** is nystagmus induced by a visual pattern moving across the visual field at a constant velocity. OKN an be used to determine visual acuity. OKN is an eye movement that follows the pattern slowly for the slow phase and then jerks back in the opposite direction for the fast phase to pick up the pattern at the other side of the visual field.

2. Supranuclear Control of Eye Movements

- Conceptually, the control mechanisms for eye movements fit into five functionally distinct groups. These are as follows:
  - Saccadic system
  - Smooth Pursuit system
  - Vestibular system
  - Vergence system
  - Position maintenance system
- Eye movements are categorized by their triggering stimulus and movement response. **Supranuclear centers** specify the function of coordinated muscle groups and not of individual muscles. Destruction of supranuclear centers or pathways results in a loss of gaze function, not in diplopia.
- **Dual modal control**: The output of these systems is translated into action in one of 2 modes: rapid eye movements or slow eye movements. <u>Rapid eye movements</u> are due to a **pulsatile output** whose output is determined by **burst activity**. <u>Slow eye movements</u>, on the other hand, are mediated by a **continuous graded response**. The slow system can be analyzed in terms of a **closed loop continuous feedback** monitoring system that can function smoothly at **speeds up to 40 degrees/second**. At speeds exceeding this, the target will fall on non-foveal points and a corrective saccade will result in foveation.

3. Agonist-Antagonist Relationships

- **Agonist/synergist**: when the primary action of a muscle is helped by another muscle ie. Inferior rectus and superior oblique working together to depress the eye.
- **Antagonist**: two muscles working against each other (ex. superior rectus and inferior rectus)
- According to **Sherrington's Law** (of reciprocal innervation), contraction of one muscle is accompanied by the simultaneous relaxation of its antagonist

4. Primary Action and Secondary Action and Tertiary Action

- **Primary Action** is the main action
- **Secondary Action** is the subsidiary action

Muscle	Primary action	Secondary Action	Tertiary Action
Lateral Rectus	Abduction	None	None
Medial Rectus	Adduction	None	None
Superior Rectus	Elevation	Intorsion	Adduction
Inferior Rectus	Depression	Extorsion	Adduction
Superior Oblique	Depression	Intorsion	Abduction
Inferior Oblique	Elevation	Extorsion	Abduction
Levator Palpebrae Superioris	Elevation (eyelid)	Elevation (eye, via association with SR sheath)	

5. Fields of Action

- **Vergence movements** are when the eyes move in the opposite left-right directions = disjunctive movements
    - **Convergence** – each eye is adducted
    - **Divergence** – each eye is abducted
- **Version movement** are when the eyes move in the same left-right direction = conjugate movements
    - **Dextroversion** – right gaze
    - **Levoversion** – left gaze
    - **Supraversion** – both eyes are elevated
    - **Infraversion** – both eyes are depressed

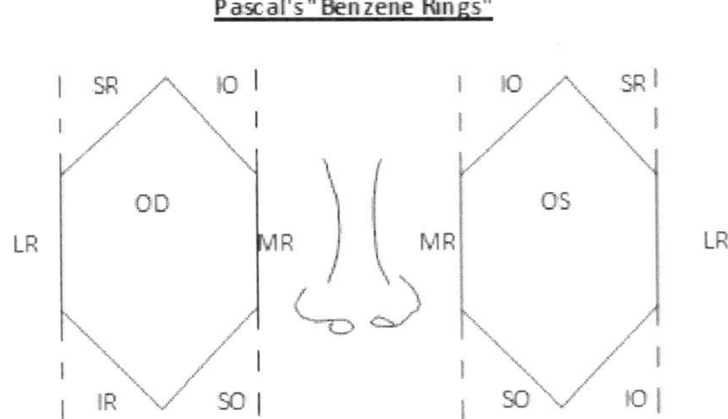

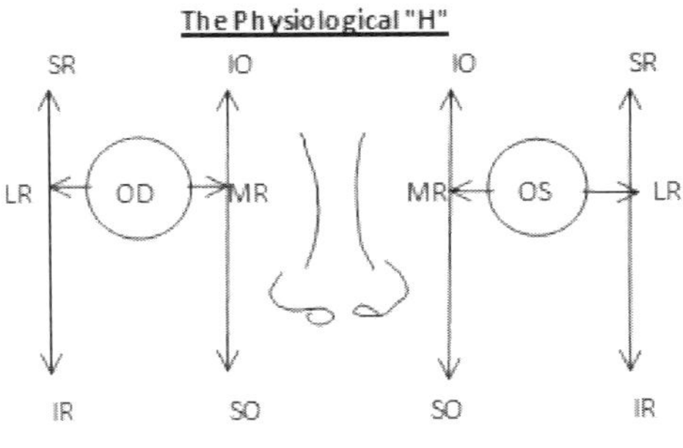

6. Conduction and Contraction

- Traditionally, EOMs have been characterized as being **weak, fast**, and **fatigue resistant**
- Under **isometric** conditions, EOM have **short contraction** (time required to reach peak twitch force) **and half-relaxation** (time from peak to half-peak twitch force) times compared with prototypical fast muscles.

Chapter 12 – Conjunctiva/Cornea/Refractive Surgery

CORNEA (GROSS ANATOMY)

1. Normal Dimensions Including Diameter, Radii of Curvature and Thickness

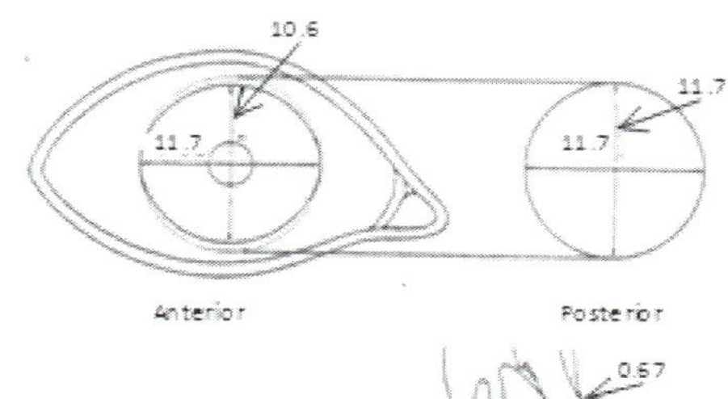

- Diameter:
  - **Anterior:** elliptical --12 mm horizontally & 11 mm vertically
  - **Posterior:** circular – 11.7 mm
- Radius of curvature:
  - **Anterior** 7.8 mm
  - **Posterior** 6.5 mm
- Thickness:
  - **Centrally** 0.52 mm
  - **Peripherally** 0.67 mm
- Temperature:
  - The cornea is avascular and is cooled by the air. It is cooler than the iris. The aqueous behind the cornea is cooler than the aqueous in front of the iris. Convection currents are thus set up, the aqueous sinking behind the cornea and rising in front of the iris.

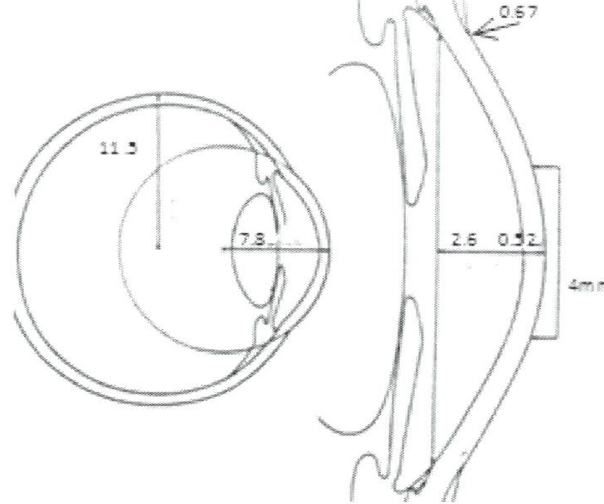

2. Epithelium (Histology and Ultrastructure)

- The epithelium (50μm) is 5-7 layers of stratified epithelial cells that connect to each other through desmosomes and gap junctions. It makes up 10% of the total thickness of the cornea and is the outermost layer
- Rich in nerve endings and continuous with the conjunctival epithelium
- Consists of 3 groups of cells (anterior to posterior):
  1) **Surface cells**:
     - 2 layers of flat non-keratinized cells.
     - Have microvilli to help hold up the mucin layer of tear film against the cornea as well as the ability to secrete the glycocalyx.
     - Tight junctions connect the cells laterally and prevent the uptake of excess fluid from the tear film, allowing passage of molecules and fluid through but not between cells. The tight junctions also create a protective barrier to infection and the atmosphere.
     - As the cells age they get larger and darker and slough off into the tear film
     - Mitosis occasionally occurs
     - Lymphocytes, macrophages, nerve fibers, and nerve endings are also found here

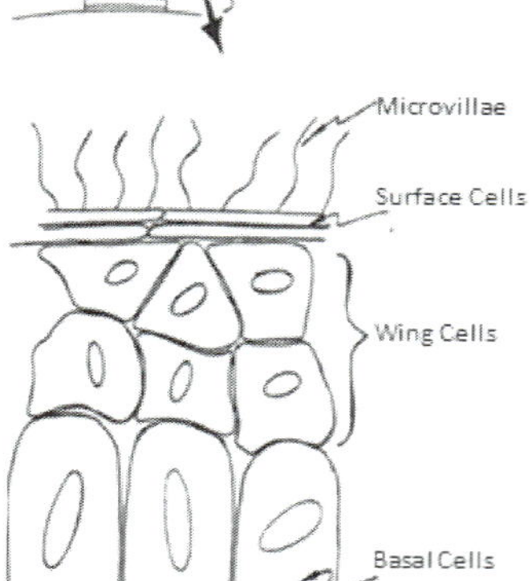

  2) **Wing cells:**
     - 2-3 layers of wing-shaped epithelial cells (polyhedral) are joined by gap junctions and desmosomes

3) **Basal cells**:
   - Single layer of columnar cells that have flat bases and rounded tops.
   - It is the germinal layer of the epithelium where most mitosis occurs. The basal cells become wing cells which become surface cells, that eventually slough off.

3. Basal Lamina (Relationship to Epithelium)

- The **basal lamina** is the underlying basement membrane secreted by the basal cells. The basal lamina attaches the epithelium to the underlying connective tissue through hemidesmosomes.
- The basal lamina also contains 70nm pores, which are much smaller than 1um bacteria, and function as a barrier to bacterial infection into the stroma.

4. Anterior Limiting Lamina (Bowman's Layer)

- **Bowman's layer (8-14μm),** also called anterior limiting membrane and anterior elastic lamina, is not a true membrane but rather a transitional layer to the stroma. It is made of very dense interwoven network of thin 20-25nm collagen fibers, mucopolysaccharides, and glycosaminoglycans.
- While indistinguishable from the stroma visually, it differs from the stroma by being acellular and having smaller diameter collagen fibers (1/3 thinner), which are irregularly arranged.
- It is an anchoring matrix to which the basal lamina of the epithelium attaches through anchoring fibrils, hemidesmosomes, and anchoring plaques. It ends at the limbus and does not have a counterpart in the sclera or conjunctiva.
- Has numerous pores that transmit epithelial branches of the corneal nerves, which lose their Schwann cell covering and pass into the epithelium as "naked" nerves.
- On the stromal side the collagen fibers begin to become more organized as the layers transition
- Bowman's layer is prenatally produced and cannot regenerate. If it is injured the cells are replaced by epithelial cells or stromal scar tissue.

5. Stroma (Composition, Ultrastructure)

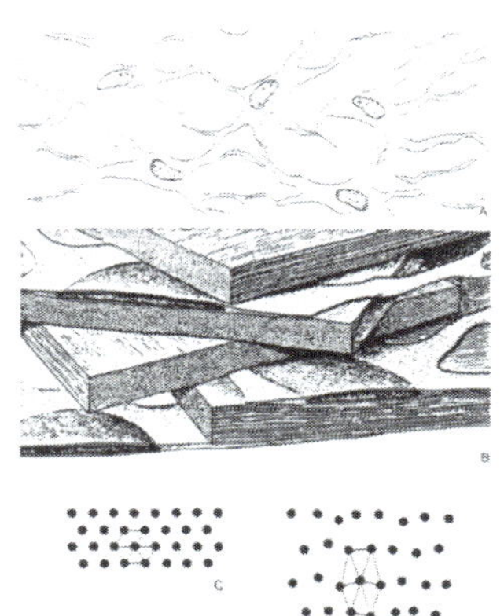

- The **stroma (470-500μm)** comprises 90% of entire corneal thickness
- Composed of lamellae and cells (see figure):
  - *Lamellae* (or layers):
    - 200-250 lamellae made of coaxial bundles of collagen fibers that lie parallel to each other and are each 2μm thick.. They extend the entire length of the cornea. Glycoproteins (GAGs) and mucopolysaccharides (i.e. ground substance) attract water and maintain fibril spacing and corneal hydration.
      - If too much ground substance is produced, too much water enters the stroma and the layers are separated from each other more than normal, causing decrease in transparency of the tissue.
    - Adjacent lamellae are oriented in different directions so as to crisscross over each other at approximately 60°, allowing for a transparent organized layer of stromal tissue.
    - The half-life of each lamella is 100 days.
  - *Cells*:
    - 2-5% of the stromal volume is cellular.
    - 2.4 million Fibroblasts (or keratocytes) that are 2μm thick are scattered throughout the lamellae scarcely enough to maintain transparency. They have a spidery-like appearance and maintain the stroma by synthesizing collagen fibers and mucopolysaccharides
    - Other cells that may be present in the stroma are lymphocytes, macrophages, and PMN's, which may increase with pathological infections.
- **Maurice Theorem**: collagen fiber bundles are separated from each other by 500 nm. This spacing, and their highly regular organization, aids in destructive interference of light and maintains corneal transparency. The irregularly arranged collagen fibers in Descemet's and Bowman's layer scatter particles minimally due to their minimal separation between fibers and smaller fibers.

6. Posterior Limiting Lamina (Descemet's Membrane)

- **Descemet's Membrane (10-12μm)** is also called the posterior limiting membrane or posterior elastic membrane.
- It is a true membrane made by the endothelial cells and is considered the basement membrane of the endothelium. Like Bowman's membrane, it ends at the limbus and forms a thickened area of collagenous tissue called **Schwalbe's line**.
- Unlike Bowman's layer it is produced constantly (can regenerate) and thickens throughout life. The fetal Descemet's membrane is thinner than endothelium, while the adult Descemet's membrane is 2/3 thicker than endothelium. A child's Descemet's membrane is 5μm thick, while an adult's is 15μm thick.
- The membrane's structure is sharply differentiated from the stroma. Descemet's membrane has two laminae, an anterior lamina composed of a latticework of collagen fibrils that is embryonically developed and maintains corneal structure, as well as a posterior lamina that is homogenous and grows throughout life.
    - Sometimes the endothelium can over secrete basement membrane locally, causing localized thickenings in Descemet's membrane that protrude into the anterior chamber. When located in the peripheral cornea they are called **Hassall Henle bodies** and normally increase with age. When located in the central cornea, they are called **corneal guttata** and indicate endothelial dysfunction. Both appear as dark spots or holes in endothelium when viewed using specular reflection upon slit-lamp examination.
- The membrane is a barrier against infection from the stroma to the anterior chamber, is resistant to inflammatory processes, provides elasticity, filtration and toughness to the cornea, and also constantly pumps water out of the eye.

7. Endothelium (Composition, Ultrastructure)

simple squamous

- The **endothelium (5μm)**, is a single layer of polyhedral cells which are 5μm thick and 20μm wide
- The endothelial cells have a very irregular arrangement known as the **endothelial mosaic.** The cells tend to be larger in the periphery, and they do not regenerate, so when cells are lost adjacent endothelial cells must thin and stretch to cover the area of missing cells. Thus, the total number of cells (500,000) decreases normally with age. These disruptions can cause **polymegathism** (cell size variability) and **pleomorphism** (cell shape variability).
- The basal side of the cells is attached to Descemet's membrane while the apical side lines the anterior chamber. The basal-Descemet's interface is not connected by traditional hemidesmosomes but rather by interdigitations which allows for an incomplete barrier that allows the entrance of nutrients (glucose and amino acids) from the aqueous humour. The apical side of the cells have microvilli attached that protrude into the anterior chamber as well as marginal folds at intercellular junctions which also project into anterior chamber. The endothelium also has channels that transport fluids and ions.
- The endothelium functions to secrete Descemet's membrane, and metabolically pump ions to maintain proper hydration of the cornea. The tissue is metabolically very active and has more mitochondria than any other ocular components except retinal receptors. Proper hydration maintains corneal transparency and thickness. Damage to the endothelium can cause leakage and opacification.

8. Limbus

- The limbus is the transition zone between the cornea and sclera and the cornea and conjunctiva. It is where the very regular squamous corneal epithelium (5-6 layers) becomes thicker conjunctival epithelium (10-15 layers) and the regularly arranged corneal stroma becomes the irregularly arranged scleral stroma. It is 2mm wide and encircles the corneal periphery. The transition between the layers is so gradual no exact demarcation line can be distinguished.
- The corneal endothelium becomes discontinuous, and Bowman's and Descemet's membrane terminate at its anterior border.
- The conjunctival stroma, episclera, and Tenon's capsule all begin within the limbal area.

- The basal layer may contain melanocytes and be pigmented in darker pigmented individuals.
- The limbus is highly vascularized by the anterior ciliary artery, long posterior ciliary artery, and the anterior ciliary vein. Capillary loops from vessels in the conjunctiva and episclera form networks in the limbus that surround and nourish the avascular cornea.
- It functions to provide nutrients to adjacent tissue and provide a pathway for drainage of aqueous humor from the eye (internal sclera sulcus, trabecular meshwork, canal of Schlemm).

9. Innervation

- The cornea is densely innervated with sensory fibers and is the richest sensory innervation in the body with the nerve density greatest in the central 5mm of the cornea. 70 to 80 nerve fibers (branching from the **posterior ciliary nerves**) enter the peripheral cornea and run radially into both the epithelium and anterior 2/3 of the stroma. These nerves enter the cornea via the scleral stroma and conjunctiva.
- These peripheral nerves are myelinated for 2 to 3 mm in the cornea then lose their myelin sheath. The Schwann cells remain until they are lost as the nerves pass through Bowman's layer into the epithelium.
- The cornea is also innervated by sympathetic nerve fibers that aid in regulation of corneal epithelial metabolism, proliferation, and wound healing.
- Descemet's membrane and endothelium are not innervated.

10. Regeneration

Summary of Corneal Regeneration	
Corneal Tissue Layer	**Regenerates?**
Epithelium	Yes – 7 Days
Bowman's Layer	No
Stroma	Yes- Weeks
Descemet's Membrane	Yes
Endothelium	No

- Mitosis occurs at the basal cell layer of the epithelium. The epithelial cells migrate outward toward the surface. As cells migrate, they flatten and become wing cells, and then finally surface cells. This process allows corneal epithelium to regenerate completely every 7 days
- Bowman's layer cannot regenerate
- Collagen in the stroma is maintained by the keratocytes. Stroma may take weeks to regenerate and may leave scars due to irregularly arranged lamellae.
- Descemet's membrane regenerates through the constant secretion by the endothelium.
- Endothelial cells do not regenerate but rather migrate and stretch to cover areas of cell loss leading to endothelial thinning.

CORNEA (DEVELOPMENTAL ANATOMY)

1. Inductive Mechanisms

- Prior growth and development of the optic cup is the primary inductive mechanism for corneal differentiation. The cornea will not form if the optic cup is missing.

2. Ectodermal Components (Epithelium, Primary Stroma)

- Corneal epithelium is derived from **surface ectoderm**.
- At the 6th week the surface epithelium forms a double layer of cells consisting of an inner cuboidal layer and an outer flattened layer.
- At the 8th week, a polyhedral cell layer forms between the first two layers.

3. Mesenchymal Components (Waves)

- Stroma (substantia propia), Descemet's membrane, corneal endothelium and Bowman's layer are derived from mesenchyme.
- Development of corneal layers:

- During the 5th-6th week a layer of cells is laid down between the surface ectoderm and the lens vesicle forming the posterior corneal surface.
- During the 8th week corneal stroma begins to develop when a second layer of mesenchyme invades the acellular fibrous layer the corneal epithelium and endothelium.
- By the 5th month Bowman's layer derived from corneal endothelium is present.
- Between 6-9 months, Descemet's membrane forms from corneal endothelium.

4. Corneal Nerve Development (Origin)

- During the 3rd month developing nerves enter the cornea and approach the corneal epithelium by the 5th month.
- Rapid arborization (branching) occurs throughout the anterior stroma between the 6th and 9th months.

5. Factors Affecting Corneal Size, Curvature, Transparency

- Corneal size
  - At birth the transverse diameter of the cornea is 10 mm.
  - Most of the growth occurs in the first 6 months.
  - By the 2nd year the cornea reaches its adult size of 12 mm.
- Corneal curvature
  - The growth of the anterior chamber and of the cornea itself causes the curvature of the cornea to differ from that of the globe.
  - At birth the corneal curvature is flatter than the adult's.
- Corneal transparency
  - By age 2 or 3 the corneal transparency improves as the number of stromal fibers increases.

CORNEA (PHYSIOLOGY)

---

1. Physical Characteristics (Water Content, Protein Content, Cells, Resistance to Trauma)

- **Water content**: Water makes up 78% of corneal weight, while collagen makes up 75% of corneal dry weight

Cells

- Epithelium
  - 5-10 cell layers thick. Approximately 50μm thick.
  - Innermost layer of epithelial cells are columnar closely packed cells that adhere to the basement membrane. They migrate and flatten out creating the wing cells of the next layer, which flatten to create the squamous cells of the superficial layer.
- Bowman's layer
  - Approximately 12μm thick.
  - Composition: randomly oriented fibrils, probably collagenous material.
  - Acellular, uniform and homogenous.
  - Resistant to deformation, trauma and foreign bodies, will scar if damaged.
  - Ends at limbus.
- Stroma
  - 90% of corneal thickness.
  - 75-80% water.
  - 20-25% solids.
  - Composed of lamellae of parallel collagen fibers that run at various angles from limbus to limbus.
  - Lamellae lie flat, one on top of the other. Human stroma is about 200 lamellae thick. Space between the fibers is completely filled with mucopolysaccharides (MPS). The hydrophilic characteristic is responsible for the high water content of the stroma.

- Descemet's membrane (posterior limiting membrane)
  - Secreted by endothelial cells, acts as true basement membrane of endothelial cells.
  - 5 -10μ thick; thickens with age.
  - Composed of collagen fibers organized into a meshwork with MPS ground substance.
- Endothelium
  - Single layer of cells which are not able to reproduce in an arranged hexagonal mosaic.
  - 4 - 5μ thick, approximately 20μ across (per cell).
  - Cells characterized by large nuclei and large numbers of mitochondria and golgi bodies.
  - Acts as the dehydrator of the stroma.

Proteins

- Glycosaminoglycans/MPS: (4-4.5% dry weight vs. 1.5% in the sclera)
- Keratin sulfate
- Chondroitin
- Keratocytes comprise 2-3% of the total stromal volume.
  - There are relatively few cells per unit volume.
  - They are non-reproducing fixed cells.
  - In the posterior layer they are found between lamellae, whereas in the anterior layer they can be found within or between lamellae.
  - Keratocytes are characterized by large nuclei and long, thin processes that appear to touch though they actually maintain their individuality.
  - Their metabolic activity is about the same as that of other corneal cells.

Resistance to Trauma

- Descemet's membrane is involved.

2. Permeability Characteristics of Various Layers

- Layers rich in lipid are traversed by non-polar compounds:
  - Epithelium: multi-cellular and hydrophobic.
  - Endothelium: lipid membranes, but weaker barrier than epithelium as it is only 1 cell layer thick.
- Layers rich in water are easily traversed by polar compounds. (Stroma: high water content)
- Molecules with both lipid and water soluble characteristics have potential to enter the eye, whereas those that are strictly water soluble do not. Weak acids or weak bases do not readily dissociate when dissolved in water. In the uncharged form, they are lipid soluble.
- Epithelial cell outer membranes are relatively impermeable to the passage of ions and the epithelial cells are connected to surrounding cells by tight junctions which impede ion flow. Endothelium is 20 times more permeable to electrolytes than the epithelium but is still 10 times more resistant than the stroma. If the epithelium is removed, uptake of water soluble drugs is substantially enhanced. In contrast, highly lipid soluble materials typically penetrate both an intact and denuded cornea equally well.
- High concentrations of some drugs are used because only a small percentage reaches the anterior chamber through the cornea.

3. Metabolic Characteristics of Various Layers

- The catabolism of glucose and glycogen is the main energy source for the epithelial cells. Most of the glucose is derived from the aqueous humor with smaller contributions from the tears and capillaries. The epithelium is also able to store large amounts of glycogen, which can be mobilized when the supply of free glucose is insufficient (i.e., in hypoxia and trauma). ATP is generated from glycolysis and the Kreb's cycle. It is thought that the Kreb's cycle is not very active because it takes place in mitochondria which are not very abundant in the epithelium. The catabolism of glucose yields ATP and NADPH, high energy compounds, which are then used in cellular processes.
- CO_2 is produced under aerobic conditions and eliminated by diffusion or conversion to bicarbonate.
- Anaerobic glycolysis yields pyruvate and lactic acids. Since lactate cannot pass through the epithelium it must diffuse through the stroma and endothelium into the aqueous. During hypoxia or

other times of corneal stress, lactate can build up and cause localized acidosis. This can cause epithelial and stromal edema and endothelial functional alterations.

- The endothelium and the epithelium consume most of the O_2 taken in by the cornea. When comparing equal weight portions of the epithelium or endothelium and the stroma, the epithelium and endothelium contain 15 - 20× the number of cells as the stroma and consume 25 - 30× more oxygen than the stroma. The epithelium gets most of its oxygen from either the limbal capillaries (minor source) or from oxygen dissolved in the tears (major source) while the endothelium gets most of its oxygen from the aqueous. The endothelium appears to contain the same aerobic and anaerobic glycolytic pathways as the epithelium, although their activities are lower.
- The ability of the endothelium to store glycogen is not known. Glutathione is also important for normal endothelial function. Most likely it plays a role in elimination of free radicals and toxic peroxides formed during light exposure.

4. Theories of Corneal Transparency

- The control of stromal hydration is essential for transparency. The lack of blood and lymph vessels and absence of myelin sheaths around corneal nerves are also aids in transparency. The diameter of the collagen fibrils is about 300A and the fibers are closely spaced (approximately 550A), these are the 2 most important factors determining corneal transparency.
- Corneal collagen fibrils form a lattice structure arranged so that scattering of light is eliminated by mutual, destructive interference from individual fibers.
- Goldman and Benedek suggested that the cornea is transparent because fibrils are small relative to the wavelength of light. Consequently, incident light is not scattered as much as if larger particles were dispersed through the cornea.
- To maintain transparency, the cornea must be bathed with a fluid having an osmotic pressure as high as interstitial fluid. If the cornea was bathed in a hypotonic solution, it would become cloudy due to loss of osmotic forces acting at the corneal epithelium. Corneal clouding due to swelling can be temporarily cleared by bathing eye with a hypertonic solution such as a 10% salt/glycerin solution.
- Epithelium is much more resistant to water movement than stroma. Thus, although aqueous easily passes through the stroma, its escape is retarded by the epithelium, which becomes edematous. Normally, tear film is concentrated by evaporation. When evaporation does not occur, edema becomes considerably worse.

5. Factors Influencing Corneal Thickness/Hydration

- Evaporation of H_2O from the tear film results in hypertonicity (osmolarity) of the tears and draws H_20 from the epithelial cells and subsequently the stroma. Both the epithelium and the endothelium act as barriers to the movement of H_20 and ions into the stroma.
- The endothelium pumps play the major role in active dehydration of the cornea, providing >90% of the dehydration. The endothelium actively transports bicarbonate and probably sodium from the stroma to the aqueous. This ion transport creates an osmotic gradient (2 to 3 mOsm), which balances the swelling pressure of the corneal stroma which is caused mainly by the GAG's affinity for the cations and water.
- The epithelium pumps play a smaller role in the dehydration process. Epithelial cells secrete chloride into the tears by active transport, which is regulated by a beta-adrenergic receptor and is mediated intracellularly by adenylate cyclase.
- The integrity of the epithelium and endothelium differ such that damage to the endothelium causes more and often permanent swelling than damage to the epithelium.

6. Physiological Parameters Necessary to Maintain Corneal Integrity

- **Oxygen level:** When oxygen tension at the epithelial surface is reduced to 10-20 mmHg, the cornea begins to swell. Oxygen is mainly supplied by the tear film. The oxygen tension of the aqueous humor is 30-40 mm Hg and is not high enough to meet the epithelial metabolic needs. In the open eye the partial pressure of oxygen in the tears is approximately 155 mm Hg. When the lids are closed, oxygen enters the tears only by diffusion from the conjunctival vessels and the partial pressure falls to about 55 mm Hg. Unlike the epithelium, the endothelium oxygen need is supplied by the aqueous.

- **Glucose levels:** The epithelium gets its glucose primarily from the aqueous humor—10% or less comes from the limbal vessels or tears. The major energy source of the endothelium is glucose and is derived from the aqueous humor.
- **pH:** The pH of tears is approximately 7.4. In general, solutions with pH ranging from 6.0 – 8.2 are well tolerated.

7. Epithelial Regeneration (Normal and Response to Trauma)

- The epithelium regenerates completely every 7 days. Normal wound healing is a process of cell migration, mitosis, and adhesion. Small defects are covered by migration of adjacent epithelial cells, and this is followed by cell division until the thickness of the epithelium returns to normal. With larger defects both migration and mitosis are involved in covering the defect and more time is required.
- After epithelial wounding, a temporary layer of fibrin and fibronectin forms on the denuded surface and facilitates epithelial migration and attachment. The process of cell sliding involves detachment from underlying fibronectin through activation of plasmin, a proteolytic enzyme, and advancement to adjacent fibronectin. Epithelial cells are stimulated by fibrin and fibronectin to release plasminogen activator. Plasminogen activator then causes the conversion of plasminogen into plasmin. The active plasmin decreases epithelial adhesion to the fibrin and fibronectin, allowing advancement of the cell.
- Once epithelial integrity is restored, the temporary matrix of fibrin and fibronectin is reabsorbed. After the epithelial layer is intact, basement membrane and anchoring filaments are formed. If stroma has been removed, collagen is laid down beneath the epithelium and new anchoring fibrils may constantly be reformed until normal stromal thickness is achieved.

8. Physiological Characteristics of Corneal Nerves

- The cornea has the richest sensory innervation in the body, with sensory nerves derived from the anterior ciliary nerves and the long posterior ciliary nerves which are the end branches of the ophthalmic division of the trigeminal nerve. The nerves pass into the cornea as 60 to 80 myelinated trunks at the limbus. They enter in the anterior and middle stromal layers and run forward in a radial fashion toward the center of the cornea. They normally lose their myelin sheaths 2 to 4 mm into the cornea and divide into anterior and posterior groups.
- The anterior group runs through the stroma and then perforates Bowman's membrane to form a plexus beneath the epithelium. The fibers then become free nerve endings, which run between the epithelial cells. These anterior nerve endings are stimulated when the normal corneal integrity is affected by a foreign body, abrasion, or bacterial corneal ulcer. The posterior division passes posteriorly and innervates the posterior stroma and endothelium.
- It is generally agreed that the cornea is highly sensitive to both touch and pain, with pain threshold about ten times higher than the touch threshold. The degree of sensitivity corresponds to the distribution the corneal nerves, being the greatest in the center and falling off toward the periphery. It is not, however, sensitive to both heat and cold. The cornea contains many cold sensing spots, but the sense of heat is almost entirely absent. This explains why it is usually more comfortable for a hard contact lens wearer to rinse his lenses in warm water, whereas cold water produces discomfort when the lens is placed upon the eye.

9. Aging Changes of the Cornea

- Decrease in corneal sensitivity.
- Increase in light scatter.
- Stippling of Bowman's membrane.
- White limbal girdle.
- Thickening of Descemet's membrane.
- Localized thickening of Descemet's membrane (Hassall-Henle bodies).
- Endothelial cell loss, cells cannot regenerate in adults.

CORNEA (PATHOLOGY)

1. Observation, Inspection, Recognition of Signs, and Techniques and Skills

Biomicroscope

- Functions:
  - Examine the anterior segment of the eye, specifically: tear film, cornea, eyelids, conjunctiva, anterior chamber, iris, and lens.
  - Grading the anterior chamber angle.
  - Applanation tonometry (with the Goldmann tonometer).
  - Fundus examination (with addition of the Hruby lens or other condensing lens).
  - Tear break-up time determination.
- Principles of operation:
  - The biomicroscope consists of an illumination system and observation system (a microscope). The two can be coupled (thus focused at the same time) or dissociated to obtain different types of illumination.
- Methods of illumination
  - Size of light beam can change from parallelepiped to an optic section.
  - Direction of beam and microscope can vary, creating different types of illuminations.

2. Dystrophies

- In general:
  - Most dystrophies are relatively rare and are seen infrequently in primary care optometry.
  - Most are discovered during a routine slit lamp exam.
  - Almost all are autosomal dominant.
  - No associated systemic or ocular disease is usually in history.
  - Usually early findings (by age 20).
  - Bilateral.
  - Slowly progressive.
  - Centrally located.
  - Involve only one corneal layer.

Epithelial Layer Dystrophies

- **Epithelial Basement Membrane Dystrophy (EBMD)** aka **Anterior Basement Membrane Dystrophy**
  - A term given to a group of disorders of the epithelial membrane, all of which can cause recurrent corneal erosion and foreign body sensation.
  - Prevalence is believed to be around 2-5 % of population, with most observing autosomal dominant nature of dystrophies, and increasing in the older populations. Nature and severity of presentation is probably also affected by risk and severity of ocular trauma (PMMA wearer) as well as environment.
  - Symptoms range from asymptomatic to moderate photophobia, pain and reduction best corrected visual acuity.
  - History of recurrent corneal erosion (RCE) often.
  - Slow epithelial healing time (weeks) with chronic erosion.
  - Usually bilateral, negative fluorescein staining usually except in later, more severe stages, where epithelial cells may rupture. Also, there may be very short TBUT times (often instantaneous)
  - Treatment can include hypertonic saline drop AM and ung PM. Bandage contact lenses or patching with gentamicin can be used for severe case.
- **Cogan's Microcystic Epithelial Dystrophy**
  - Occurs more in females and presents as gray white round or comma shaped deposits in epithelium. The deposits are cysts which are the result of re-malforming epithelial cells which eventually migrate to the surface and may cause rupturing.

- **Map Dot Fingerprint Dystrophy**
  - Presents as patterns of its namesake as seen in indirect or retro illumination. It is the result of the basement membrane growing over basal cells. Usually not associated with visual symptoms though recurrent erosion may be a problem.
- **Meesmann's Dystrophy**
  - Presents as very small cyst like vesicles and are seen best with indirect retro illumination. Lesions occasionally extend to limbus and are most numerous in the interpalpebral area, which may cause irregular astigmatism and erosion.

Bowman's Layer Dystrophies

- **Reis Buckler's Dystrophy**
  - "Fishnet" swirl pattern opacities at level of Bowman's thought to be due to destruction of Bowman's layer and subsequent scarring. Best seen with tangential illumination.
  - Most dense in the center, gives cornea a "honeycomb" appearance.
    - Painful recurrent erosion but decreased corneal sensation when epithelium is intact.
- **Anterior Mosaic Dystrophy** (anterior crocodile shagreen)
  - Central, gray polygonal opacities which look like crocodile skin.
  - Not pathological, usually asymptomatic and thus no TX.
- **Vortex Dystrophy** (associated with Fabry's disease)
  - Pigment lines in a whorl like pattern located between Bowman's and stroma. Asymptomatic.
  - Also associated with several drugs: phenothiazines, chloroquines, indomethacin, amiodarone, tamoxifen.

Stromal Dystrophies

- **Granular Dystrophy** (Groenouws Type I)
  - Small, granular, hard, white deposits, thought to be hyaline, are located more axially and usually appear in first decade of life but do not become symptomatic until VA is reduced in 50's 60's.
- **Lattice Dystrophy** (Biber Haab Dimmer)
  - Branching filaments within the anterior or mid stroma forming a lattice network with central haze and anterior stromal refractile lines.
  - Spares the corneal periphery.
  - Thought to be accumulation of amyloid.
- **Macular Dystrophy** (Groenouw Type II)
  - Autosomal recessive; causes severe symptoms of decreased vision, irritation, and photophobia.
  - Central, grey white, poorly delineated opacities consisting of glycosaminoglycan; diffusely cloudy stroma.

Posterior Corneal Dystrophies

- **Fuch's Dystrophy**
  - Seen more often in females in old age.
  - A disorder of the endothelial cells, guttata.
  - Asymptomatic (ages 20-30's).
  - Early endothelial dystrophy (more guttata).
  - Late corneal edema and bullous keratopathy.
  - Painful epithelial breakdown with recurrent erosion can then occur.

3. Degenerations

- In general:
  - Seen more often in optometry than dystrophies.
  - Unlike dystrophies, usually there is later onset.
  - Generally more acute, progressive than dystrophies.
  - Though can occur bilaterally, will often occur unilaterally.
  - Are not autosomal dominant and usually not genetically determined.

- Are not primarily centrally located.
- May easily affect more than one corneal layer.

- **Arcus**
  - Asymptomatic, presents as whitish ring of lipid concentric to limbus. More common in blacks, occurring in 50% of population by 50 yrs. and 100% over 80 yrs. Bilateral Begins inferiorly, then superiorly, finally forming a ring.
  - Treatment: blood work up if under 40 or with risk factors (hypertension, smoker, obesity). Over 40 may not be indicative of hyperlipidemia, but if patient has not had recent medical check-up, refer.
- **Band Keratopathy**
  - Calcium accumulation in area of palpebral fissure presents as whitish yellow haze in the subepithelial space and anterior portion of Bowman's membrane. Starts at nasal and temporal limbus and eventually spreads centrally over months to years.
  - Treatment: Possible hyperparathyroid workup in adults. Lubrication if surface problems, monitor every 3-4 months for resolution; chelation or excimer laser keratectomy.
- **Bullous Keratopathy**
  - Acute, subacute, or insidious formation of blister (bullae) due to recurrent epithelial breakdown, often associated with Fuch's dystrophy or similar syndrome which causes loss of endothelial cells. May present with edema.
  - Treatment: Hypertonics for edema, Soft CL as bandage with prophylactic, possibly keratoplasty.
- **Coat's White Ring**
  - A response to a foreign body will present as an infiltrative, edematous ring seen with direct and indirect illumination.
  - Treatment: Removal of foreign body will resolve ring in a week. In old foreign body or one where removal is not indicated, ring will usually not cause symptoms.
- **Dellen (Gaule Spot)**
  - Focal, peripheral corneal thinning adjacent to limbus, usually 0.5 mm to 1.0 mm in diameter and seen more frequently at 3 and 9 o'clock. Associated with other raised entities like pinguecula, chemosis, and subconjunctival hemorrhage. No staining with fluorescein and no threat of perforation.
  - Treatment: None if asymptomatic. If large enough to disrupt CL wear, adjust fitting, or removal or patching to get rid of. Lubrication for 1 week may also remove.
- **Mooren's Ulcer**
  - Peripheral ulcerative keratitis due to ischemic necrosis resulting from vasculitis of limbal vessels. A severe inflammatory ulcerating disease with a painful and progressive course. Seen as advancing edge of epithelial defect with vascularization at the base of the ulceration.
  - Two forms:
    1) Limited form: Older patients (males) affected, unilateral; more benign
    2) Progressive form: Younger patients affected, bilateral and relentless; more severe.
  - Treatment: Immunosuppression topical therapy (steroids), systemic therapy (steroids, cyclosporins, cytotoxic drugs); Conjunctival excision and recession, Cryotherapy. Refer to corneal specialist.
- **Pellucid Marginal Degeneration**
  - Rare, bilateral idiopathic thinning of inferior cornea which is asymptomatic and which does not present a threat of perforation.
  - Onset 20-40years old.
  - Irregular astigmatism common. May show keratoconus changes.
  - Treatment: None except monitor for possible keratoconus.
- **Posterior Crocadile Shagreen**
  - Diffuse, grayish polygonal degeneration of posterior corneal surface.
  - No associated visual or ocular complications.
  - Treatment: None indicated.

- **Salzman's Nodular Degeneration**
  - Bilateral formations of elevated, grayish blue stromal opacities, which form nodules elevating corneal epithelium either centrally or peripherally. Nodules are thought to be due to excess collagen from an overactive healing process to some external insult (infection, inflammation, trauma). Asymptomatic or acute epithelial breakdown may be confused with Bullous keratopathy, which is more painful.
  - Treatment: Bandage soft CL and prophylactic for epithelial erosion, corneal epithelial debridement or superficial keratectomy, lamellar or penetrating keratoplasty for permanent repair.
- **Terrien's Marginal Degeneration**
  - Superior nasal thinning of peripheral cornea near limbus with yellow white punctuate stromal opacities. Usually bilateral; more common in males over 40 years of age. Progressive course results in distortions in the cornea, secondary inflammation, neovascularization, and loss of vision due to severe astigmatism. Lipid is material in superior deposits.
  - Treatment: Topical steroids usually marginally effective, Penetrating Keratoplasty to replace thinned cornea. There is threat of perforation, so warn about it and monitor for trauma.
- **White Limbal Girdal of Vogt**
  - Narrow band of fine crystal like opacities lined up along nasal or temporal borders seen bilaterally and always asymptomatic. Thought to be due to exposure to UV light, as in pinguecula or pterygium. Commonly seen in women over age 50.
  - Two types:
    1) An early from of band keratopathy, seen as circumferential band with a narrow, clear interval separating it from the limbus.
    2) An elastic degeneration of subepithelial collagen, extending from limbus without a clear zone.
  - Treatment: None indicated.

4. Keratoconus

- **Aka Corneal Ectasia**
- Idiopathic bulging of cornea with thinning, producing high astigmatism which can result in a painless loss of vision through high RE, though glare and photophobia is usually evident. Patient begins to show slow, insidious change in RE at 15 to 25 yrs, progressively changing for 5-6 years with stabilization subsequent. No perforation.
- Changes are seen centrally or paracentrally.
- Usually no familial pattern, though history of asthma, allergies, and chronic eye rubbing or mechanical pressure is common.
- Associated with Down's Syndrome, Ehlers Danlos syndrome, Marfan's, Addison's, Neurofibromotosis (Von Recklinghausen's Disease), Apert's Anomoly, vernal conjunctivitis and atopic eczema.
- Signs: Scissor type reflex seen with retinoscopy, keratometer shows steepening of cornea and distortion of mires. Placebo disc shows irregular pattern, and maximum corrected VA is reduced. Munson's Sign: in down gaze will see central or inferior cornea bulging profile of the lower lid. Vogt lines are vertical lines seen in posterior cornea. Stromal nerve fibers more prominent. Fleischer's Ring is a brownish orange ferrous ring surrounds the base of the cornea cone.
- Treatment: Spectacle lenses or CL in early or mild cases, RGP CL's or keratoplasty with good prognosis in advanced cases.

5. Corneal Pigments

- **Ferry's Line** (Orange brown)
  - Ferric ions around a surgical bleb, not pathognomonic.
- **Fleischer's Ring** (Orange brown)
  - Ferric ions around base of cone in keratoconus.

Corneal Pigments	Etiology/Association
Ferry's Line	Bleb
Fleischer's Ring	Keratoconus
Hudson Stahli's Line	Tear Deposit
Kayser Fleischer Ring	Wilson's Disease
Kruckenburg's Spindle	Uveitis Pigmentary Dispersion Syndrome
Stocker's Line	Pterygium

- **Hudson Stahli Line** (Orange brown)
    - Faint or continuous lines, possibly surrounded by opacities at level of Bowman's along palpebral fissure. Due to migration of ions. Frequent site of spontaneous or recurrent corneal erosions. More frequent in males.
- **Kayser Fleischer Ring** (Orangish)
    - Brownish, orangish ring in posterior cornea (Descemet's membrane) due to deposition of copper, as seen in Wilson's Disease. Best seen with gonioscopy or indirect illumination.
- **Krucknburg's Spindle** (Brownish)
    - Vertical deposition of pigment on posterior cornea. Sign of old uveitis or pigment dispersion syndrome (pattern caused by convection current in aqueous).
- **Stocker's Line** (Orangish brown)
    - Deposits at the head of pterygium at the epithelium layer.

6. Superficial Keratitis

- General things to remember:
    - This is a category of corneal disorders which affect the epithelium and the anterior stroma.
    - The etiologies of the various infections and inflammations include infective (viral and bacterial), toxic, degenerative, and allergic processes.
    - Subjectively, patients commonly complain of sandy gritty feeling, foreign body sensation, or "something under upper lid".
    - Objectively, a classic sign of superficial keratitis is Superficial Punctate Keratitis (SPK), superficial irregularities in the epithelium, infiltrates (white blood cells) can be in superficial epithelium or deeper.
    - Treatment:
        - For prevention of infection (prophylaxis): Aminoglycosides (gentamicin, tobramycin).
        - Topical steroids are used for superficial involvement or keratitis caused by immune response.
        - Lubricants and hypertonic saline solutions and ointments to relieve subjective complains and edema.
        - Cycloplegia and dilation are used to reduce risk of secondary anterior uveitis.
- **Filamentary Keratitis**
    - Dead epithelial cells combine with mucin debris to form filaments which adhere to surface of cornea and cause foreign body sensation. A number of disease processes, including atopic keratoconjunctivitis, burns, dry eye, Herpes Simplex, Herpes Zoster, and recurrent corneal erosion, can cause the epithelium to be compromised to begin with. Filaments stain with both fluorescein and Rose Bengal.
    - Treatment: Treat underlying disease process causing epithelial breakdown, Heavy lubrication, and mechanical removal of filaments with jeweler's forceps or cotton swab applicator.
- **Marginal Keratitis**
    - Corneal lesions caused by an infiltrative response to staphylococcal exotoxins. The lesions always present as "islands" with a clear interval (of Vogt) between the limbus and the distal border of the island. Islands seen at 2, 4, 8, 10 o'clock. Painful, watery eye with or without photophobia with acute or subacute presentation upon awakening.
    - Culture of lesion will be negative since no Staph organisms are actually present. It is a response to their exotoxin. Fluorescein, however, will stain the island brightly.
    - Treatment: Depends on severity of symptoms and risk for infection:
        - <u>Mild:</u> Hot packs, Gentamicin or Bacitracin. RTC 3-5 days.
        - <u>Moderate:</u> Cycloplege, dilate with higher doses of Gentamicin and Bacitracin. RTC 2-3 days.
        - <u>Severe:</u> Cycloplege and dilate with higher and more frequent doses of Gentamicin and Bacitracin. RTC 24 hrs.
- **Staphylococcal Superficial Punctate Keratitis (SPK)**
    - Variable degrees of SPK staining (fine dots to patches) due to Staphylococcus infection. Usually seen bilaterally and more often in dry eye patients. Most frequent presentation is staining on inferior corneal surface.

- No discharge except in severe cases, in which there will be a mucopurulent discharge. Patient complains of sandy, gritty sensation.
- Treatment: Ocular lubricants, Anti Staph drugs including Bacitracin and Gentamicin.

- **Superficial Punctate Keratitis of Thygeson**
  - An idiopathic, generally mild and self-limiting SPK which affects more young adult females (15-40). Patients are generally asymptomatic, may have sandy, gritty sensation. Variable SPK staining pattern. Infiltrates may appear in exacerbations of the disease, but the eye remains clear even in presence of keratitis (normally eye produces secondary conjunctival inflammatory response).
  - Treatment: Ocular lubricants for sandy, gritty feeling. Topical steroids and soft CL for more severe SPK.

7. Infectious Keratitis

- Some general things to consider:
  - Infectious keratitis by definition is a keratitis caused by the presence of live infectious organisms in the cornea. Whereas a superficial keratitis causes an epithelial response to the toxins of an organism, an infectious keratitis is the result of the body's response to the actual organism, and occurs in the stroma. The body responds to the live organism via an inflammatory response. This can cause lid edema, conjunctival hyperemia, corneal edema, infiltrates (WBCs in stroma), neovascularization, posterior corneal keratitic precipitates, Descemet's folds, uveitis, and increased IOP. A diagnostic sign of infectious keratitis is an ulcer, which is a local excavation of the cornea produced by sloughing of inflammatory necrotic tissue. The patient's complaints will have more of an acute onset, and typically consist of corneal irritation or deep pain. Poor contact lens care or health related risk factors such as recurrent Staph infections, chronic use of steroids, post corneal surgery, or AIDS contribute to risk. Pupils may be miotic, and VA is reduced.
  - Treatment: For all ulcers hospitalization is required since medication must be closely monitored. Typically, topical drugs are given to kill the invading organism. Immunosuppressives are then typically given. Corneal scarring and possible permanent vision deficit are inevitable consequence of ulcer treatment.
- **Acanthamoeba Keratitis**
  - The worst form of keratitis to get.
  - It is caused by a protozoan found in many sources of water (stagnant, pools, hot tubs, homemade saline CL solutions). History of patient with it usually involves some form of corneal trauma or compromise. Very painful, and present with very dramatic signs.
  - May start with epithelial disruption, but as condition advances you will see hypopyon, hyphema, edema, infiltrates which begin as localized but then progress to stromal rings, ulcers, stromal "melt", and descematocele which can lead to perforation. All this can occur in days.
  - Standard bacterial cultures will be negative.
  - Treatment: Non responsive to medical therapies. Refer to corneal specialist/hospitalization Ketoconazole, Miconazole, Neomycin, Propamadine have all been suggested, along with Topical steroids, bandage soft CL, but Penetrating keratoplasty is generally the treatment.
- **Bacterial Keratitis** aka (**Bacterial Ulcer, Central Corneal Ulcer, Corneal Ulcer**)
  - Can be due to gram positive or gram negative organism. Most common cause of all bacterial ulcers is Pseudomonas. (Clinical rule of thumb: **Assume pseudomonas until proven otherwise**). Seen more in warmer climates. CL wearers are at greater risk of getting (0.5% risk for daily wear soft, 3.5% risk of extended wear pts.).
  - Subjectively, patients usually complain of irritation, progressing to increased lacrimation, photophobia, reduced VA due to edema and infiltrates, and finally deep seated pain. Ulcer is main thing, and causes acute, unilateral problems. Objectively, will see ulcer usually located centrally, edema, infiltrates, Descemet's folds, keratic precipitates, and will always see anterior uveitis during the active ulceration stage. Dx is conclusive with culture, but should assume *Pseudomonas* until proven otherwise.

- All ulcers require immediate medical attention, usually requiring hospitalization with close monitoring of drug therapy. Usually intensive treatment with broad spectrum antibiotic and anti pseudomonal emphasis to begin with, to be modified once invading organism is identified.
- **Gram Positive Ulcers**
  - Most commonly due to Staphylococcus and Streptococcus pneumoniae or pyogenes. Staph tends to produce a slower and less intense developing ulcer (due to exotoxic nature) than Streptococcus or gram negatives, which produce acute and aggressive ulcers due to their endotoxive nature.
  - Staphylococcus ulcers tend to have well defined borders, whereas Strep and gram negative ulcers tend to have fuzzy borders. Cornea Staph infiltrates tend to be more circumscribed, whereas gram negative infiltrates are more diffuse and hazy.
  - Streptococcus can enter an intact epithelium.
- **Gram Negative Ulcers**
  - Commonly due to (from most to least):
    - *Pseudomonas aeruginosa*
    - *Neisseria gonorrhoeae*
    - *Hemophilus influenzae*
    - *Morax axenfeld (assoc. with alcoholics)*
    - *Serratia marcescans*
    - *Proteus vulgaris*
    - *Klebsiella*
    - *Escherichia coli*
    - *Corenybacterium*
  - Gram negative bugs tend to produce a more acute reaction than gram positives with greater risk of corneal damage. Pseudomonas does not require a broken epithelium to enter the cornea; but once it has it can destroy the stroma within minutes to hours! Pseudomonas and Neisseria can enter an intact epithelium. Ulcers caused by gram negative bugs tend to have fuzzy borders; infiltrates tend to be more diffuse.

- **Fungal Keratitis (Fungal Ulcer, Mycotic Keratitis)**
  - This is a serious condition because fungi can cause extensive damage to the eye.
  - There are a small number of effective medications. Fungal infections do not respond to steroids.
  - Most commonly due to Fusarium or Aspergillus (filamenous fungi) or Candida (yeast).
  - Relatively rare, but you should look for three risk factors: Southern or farming communities for most fungal keratitis.
  - Candida commonly seen in northern and coastal regions. Most common history is injury to cornea by a plant.
  - Ulcer seen is "creeping" along peripheral cornea, with feathered edges and branching with spores at the tips. The characteristic appearance is a gray or dirty white dry, rough, textured surface with elevated margins
  - May also see Descemet's folds, cells and flare, hypopyon.
  - The most important thing to do is to culture the fungus with cultures and scrapings, since often this is the only means of trusty diagnosis.
  - Treatment: Antifungal meds by a corneal specialist. These include Nystatin, Amphotericin B, and Natamycin, all of which are extremely toxic. Do not respond to Steroids. Often complete corneal grafts (penetrating keratoplasty) must be done (fungi are difficult to isolate) and to prevent losing the cornea.
- **Herpes Simplex Virus**
  - The most common virus found in humans, the virus is responsible for more than 1.5 million cases of blindness in the U.S. each year (leading infectious cause of blindness).
  - Two forms of the virus;
    - Type 1 (HSV 1): oral
    - Type 2 (HSV 2): genital
  - Previously it was thought most ocular infections were from Type 1, but recent statistics show dramatic increase due to the Type 2 genital variety.

- Infection by the Herpes virus occurs via a primary, recurrent, or transmission from a carrier. Transmission is through direct contact, mostly saliva or mouth contact, or from skin lesions. Primary Herpes Infection/Keratitis.
- By the age of 5, 70% of kids have been inoculated with the virus, commonly showing the classic sign of a fever blister or cold sore.
- The primary infection usually does not involve the eye, though when it does it is dramatic. After self-resolution, sometimes with the help of antivirals, the virus retreats to reside along the Trigeminal Nerve ganglion and its route in a dormant state.
- Recurrent infection occurs later in life that can have profound ulcerative and destructive changes (mainly due to inflammatory response of eye) on the epithelium, stroma, and iris.
- Subjectively, the primary infection usually is seen in young children who present with fever, malaise, mild foreign body sensation, photophobia, and burning irritation. Objectively will see: Classic skin lesions, especially near mouth. Enlarged preauricular lymph node (ipsilateral to lesions) moderate to severe adenopathy, follicular conjunctivitis.
- In the cornea, may see: Fine to coarse diffuse SPK, dendrites (corneal patterns which have the appearance of branches with round buds at the terminal edges and which stain with both fluorescein and Rose Bengal).
- Treatment: Co-manage with pediatrician. Acyclovir ointment for skin lesions and Viroptic drops for eyes.

- **Herpes Simplex**
  - Conjunctivitis and scleritis occur in about half the cases.
  - Watery hyperemia, follicular conjunctivitis, and regional adenopathy.
  - Scleritis may cause scleral thinning. Keratitis occurs in about 40% of cases and may precede skin lesions.
  - May present as fine or coarse SPK with or without edema. SPK may take on dendritic shape, which mimics Herpes Simplex keratoconjunctivitis.
  - Corneal sensation is more reduced in Zoster than in Simplex.
  - Melting or corneal perforation may occur if persistent epithelium defect is present. Interstitial keratitis in diffuse or disciform may be present. Iridocyclitis frequently occurs.
  - After resolution of an attack, atrophy of iris may be seen. Hypopyon may also be seen. Glaucoma may occur in acute form following trabeculitis.
  - Treatment: Refer to corneal specialist. Treatment varies from warm or cold packs, cycloplegia, to oral and systemic antivirals (Acyclovir). Steroid to be delayed if possible and Keratoplasty in severe cases.
- **Recurrent Infection/Keratitis**
  - History of previous attacks is most useful diagnostic tool.
  - Factors which aggravate or incite recurrence: Sunlight, trauma, extreme heat or cold, fever, steroids, infectious disease, or surgery. Manifestation of recurrent infection can occur as epithelial infection, stromal interstitial keratitis, iridocyclitis, or combinations thereof. Epithelial infection. Unilateral follicular conjunctivitis, dendrites, ulcers which may take on an ovoid or linear shape, corneal hypoesthesia (decreased corneal sensitivity).
  - Ulcers indicate a defect in the basement membrane. Dendrite presence usually indicates epithelial involvement. HSV is the only condition that will produce a true ulcerative dendritic keratitis.
  - Treatment: Mechanical removal of dendrites (debridement) and antiviral therapy (Vidarabine 3% OR Idoxuridine 0.5%) Steroid use is to be avoided. Soft CL or patching can be used to treat ulcer.
- **Stromal Interstitial Keratitis**
  - Present usually in conjunction with epithelial infection as necrotic, blotchy, cheesy white infiltrates which lie in the stroma. This is due to inflammatory response of the eye, and in severe cases may see neovascularization. Wessley rings (sites of antigen antibody reactions) are often seen in anterior stroma.
  - Classic signs are:
    - Infiltration
    - Neovascularization
    - Stromal thinning

    - May also present in disciform type as stromal disc believed to be the result of a type IV (delayed hypersensitivity) response.
    - May see edema, keratic precipitates. Usually see uveitis with increased IOP and hyphema and/or cells, flare.
  - Treatment: Refer to corneal specialist, steroids only if necessary, cycloplegia to prevent iris involvement, penetrating keratoplasty.
- **Iridocyclitis**
  - Uveitis due to inflammatory response of the body. It is often seen concomitant with interstitial keratitis.
  - Treatment: Cycloplegic and non-steroidal anti-inflammatory drugs to prevent structural damage to eye from HSV infection. Oral acyclovir and Pred Forte may also be used.
- **Herpes Zoster Virus (Ophthalmicus)**
  - Varicella or chicken pox virus which makes a primary infection of the dorsal root ganglion or first division of Trigeminal (V) nerve.
  - Virus attacks frontal, nasal, and less commonly the maxillary or mandibular branch.
  - The result is vesicle skin lesions over area of skin innervated by infected branch.
  - **Hutchinson's sign** (vesicle on tip of nose) indicates nasociliary branch involvement and likelihood of ocular involvement (ophthalmicus).
  - A secondary eruption of vesicles may occur as a result of inflammatory or neoplasis in ganglion. Regional lymphadenopathy with pain is present with the primary form but not in secondary.
  - Ocular signs are combinations of conjunctivitis, episcleritis, scleritis, punctuate epithelial keratitis, iridocyclitis, and glaucoma. Often mimic other entities, esp. herpes simplex.
- **Molluscum Contagiosum**
  - This virus causes characteristic epithelial tumor-like lesions on the eyelids which have umbilicated centers and "cheesy" caseous material. Often these lesions are located near the lid margins. Corneal involvement is diffuse SPK thought to be due to a toxic reaction by the cornea to the contents of the lesions, which somehow get into tears or cul de sac.
  - Treatment: Removal of the lesions results in rapid clearing of keratitis. Lesions may be expressed first, then excision, cauterization, or cryotherapy removes them.
- **Acne Rosacea**
  - A common idiopathic sebaceous gland disease which has skin and ocular presentations.
  - "Butterfly" rash across face is classic skin sign. This is made up of smaller, macular, slightly scaly lesions on an erythematous base. There are telangiectal vessels and patient may have history of prominent blushing.
  - Seen more in fair complexion, specifically Scottish Irish/Northern European descent.
  - Ocular signs: Blepharitis is usually non ulcerative, bilateral, and can be from history of chronic chalazion, styes, or hordeolums. Conjunctivitis is low grade and produces burning and nonspecific irritation. Keratitis may present as marginal infiltrate with neovascularization with migration across the cornea.
  - Treatment: Lid scrubs/hygiene for blepharitis and systemic Tetracycline is primary treatment
- **Chlamydial** (Adult inclusion and Inclusion Gonorrhea)
  - The adult form is called “Inclusion,” and affects sexually active adults.
  - When transmitted to newborns from an infected mother, it is called “Inclusion Gonorrhea” which is the most frequent cause of conjunctivitis in infants.
  - The sexual keratitis caused by intracellular parasite is similar to trachoma, which is transmitted from eye to eye, hand to eye, or maternally by infected mother to newborn.
  - It presents with both bacterial and viral signs:
    - Bacterial unilateral mucopurulent discharge
    - Meaty red bulbar hyperemia
    - Diffuse SPK
    - Viral follicular conjunctivitis
    - Chemosis
    - Preauricular lymph node enlargement
    - Pseudomembrane and marginal infiltrates
  - The key to diagnosis is a history of sexual activity and a recent urinary tract infection.

- Another tip off is non-response to standard topical antibiotics (patient still has signs after 24 weeks).
- Confirmation of diagnosis is by lab culture.
- Treatment: Oral and topic tetracycline, except for infant inclusion gonorrhea, in which sulfa or erythromycin are used as alternatives.

- **Syphilis Interstitial Keratitis (IK)**
  - 90% of all IK seen is due to syphilis
  - Two forms of Syphilis:
    1) Congenital - much more common, onset is usually between 5 and 20 years. Bilateral
    2) Acquired - much less common, later onset, unilateral
  - The keratitis seen is due to an infiltrative inflammation of the stroma, especially deeper layers, which is chronic and which may accompany inflammation of the anterior uveal tract.
  - Clinical course begins with edema of endothelium and deeper layers of stroma with pain, lacrimation, photophobia, and blepharospasm.
  - There is circumcorneal injection and the cornea is hazy. As neovascularization progresses, the edema and inflammation subsides, leaving behind deep opacities and ghost vessels. Guttata due to excess hyaline may be present in the resolved cornea.
  - Treatment: Topical steroids are usually effective.
- **Trachoma**
  - Caused by TRIC organism (chlamydial trachomatis species), it is endemic in underdeveloped countries in Asia, Africa, South America, and in American Indians. Usually presents with genitourinary involvement/infection.
  - See conjunctival and corneal involvement, without which patient is usually asymptomatic. Conjunctival: Follicles or papillae with and without scarring.
  - Cornea: Superior lid and cornea is scarred (most likely to see old, resolved scars). Will also see superficial epithelial keratitis, ulceration, limbal follicles, and depressed scars (Herbert's Pits). Scarring on tarsus are Arlt's Lines. Rule out Chlamydial (no heavy sexual activity; check ethnic background.
  - Treatment: Oral and Topical tetracycline ointment; topical steroids if active corneal involvement.
- **Dry Eye (Keratitis Sicca)**
  - One of the most common causes of minor irritation, especially in the elderly population (postmenopausal women). Almost always bilateral, the classic symptoms are "sandy, gritty feeling", foreign body sensation, dryness or irritation. Paradoxically, the eyes may by very watery due to continual reflex tearing. Vision may fluctuate.
  - Etiologies include:
    1) Idiopathic (many have no ocular or systemic cause).
    2) Environmental: Air conditioning, dust, smoke, near work
    3) Drugs: Antihistamines, decongestants, diuretics, steroids, birth control pills, alcohol.
    4) Ocular: Lagophthalmos, Blepharitis, Meibomitis, Contacts.
    5) Systemic Conditions: Infectious or inflammatory disease, Sjogren's syndrome, Rheumatoid arthritis, Lupus, Pemphigoid, Steven Johnson's, Sarcoids,
  - Staining: Characteristic of KCS is a band of staining with either fluorescein or Rose Bengal in palpebral fissure region.
  - Slit lamp: Low grade hyperemia, debris in tear film, dellen, filamentary keratitis, usually no discharge.
  - TBUT: Low (< 10 sec) but not instantaneous (diagnostic for basement disorder) TBUT time means mucin deficiency.
  - Schirmer: less than 10 mm is abnormal and less than 5 is (+) for KCS in I, 15 mm in II aqueous test.
  - Defect in Tear Layer:
    1) Lipid layer: infectious blepharitis, meibomitis, Staph toxin.
    2) Aqueous: Lacrimal and accessory gland disorders, Sjogren's, drug related, neurological.
    3) Mucin: Goblet cell disorder, Vitamin A deficiency, Steven Johnson's syndrome, conjunctival disease, drug related.

- Treatment: **Mild to moderate**: Lubricants, eye drops, ointments, Inserts (Lacrisert). No specific regime, trial and error basis with recheck every 1-3 weeks. **Severe**: Maximal levels of lubricants, eye drops, etc. Bandage soft CL, goggles, punctal plugs.

- **Recurrent Corneal Erosion**
  - Basically caused by deficiency in the basement membrane which causes epithelial cells to slough off, sometimes in large patches. Epithelium grows back but erosion then occurs, resulting in a vicious cycle.
  - Two classic histories:
    1) Secondary to corneal injury (may have involved basement membrane, epi is not healing properly).
    2) Spontaneous (no obvious cause). Recurrent nature is key.
  - Symptoms are commonly seen in corneal irritation (sandy, gritty, FB, photophobia), usually seen unilaterally. The key is morning discomfort (epi. is sheared off by lids as patient awakes, may be due to edema during sleep).
  - Slit Lamp exam with fluorescein will show staining, sometimes in large patches. In smaller deficits, there may be no staining if the patient sees you late in the day (epi has sealed itself).
  - Treatment:
    - Try to determine etiology:
      - Injury will heal if given the chance
      - Dystrophy/Degeneration; variable prognosis
      - Chronic; no cure, patient education to self-management.
    - Warm packs, hypertonic drops/ointments, especially before bedtime. Stress that it takes 6-8 weeks for basement membrane to completely heal, thus patient has to be careful during this period.
    - Patching, therapeutic soft CL in more severe cases.

CONJUNCTIVA (GROSS ANATOMY)

1. Location

- The conjunctiva is a clear mucous membrane that lines the lids, fornix, and anterior sclera allowing movement of the eyelids over the globe. The **bulbar conjunctiva** extends from the limbus to the fornix covering the sclera and limbus, and the **palpebral conjunctiva** extends from the fornix to the lid margin, covering the marginal, tarsal, and orbital regions. Merges with naso-lacrimal system at the lacrimal punctum, forming a sac.

2. Composition

- Layers:
  - Epithelium: 10-15 **stratified squamous epithelial cells** thick, continuous with the corneal epithelium. Melanin granules present in cell cytoplasm, especially cells near the limbus.
    - **Goblet cells** located in epithelium
  - Substantia propria (Stroma) – vascularized loose collagenous connective tissue network that contains collagen elastin fibrils, and ECM
    - This layer also contains lymphoid tissue containing macrophages, mast cells, PMNs, eosinophils and lymphocytes providing immunological defense
- Glands:
  - Accessory lacrimal glands of **Krause** and **Wolfring**: Secrete serous fluid and tears.
  - **Goblet cells**: Secrete mucus (making up the lowest layer of tears).
- **Palisades of Vogt** are radial projections of limbal epithelium and stroma that extend into the cornea. This area is suspected to be the source of corneal epithelial basal cell replication and stem cell origin as well as the location of stem cells for the bulbar conjunctiva.

3. Relationship to Tarsal Plate, Extraocular Muscles, Sclera, Vagina Bulbi (Tenon's Capsule), Cornea

- The stroma of the palpebral conjunctiva is very thin near the **tarsal plates** but thickens in the orbital portion. The posterior surface of the tarsal plates are adherent to the Palpebral conjunctiva.
- The palpebral conjunctiva is attached loosely to the levator, tarsal muscle of Muller, and extraocular muscles at the fornices to allow for coordinated muscle movement of the globe and lids.
- The bulbar conjunctiva is attached loosely to the underlying tissue up to within 3mm of the cornea, where it then becomes tightly attached and merges with the sclera and Tenon's Capsule.
- **Tenon's Capsule (Vagina Bulbi)** is a thin but dense fibrous sheet that encases the globe. It acts as a barrier to prevent the spread of orbital infections into the globe.
    - It lies between the episclera and the conjunctiva and merges with them anteriorly in the limbal area.
    - It merges posteriorly with the dural sheath of the optic nerve.
    - It is pierced by the optic nerve, vortex veins, ciliary vessels and nerves, and extraocular muscles.
- In relation to the cornea, the thicker conjunctival epithelium becomes the thinner very regular squamous corneal epithelium in the limbal area.
- The conjunctival stroma, episclera, and Tenon's capsule begin within the limbal area.

4. Blood Supply and Venous Drainage, Lymphatic Drainage

- Blood Supply
    - The palpebral conjunctiva receives blood from the palpebral arcades.
    - The fornices receive blood from the peripheral arteriole arcades.
    - The bulbar conjunctiva receives blood from the posterior conjunctival arcades, which anastamose with the anterior conjunctival arcades which arise from the anterior ciliary artery.
- Venous drainage
    - Veins follow arteries by way of the superior and inferior palpebral plexus, which drain into the palpebral and ophthalmic veins.
- Lymphatic drainage:
    - Conjunctival lymphatic vessels in the submucosa drain into the lymphatics of the eyelids.
    - The medial area drains into the submandibular lymph node.
    - The lateral area drains into the parotid lymph node.

5. Innervation

- All sensory innervations is from the Trigeminal nerve (CN V)
    - The bulbar conjunctiva has sensory innervations from the long ciliary nerves.
    - The superior palpebral conjunctiva has sensory innervations from the **frontal** and lacrimal branches of the **ophthalmic nerve** while the inferior palpebral conjunctiva has sensory innervations from **lacrimal** nerve and **infraorbital** branch of the **maxillary nerve**.
- Parasympathetic innervation via the **Long Ciliary** nerves.

6. Plica Semilunaris

- The **plica semilunaris** is a moon-shaped conjunctival fold at the medial canthus.
- The epithelial layer is 8-10 cells thick and contains goblet cells
- The vascularized stromal layer has smooth muscle and adipose tissue.
- Its believed function is to allow full lateral movement without stretching the tissue of the eye

7. Caruncle

- The **caruncle** is a mound of tissue that overlies the medial edge of the plica semilunaris.
- It has components found in the conjunctiva (non-keratinized epithelium, accessory lacrimal glands) as well as the skin (hair follicles, sebaceous and sweat glands).

CONJUNCTIVA (DEVELOPMENTAL ANATOMY)

1. Ectodermal Specialization Forming Conjunctiva and Glands

- Conjunctival epithelium which covers the anterior surface of the globe and inner surface of the lids is derived from **ectoderm** that folds in during the formation of the lid folds.
- The glands of Moll and Zeiss are formed during the 4th month as epithelial ingrowths.
- The Meibomian (tarsal) glands are also formed at this time by basal epithelial budding of the inner part of the fuse lid margins.
- The accessory lacrimal glands (Krause) are formed from epithelial conjunctival ingrowth approximately during the 6th - 7th month.

CONJUNCTIVA (PATHOLOGY)

1. Pterygium

- Thick, fleshy triangular mass of tissue (apex toward cornea) which takes decades to develop as a tissue response to UV exposure and arid climate. Usually asymptomatic though sometimes may have hyperemic appearance, irritation, foreign body sensation, and reduction of vision if it grows into visual axis. Frequently bilateral and relatively rich in vascularization
- A pinguecula is a pterygium which has not yet grown onto the cornea.
- Treatment: Prevention with UV tints is the key, otherwise usually no treatment if stable and asymptomatic. Lubricants for foreign body sensation, vasoconstrictor for hyperemic appearance. Surgery to remove if on visual axis, but patient must be warned of aggressive nature of regrowth.

2. Keratoconjunctivitis

- **Atopic Keratoconjunctivitis**
  - Greater prevalence in men ages 20-50 with history of atopic dermatitis.
  - Presents as severe itching all year around with moderate to severe SPK. Chronic forms will show limbal arcades with stromal haze and scarring. Keratopathy is the main cause of visual impairment
  - Treatment: Cold packs, Antihistamines and OTC decongestants. Prednisolone 1% Topically is very effective.
- **Phlyctenular Keratoconjunctivitis**
  - Raised, circumscribed, infiltrative nodules of cells and debris thought to be a result of a delayed type hypersensitivity reaction, often associated with Staphylococcus infection.
  - Key sign is "leash" of vessels present when the "phlyctenule" nodule migrates onto the eye. Patients will complain of classic symptoms of superficial keratitis: a sandy, gritty feeling, a foreign body sensation, or something under the upper lid. Often seen in young patients
  - Treatment: Topical Steroids the drug of choice (Prednisolone 1% or Dexamethasone 0.1%)
- **Viral Keratoconjunctivitis (Adenovirus)**
  - Two Types
    1) Pharyngoconjunctival Fever
    2) Epidemic Keratoconjunctivitis
  - They are diseases of the cornea and conjunctiva as a result of adenovirus infection.
  - Classic signs are acute follicular conjunctivitis (follicles on the palpebral conj.) and preauricular adenopathy (swollen lymph nodes).
  - Symptoms may be relatively asymptomatic to irritation, watery discharge, and hyperemia.
  - They are differentially diagnosed from Herpes Simplex Keratitis by corneal esthesiometry test (test for corneal sensitivity).
  - Subjective rating of 1-10 (1=no sensation, 10=patient jumps out of chair) is accomplished by taking wisp of cotton ball and brushing across the cornea. Doctor judges patient response, then repeat and ask patient to judge.

- Quantitative measurements using different amounts of force can be determined by commercially available Cochet Bonnet or Schirmer esthesiometers. If the response is judged to be less than or equal to 7, or very low, this is suggestive of keratitis due to Herpes virus and not adenovirus.
- Generally no treatment except supportive for comfort since condition is self-limiting (about 2 wks).
- **Pharyngoconjunctival Fever (PCF)**
  - Associated with adenovirus 3 and 7; almost always as a result of recent history of upper respiratory infection (URI). Seen in younger patients (5-15). Purplish pinkish bulbar hyperemia, serous discharge, and a quick TBUT along with classic signs of adenovirus of follicles on palpebral conjunctiva and enlarged lymph nodes. Cornea itself shows fine, diffuse SPK and possibly small subepithelial infiltrates uncommon.
  - No cure, self-limiting within 10-14 days. Supportive measures of warm or cold packs, ocular lubricants, and decongestants for discomfort.
- **Epidemic Keratoconjunctivitis (EKC)**
  - The most common contagious clinical condition seen in primary care optometry. It is associated primarily with adenovirus 8, though 4, 11, 13, 19, and 37 which are transmitted by direct or indirect contact (towels, hands, instruments). Can be very contagious! Unlike PCF, seen in older patients (over 15), and is not associated with URI or systemic infection.

EKC Rule of 8's
Adenovirus 8
First 8 days conjunctivitis and very contagious
8 day corneal SPK is present
8 days later (16th day) subepithelial infiltrates

  - Patient complains of nonspecific irritation and burning sensation with slightly reduced VA. Objectively same signs as PCF. Pseudomembranes (infiltrative cells combined with fibrin and mucin) may be present. Differentiate from PCF by age of onset (older) and lack of systemic disease.
  - Treatment: Advise pt. of contagious nature (don't touch or rub eyes, don't share towels). Otherwise no treatment other than lubricants or warm and cold packs for discomfort. Condition usually resolves itself in 25-30 days. Removal of pseudomembranes by jeweler's forceps.

- **Superior Limbic Keratoconjunctivitis (SLK of Theodore)**
  - Idiopathic, associated with hyperthyroidism (20-50%, it occurs more in middle aged women who present with complaints of generalized ocular irritation and discomfort.
  - Bilateral, prominent superior bulbar hyperemia, superior tarsal palpebral papules (smaller than those seen in GPC), superior fine SPK, papillary hypertrophy at the limbus, punctuate epithelial erosions of superior cornea, and possibly pseudodendrites.
  - Self-limiting over 5 to 10 years.
  - Treatment: Cold packs, NSAIDs, antihistamines, decongestants, and Cromolyn Sodium for anti-inflammation, Topical steroids for subjective and objective signs.
- **Contact Lens Related SLK (CL SLK)**
  - A condition which is similar to SLK of Theodore in having superior hyperemia, papillae, and SPK. However, CL SLK occurs at any age, does not occur more in females, and is directly related to thimerosol use and soft CL wear. TX is removal of thimerosol from regimen and stoppage of CL wear until resolution.
- **Vernal Keratoconjunctivitis**
  - A seasonal, allergic reaction affecting young people who complain of itching, tearing, foreign body sensation, and photophobia.
  - It is a bilateral production of giant papules on the superior tarsus similar to GPC but having a "Cobblestone" appearance. May see white, chalky concretions on the limbal conjunctiva known as Tranta's dots. The key, though, are very thick, ropy, whitish yellow strands of mucus which cover superior tarsus, conjunctiva, and cornea. Rule out atopic keratoconjunctivitis (year round vs. seasonal) SLK (usually a milder, less symptomatic presentation). GPC (less symptomatic, GPC due to soft CL not allergy).
  - Treatment: Topical Steroids and/or aspirin to help with inflammation.

Chapter 13 – Lens/Cataract/IOL/Pre- and Post-Operative Care

LENS, ZONULES (GROSS ANATOMY)

1. Zonules

- Location
    - Originate in the pars plana basement membrane and insert into the lens.
        - Appear 1-1.5mm anterior to the ora serrata.
    - Forms a thin sheet that lies on the surface of the pars plana.
    - Splits into bundles at the ciliary processes that run in the valleys.
- 3 parts:
    1) Tension fibers
        - Small fibers that anchor the zonule fibers to the sides of the ciliary processes.
    2) Zonular plexus
        - The vertical plane of bundles between the ciliary processes.
    3) Zonular fork
        - The plexus splits into an anterior and posterior branch.
        - The anterior fork inserts into the lens anterior to the equator.
        - The posterior fork inserts into the lens posterior to the equator.

2. Location of Lens

- The lens is located in the posterior chamber, anterior to the vitreous chamber and posterior to the iris and anterior chamber.
- It is suspended in its locations by zonule fibers from the ciliary body.
- The lens is centered downward and nasally.

3. Epithelium (Capsule, Ultrastructure)

- Capsule
    - Transparent, thick basement membrane of the lens epithelium.
    - Elastic membrane that surrounds the entire lens.
        - The capsule's elasticity is attributed to its laminar arrangement rather than elastic fibers. There are no elastic fibers in the capsule.
    - Composed of very fine collagen fibers.
    - The capsule is thickest anterior and posterior to the equator where the zonules insert and thinnest at the posterior pole.
    - Curvature of anterior and posterior capsule increases towards poles.
        - The anterior capsule curvature is greater than the posterior.
        - Optically significant because the posterior pole is the nodal point of the lens .
- Epithelium
    - Just internal to capsule in equatorial and anterior part of the lens.
    - 3 zones:
        1) *Central zone* - cuboidal cells in the center of the lens on the anterior surface.
        2) *Intermediate (Pre equatorial) zone* - mitotically active cells between the center and equator.
        3) *Equatorial zone* - very columnar, elongated cells.

4. Cortex (Composition of Lens Fibers, Ultrastructure)

- Cortex Fibers
  - Mass of elongated cells
    - Epithelial cells are considered fibers when the nuclei disappear.
  - The mature fiber has a long, thin ribbon shape with a roughly hexagonal cross section. The ribbon is 8-12mm long, 8-10μm wide, and 2-5 μm thick.
    - Among the longest non-neuronal cells in the body
    - The adult lens has approximately 2000 fibers.
  - All the cells in 1 layer of the lens are of the same generation of growth.
  - Interdigitations between lens fibers are extremely well attached.
  - The fibers fit together to form smooth lamellae parallel to the curved surfaces.

5. Nuclei (Various Names and Locations)

- Nuclei (from most internal to most external)
  - Embryonic nucleus
    - Optically clear central area
    - Primary lens fibers grow from the posterior to the anterior surface.
  - Fetal nucleus
    - Encircles previous nucleus (includes embryonic nucleus + fibers added to lens before birth)
    - Secondary fibers
    - Has distinctive Y sutures
  - Infantile nucleus
    - Embryonic + fetal nucleus
  - Adult nucleus
    - All 3 previous nuclei + fibers added before sexual maturation
    - Central part of mature lens

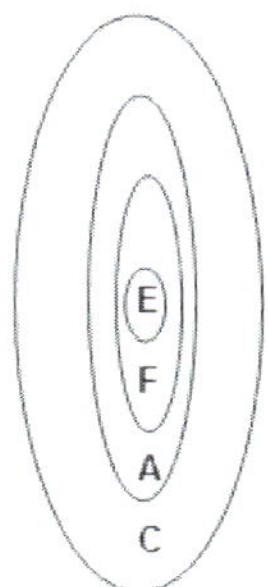

E=Embryonic Nucleus
F=Fetal Nucleus
A=Adult Nucleus
C=Cortex

6. Sutures (Location)

- Insertion lines of lens fibers
- Formation of sutures enables lens shape to change from spherical to flat biconvex.
- Fetal sutures are an erect Y shape on the anterior surface and an inverted Y on the posterior surface.
  - The fibers of the fetal sutures are all equal in length.
- Cortical sutures have a more complex star pattern.
  - The fibers of the cortical sutures are all equal in length.

LENS, ZONULES (DEVELOPMENTAL ANATOMY)

---

1. Zonule Development

- Zonule fibers develop between the 3rd and 6th month
  - The 1st sign of these fibers emerges when the thickened basement membrane of the ciliary epithelium breaks up into minute fibrils.
- Zonular formation by fusion of fibers termination over the lens capsule
  - During the 6th month, well-formed fibrils can be seen running forward from the ciliary processes towards the lens.
  - First, the fibers run parallel to the ciliary epithelium for a short distance before they inwardly transverse the triangular zone of the vitreous.
  - At this point, they run perpendicularly to the main mass of fibers and eventually reach the lens. Here, their terminations unite to form fine lamella on the capsule surface.
  - As the eye grows in size, the developing ciliary body and the cup margin become increasingly withdrawn from the lens equator. As a result, the fibrillae become longer, stronger, and more defined.

- Eventually, the fibers become grouped in two bundles:
  - An anterior group that runs behind the iris.
  - A posterior group that runs parallel to the membrane.
- These compact and well defined bands of fibers form the adult zonular system.

- Other theories of zonular formation:
  - The entire capsule including this lamella is a secretory product of the epithelial cells of the lens.

2. Tissue Origin

- Zonule fibers develop from the tertiary vitreous (neural ectoderm).
- The entire capsule is derived from the basement membrane.

3. Tissue Induction and Interaction (Effect on Development of Vitreous, iris, Cornea, Retina)

- Tissue Induction
  - Development of the lens is dependent on an induction emanating from the (1) head mesoderm and (2) the optic vesicle. Without induction, lens development is defective or does not occur at all.
  - The first sign of the development of the lens vesicle is the **lens placode**.
  - As the optic cup touches the surface ectoderm, it gives off a stimulus that causes the epidermal cells to develop into the lens rudiment.
  - Experiments have suggested that the inducing agent is a chemical substance, possibly RNA.
- Tissue Interaction
  - Evidence suggests that chemical induction from the developing lens is a necessary factor in the normal development of the neural ectoderm and mesodermal elements of the eye.
  - Removal of the lens vesicle results in:
    - Thickening and folding of the retina
    - Reduction of vitreous
    - Failure of invagination of the optic vesicle results in failure of optic cup formation
    - Failure of induction of the epidermis developing into the cornea

4. Mechanism of Lens Fiber Orientation

- Primary fibers
  - Extend from the surface of the lens along the antero-posterior plane.
  - Early on, straight suture lines are seen in the fetal nucleus. On the anterior surface of the lens is an erect Y and on the posterior surface an inverted Y.
  - Addition of new fibers from the equatorial cells compress of the central fibers. As the lens increases in size, sutures become more complex. Y-suture arrangement becomes merged into a star shape, which may be found on the surface of the lens at or soon after birth.
- Secondary Fibers
  - Unlike the earliest fibers that run antero-posteriorly, the later fibers are circumferentially oriented.
  - The secondary lens fibers are thick at the equator but taper as their ends extend toward the front and back of the lens.
  - Secondary fibers do not become thin enough to meet other fiber ends at a single point and form a star pattern. As a result of this arrangement, the fibers are never long enough to completely reach from pole to pole.
  - Because the secondary fibers are successively laid down on top of each other with the thickest parts at the equator, the lens becomes less spherical.

5. Stages of Lens Development (Lens Placode, Lens pit, Lens vesicles)

- Lens Placode (or plate)
    - Formed from the portion of surface ectoderm that is in direct contact with neural ectoderm of the optic outgrowth.
    - When the optic vesicle contacts the surface ectoderm, it induces mitotic division of the columnar surface cells.
    - The thickening of the epithelium results in the formation of the lens plate, which subsequently invaginates.
- Lens Pit
    - The earliest sign of the lens pit is when the lens placode starts to show a slight depression (fovea lentis).
- Lens Vesicle
    - The lens pit then deepens to form a sac then a pore. When its opening constricts, it becomes the lens vesicle.
    - The lens is still connected to the surface ectoderm by a stalk.
    - The lens is now a hollow sphere with its wall composed of a single layer of short columnar cells.
    - As soon as the vesicle separates from the surface ectoderm, mesoderm grows in between the surface ectoderm and the lens. All trace of the point of attachment of the vesicle to the surface ectoderm is immediately lost.

6. Stages of Lens Fiber Development

- After the lens vesicle separates from the surface ectoderm, the inner cells of the lens vesicle wall begin to differentiate.
- Anterior cells
    - A single row of cubical cells increases in number. They form the anterior capsule and remain as a simple cubical epithelial layer.
- Posterior Cells
    - The columnar cells of the posterior wall form the first lens fibers. Except for the anterior epithelium, the entire adult lens is formed from cells from the posterior wall and equatorial region.
    - The columnar posterior cells lengthen in the antero-posterior direction. The circular lumen of the vesicle becomes more crescent-like and eventually is obliterated.
    - Nuclei of cells migrate slowly during growth so that they are always closer the anterior end of the cells.
- Primitive Lens Fibers
    - The primitive lens fibers are longest and straightest at the posterior pole. They decrease regularly in length and increase in curvature as they approach the equatorial region. Here, they merge into the cubical anterior wall cells.
    - Primitive lens fibers remain at the exact center of the lens throughout life.
- Secondary lens fibers
    - Secondary lens fibers begin to proliferate in both directions from the equatorial region of the anterior layer of the lens vesicle. These fibers originate from the cuboidal cells at their junction with the columnar cells at the equator.

7. Developmental Nuclei (Embryonic, Fetal, Infantile)

- Earlier fibers become more sclerosed than the later superficial ones. In the adult lens, a stratification of zones can be observed.
- Embryonic nucleus: Formed in 1st 3 months of embryonic life
- Fetal nucleus: Formed from the secondary fibers during 3rd to 8th month of fetal life
- Infantile nucleus: Formed between the last weeks of fetal life and 4 years of age
- Adult nucleus: Formed up until to puberty
- Cortex: Includes all secondary fibers added after sexual maturation

8. Zones of Development of Lens Epithelium

- The anterior cuboidal cells of the lens capsule form the lens epithelium monolayer, which covers only the anterior surface of the primary fiber mass.
- The progenitor cells are distributed only in the **germinative zone**, a small, narrow, peripheral, latitudinal band of the lens epithelium at the equator. Only these cells undergo mitosis and differentiate into secondary fibers.
- Secondary fiber cells grow and move towards the **central zone** of the lens epithelium.

LENS (PHYSIOLOGY)

1. Function of Lens

- Maintain its own clarity
- Refract light entering the optical system of the eye
  - Light rays that pass through the peripheral part of an optical lens have a shorter focal length than through the center.
  - Crystalline lens compensates for this by having an refractive index gradient. The refractive index increases from the periphery to the center due to the varying protein content throughout lens.
    - Increased protein concentration is correlated with increased refractive power.
- Absorb UV light
  - Cornea absorbs UVC (λ<295nm).
  - Lens absorbs UVB and UVA (295< λ<400).
  - The lens transmits 90% visible light when young.

Structure	Absorb UV	Wavelength
Cornea	UVC	<295 nm
Lens	UVB and UVA	295 - 400 nm

- Accommodation
  - Allows the eye to clearly focus objects within a 6M range.
  - When the lens is accommodating:
    - The ciliary muscles contract and the choroid moves anteriorly.
    - The tension on the zonule fibers is released. The lens bulges.
  - When the lens is not accommodating:
    - Ciliary muscle is relaxed.
    - Zonules pull on the lens.
    - Capsule is under tension.
    - The lens is flat.
  - Radius of curvature of the anterior and posterior surface changes during accommodation.
    - Most of the change is due to the anterior surface.
    - The anterior pole of the lens moves forward.

2. Composition of Lens

- The lens is composed of a mass of lens fibers enclosed in a capsule.
- The lens has the highest protein content (33%) compared to of all body tissues.
- Types of lens proteins:
  - Soluble
    - α, β, and γ crystalline mostly in lens cortex
  - Insoluble
    - Albuminoid mostly found in nucleus

Composition	
Water	66%
Proteins	33%
Insoluble	-15%
Soluble	-85%
α-crystallin	-15%
β-crystallin	-55%
γ-crystallin	-15%
Lipids, Salts, Carbohydrates	1%

3. Difference in Composition between Lens and Aqueous

- Greater change in refractive index at the air-cornea interface than at the aqueous-lens and the lens-vitreous interfaces. Thus, the lens has less refractive power than the cornea.
- The lens alters the aqueous by using glucose, amino acids, and other solutes as metabolites and produces and releases lactic acid back into the aqueous.
- The aqueous is 98.7% water, while the lens is 66% water.
- Some of the lens proteins are in low concentration in the aqueous. Patients with senile cataracts have higher concentrations of these proteins suggesting the proteins leak from the lens.

4. Metabolism of Lens (Various Pathways Essential to Lens)

- The lens is avascular and receives all its nutrients from the aqueous.
- The lens requires a steady supply of glucose and oxygen to support:
  - The high energy demands of protein synthesis for reproduction and growth
  - The active sodium water pump in the epithelial cell membranes that maintain lens dehydration
    - 1 molecule glucose = 2 ATP molecules
- Metabolic pathways used by the lens include
  - Glycolytic pathway – 80%
    - Main lens pathway used for energy production.
  - Krebs (oxidative) cycle
  - Hexose monophosphate (pentose) shunt – 15%
    - Used to produce pentose for RNA synthesis and NADPH to maintain lens glutathione.
  - Sorbitol pathway
    - Insignificant contribution to energy, but important in production of diabetic and galactosemic cataracts.
- Glucose metabolism end products include lactic acid, CO_2, and H_2O. Lactic acid diffuses into the aqueous.

5. Types of Lens Proteins

- The human lens has the highest protein concentration (33%) of any tissue in the body.
- The proteins are synthesized in the anterior epithelium and equatorial zone. The anterior lens epithelium also transports the amino acids from the aqueous, which are synthesized into proteins.
- The initial separation of lens proteins is based on their solubility (15% insoluble, 85% soluble).
  - Water insoluble proteins (albuminoid) include membrane bound proteins and aggregated crystallins.
  - Water soluble proteins include alpha, beta, and gamma crystallins.

6. Factors which Regulate Size and Solubility of Lens Proteins

- Ascorbic acid (vitamin C)
  - Present in high concentrations in the lens and its environment.
  - Function: Reducing agent and free-radical scavenger, which generates hydrogen peroxide in the process.
  - It is also known that ascorbic acid in the presence of light and a metal ion (or riboflavin) spontaneously forms hydrogen peroxide.
- Glutathione
  - Present in high concentration, actively synthesized in the lens.
  - Function:
    - Contains sulfhydryl groups which preserve the physiochemical equilibrium of lens proteins by reducing disulfide bonds.
    - Maintains transport pumps (amino acid, xenobiotic removal, Na^+/K^+ pump) and the molecular integrity of lens fiber membranes.
    - Detoxifies hydrogen peroxide.
- Ion transport
  - Na/K current loops cycle nutrients in the lens.

- Na concentration greater posterior (net movement of Na from posterior to anterior).
- K concentration greater anterior (net movement of K from anterior to posterior).

7. Theories of Lens Transparency

- Lack of light scattering particles
  - Loss of vascular components during development
  - Absence of visible light absorbing chromophores.
  - When new epithelial cells are elongating and still have organelles, they are not in the visual axis.
- Regular arrangement of crystalline protein within the fiber cells
  - Highly organized structure gives minimal light scatter.
  - This minimizes small particle scatter (SPS) in the lens fiber cell by destructive interference, which means scatter from 2 neighboring molecules cancels out
- Small spacing between lens components
  - Refractive index between protein molecules is close to zero.

8. Mitotic Activity of Lens Epithelium

- Mitosis mostly occurs slightly anterior to the equator. There is no mitotic activity in the central zone.
- There is continuous regeneration and migration throughout life.
- The lens fibers originate in the epithelium.
  - The new cells near the anterior pole are cuboidal. As the cells migrate towards the equator from the pre-equatorial region, they elongate and form into lens fibers.
- The younger fibers are laid down on top of the older ones. Epithelial cells are pushed around the equator to the posterior side of the lens. Posterior cells get pushed more posterior and then elongate.
- The older fibers become tightly packed to form the nucleus of the lens. The younger fibers near the surface form the cortex.
  - The result is a soft cortex with a hard nucleus and a continual change in refractive index from cortex to nucleus.
- The lens bow is the swirl of nuclei as they are displaced in mitosis and the lens grows in diameter in all directions like an onion skin.

9. Aging Changes in Composition of the Lens

- Physical features
  - Lens yellowing and brunescence, which decreases the transparency
  - Increased weight and volume
  - No change in refractive power due to cancellation between:
    - Increased thickness and curvature
    - Increased refractive index
- Physiology
  - Enzyme activity
    - Decreased for most enzymes
    - Increased for proteolytic enzymes and glycosidases
  - Increased Na:K ratio
    - Gain Na^+ ions and water
    - Slight loss of K^+ ions
    - Corresponds to increased lens optical density
- Composition
  - Decreased:
    - Soluble lens protein
    - Glutathione
    - Amino acids
    - Inositol
    - ATP content

- Increased:
  - Insoluble lens protein
  - Calcium ions

LENS/CATARACT (PATHOLOGY)

1. Epidemiology, History, and Symptom Inventory

- Epidemiology
  - One of the greatest causes of blindness worldwide
  - Defined as any lens opacity
  - Risk factors
    - Age is the major contributor
    - UV exposure
    - Nutritional & metabolic deficiencies
    - Trauma
    - Genetics
- History
  - Attention to systemic diseases, medications, functional visual status and risk factors
    - Associated ocular diseases: uveitis, retinitis pigmentosa
    - Systemic medications: corticosteroids
    - Systemic disorders: diabetes
    - Congenital developmental syndromes: Down syndrome
  - May be found at birth or develop through the life of the patient
- Symptom inventory
  - Painless, progressive vision loss unless the cataract is due to trauma
  - Reduced contrast sensitivity
  - Glare
  - Reduced vision

2. Observation, Inspection, Recognition of Signs, and Techniques, and Skills

Observation, Inspection

- DFE
- Refraction
- Slit lamp examination
  - Use a 45° angle between microscope and light beam.
  - Examine lens with overall view, optic section with bright illumination, and then with retro-illumination.
  - Begin with examination at center of lens and work backwards toward the anterior capsule.
  - Attention should be given to the zones of discontinuity.
- Pre-cataract extraction and IOL implant
  - Potential acuity meter (PAM) to analyze posterior segment quality if cataract is present.
  - Keratometry and A scan biometry to calculate the power of the IOL implant.

Techniques Using SLE		
Cataract Type	**Illumination**	**Beam**
Nuclear	Diffuse	Optic section Oblique beam for NS
Cortical	Retro	
PSC	Retro	Oblique beam

3. Developmental Anomalies

- Disorders may involve abnormalities in shape and size of lens, position in the eye, and clarity.
- **Mittendorf Dot**
  - Part of hyaloid system.
  - Circular white opacity located inferior nasal on posterior lens capsule.
  - Typically small with no reduction in vision.
- **Vogt's Reflex Line**
  - Part of hyaloid system.
  - Faint grayish reversed C-shaped thin line on posterior lens surface

- No affect on vision
- **Coloboma**
  - Incomplete lens development
  - A notch in the lens edge may be associated with iris and retinal colobomas
- **Lens Luxation**
  - Can be acquired from trauma or part of syndromes (**Marfan's** - luxated up, **Homocystinuria** - luxated down)
- **Lenticonus**
  - Conical deformity with projection of either the anterior or posterior lens surface
  - Usually unilateral with irregular astigmatism, myopia or reduced acuity
  - Anterior lenticonus → **Alport's Syndrome**
  - Posterior lenticonus→ **Lowe's Syndrome** (also associated with glaucoma and mental retardation
- **Microphakia**
  - Abnormally small lens
  - May be associated with other lens abnormalities, extreme myopia, and **Marchesani Syndrome** (short stature, stubby fingers and toes)

4. Congenital Cataracts

- Congenital cataracts are present at birth or develop within 3 months after birth. May be unilateral or bilateral, stable or progressive, and vary in location and severity.
- Etiology
  - Duration and timing of exposure to cataractogenic agent during pregnancy is key to development
  - 25% of congenital cataracts are inherited and part of syndromes
  - Most congenital cataracts are idiopathic
  - Bilateral congenital cataracts are frequently inherited with autonomic dominant transmission
- Common causes of abnormal lens development and congenital cataracts:
  - Ionizing radiation – 1st trimester, X-irradiation involving pelvis region
  - Drugs – 1st trimester, corticosteroids, certain antibiotics, sulfonamides
  - Metabolic diseases – diabetes, galactosemia, hypocalcaemia, parathyroid disorders
  - Maternal malnutrition
  - Intrauterine infection – toxoplasmosis, rubella, cytomegalovirus
- **Embryonic Nuclear Cataract** – grainy, axial central opacity
- **Cataracta Centralis Pulveralenta** – granular central opacity
- **Sutural Cataract** – usually bilateral, about 30% of congenital cataracts. Opacities described as stellate, stalagmite, or coral in shape. Vision usually good
- **Anterior Polar** – Cotton ball-like opacity in the anterior sub-capsule.
  - Little or no visual decrease
  - Composed by hyaline material, calcium, cholesterol, and degenerating lens fibers
- **Posterior Polar** – Same as anterior polar except under posterior capsule
  - May be associated with hyaloids remnant
  - Greater decrease in vision due to posterior location
- **Pyramidal** – cone-shaped opacity
- **Zonulae-Lamellar** – most common congenital cataract (40%) – usually bilateral
  - Affects one lamella of zone of lens fibers
  - Seen as a circular zone with a clear center
  - May have spokes or "riders" of overlying affected fibers
  - Opacity appears disc shaped when viewed frontally
  - Associated with abnormal calcium metabolism so abnormalities of tooth enamel and formation
- **Total** –diffuse, frequently inherited, all fibers affected, seen as a white mass within the pupil

5. Age-Related Cataracts

- **Juvenile Cataracts** – involve the juvenile nucleus and present **after 3 months** of age and into adolescence or mid teens. Visual acuity is usually minimally affected
- **Pre-senile Cataracts –** involve adult nucleus or cortex and are usually considered premature onset of "senile" or age related cataracts
- **Age Related "Senile" Cataracts** – cataracts related to oxidative stress and resulting in protein modifications
  - Risk factors include aging, smoking, corticosteroid use, diabetes, and UV light
  - **Cortical Cataracts**
    - Involve the cortex of the lens, considered "soft" due to fluid component of development.
    - Changes are from hydration and intumescence (swelling). Fluid is absorbed into the lens from the aqueous due to increasing permeability of the lens capsule. There is an imbalance of electrolytes with increased lens hydration and liquefaction of fibers. Opacification develops with breakdown and coagulation of protein.
    - Incidence: 2.7% ages 43-54, 26% of patients >75 years
    - Symptoms: glare, decreased acuity, decreased contrast, monocular diplopia, slight increase in hyperopic refraction
    - Clinical features and stages
      - Vacuoles – circular pocket of fluid
      - Water clefts – linear fluid filled regions
      - Spokes (cuniform) – wedge shaped opacities
      - Lamellar separation – fine separations of lamellae by fluid
      - Diffuse opacification – mature – entire cortex is hazy and eventually more gray to white in color
      - Hypermature – entire cortex is completely opaque and white
      - Phacotoxic – pancoanaphylactica – escape of lenticular amino acids into aqueous may incite lens induced uveitis and phacolytic glaucoma
      - Swelling of cortex increases its size which may shallow the anterior chamber with secondary narrow angle glaucoma a complication

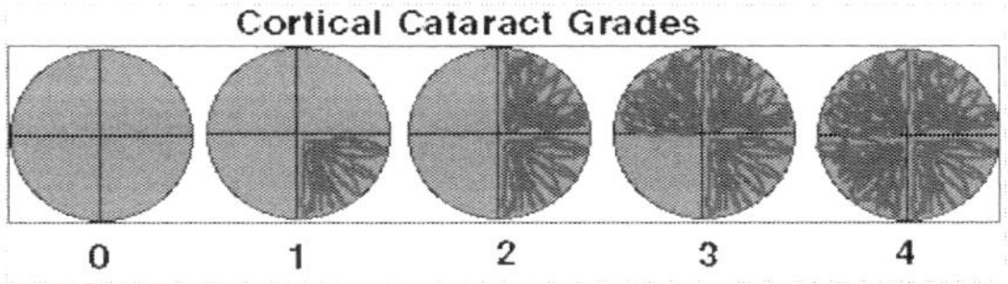

  - **Nuclear Cataracts**
    - Located in embryonic or fetal nucleus
    - Newly formed fibers push and compress the older fiber into the center of the lens. This compaction produces a hardening (**sclerosis**) of fibers and an increase in the optical density of the nucleus and a higher refractive index.
    - Modification of proteins and the formation of urochrome pigment in nuclear cataracts accounts for their golden color in more advanced stages. Nuclear sclerosis involves any of the nuclear layers.
    - Considered "hard" cataracts
    - Incidence: 4.8% ages 43-54, 55% of patients >75
    - Symptoms: distance blur, myopic refractive shift, improved near vision (second sight), loss of color discrimination, diplopia
    - Clinical features and stages
      - Slight yellow color from posterior nuclear fibers with central lens lines visible
      - Increase in yellowing with loss of central lens lines
      - Entire nucleus is golden in color with central zone a pearly opalescence color
      - Mature – entire nucleus is brown to dark brown or black in color
  - **Posterior Subcapsular Cataracts**
    - Located at the nodal point of the eye. Two main types:
      - Cupuliform (cup or saucer shape)- associated with aging, myotonic dystrophy, atopic dermatitis, corticosteroids, more common
      - Complicated – less common, associated with longstanding intraocular disease
    - Incidence: 1.7% ages 43-54, 11% of patients > 75 years

- Symptoms: decrease in vision especially in bright light or reading
- Clinical features
  - Cupuliform cataracts are saucer shaped granular opacification under posterior subcapsular region – the opacification spreads along this region (not into the overlying cortex). Faint iridescence of blue/green colors may be associated with this type
  - Complicated cataracts also involve the subcapsular region as well as the adjacent cortex and may spread axially. Polychromatic colors of blues, reds, and greens are highly associated with this type of cataract
- Risk factors: Renal failure, Glaucoma surgery, Diabetes, Chronic corticosteroid use

6. Miscellaneous Types

- **Traumatic Cataract** – stellate or "rosette" (shaped like a rose or flower) in shape especially seen in blunt ocular trauma, typically involves the anterior or posterior subcapsular region and may develop within hours of injury or years following. Trauma where the lens has been directly touched from penetration may result in rapid opacification of most of the lens fibers. Examples of traumatic insult: electric shock, concussion.
- **Coronary Cataract** – crown-shaped opacification arranged in a radial distribution around the periphery of the adult nucleus or cortex. No significant visual decrease, etiology unknown.
- **Cerulean (Blue dot) Cataract** – Bluish punctate opacities within adult nucleus or cortex. No significant visual decrease, etiology unknown.
- **Diabetic Cataract** – white punctate or snowflake-like opacities within anterior or posterior subcapsular regions. Associated with diabetes – caused by elevated glucose levels from glucose in the aqueous. Rapid development. Glucose goes through sorbitol pathway, leading to an increase in sorbitol concentration within the lens fiber. This draws water into the fiber, causing swelling of the lens fibers and increases the risk of rupture.
- **Crystalline Cataract** – multicolored crystalline-like opacities within adult nucleus or cortex – no significant visual decrease, etiology unknown.

7. Cataract Extraction

- Cataract surgery is the most frequent surgical procedure in those 65 years or older and represent 80% of ocular surgery.
- Cataract surgery should be considered when the quality of vision resulting from cataracts begins to affect a patient's daily activities.
- The procedure can be done at any stage of cataract development with the specific timing varying from patient to patient depending upon their visual requirements.
- **ICCE (intracapsular cataract extraction)** technique – involves the removal of the entire lens capsule, required very thick glasses or later on contact lenses for patients to recover vision.
- **ECCE (extracapsular cataract extraction)** technique – suture-less clear corneal incisions and intraocular lens implants or IOLS.
- Surgical ocular complications of cataract extraction:
  - Corneal edema
  - Infection – enophthalmitis
  - Prolonged inflammation – uveitis, glaucoma, hyphemas **(UGH Syndrome)**
  - Iris prolapsed – secondary to trauma, Valsalva maneuver
  - Iris "capture" or IOL
  - Iris atrophy
  - IOL decentration
  - Posterior capsule tear with vitreous loss, loss of lens fragments into vitreous can result in chronic inflammation, uveitis, glaucoma, cystoids macular edema
  - Retained cortical material with chronic inflammation
  - Retinal detachment
  - Opacification of posterior capsule by residual epithelial cells and regeneration of lens fibers – aka **Elschnig's pearls** result in decreased vision. YAG laser creates central opening incapsule (**YAG capsulotomy**)

Chapter 14 – Episclera/Sclera/Anterior Uvea

SCLERA (GROSS ANATOMY)

- A thick, dense connective tissue layer that is continuous with the corneal stroma at the limbus. The stroma maintains the shape of the globe, offers resistance to internal and external forces, and provides an attachment for the extraocular muscle insertion.

1. Size

- Sclera runs from the limbus of the cornea to the optic nerve.
- Forms the posterior 5/6 of the connective tissue of the globe.
- 80% of the surface area of the globe is sclera.

2. Radius of Curvature

- Radius of Curvature: 11 mm

3. Thickness

- It is thinnest posterior to the insertion of the four recti muscles (0.3mm).
- The anterior sclera near the limbus is 0.8 mm thick.
- Thickness at the equator varies between 0.4-0.6 mm.
- Sclera is thickest near the optic nerve.

4. Color

- Anterior sclera visible through a healthy conjunctiva and appears opaque and white.
- Becomes yellow with age, sclerosis, fatty deposits, and liver disease.
- Becomes blue with thinning:
    - Infant sclera have a blue tint because it is almost transparent and the underlying pigmented vascular uvea can show through.

5. Relationship to Conjunctiva, Tenon's Capsule, Suprachoroidal Space

- Conjunctiva:
    - Anteriorly, the episclera is in contact with loose subconjunctival tissue and the cornea.
- Tenon's capsule:
    - Outer to the sclera, but not a part of the sclera.
    - Is a dense collagenous layer which is found between the superficial conjunctival stroma and the underlying episcleral tissue.
    - Is thickest in the regions of the extraocular muscle insertion.
    - The episcleral space is the potential space between Tenon's capsule and the episclera.
- Suprachoroidal space:
    - Space between the sclera and choroid where the long and short posterior ciliary nerves travel.
    - On its internal surface, the sclera is adjacent to the choroid and the ciliary body.
    - The suprachoroidal tissues lie close to, and to a certain extent, blend with the internal collagen lamina fusca of the sclera.

6. Emissaria (Contents, location)

- There are channels in the sclera for the passage of arteries, veins, and nerves into or out of the eye. These are divided into anterior and posterior groups:
    - Anterior channels:
        - Found in the limbus and consists of venous branches of the deep and intrascleral plexus.

- Join the episcleral venous plexus and small vessels from the anterior ciliary arteries, which supply the limbal and peripheral corneal tissues.
  - Posterior channels:
    - The optic nerve
    - Lamina cribosa
    - The four vortex veins
    - The long posterior ciliary arteries and nerves (they enter at the back of the eye and run anteriorly through the choroid and ciliary body to the cornea without branching).
    - The short posterior ciliary arteries and nerves
- Contains 65% water (compared to the cornea which contains 72% to 82% water). This difference allows for tighter packing of collagen fibers, irregular fiber arrangement, and opaque color.

7. Composition

- Episclera (superficial layer):
  - Anterior episclera is a loose, vascular connective tissue which is really a part of the superficial sclera stroma.
  - The equatorial episclera posterior to the rectus muscle insertions is thinner than the anterior portion, is loosely joined with Tenon's capsule by fine strands of collagen, and is relatively avascular.
  - Has spaces providing passage for arteries, veins, and nerves.
- Scleral stroma (middle layer):
  - Composed entirely of bundles of collagen and fibroblasts with moderate amount of ground substance.
  - Lamellae and fibrils are in a disarrayed pattern, which aids destructive interference. This is why the sclera is opaque or white.
- Lamina fusca (deep layer):
  - Consists of modified internal scleral lamellae which merge with the underlying suprachoroidea (or supraciliaris).
  - There is a marked increase of pigment in the area due to the presence of increased numbers of melanocytes and pigmented macrophages.

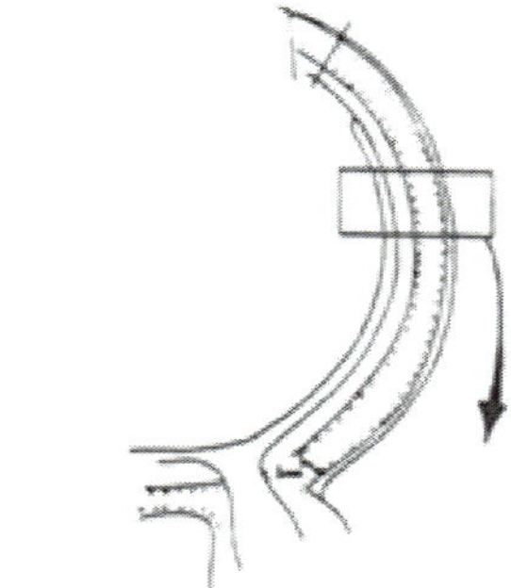

8. Lamina Cribrosa (Structure)

- Highly perforated part of sclera through which the optic nerve passes.
- Formed from sclera with many perforations (holes)
- 1.5 mm in diameter.
- Firm attachment for the optic nerve to the back of the eye.
- The principal part of the lamina cribosa is formed by an extension of collagen bundles and elastic fibers from the inner two thirds of the sclera across the optic nerve canal.
- **Lamina cribrosa, or cribriform plate**, serves two functions:
  - It forms a scaffold for the passage of bundles of optic nerve axons, anchoring the bundles to each other and to the sides of the optic nerve canal.
  - It reinforces the posterior eye, protecting it from injury at the site of the nerve exit.

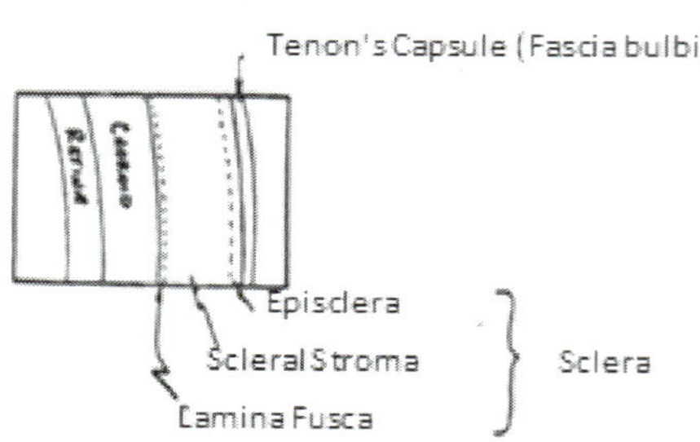

SCLERA (DEVELOPMENTAL ANATOMY)

1. Inductive Mechanisms

- Development of the pigmentary epithelium. The structural growth is dependent upon interactions amongst other differentiating tissues.
- The RPE is the driving element within the optic cup to induce scleral cartilage formation.

2. Tissue Origin

- Sclera forms from the mesodermal germ layer.
- By the 4th week, mesenchyme forms an anterior scleral condensation around the front edges of the optic cup.
- By the 7th week, the posterior-developing sclera is halfway to the posterior pole completing its development by the 8th week.
- By the end of the 3rd month the sclera has surrounded the choroid.
- The sclera thickens during the 5th month and by 6th month scleral tissue penetrates the optic nerve forming the lamina cribrosa.

3. Comparison with Cornea

- Curvature:
    - During early development the cornea and sclera have the same radii of curvature.
    - By the 3rd month as the anterior chamber develops the corneal curvature increases compared to the sclera.
    - Mesodermal ingrowth is the primordium of the anterior chamber.
- Transparency:
    - Until the 4th month the cornea and sclera are both transparent.
    - After the 4th month the sclera loses its uniform collagen fiber arrangement and becomes opaque.

ANTERIOR CHAMBER AND ANGLE (GROSS ANATOMY)

1. Shape and Volume

- The shape is roughly ellipsoidal with the posterior surface of the ellipsoid flattened because of the iris.
- Volume is 0.25 mL.
- Anterior chamber angle is formed at the peripheral meeting of the corneosclera and uvea. This is where the aqueous leaves the anterior chamber.

2. Boundaries

- **Anteriorly** by the corneal endothelium.
- **Posteriorly** by the anterior surface of the iris and the pupillary portion of the lens capsule.
- **Peripherally** by the trabecular meshwork on the anterior side, and by the ciliary body and iris root on the posterior side.

3. Depth

- **Diameter:** 12 mm (which is the same as the cornea and iris)
- **Depth:** 3.61 to 3.70 mm for males and 3.41 to 3.65 for females
    - The chamber is deeper in the center than the periphery.

4. Trabecular Meshwork (Components, Ultrastructure)

- It occupies most of the **internal scleral sulcus.**

- It is triangular in shape. The apex is near the end of Descemet's membrane (Schwalbe's line) and the base is formed by the scleral spur and the ciliary body.
- At the apex near the cornea, it is 3 to 5 layers thick.
- At the base, it is 15 to 20 layers thick.
- There are 3 sections of trabeculum:
    - **Corneoscleral meshwork:**
        - A major component which consists of flat fenestrated sheets of tissue (collagen fibers surrounded by endothelium) having filtering holes called "intratrabecular spaces".
        - There are larger filtering holes, (6 to 12 microns in diameter), called the "spaces of Fontana." These holes are large near the anterior chamber angle and decrease in size towards the canal of Schlemm.
    - **Uveal meshwork:**
        - Is the most internal component of the trabecular meshwork, and is very thin
        - Is derived from the iris and ciliary body
        - Is the most anterior extension of the uvea
        - Sometimes called "uveal chords"
        - Muscular extensions from the ciliary body attach to the uveal meshwork and open up trabecular spaces, which increases aqueous outflow.
        - The scleral spur can be found in between the uveal and corneoscleral meshwork.
    - **Pectinate fibers or iris processes:**
        - Extend from the iris root to the uveal meshwork and bridges the anterior chamber angle
        - There are about 100 per eye.
        - They usually insert at the scleral spur region and extend as far forward as the middle of the trabecular meshwork.

5. Juxtacanalicular Tissue (Components, Ultrastructure)

- It is also called the cribriform layer.
- The region separating the endothelial cell lining the canal of Schlemm from the trabecular meshwork.
- 10 to 20 microns thick when measured between the basement membrane of the endothelium of Schlemm's canal and the nearest intratrabecular space.
- Consists of endothelial-like cells, collagen and elastic-like fibers, and ground substance.

6. Schlemm's Canal (Location, Size, Ultrastructure of Wall, Afferent and Efferent Connections)

- A circular venous channel which lies in the outer portion of the internal scleral sulcus within the limbus. It is located outside the trabecular meshwork and anterior to the scleral spur.
    - The external wall of the canal lies against the limbal sclera, the internal wall lies against the trabecular meshwork and sclera spur
- Ring of canal has a 36 mm circumference and a flattened elliptical cross section.
- Meridional width varies between 350 and 500 microns.
- Endothelial lining surrounds the internal wall of Schlemm's canal.
    - Aside from the endothelium, there is no real wall around Schlemm's canal
    - The endothelium is strong, and only fine suspensions can pass into the canal.
    - The canal is anchored to the criboform layer (juxtacanalicular tissue) by a fibrous network that is also connected to the ciliary muscle tendon
- Internal collecting channels of Schlemm's canal are cumulatively known as the *internal collector channels of Sondermann.*

7. Scleral Spur (Composition, Location)

- Lies at the posterior edge of the internal scleral sulcus.
- The posterior portion of the scleral spur is the attachment site for the tendon of the longitudinal ciliary muscle fibers.
- The anterior portion is continuous with that of trabeculae.

- In cross section, it resembles a spur-like projection, and it provides a functionally important insertion point for the longitudinal muscle of the ciliary body and some corneoscleral chords.
- Can be observed with gonioscopy.

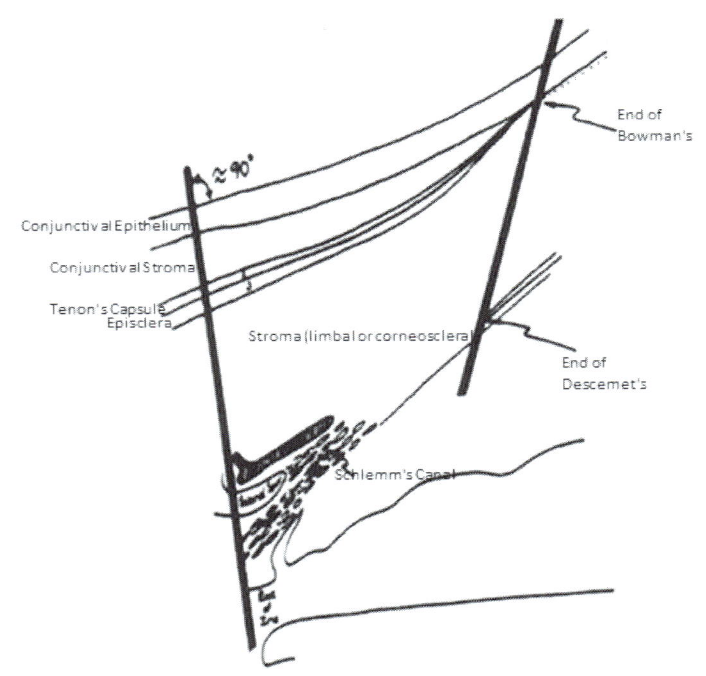

8. Schwalbe's Ring (Composition, Location)

- The termination of Descemet's membrane.
- The trabecular meshwork sheets extend posteriorly from Schwalbe's line to the scleral spur.
- Composed of collagen fibers.
- An anatomical landmark in gonioscopy used by clinicians while examining the deep corneolimbus region.
- Looks like a ring running around the inside of the eye at the anterior end of the uveal chords.

ANTERIOR CHAMBER AND ANGLE (DEVELOPMENTAL ANATOMY)

1. Creation of Anatomical Space

- One theory is that the primitive anterior chamber represented by a cleft in mesoderm appears as a result of the disappearance of mesoderm in the area between the developing cornea and iris.
- Another theory is that the anterior chamber results from 3 stages of mesodermal ingrowth.
    - The 1st ingrowth forms the corneal endothelium.
    - The 2nd ingrowth forms the corneal stroma.
    - A third wave of mesoderm forms the iris stroma.
    - The cleft between the first and third mesodermal ingrowths is the primordium of the anterior chamber.

2. Factors that Promote Growth of Anterior Chamber

- Anterior chamber begins to form at an early stage as a space surrounded by mesoderm long before the rim of the optic cup grows forward and inward to form the ectodermal basis of the ciliary body and iris. Some say the anterior chamber is present by the 6th week as a narrow chink in the mesoderm between the surface ectoderm and the anterior surface of the lens vesicle.
- The anterior chamber is present by the 5th month. It is characterized as a well-marked cleft between the corneal endothelium and the mesodermal portion of the iris. Growth of the chamber is believed to be due to the disappearance of the mesothelium and to the growth of the anterior segment.

3. Creation of Angle

- Whén the anterior chamber is small its periphery is occupied by mesodermal tissue lying between the rim of the optic cup and the surface ectoderm. The point where the anterior chamber angle does not exist is evident after the Canal of Schlemm becomes visible.
- As the angle of the anterior chamber becomes gradually deeper there are large changes in the topographical relationships between structures.

- The relationship between the Canal of Schlemm, the uveo-scleral trabeculae, scleral spur, and the major circle remains fairly constant, but their positions with regard to the anterior chamber angle changes continually as the position of the developing angle shifts posteriorly.
- At birth, the angle has reached the posterior or basal portion of the meshwork with the scleral spur and Canal of Schlemm well in front of it. The development of the ciliary muscle provides the greatest contribution to the change in topographical relationship in this area, as well as contributing to the formation of the angle.

- Four theories of the formation of the angle:
  - **Atrophy theory:** Mesodermal absorption over time in the periphery of the anterior chamber. Failure of the mesodermal tissue to separate and atrophy leads to congenital glaucoma.
  - **Cleavage theory:** Separation of two dissimilar layers of mesodermal tissue, which grow unequally. The cleavage occurs along the line of the inner layer of the uveal trabeculae. The displacement caused by the growth of the ciliary muscle aids this process.
  - **Rarefaction theory** (not found in any text).
  - **Reorganization theory:** Rearrangement, expansion and dilation of spaces between cells.

4. Differentiation of Schlemm's Canal, Scleral Spur, Trabecular Meshwork

- During the latter part of the 3rd month, the **Canal of Schlemm** (COS) appears as a small plexus of venous channels within fibers of the corneo-scleral condensation. By the 8th month of gestation an outflow path exists connecting the COS with the scleral veins.
- Sondermann considers the development of COS as depending on the alterations of IOP, which occur as the fetal eye differentiates.
  - At first the canal is present not as a single vessel but formed from radial veins, which at the end of the 3rd month conveys blood from the margin of the optic cup to the anterior ciliary vessels.
  - During the 3rd month considerable hardening of the anterior part of the sclera occurs which causes the pressure to slowly increase on the penetrating veins.
  - This increased pressure results in the development of stasis pressure and in dilation of the distal parts of the veins.
  - The dilation is so great that anastomoses between the vessels occur thus forming COS.
- During the 4th month a triangular wedge of dense scleral condensation appears immediately behind the COS. It is continuous with the meridional fibers of the ciliary muscle and gradually consolidates to form the **scleral spur.**
- The ciliary muscle is slow to reach full development which is not achieved until shortly after birth.
- During the 5th to 6th month the angle deepens and the loose mesodermal tissue lying between the COS and the root of the iris differentiates into a fan-like bundle of widely spaced anastomosing strands which ultimately constitutes the scleral and uveal portion of the **trabecular meshwork.**

5. Endothelial Membrane

- This membrane appears continuous at gestational month 7 but is discontinuous in the region of the meshwork by 9th month.
- During the last few weeks before birth, splits occur between cells in the membrane, and the size and number of these splits increase rapidly because of the increase in the size of the anterior ocular structures.
- The loss of continuity increases the facility of aqueous outflow.

IRIS (GROSS ANATOMY)

---

1. Gross Landmarks, Zones

- Iris is the most anterior extension of the uveal tract and divides the anterior and posterior chambers
- **Collarette:**
  - The thickest part of the iris.
  - About 1.5 mm from the pupillary margin.

- It is a slightly raised, jagged ridge that was the attachment site for the fetal pupillary membrane during embryonic development.
    - It divides the iris into 2 zones (pupillary and ciliary).
    - It is the site of the minor arteriole circle of the iris.
- **Pupillary zone:** The narrow, central region of the iris internal to the collarette that encircles the pupil.
    - The pupil is located slightly nasal and inferior to the iris center. Pupil size regulates the illumination of the retina.
- **Ciliary zone:** The region located closer to the ciliary body and is wider, stretches from the collarette to the iris root.
- **Iris root:** Thinnest part of the iris (0.5mm thick), joins the iris to the anterior aspect of the ciliary body.
- **Fuch's crypts:** Caverns that go into the anterior surface of the iris. They are in both the pupillary and ciliary portion. The walls are heavily pigmented and more common in dark eyes.

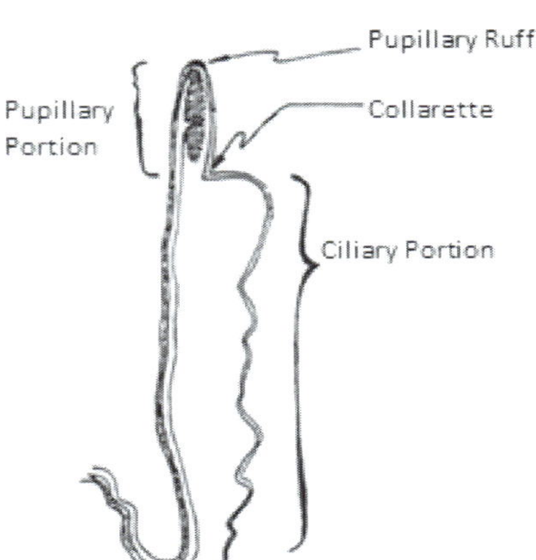

2. Diameter

- The iris is a thin circular structure 12mm in diameter and 37.5mm in circumference.
- The pupil diameter can range from 1mm to 9mm.
- Thickest at the collarette 0.60 mm thick.

3. Coloration (Factors Controlling)

- Melanin is the only pigment present. It is produced by and found in melanocytes.
- The density of pigment in the most superficial layer of the iris and arrangement of the connective tissue in the anterior border layer and stroma determines the color of the eye.
- The balance between the reflection of the blood vessels and melanocytes makes the iris color. The pigment absorbs the light.
    - Light pigment: Blue eyes
        - The lack of pigment allows light to scatter, resulting in a blue wavelength seen similar to the blue sky effect of light scattering
    - Medium pigment: Green/Hazel eyes
    - Heavy pigment: Brown eyes
    - Brown iris color is coded by dominant genes, while blue iris color is coded by recessive genes.
- Hyperpigmentation (accumulation of melanocytes) may occur as a freckle or nevus in the anterior border layer.
- In all colored irises (except the albino iris) the two epithelial layers are heavily pigmented.

4. Anterior Border (Composition, Ultrastructure)

- Most anterior (surface) layer of the iris, ends at the iris root.
- Condensation of stromal tissue.
- Composed of 2 cell types: Fibroblasts & pigmented melanocytes as well as collagen fibrils.
- Fibroblasts form a relatively continuous single layer of cells over the surface of the iris from the base to the pupillary margin.
- Melanocytes are deep to fibroblasts. The thickness of the melanocyte layer may vary forming freckle-like masses and contribute to iris colors.
- The collagen fibrils are radially arranged in columns and seen as the visible white fibers in lighter-colored irides.
- Source of iris processes near root which attach to the trabecular meshwork.

5. Stroma (Composition)

- The iris stroma is continuous with the stroma of the ciliary body.

- Consists of loose collagen fibrils, ground substance, elastin fibrils, pigmented, and non-pigmented cells.
- The thickest portion of the iris.
- Cells in the stroma:
    - Non-pigmented:
        - Lymphocytes
        - Fibroblasts:
            - Most common cell type.
            - Produce collagen fibers, ground substance, and elastin.
        - Macrophages
        - Mast cells:
            - Part of the immune system.
            - They release histamine if there is an ocular inflammation. This stimulates iris blood vessels and can result in iritis.
    - Pigmented:
        - Melanocytes
        - Clump cells (Pigmented Macrophages):
            - Found mostly in pupillary region.
            - They are large, round cells that eat other cells, debris, and also melanin granules which they digest and break down.

6. Sphincter Muscle (Type, Composition, Innervation)

- Smooth muscle confined to the pupillary portion of the stroma, and is circular in shape.
- Measures 0.75 to 1.0 mm in diameter and 0.10 to 0.17 mm thick.
- The bundles of muscle cells are closely packed, connected by gap junctions, and are separated by a thin but dense layer of collagen which runs from the stroma anterior to the dilator muscle.
- The sphincter is anchored firmly to the adjacent stroma and retains function even if severed.
- Contraction of the sphincter causes the pupil to constrict (**miosis**).
    - Its action is like a purse string; it reduces the size of the pupil evenly and uniformly when stimulated. The muscle is able to shorten by 87%.
- Innervation is by the parasympathetic system:
    - Motor nerves which supply the sphincter enter the eye via the Short Ciliary nerves.
    - The sphincter constricts in response to drugs such as parasympathomimetics and anticholinesterases.

7. Anterior Epithelium (Ultrastructure)

- Located posterior to the stroma and anterior to the posterior epithelial layer.
- Somewhat pigmented, but less than the posterior pigmented epithelium.
- Continuous with the external pigment epithelium layer over the ciliary body.
- Consists of **myoepithelial cells** with epithelial apical sides against the apical surface of the posterior pigment epithelium, and a muscular basal side.
- The basal side has muscular processes that make up the dilator muscle.
- The muscular processes are surrounded by the basement membrane.
- Most of the fibers are found in the ciliary portion and point toward the pupil. They extend about halfway through the width of the sphincter.
- The fibers interdigitate with the sphincter fibers at the termination of the dilator (Fuch's Spur) and about halfway (Michel's Spur) between the papillary border and collarette.

8. Dilator Muscle (Type, Composition, Innervation)

- Developed from and is an integral part of the anterior iris epithelium.
- The muscular basal processes have the histologic and pharmacologic characteristics of smooth muscle and are arranged radially.

- Constriction of the dilator muscle causes the pupil to enlarge (**mydriasis**).
- The innervation is by sympathetic nerve fibers (Adrenergic) that originate in the Superior Cervical ganglion. The fibers innervate the dilator at the apical side.
- There are also parasympathetic nerve endings in and around the dilator, but they probably are extensions of those to the sphincter muscle.
- The muscle fibers are all coupled together with direct electric contact between them. So, if any potential propagates down one fiber, the potential will go through the whole network of fibers, resulting in the muscle acting as a whole unit. This way the iris accomplishes the uniform dilation of the pupil.

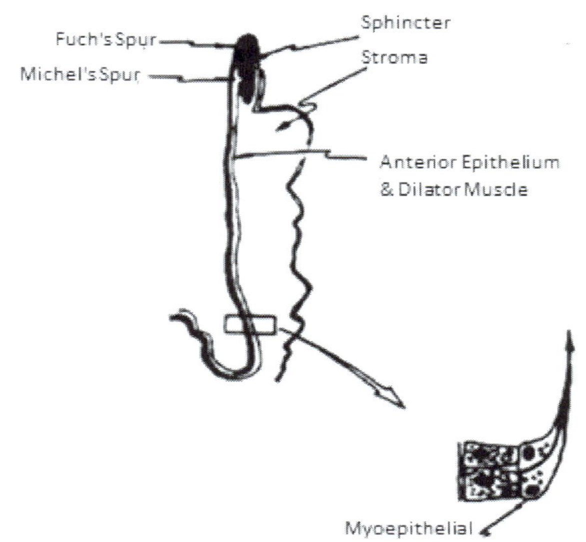

9. Posterior Epithelium

- Single row of tall, heavily pigmented, columnar epithelial cells in which the apical surface is against the apical side of the anterior epithelial cells.
- The basal surface contacts with the aqueous humor of the posterior chamber.
- As you move from the iris to the ciliary body, the pigmented epithelium loses pigment and becomes the non-pigmented epithelium of the ciliary body.
- The basement membrane of the posterior pigment epithelium is adjacent to the aqueous at the pupillary margin of the iris. These cells curl around the posterior iris to the anterior surface at the pupillary margin forming the **pupillary ruff**.
- The posterior epithelium lies but is normally not adherent posterior to the anterior lens. An abnormal adherent attachment between the posterior iris surface and the anterior lens is known as a **posterior synechiae.**

10. Blood Supply, Venous Drainage

- Iris has 2 main circular distributions for blood
    - **Major arterial circle:**
        - Lies in the ciliary body along the root of the iris
        - Made by anastomoses between the anterior ciliary (branch from muscular artery) and long posterior ciliary Arteries
    - **Minor arterial circle:**
        - Located toward the pupil at the level of the collarette
        - Formed by anastamoses of the radial branches from the major circle
- Sources of Blood to the Iris
    - **Long posterior ciliary arteries:**
        - Run anteriorly in suprachoroidal space and enters the ciliary body to anastomose with anterior ciliary arteries.
    - **Anterior ciliary arteries:**
        - Branch from muscular arteries and send their perforating branches down the limbus and join the Major Arterial Circle.

11. Innervation

- Dually innervated by Sympathetic and Parasympathetic Autonomic Nervous Systems.
- Sympathetic comes from the Superior Cervical ganglion and follows the internal carotid artery to the cavernous and/or carotid sympathetic plexus and leaves with long posterior ciliary nerves (branch from nasociliary nerve)

- Parasympathetic travels with the oculomotor nerve (CNIII) to the ciliary ganglion and enters the eye with the short posterior ciliary nerve.
- Sensory innervation goes to the brain by way of the ophthalmic division of the trigeminal nerve (CN V).

12. Size and Location of Pupil

- The diameter varies from 1 mm to 9 mm depending on lighting conditions.
- The pupil is located slightly nasal and inferior to the iris center.

IRIS/PUPIL (DEVELOPMENTAL ANATOMY)

---

1. Development of Iris Stroma (Anterior Leaf, Posterior Leaf)

- The iris stroma is derived from the neural crest cells which are mesodermal in origin.
- By the end of the 3rd month, the lip of the optic cup elongates and grows forward between the lens and the cornea.
    - The outer layer of the optic cup becomes the anterior iris epithelium.
    - The inner layer of the optic cup becomes the posterior iris epithelium.
- The iris stroma is originally continuous with the pupillary membrane.

2. Development of Pars Iridica Retinae (Epithelial Layer)

- The ectodermal iris begins development about the latter part of the 3rd month and can be seen as a small, blunt margin just anterior to the folds of the primitive ciliary processes. It then grows steadily forward over the anterior surface of the lens so that by 8 months it is practically complete and the pupil fully formed.
- The pars iridica retinae includes the double layer of pigmented epithelium which covers the posterior surface of the adult iris and also includes derivatives of the pigmented epithelium, the sphincter and dilator muscles.
    - The anterior layer of iris epithelium is directly continuous with the outer wall of the optic cup further back (pigmented layer of the retina).
    - The posterior layer of the iris is continuous with the wall of the optic cup.
- Differentiation of the anterior and posterior layers of ectodermal iris continues with the forward growth of the whole margin of optic cup.
    - Columnar cells of anterior layer are pigmented.
    - Those of the posterior layer are not pigmented at this stage.
- Marginal ring sinus:
    - At the extreme edge, just where the anterior layer turns over to become posterior layer, a space between the two layers of the optic cup exist, a circular channel called marginal sinus.
    - The marginal sinus increases as the iris grows and at 5 months, the time most active growth and differentiation at the edge of the cup, the marginal sinus is very large.
    - With time the marginal sinus gets smaller and disappears by 7 months.
    - This channel represents the last trace of the cavity of the optic vesicle.
- Pigmentation of the posterior layer of the ectodermal iris occurs gradually and extends from the anterior layer around the marginal sinus and backwards along the posterior layer from the pupil border towards the ciliary region. Pigmentation begins to appear in the 10th week and is completed during the 7th month.
    - The color of the iris can continue to darken for the first 6 postnatal months

3. Development of Dilator and Sphincter Muscles

- Dilator:
    - Appears in the 6th month.
    - Fine longitudinal fibrils form the most anterior layer of the epithelium, peripheral to Micheal's spur; while the nuclei and pigment are posteriorly displaced.

- The contractile muscle thus represents a direct transformation of the cytoplasm of the epithelial cells to form a myoepithelial unit.
- The dilator is not fully formed until after birth.
- It is not invaded by mesoderm nor is it vascularized, and it remains permanently in close association with the epithelium.

- Sphincter:
  - Earliest appearance is at 4th month (earlier than dilator).
  - In the small cubical cells lining the anterior wall of the marginal sinus, fine myofibrils are seen and a compact mass of muscle cells develops. These gradually increase in area down the anterior wall of the sinus as the iris continues to grow.
  - Peripheral limit of the muscles marked off by a spur of pigment, Michael's spur.
  - At first, the muscle forms a compact mass of fibers lying in close apposition with the anterior surface of the ectodermal layer. However, at the 6th month capillaries and connective tissue begin to grow into it, dividing it into bundles finally separating it from the parent epithelium except at the pupillary border where the two remain permanently associated (8th month).
- Most muscle comes from mesenchyme, but the iris dilator and sphincter come from **neural ectoderm**.

4. Pupillary Membrane (Atrophy)

- Pupillary membrane is the whole of the mesodermal layer stretching across the opening of the optic cup. At an early stage it includes a portion of mesoderm which will eventually be backed by the ectodermal iris as it grows forwards and will then form part of the mesodermal iris stroma.
- Pupillary atrophy:
  - Allows communication between anterior chamber and the posterior chamber.
  - If atrophy fails, the condition that exists is called persistent pupillary membrane.
  - Pupillary membrane atrophies as its blood supply diminishes.
  - During the 7th month, while vascularization of the mesodermal portion of iris is attaining its definitive condition, atrophy begins. Atrophy only involves the central part and consists of gradual shrinkage of vessel walls and cessation of blood flow.

5. Cilio Iridic Circulation

- The nasal and temporal long posterior ciliary arteries run forward on either side of the optic nerve, traverse the scleral condensation, and continue between it and the choroid towards the margin of the optic cup. Here each divides into 2 terminal branches. They form the peripheral vessels of the anterior portion of the vascular tunis of the lens and eventually form the greater Circle of the Iris (major) in the deeper layer of mesoderm (6th month completed).
- From this vascular circle three sets of vessels are given off:
  - Superficial branches to the iris, combining with those of the pupillary membrane to supply the vascular arcades.
  - Intermediate branches running deeply into the peripheral portion of the mesoderm to form a network in the deep layer of the iris stroma.
  - Recurrent vessels to the ciliary body.
- Taking mesodermal tissue with them, these vessels grow from the periphery running in an axial direction underneath the superficial layer of the stroma, keeping in step with the ingrowth of the optic cup.
- These vessels participate with the sphincter via branches invading the muscle itself, carrying with them mesodermal elements so that the muscle is divided into bundles by vascularized connective tissue.
- At this time, 7th month, there are four layers of vessels present in the iris near the pupillary margin: (1) arcades of pupillary membrane lying near the pupil margin, (2) radial vessels of the iris stroma, (3) inter-sphinteric and (4) sub-sphinteric recurrent ciliary branches formed by the 8th month.

6. Development of Iris Pigmentation

- A sparse distribution of collage fibers begins to accumulate to form the iris stroma.

- Stromal melanocytes continue to produce more pigment, and the color of the iris continues to darken for the first 6 postnatal months, with some stromal organization not complete until 7 years old.

POSTERIOR CHAMBER (GROSS ANATOMY)

1. Size and Volume

- Normally annular in shape.
- During accommodation, the chamber gets smaller.
- During dilation, the chamber also gets smaller.
- Volume = 0.06 mL
    - The ciliary processes that secrete aqueous project into the posterior chamber.

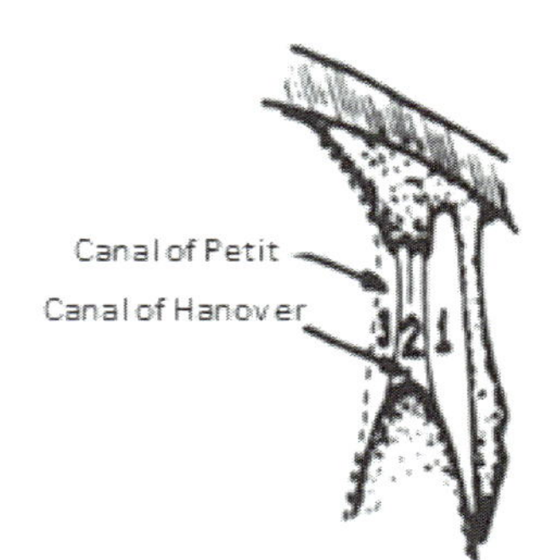

1. Posterior Chamber Proper
2. Tonular Portion
3. Retrozonular Portion

2. Boundaries

- Anterior limit: Posterior pigment epithelium of the iris.
- Posterior limit: Anterior hyaloid of the vitreous.
- Lateral limit: Non-pigmented epithelium of the ciliary processes.
- Medial limit: Lens capsule.

Divisions:

- Posterior Chamber Proper: Posterior to the iris and anterior to the zonule fibers.
- Zonular Portion (**Canal of Hanover**): The space in between the zonule fibers themselves.
- Retrozonular Portion (**Canal of Petit**): The space posterior to the zonular fibers and anterior to the anterior hyaloid of the vitreous.

POSTERIOR CHAMBER (DEVELOPMENTAL ANATOMY)

- With the formation of the pupillary membrane the anterior chamber is separated from the posterior chamber; however, with the subsequent atrophy of the pupillary membrane, communication between the two chambers is restored (14th week).

CILIARY BODY (GROSS ANATOMY)

1. Gross Morphology

- A ring-shaped structure when viewed from the front of the eye.
- Its width is about 5.9 mm on the nasal side and 6.7 mm on the temporal side .
- The posterior side appears flat while the anterior side contains numerous folds and 70-80 processes which extend into the posterior chamber.
- Divided into two parts:
    - **Pars plicata (corona ciliaris)**- thicker, anterior portion, contains ciliary processes.
        - Regions between the ciliary processes are called **valleys of Kuhnt**
        - Each ciliary process measures 2mm long, 0.5mm wide, and 1mm high
    - **Pars plana (orbicularis ciliaris)** – flatter region, extends from the posterior pars plicata to the ora serrata.
- 4 layers of the ciliary body:
    - Non-pigmented epithelium
    - Pigmented epithelium

- Stroma
- Supraciliaris

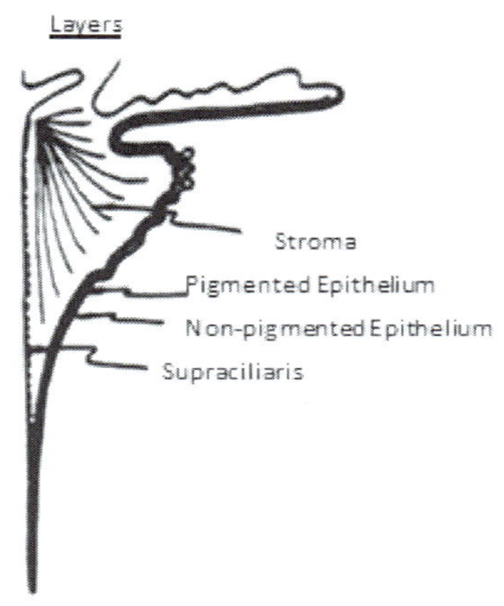

2. Dimensions

- Anterior limit is the scleral spur – 1.5 mm posterior to the termination of Descemet's Membrane.
- Posterior limit is the Ora Serrata – 7.5 mm posterior to the termination of Descemet's on the temporal side and 6.5 mm posterior on the nasal side.

3. Relationship to Sclera, Anterior Chamber, Iris, Posterior Chamber, Lens and Retina

- In sagittal section, the ciliary body has a triangular shape, the base of which is located anteriorly.
- The outer side of the triangle lies against the sclera.
- The portion of the base borders the anterior chamber.
- The anterior aspect of the ciliary body is joined to the iris by the iris root.
- The inner side of the triangle lines the posterior chamber.
- The zonule fibers course from the ciliary body to the lens.
  - The fibers insert either into the internal limiting membrane of the pars plana or the internal limiting membrane of the valleys of the pars plicata.
- The apex is located at the ora serrata.
- The attachment to the vitreous, vitreous base, extends forward 2mm over the posterior pars plana.

4. Pars Plana (Location, Components)

- aka Orbicularis ciliaris
- Posterior portion
- Runs from the ora serrata to the ciliary processes
- Flat, most posterior portion of the ciliary body
- Composed of bays and dentate processes
- Produces mucopolysaccharides for vitreous humor

5. Pars Plicata (Location, Components)

- aka Corona ciliaris or ciliary processes
- Anterior portion
- Composed of 70-80 folded processes
- Produces aqueous humor

6. Stroma (Components)

- Highly vascularized inner connective tissue layer:
  - Loose tissue external to the basement membrane
  - Has collagen fibers, blood vessels, nerves, fibroblasts, and mast cells
    - Major arterial circle of the iris is located in the ciliary stroma
    - Stromal capillaries are large and fenestrated
  - Lies between the muscle and the epithelial layers and forms the core of each of the ciliary processes.
- Bruch's Membrane:
  - Ciliary body stromal basement membrane becomes Bruch's Membrane at the Ora Serrata.

7. Ciliary Muscle (Components, Relations, Action, Innervation)

- Composted of smooth muscle fibers in longitudinal, radial, and circular directions.
- **Longitudinal portion** (Brucke's muscle or Meridional fibers):

- Origin at the scleral spur
    - Insertion into choroid (epichoroidal muscle stars)
    - Moves choroid anteriorly
- **Radial portion** (oblique fibers):
    - Origin at the scleral spur
    - Inserts at base of the ciliary processes and the Pars plana
    - Action pulls pars plana anteriorly
- **Circular portion** (Mueller's muscle of Ciliary sphincter):
    - Innermost region of the muscle. Origin at scleral spur
    - Insert into anterior part of ciliary processes
    - Action is to constrict lens aperture
- Action:
    - Ciliary body constricts anteriorly re.leasing the tension on the zonules, allowing for the lens to bow forwards (accommodate).
- Dually innervated by autonomic nervous system:
    - Parasympathetic stimulation activates the muscle for contraction.
    - Sympathetic innervations likely have an inhibitory effect that is function of the level of parasympathetic activity.

8. <u>Pigmented Epithelium (Basal Lamina, Ultrastructure)</u>

- Layer of pigmented cuboidal cells anterior to the non-pigmented epithelium.
- Continuous anteriorly with the anterior epithelium of the iris and posteriorly with the retinal pigmented epithelium at the ora serrata.
- Basement membrane firmly anchored to the stroma of the ciliary body.
- Thickens with age.

9. <u>Non-pigmented Epithelium (Basal Lamina, Ultrastructure, Relationship to Pigmented Epithelium)</u>

- Most internal layer – one (columnar) cell thick.
    - Cells are interconnected by desmosomes, gap junctions, and zonula occludens forming one site of the blood-aqueous barrier.
    - Cells are metabolically active in the secretion of aqueous humor components.
- Continuous anteriorly with the pigmented epithelium of the iris and posteriorly with the neural retina at the ora serrata.
- Has heavily folded basement membrane on the internal surface to increase the surface area. Important transport epithelium due to its production of aqueous humor.
- External surface is the apical surface, which is against the apical side of the pigmented epithelium.

10. <u>Blood Supply and Venous Drainage</u>

- Arterial:
    - From the two **long posterior ciliary arteries** and the seven **anterior ciliary arteries** that make up the major arterial circle.
- Venous:
    - Anteriorly, through the ciliary plexus and ultimately to episclera and anterior ciliary veins.
    - Posteriorly, directly into the choroid, which drains into the four vortex veins.

11. <u>Innervation</u>

- Sensory:
    - Via the ophthalmic division of CN V (Trigeminal). Leaves the eye with the long posterior ciliary nerves.
- Motor:
    - Sympathetic – Superior cervical ganglion
    - Parasympathetic – Oculomotor (III)

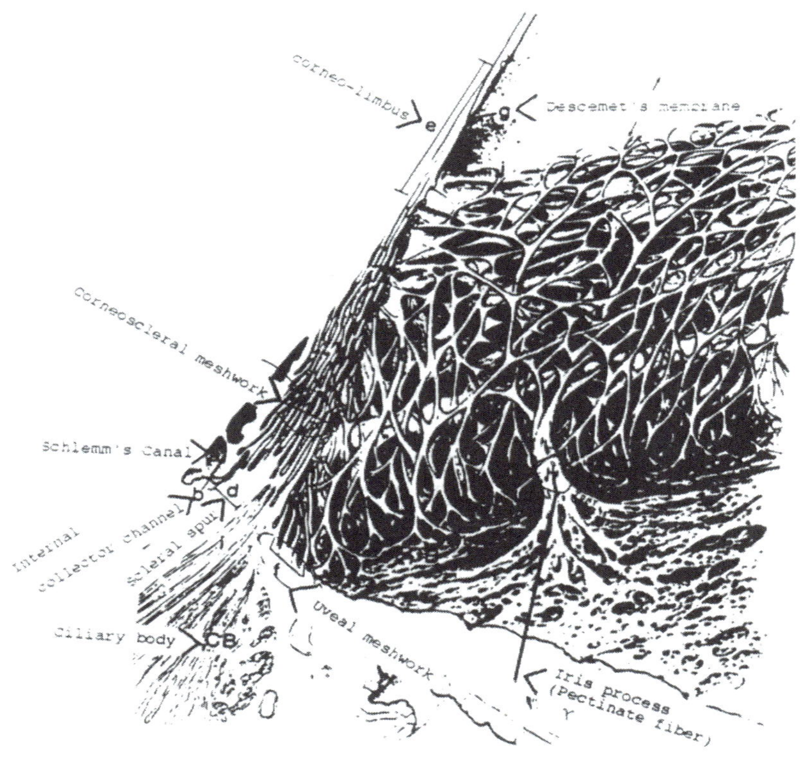

CILIARY BODY (DEVELOPMENTAL ANATOMY)

1. Tissue Origin (Mesoderm, Neural Crest)

- The mesoderm condenses to form the ciliary muscle and the mesodermal cores of the ciliary processes. Ciliary vessels are also created from mesoderm.
- Both layers of epithelium of the ciliary body are derived from neural ectoderm of the optic cup.

2. Development of Pars Ciliaris Retinae (Epithelial Layers)

- At 10 weeks the inner wall of the optic cup everts itself over the edge. A number of radial folds appear around the circumference of the cup, at first involving only the inner layer of the cup but eventually involving both layers. As the growing edge of the cup advances to form the ectodermal part of the iris, the folds are left behind to form the ciliary processes.
    - Each fold is formed of two fused layers of neural epithelium, the outer neural epithelium pigmented like the RPE, from which it is derived, and the inner composed of non-pigmented short columnar cells.
    - These folds increase slowly in size, depth, and into each projects a mesodermal core determined to be the ciliary muscle, carrying with it the vascular elements.
- In accordance with the progressive increases in size of the eye, ciliary processes move farther forward, leaving behind a smooth region composed of 2 fused epithelial layers (pars plana). Tips of the processes become further removed from the lens after 4 months.
- Ciliary epithelium begins to secrete aqueous 7 to 9 days after birth.

3. Development of Ciliary Processes, Ciliary Muscles, Ciliary Vessels

- Ciliary processes:
  - The inner non-pigmented epithelium from the inner optic cup layer grows and folds with it.
  - These folds (almost 70 in number) become the ciliary processes.
- Ciliary muscles:
  - In contrast to muscle of the iris, ciliary muscle is mesodermal in origin, developing from mesoderm between the ciliary body and the sclera.
  - During the 3rd month mesodermal cells become more regularly arranged in longitudinal formations.
  - By the 5th month the meridional portion of the muscle is evident. They are continuous with a dense condensation of scleral fibers which grow obliquely inwards to form the scleral spur (from which meridional fibers of the muscle originate).
  - Other muscle fibers appear at 6 months (e.g. circular). Other fibers are well formed by the 7th month and continue to develop after birth unlike the meridional.
- Development of ciliary vessels:
  - The capillary-venous system develops first.
  - The anterior portion of the choroidal net shows a parallel arrangement of large vessels which run a fairly straight course forwards to the iris region where they form a net. Most of these vessels are veins.
  - These vessels pass forward and run beneath the ciliary folds.
  - At the beginning of the 6th month the major circle is complete and the following three branches from it are recognizable (1) large superficial vessels of the pupillary membrane, (2) small vessels to the iris stroma, and (3) recurrent vessels to the ciliary region. The recurrent vessels extend back and one reaches each ciliary process and vascularizes it at the end of the 8th month. Little change beyond this occurs except that the size of the arteries increases.

UVEA (PHYSIOLOGY)

---

1. Functions of Ciliary Body

- Accommodation: Contraction of ciliary muscles releases tension on the zonule fibers and allows the lens capsule to adopt a more spheric shape. Also, ciliary muscle contraction changes the configuration of the trabecular meshwork, facilitating aqueous movement.
- Aqueous humor production: The large capillaries are fenestrated, facilitating the movement of substances into and out of the vessels. The non-pigmented epithelium actively secrets aqueous humor components into the posterior chamber.
- Production and maintenance of the lens zonules.
- Vitreous production: Tthe epithelium in the pars plana produces and secretes macromolecules for the vitreous body.
- Blood-aqueous barrier: The tight zonular junctions of the non-pigmented epithelium prevent the molecules from passing between the cells.

2. Functions of Iris

- Control the amount of light entering the eye.

3. Functions of Choroid

- Nutritive: Capillaries of choriocapillaris serve to nourish the outer receptor layers of the retina.
- Heat sink: Removes heat produced from light striking the retina.
- Structural: Provides attachment for the retina; soft pathway for vessels from posterior to anterior region of eye.
- Pigment reduces light scatter by absorbing excess light.
- Regulation of IOP via blood flow in choroidal arteries.

4. Uveal Blood Flow: Choroid, Ciliary Body, Iris (Unique Characteristics of Each, Functions of Each)

- The short posterior ciliary arteries enter the globe in a circle around the optic nerve, and their branches form the choroidal vessels.
- The long posterior ciliary arteries and the anterior ciliary arteries join to form the major circle of the iris, which supplies vessels to the iris and ciliary body.
- Venous return for most of the uvea is through the vortex veins.

UVEITIS, SCLERA/EPISCLERA (PATHOLOGY)

---

1. Uveitis

- Epidemiology and history:
  - In one year, 15/100,000 develop uveitis (12/15 get anterior uveitis). Usually affects ages from 20 to 50.
  - Most commonly in younger patients due to: congenital toxoplasmosis, toxocariases, peripheral uveitis (cyclitis), HLA B27 diseases.
  - In elderly patients, most common are toxoplasmosis, herpes zoster, aphakic uveitis.
- Symptoms:
  - (Acute) pain, redness, photophobia, consensual photophobia, excessive tearing, decreased vision; (Chronic) less symptomatic, possibly decreased vision.
- Observation, inspection, techniques, and skills:
  - VA: decreased if CME present.
  - SLE: cells and flare in the anterior chamber, ciliary flush, keratic precipitates (KP) (fine or mutton fat), hypopyon, iris nodules, iris atrophy, iris heterochromia, iris synechiae, band keratopathy.
  - Gonioscopy: PAS.
  - IOP: low (most cases) or high (i.e. herpetic, Posner-Schlossman syndrome).
  - DFE: vitreous spill over (i.e. formation of snowballs and/or snowbank).
- Diagnostic testing:
  - Child (<5 years old): ESR (+ if systemic inflammation), ANA (+ if JRA associated with iridocyclitis), VDRL (+ if active syphilis infection), FTA ABS (+ if exposure to syphilis) .
  - Adult: ESR, chest X-ray (+ if sarcoid), TB skin test and PPD (+ if TB), VDRL, FTA ABS, HLA-B27 (+ if ankylosing spondylitis, Reiter's syndrome), Sacroiliac X-ray (+ if ankylosing spondylitis), ACE and Gallium scan (+ if sarcoid), Lime titer (+ if Lime disease).
- Pathophysiology and disease:
  - Systemic associations:
    - Musculoskeletal: Arthritis rheumatoid, gout, Reiter's Syndrome, ankylosing spondylitis, psoriatic arthritis, and JRA.
    - Genitourinary: Reiters Syndrome, Behcet's.
    - Gastrointestinal: Crohn's or ulcerative colitis.
    - Skin: Behcet, sarcoids, syphilis, Lyme disease, psoriatic arthritis, VKH, herpetic.
  - Ocular associations:
    - Acute: Ankylosing spondylitis, Reiter's, inflammatory bowel disease, syphilis, H simplex, H. zoster, idiopathic (most common), psoriatic arthritis, Behcet's.
    - Insidious: JRA, Fuch's heterochromic iridocyclitis, sarcoid, masquerade syndrome (retinoblastoma, leukemia, intraocular FB, peripheral retinal detachment, melanoma).

2. Episcleritis

- Epidemiology and history:
  - Affect women > men (2:1), typically in young adults, history of recurrent episodes is common.
  - History: rash, arthritis, venereal disease, recent viral illness, general systemic health.
- Symptoms:
  - Acute onset of redness and mild pain in one or both eyes, no discharge, no decreased vision.

- Observation, inspection, techniques and skills:
  - External examination in natural light: look for the bluish hue of scleritis
  - SLE: determine depth of injected blood vessels, clear cornea, deep and quiet anterior chamber
  - IOP: normal
- Diagnostic testing:
  - Phenylephrine (2.5%) test: instill 1qtt in the affected eye and re-examine after 10 to 15 minutes. Look for blanched blood vessels.
- Pathophysiology and disease:
  - Idiopathic: most common
  - Infectious: herpes zoster virus
  - Others: rosacea, atopy, thyroid disease

3. Scleritis

- Epidemiology and history:
  - Affect women > men, typically in their 40's to 50's, history of associated systemic disease in 50%.
  - History: previous episodes, medical problems.
- Symptoms:
  - Severe and boring pain, which radiates to the forehead, brow, or jaw. Gradual or acute onset with red eye and decrease in vision, recurrent episode is common.
- Observation, inspection, techniques and skills:
  - Gross inspection of sclera in all direction of gaze.
  - SLE: red-free filter to determine avascular area of sclera.
  - DFE: rule out posterior involvement.
  - Complete physical examination by an internist or rheumatologist.
- Diagnostic testing:
  - Complete blood count, ESR, uric acid, RPR, FTA ABS, Rh factor, ANA, fasting blood sugar, ACE, CH50, C3, C4, serum ANCA.
  - PPD with anergy panel, chest radiograph, radiograph of sacroiliac joints, B-scan ultrasonography, MRA, CT scan.
- Pathophysiology and diagnosis:
  - Most common: connective tissue disease, herpes zoster ophthalmicus, syphilis, gout.
  - Others: TB, other bacteria, Lyme disease, sarcoidosis, HTN, foreign body, parasite.

Chapter 15 – Vitreous/Retina/Choroid

VITREOUS (GROSS ANATOMY)

1. Volume

- Volume 3.9 mL (2/3 of the eye's volume).
- Refractive Index 1.33.
- Filled with gel-like vitreous body.

2. Shape

- Fills the largest portion of the globe and helps to maintain the round shape.

3. Attachments to Retina and Lens (Ultrastructure)

- Attachments to the retina:
  - Vitreous base (the strongest attachment): located at the ora serrata.
    - Extends from 1.5 to 2mm anterior to the ora serrata, 1 to 3mm posterior to it and several mm into the vitreous.
  - Optic nerve head.
  - Fovea (Maxwell's spot).
  - Retinal blood vessels: weak attachment.
    - Fine strands extern through the internal limiting membrane to surround the larger retinal vessels.
    - These weak attachments might be the cause of hemorrhages from vitreal traction on the retina.
- Attachments to the lens:
  - **Wieger's ligament** (a.k.a. Hyaloideocapsulary/pectinate ligament)
    - Extends from the posterior surface of the lens and the anterior face of the vitreous
    - Anterior hyaloid is lightly attached all around the lens surface.
    - Strength of this attachment decreases with age.
  - **Retrolental space of Berger** – present where lens and vitreous are juxtaposed but not joined.

4. Patellar Fossa (Location)

- **Cloquet's Canal** is the remnant embryonal hyaloids system that extends from the lens to the optic nerve head. The canal widens anteriorly, forming the **patellar fossa** (depression in the vitreous that the lens fits into). **Berger's space** lies between the patellar fossa and the lens.
- Inside the circle of Wieger's ligament.

5. Anterior Hyaloid (Location)

- The **Anterior Hyaloid Membrane** separates the vitreous from the lens. It shares its attachment with the posterior zonule via the circular **Wieger's ligament**, also known as **Egger's line.**

6. Posterior Hyaloid (Location)

- The **Posterior Hyaloid Membrane** separates the posterior vitreous from the retina. It adheres to the internal limiting membrane of the retina.
- During a posterior vitreous detachment the posterior hyaloid membrane separates from the retina.
- The posterior hyaloid membrane meets in a ring of adhesion with the posterior end of Cloquet's canal. During a PVD, this tissue is torn from the optic nerve head forming **Weiss' Ring**.

7. Cortex (Composition)

- The **cortex** is also called the hyaloid surface and is the outer surface layer of the vitreous
    - 100 microns wide, composed of tightly packed collagen fibers
    - Contains transvitreal channels (pre-papillary hole, pre-macular hole, pre-vascular fissures)
- Anterior = anterior to the vitreous base. Overlies most of the ciliary body
- Posterior = posterior to the vitreous. Overlies the internal limiting membrane of the retina.

8. Hyaloid Canal (Location, Origin)

- Aka **Cloquet's canal**
- An empty channel that extends from the optic nerve to the lens through the center of the vitreous body. It is the remnant of the primary vitreous
- Shaped like a trumpet (S shape)- dip downward at the former area of the hyaloids artery system
    - Flaring out at both ends
    - Flare much more at the optic nerve - called the **Area of Martegiani**

VITREOUS (DEVELOPMENTAL ANATOMY)

---

1. Primary Vitreous

- Hyaloid canal:
    - Forms by the end of the 8th month.
    - Hyaloid artery atrophies and leaves the hyaloid canal in its place.
- Hyaloid vasculature remnants:
    - Central retinal artery and vein develop from the atrophy of the hyaloid system.
    - Persistence of the hyaloid artery:
        - The entire vessel may remain and extend from the optic disc to the lens posterior surface.
        - The artery may contract and pull on the lens → congenital cataract.
        - If the artery is attached to the retina, may cause a retinal detachment.
- Tissue origin:
    - The inner wall of the optic vesicle (neural ectoderm).
    - The lens vesicle (surface ectoderm).
    - Mesodermal cells of the invaginating optic vesicle.
- Tissue characteristics:
    - Permeated with a network of fine capillaries.
    - End of the primary vitreous formation process:
        - At the 6th week
        - Marked by the appearance of the hyaline capsule of the lens
    - The presence of blood vessels in the primary vitreous distinguishes it from the avascular secondary vitreous.

2. Secondary Vitreous (Tissue Origin, Tissue Characteristics)

- Tissue origin:
    - Forms between the 6th week and 3rd month.
    - Composed of neural ectoderm.
- Tissue characteristics:
    - Fine, fibrils that are densely packed in an orderly arrangement.
    - Surrounds the primary vitreous in the area of the atrophying hyaloids vessels, forming the funnel-shaped **Cloquet's Canal.**
    - Avascular.
    - Contains fibril network and primitive hyalocytes.
    - Forms attachment to the vitreous base and at the hyaloidocapsular ligament during the 3rd month.

3. Tertiary Vitreous

- Tissue origin:
  - Develops from the neuroepithelium of the ciliary body.
  - Forms at the 3rd month.
- Tissue characteristics:
  - Zonular fibers grow from ciliary processes of the tertiary vitreous

---

VITREOUS (PHYSIOLOGY)

---

1. Functions

- Fills posterior portion of eye with optically transparent media, absorbs "shock" from the fragile retina during rapid eye movements and strenuous physical activity.
- Adheres and holds retina down against choroid.
- Allows nutrients to diffuse from the ciliary body to the retina.
  - Storage area for metabolites from the retina and lens.
- Transmits and refracts light.

2. Composition

- Composition:
  - Water 99%
  - Proteins 0.08%
  - Mucopolysaccharides 0.02-0.05%
- Collagen (most abundant protein):
  - Makes up the vitreous cortex, highest concentration is in the vitreous base.
  - Mostly type II.
- Hyaluronic acid (HA):
  - A type of polysaccharide glycosaminoglycan.
  - In the vitreous humor.
  - Responsible for the viscosity and viscoelastic properties of the vitreous.
- Hyalocytes (Vitreous Cells):
  - Located in a single, widely spaced layer in the cortex near the vitreal surface.
  - Function to synthesize HA, glycoproteins for collagen fibrils, and phagocytic properties.
  - Cells have different appearances dependent on their activity at the time.
  - Fibroblasts (<10% of cells)– located in vitreous base near the ciliary body and optic disc. Synthesize collagen fibrils and are active in pathologic conditions.

3. Metabolism

- No metabolic activity that uses oxygen and carbon dioxide.
- Hyalocytes contain an enzyme that transforms glucose into hyaluronic acid.

4. Aging Changes in Composition

- Infancy – vitreous is homogenous, gel-like.
- With age gel volume decreases and liquid volume increases.
- 40 years old – 80% gel, 20% liquid.
- 70-80 years old- 50% gel, 50% liquid.
- HA and collagen detrimentally affected by free radicals.
- Liquefaction occurs due to changes in the HA molecule and alterations in the HA-collagen complex.
  - **Lacunae** – Pockets of liquid formed by changes.
- **Peripheral Retinal Traction** – vitreous base adhesion extends further posteriorly, approaching the equator causing traction on the peripheral retina. Can lead to retinal tears and detachment.

5. Physical Characteristics

- Volume:
  - Vitreous fills 2/3 of the volume of the eye, about 4mL
  - It is 98-99% water
- Light transmission:
  - Light is transmitted through the transparent vitreous due to the ordered HA-collagen complex.
  - Visible light - More than 90% of is transmitted in the normal vitreous.
  - UV light:
    - Transmission rapidly drops off between 350 and 300 nm.
    - Zero below 300 nm.
  - Infrared light -Transmission drops off at 800 nm.
  - Wavelengths longer than 1600 nm – There is no transmission (complete absorption).

VITREOUS (PATHOLOGY)

- **Posterior vitreous detachment (PVD)**
  - Pathophysiology:
    - Syneresis and liquefaction (normal age related change) create pockets of fluid.
    - May cause collapse of vitreous and separation from macula and optic nerve head.
    - The thin remaining coat of the cortical vitreous breaks.
    - Collected fluid empties itself into the pre-retinal space.
      - Causes symptoms of flashes and floaters.
  - Epidemiology:
    - Acute PVD is found in 65-75% of patients over age 65.
  - Symptoms:
    - Acute onset of floaters and flashes.
    - 50% asymptomatic.
  - Signs:
    - Vitreal opacities
    - Weiss ring
    - Displacement of vitreal cortex
  - Observation, inspection, techniques:
    - Careful examination of peripheral retina for holes or tears
    - NCF for Weiss ring
  - Complications:
    - Primary cause of retinal detachments and retinal tear formation
      - 10% risk
      - If vitreal hemorrhage present, 75% risk
    - Fellow eye usually has PVD within 2 years
- **Vitreal hemorrhage**
  - Common causes:
    - Retinal break
    - PVD
    - Trauma
    - Neovascularization
  - Symptoms:
    - Acute onset of floaters
    - Reduced vision
  - Signs:
    - Cells or blood in vitreous
    - Tobacco dust aka Shafer's sign (Pigment & vitreal cells in the anterior vitreous)
  - Observation, inspection, techniques:
    - Careful examination of peripheral retina for holes or tears
    - IOP

- B-scan ultrasonography if poor view of the retina

Vitreal opacities – Differential diagnosis

- Asteroid hyalosis:
  - Calcium phosphate particles attached to vitreal strands
  - Epidemiology
    - Elderly patients
    - 0.5% of population
  - Clinical significance - affects view of fundus
- Tobacco dust
- Persistent hyperplastic primary vitreous
  - Abnormal regression of the hyaloid artery
- Posterior uveitis or vitritis
- Synchesis scintillans:
  - Golden refractile cholesterol crystals
- Vitreal syneresis
- Tumor cells
- Amyloidosis (rare)
- Abnormal protein deposition

CHOROID (GROSS ANATOMY)

---

1. Extent

- The choroid extends from the ora serrata to the optic nerve.
- Located between the sclera and the retina.

2. Thickness

- About 0.1-0.15 mm anterior and 2.2 mm posterior.
- The choroid thins with age due to:
  - Decreased number of vessels
  - Decreased caliber
  - Sclerosis

3. Relationship to Lamina Fusca of Sclera

- Suprachoroidia (lamina fusca):
  - Thin, pigmented, ribbonlike branching bands of connective tissue that is a transition between sclera and choroid, traversing the **suprachoroidal space** (carries the long posterior ciliary arteries and nerves from the posterior to the anterior portion of the globe).
    - Lamina suprachoroidia: comes from direction of the choroid.
    - Lamina fusca: comes from direction of the sclera.
  - The suprachoroidia contains many collagen fibers, fibroblasts, and melanocytes that absorb light from passing through the choroid from outside.
    - The darkly pigmented choroid absorbs excess light that passes through the RPE layer.
- The tissue is loose and allows the vascular net to swell without causing a detachment of the choroid to the sclera.

4. Choriocapillaris (Ultrastructure, Type of Capillaries)

- The **choriocapillaris** is a single layer of capillaries with large lumens and many **fenestrations**.
  - The lumens are 3-4x larger than ordinary capillaries (2-3 blood cells can pass through vs. 1)
  - It is densest in the macular era (only blood supply to the macula).
  - Does not continue into the ciliary body.
- Rapid changes in size of the arteries to capillaries

- Blood flow is increased here which keeps the blood pressure high in the choriocapillaris.
  - There are some **pericytes (Rouget cells)** around the capillary cells that contract to alter local blood flow.
- The vascular choroid provides nutrients to the outer retina and removes catabolites from the retina.

5. Stroma

- The **choroidal stroma c**onstitutes the bulk of the choroid. It is a pigmented, vascularized, loose connective tissue layer that contains fibroblasts, melanocytes, macrophages, mast cells, plasma cells, lymphocytes, and unmyelinated nerves.
- Collagen fibers circularly surround the blood vessel branches from the short posterior ciliary arteries which are organized into two tiers.
  - Large vessels = **Haller's Layer**
  - Medium vessels = **Sattler's Layer**
- Cells in the outer 2/3 of the stroma.

6. Blood Supply

- **Long posterior ciliary arteries** (two) supply the anterior ½ of the choroid to make up the Greater Circle of the Iris or Major Arterial Circle (MAC).
- **Anterior ciliary arteries** (seven) are not major suppliers.
- **Short posterior ciliary arteries** supply the posterior ½ of the choroid make up the circle of Haller-Zinn.

7. Venous Drainage

- Vortex veins (four):
  - Major drainage route
  - Diameter 1.0 – 1.5mm
  - Come together at the ampulla
- Anterior ciliary veins drain the anterior ½ of the choroid via the limbal plexus.
- Pial veins drain the optic nerve meninges and small part of posterior choroid.

8. Innervation

- Sympathetic causes vasoconstriction.
- Parasympathetic causes vasodilation.

9. Bruch's Membrane (Location, Composition)

- **Bruch's membrane** (basal lamina) is the innermost layer of the choroid. It lies between the choroid and the RPE, and runs from the optic nerve to the ora serrata, and continues into the ciliary body
- It is a multilaminated sheet containing a center layer of elastic fibers
- It is composed of 5 layers:
  1) Interrupted basement membrane of the choriocapillaris
  2) Outer collagenous zone
  3) Elastic layer
  4) Inner collagenous zone
  5) Basement membrane of the RPE cells
- The merging of RPE basement membrane filaments with the inner collagenous zone fibers allow for tight adhesion between the choroid and RPE.

CHOROID (DEVELOPMENTAL ANATOMY)

1. Tissue Origin (Paraxial Mesoderm, Neural Crest Cells)

- The primitive choroid develops from the neural crest cells and paraxial mesoderm.
- To differentiate, the mesenchyme that forms choriocapillaris must be in contact with developing pigment epithelium.
- Vessels appear during 2nd month.
- Bruch's membrane is present at midterm.
- Choroidal stroma is pigmented by term.

2. Development of Choroidal Vasculature (3 stages)

- **Stage 1:** Formation of a plexus with vascular channels next to the outer surface.
  - A rich plexus of endothelial blood spaces develops in the undifferentiated mesoderm.
  - The outer layer of the optic cup is not vascularized until pigment appears within its cells at around 5 weeks. Thereafter the development of vascular spaces rapidly proceeds.
  - At 5-6 weeks, the outer layer of the optic cup is covered by small vessels. By the end of the 6th week the **choriocapillaris** is complete.
  - As development proceeds, the plexus becomes denser and richer. At the anterior rim of the optic cup, the vessels coalesce to form the annular vessel around the margin.
- **Stage 2:** Precursor of large choroidal vessels: formation of the second plexus.
  - Before the 3rd month, the loose venous channels drains the choriocapillaris into the supra and infra-orbital venous plexuses. During the 3rd month, the channels aggregate into a wide meshed network between the capillary layer and the mesodermal condensation that is developing around the sclera.
  - From the channels, a few large trunks emerge and perforate the sclera to form the **vortex veins**.
- **Stage 3:** Precursor of the intermediate layer of small choroidal vessels: Arterial intrusion between the capillary and venous layers.
  - Before the 7th week, the primitive dorsal ophthalmic artery gives off the common temporal ciliary artery. The primitive ventral ophthalmic artery gives off the common nasal ciliary artery.
  - **Long posterior ciliary arteries**: Run anteriorly to form a terminal anastomosis (the MAC)
  - **Short posterior ciliary arteries**:
    - Develop from the ophthalmic artery close to the origin of the long posterior ciliary artery.
    - Five or 6 small branches run forward around the optic nerve and break up into 12-15 small branches.
    - These vessels supply the choriocapillaris encircling the optic nerve head.
  - By the 5th month, all layers of the choroid are visible.
  - By the 7th month, the choroid is fully differentiated.

3. Development of Bruch's Membrane

- Composition:
  - Inner ectodermal lamina
  - Outer mesodermal lamina
- During the 6th week, Bruch's begins to form as randomly oriented elastic and collagen fibers.
- During the 12th week, the outer elastic lamina of Bruch's membrane becomes histologically visible when the elastic elements of the choroidal stroma are sufficiently condensed.

CHOROID (PATHOLOGY)

- **Choroidal neovascularization (CNV)**
    - Etiology:
        - Growth of new choroidal vessels into retina
        - Any alteration of Bruch's membrane
    - Causes of CNV:
        - Diabetic retinopathy
        - Wet ARMD
        - Histoplasmosis
        - Angioid streaks
        - High myopia
        - Retinal telangiectasia
    - Symptoms:
        - Metamorphopsia
        - Decreased vision
    - Signs:
        - Subretinal fluid
        - Subretinal exudates
        - Subretinal hemorrhage
        - Dirty gray membrane (blood accumulation between Bruch's and RPE)
    - Observation, inspection, techniques:
        - Stereoscopic observation
        - Fluorescein angiography
    - Complications:
        - Sensory RD
        - Cystoid edema
        - RPE detachment
        - Fibrosis of new vessels
        - Fibrotic or disciform scarring
- **Choroidal effusion/detachment**
    - Signs:
        - Orange-brown elevation
        - More solid appearance than RD
        - Often 360 degrees
        - Hypotony
- **Angioid streaks**
    - Pathological changes in RPE, Bruch's and choroid
    - Streaks represent breaks on thickened and calcified Bruch's
    - Causes:
        - Pseudoxanthalasma elasticum
        - Paget's disease (Osteitis deformans)
        - Ehlers-Danlos syndrome
        - Sickle cell disease
        - Hemolytic anemia
        - Cardiovascular disease
        - High myopia
        - Neurofibromatosis, Sturge-Weber, Tuberous sclerosis
        - Trauma
        - Ocular melanocytosis
        - Optic disc drusen
    - Signs:
        - Bilateral but asymmetric
        - Colored lines surround ONH (gray, red gray, red brown, or red)
        - Radiate peripherally like irregular spokes

- Complications:
  - Dry AMD
  - CNV

White Dot Syndromes

- **Birdshot Choroidopathy**
  - Epidemiology:
    - More common in females
    - Age 40-60 years
    - HLA A29
  - Signs:
    - Ovoid lesions
    - Tend to be nasal
    - No anterior segment findings
  - Complications:
    - Cystoid macular edema
    - Neovascularization
- **Serpiginous Choroidopathy**
  - Epidemiology:
    - More common in males
    - Age 30-60 years
    - HLA B7
  - Symptoms:
    - Bilateral, but asymmetric
    - Severe vision loss with recurrences
  - Signs:
    - Large creamy white lesions surrounding ONH
    - Serpent like pattern
- **Multifocal choroiditis with panuveitis**
  - Epidemiology:
    - More common in females
    - Young
  - Signs:
    - Punched out appearance
    - Other white dot syndromes (see Retina Pathology)

RETINA (GROSS ANATOMY)

1. Layers (Components of Each, Ultrastructure)

- There are 10 layers. (From outermost to innermost)
- **Retinal pigment epithelium (RPE)**
  - A single layer of uniformly patterned, hexagonal shaped cells that are heavily pigmented.
  - Microvilli (Apical side) face and surround photoreceptors.
  - Basal side:
    - Adheres to Bruch's membrane (separates the RPE from choricapillaris)
    - Contains numerous infoldings for strong attachment to the choroid.
    - Acts as basement membrane of RPE.
  - Cells contain melanosomes (brown pigment)
    - More densely pigmented in the macula – melanin is used to catch stray light.
    - The cells stretch to accommodate growth of the eye and DO NOT regenerate if lost.
  - 4-6 million RPE cells in layer, each interacts with 30-40 photoreceptors.
  - Functions:
    - Zonula occludens of RPE is part of the blood-retinal barrier.

        - Cellular lysosomes phagocytose fragments from the photoreceptor outer segment discs
        - Metabolizes and stores vitamin A used in the formation of photopigment molecules
        - Pigment granules absorb light to decreases scattering
- **Photoreceptor cells**
    - Contains the outer and inner segments of rods and cones – modified cilia that contain specialized photo-labile pigments
    - 90-100 million rods and 4-5 million cones per eye
    - Outer and inner segments joined by cilium
- **External limiting membrane**
    - Not a true membrane
    - 1um thick layer at the internal end of photoreceptor cell's inner segments. Contains cell junctions between photoreceptors and Muller cells (at level of the inner segments) to function as a structural/metabolic barrier limiting the passage of larger molecules
- **Outer nuclear layer**
    - Contains the photoreceptors cell bodies
    - Thickest at the fovea – contains 10 layers of cone nuclei
- **Outer plexiform layer**
    - A wide external band of inner fibers of rods and cones and an inner band of synapses between photoreceptor and bipolar and horizontal cells
- **Inner nuclear layer**
    - Contains cell bodies of the horizontal, Muller, bipolar, and amacrine cells
- **Inner plexiform layer**
    - Synapses between the bipolar cells, amacrine, and ganglion cells
- **Ganglion cell layer**
    - Contains the ganglion cell bodies
    - Thickest at the macula, thins toward ora serrata
- **Nerve fiber layer**
    - Contains the ganglion cell axons
        - Extends from all parts of the retina towards the optic disc to form the optic nerve.
    - Papillomacular bundle
        - Fibers that radiate from macular area to disc
        - Carries visual acuity information
        - Thickest part of the nerve fiber layer
- **Internal limiting membrane**
    - Thin acellular layer
    - Lines the vitreous

2. Relationship between Retinal Pigment Epithelium and Bruch's Membrane

- The basal aspect of the RPE cells lies adjacent to the choroid. It contains numerous infoldings and is adherent to the basement membrane which forms a part of Bruch's membrane
- Although adherent to the retina, the RPE is considered part of the retina due to its common embryological germ cell layer origin (neural ectoderm)

3. Relationship between Retinal Pigment Epithelium and Photoreceptor Outer Segments

- The apical aspects of the RPE cells have microvilli that project into the outer photoreceptor layer and envelope the outer segments of the photoreceptors themselves. But, there are no intercellular junctions between the RPE and photoreceptors, as they are separated by a subretinal space (remnant of the gap formed by the two layers of the optic cup after optical vesicle invagination)

4. Synaptic Connections within Retina

- Two types of synapses
    - Electrical Synapses – rapid, found between

        - Photoreceptor and horizontal cells.
        - Occasionally between bipolar terminal and amacrine process.
    - Chemical Synapses – use neurotransmitters.
        - Found on cones and rods to the ganglion cells.

5. Glial Cells

- Function:
    - Provide structure
    - Transfer neural signals
    - Provide nutrients for the retina
- Location:
    - Nerve fiber layer
    - Ganglion cell layer
    - Inner plexiform layer
- Types:
    - Astrocytes (star-shaped):
        - Store glycogen
        - Structural support
        - Optic nerve equivalent to Muller cells for NFL
    - Muller cells:
        - Regulate GABA, glutamate, and K^+ concentrations
        - Glucose metabolism
    - Microglia:
        - Phagocytic cells
        - Respond to injury

6. Blood Supply

- Photoreceptors:
    - Choroid via the long & short posterior ciliary arteries
- Rest of the retina:
    - Central retinal artery, which bifurcates into 2 main branches within the optic nerve
    - Each of these branches bifurcates again to make a total of 4 arteries
- 2 capillary networks:
    - Deep - Between inner nuclear layer and outer plexiform layer
    - Superficial - In the nerve fiber layer
- Capillary free zone around retinal arteries and fovea
- Capillary layers:
    - Endothelium
        - Not fenestrated
        - Blood retinal barrier, joined by tight junctions
    - Pericytes
        - Contractile properties help blood flow.
- Cilioretinal arteries:
    - Present in 20% of individuals
    - Choroid supply to the inner retinal layers in the macular area
    - Enter from the edge of the optic disc

7. Anatomical Areas (Location, Size, Composition) of Area Centralis, Parafovea, Fovea, Foveola, Macula Lutea, Ora Serrata (Ultrastructure)

- **Ora serrata**
    - Extreme periphery of the retina
    - Location
        - 8.5 mm from the limbus

        - 6 mm from the equator
        - 25 mm from the optic nerve
    - Width
        - Temporally 2mm
        - Nasally 0.75mm
    - Serrated retinal termination zone
        - Dentate (teeth-like) processes that encroach the pars plana
        - Bays that lie between the teeth
    - Transition between neural retina to single non-pigmented layer of ciliary epithelium
- **Macula** (old term Area Centralis)
    - Location
        - 15.5 degrees (4mm, 28 prism diopters) temporal ONH center
        - 1.5 degrees (0.8mm, 3 prism diopters) inferior to the ONH center
    - Diameter is 18 degrees (5.5mm)
    - Characterized by increased pigment
- The macular region includes:
    - **Perifovea**
        - The outer belt surrounding the fovea
        - Location
            - The outer boundary is 2.25mm from the umbo
        - Width is 1.5 mm
        - Cone density is markedly decreased
    - **Parafovea**
        - Location
            - Inside the perifovea and closer to the umbo
        - Width 2.1 mm
        - Layer of Henle
            - Thick outer plexiform layer
        - Papillomacular bundle
            - Thickest part of the nerve fiber layer
    - **Fovea**
        - Only cones photoreceptors
        - Diameter 1.5 mm
    - **Foveola**
        - Slight dip in the foveal center
        - Diameter is 0.35mm
        - Layers present
            - RPE
            - Photoreceptors
            - External and inner limiting membrane
            - Outer nuclear layer with only cone nuclei
            - Henle's fiber layer
    - **Umbo**
        - Precise center of the macula
        - Diameter is 0.15mm

RETINA (DEVELOPMENTAL ANATOMY)

1. Development of Optic Cup

- Develops from neuroectoderm.
- Optic vesicle pushes in towards the pigmented layer and fuses at 7 weeks to form two layers of the optic cup.
- The outer layer of the optic cup → RPE, outer pigmented epithelium of the ciliary body, anterior iris epithelium.

- The inner layer → neural retinal, inner non-pigmented ciliary body epithelium, posterior iris epithelium.
    - Differentiates from glial cells.
    - Forms a single cell layer that attaches to the RPE.

2. Analogies between Development of Retina and Central Nervous System

- The retina develops from neural ectoderm of the CNS.
- Membrane barriers in the eye and brain:
    - Blood retinal barrier similar to the choroid plexus epithelium of the brain.
    - Photoreceptors morphology similar to ciliated epidymal cells that line the brain ventricle.

3. Fetal Fissure

- Formation:
    - Created by simultaneous invagination of the optic stalk and vesicle.
    - The hyaloid artery grows into the fetal fissure and provides nutrients for the developing eye.
- Function:
    - Provide the shortest passage for the ganglion cell nerve fibers to travel from the optic stalk to the brain.
- Fusion (and failure of):
    - It does not completely close to leave a canal for the hyaloid artery.
    - The cleft progressively closes. These vessels become restricted to a small opening in the center of the optic nerve head.

4. Retinal Differentiation (Stages I, II, III, proliferation, migration, differentiation)

- **Stage I*:* Epithelial**
    - Nuclear and cell division
    - The retina develops from pseudostratified neuroepithilium
- **Stage II*:* Differentiation**
    - Some cells stop dividing and differentiate into mature retinal nerve or glial cells
    - The neural retina divides into two zones during the 5th week:
        - Outer primitive zone
        - Inner marginal zone
    - The outer primitive zone then divides into inner and outer neuroblastic layers:
        - The *inner neuroblastic layer*
            - Ganglion cells: Form the nerve fiber layer and the optic nerve fibers
            - Amacrine and Muller cells
        - The *outer neuroblastic layer*
            - Cones & rods
            - Horizontal and bipolar cells
- **Stage III*:* Growth**
    - Ganglion cells develop first
    - Rods (month 7) and cones (month 4) develop last

5. Macular Differentiation

- During the first 3 months, there is rapid retinal differentiation.
- However, the development of the macula lags behind other parts of the retina.
- The macula is not complete until 3 to 4 months after birth.
- The cone population migrates (and thus increases) in the macula, elongate, and adopt an oblique orientation to form **Henle's layer**.

6. Retinal Circulation Development

- Dorsal ophthalmic artery:
    - Formed from branches of the internal carotid artery

- Branches of the primitive dorsal ophthalmic artery anastomose along the rim of the optic cup to form the Circle of Zinn.

- Ventral ophthalmic artery:
  - The ventral ophthalmic artery also branches from the internal carotid artery.
  - The ventral and dorsal ophthalmic arteries anastomose.
  - Part of the ventral ophthalmic artery develops into the nasal long ciliary artery.
  - The rest of the artery degenerates.
  - When the ventral ophthalmic artery degenerates, the dorsal ophthalmic artery becomes the future ophthalmic artery.
- Hyaloid system:
  - The hyaloid artery divides many times to forms the tunica vasculosa lentis and branches throughout the vitreous chamber (3rd month).
- Central retinal artery and vein:
  - When the hyaloids artery begins to atrophy, the central retinal vein and artery develop simultaneously.

7. Postnatal Events

- Cones - Matures a few months after
- Macula - The outer retinal layer thickens
- RPE - Pigment cell density increases

RETINA (PHYSIOLOGY)

- Rods:
  - Higher sensitivity in scotopic conditions
  - [75,000 rods:1 ganglion cell] convergence ratio
  - Regenerate in the morning
  - Visual pigment: Rhodopsin
- Cones:
  - Higher sensitivity in photopic conditions
  - [1 cone:1 ganglion cell] convergence ratio
  - Regenerate in the evening
  - Iopsin – Collectively refers to the three cone pigments (Cyanolabe, Chlorolabe, Erythrolabe)
  - Peak absorption in the blue, green, and yellow parts of the spectrum

1. Composition of Disc Outersegments

- The outer segments of rods and cones are surrounded by the microvilli of the RPE.
- The outer segments of both rods and cones contain 500 to 1000 lipid bilayer discs which have thousands of visual pigment molecules.
  - Photopigment molecules are mostly contained in the disc membrane.
- The tip of the outer segment is oriented toward the RPE and base toward the inner segment.

2. Formation of Disc Outersegments (Disc Renewal, Disc Shedding)

- **Disc Renewal** – Photoreceptor discs are constantly renewed. They are formed by invagination and evagination of the outer segment membrane at the cilium.
  - Discs detach from the membrane and are free floating in the outer segment of rods, but remain connected to the outer segment membrane in cones.
- **Disc Shedding** – The older discs are shed at the apex of the outer segment and phagocytized in the RPE. Discarded discs are called phagosomes and broken down by lysis following a diurnal cycle (cones shed at night, rods shed during the day).

3. Composition of Visual Pigments

- Composition:
  - Opsin
  - 11-cis retinal (carotenoid chromophore when bound to the protein, is a product of Vitamin A)
- The **principle of univariance**:
  - There is a threshold amount of quantal energy above which any wavelength of light must energize the photopigment for the receptor to elicit an impulse.
  - Therefore, regardless of how far above the threshold the wavelength of light hits the photopigment, it will produce the same response.
  - In other words, any wavelength of light will trigger the same response as long as it has an energy packet greater or equal to the threshold value.

4. Formation of Visual Pigments

- Opsin is manufactured in the Golgi apparatus of the inner segment of the photoreceptor. The opsin molecules are fused to the outer segment membrane of the cilium via G-proteins.
- Retinal is provided to the discs from the RPE via retinal binding protein (IRBP) carrier molecules.
  - Vitamin A is manufactured from beta-carotene.
  - Even though the eye only has 0.01% of the body's total amount of vitamin A, the eye requires a continuous supply of vitamin A.

5. Stages of Visual Cycle

- In the dark adapted eye, the chromophore 11-cis-retinal is embedded in the opsin.
- Upon absorption of a photon the retinal undergoes cis-trans isomerization from 11-cis to all-trans retinal, an unsaturated aldehyde, which dissociates from the opsin.
- When retinal bleached, all-trans-retinal is converted to retinol (vitamin A).
- Retinyl-esters and phagocytized photopigment are recycled to 11-cis-retinal.
- Rhodopsin is finally regenerated in a spontaneous reaction between 11-cis-retinal and the apoprotein

6. Photoreceptor Electrophysiology

- The resting potential of the outer segment potential is - 40 mV.
  - Membrane potential for sodium is $E_{Na} > 0$ mV
  - Membrane potential for potassium is $E_K < -70$ mV
- In the dark:
  - Na flows into the outer segment.
  - K flows out of the inner segment.
- The Na/K ATP pump uses ATP to pump out Na and bring in K to maintain the current.
- The resting conduction of the Na and K current is called the **"dark current."**
  - Net dark current: $I_{net} = I_{Na} + I_K$
  - In the dark, photoreceptor cells are partially depolarized due to the steady Na+/K+ flow. The depolarized photoreceptors release glutamate.
- Upon exposure to light and photo-isomerization in the disc membrane, the cell membrane conductance changes → blocks the inward depolarizing flow of Na by blocking cGMP gated cation channels → hyperpolarization towards the K membrane potential.
  - The hyperpolarization seizes the release of glutamate.
- Transduction: The process of converting light input to electrical impulses. The ultimate consequence of phototransduction is the modulation of the release of neurotransmitter from the rod to the bipolar cell.

7. Retinal Neurotransmitters

- Theories on transmitters between the photoreceptor disc and the cell membrane.
  - Calcium
    - Concentrated Ca^{2+} inside the discs is released into the intracellular space

      - Blocks sodium channels
  - Cyclic nucleotide cGMP
      - Phosphodiesterase attached to the photopigment is activated
      - Results in hyperpolarization

Retinal Cell Type	Neurotransmitter
Photoreceptors	Glutamate
Horizontal Cells	GABA
Bipolar Cells	Glutamate
Interplexiform Cells	GABA Dopamine
Amacrine Cells	Acetylcholine Glycine GABA peptides Dopamine

- Retinal synapses
  - Synapses:
      - Photoreceptors synapse with the bipolar cells which then synapse with ganglion cells.
      - Horizontal cells & photoreceptors
          - Provides communication between different photoreceptors.
      - Amacrine cells & ganglion cells
          - Provides communication between different ganglion cells.
  - Electrical conduction (via gap junctions)
  - Chemical (via neurotransmitters):
      - **Glutamate:** The major *excitatory* transmitter between photoreceptor, bipolar and horizontal cells.
      - **Acetylcholine:** The major *excitatory* transmitter of amacrine cells.
      - **GABA** (a derivative of glutamate): An *inhibitor* in horizontal and amacrine cells.
      - **Glycine:** An *inhibitor* in amacrine cells.
          - In the dark, neurotransmitters are constantly released, but with light stimulation, the amount of transmitter is decreased.

8. Function of Bipolar, Horizontal, Amacrine, and Ganglion cells

- **Bipolar Cells**: 2nd order neuron
  - Dendrite synapses with photoreceptor and horizontal cells.
  - Axon synapses with ganglion and amacrine cells.
  - Relay information from photoreceptors to horizontal, amacrine, and ganglion cells.
  - Receives synaptic feedback from amacrine cells.
  - 11 types, classified based on morphology, physiology, and dendritic contacts.
      - **Rod Bipolar Cell** (only 1 type): one cell synapses with 15-20 rods in central retina and up to 80 rods in periphery (improves light sensitivity). Do not synapse directly with ganglion cells, synapse with amacrine cells.
      - **Midget Bipolar Cell**: can be either flat or invaginated
      - **Diffuse Cone Bipolar Cell** (2 types)
      - **Blue Cone Bipolar Cell**
      - **Giant Cone Bipolar Cell**
- **Horizontal Cells**:
  - Transmits information in a horizontal direction.
  - Synapses with photoreceptors, bipolar cells, and other horizontal cells.
  - Can release an inhibitory transmitter, playing a role in the complex process of visual integration (inhibitory feedback to photoreceptors or inhibitory feed forward to bipolar cells.
  - 3 types: HI, HII, HIII
  - Horizontal cells can modulate the cone response, but not the rods.
- **Amacrine Cells**
  - Plays an important role in modulating the information that reaches the ganglion cells.
  - Synapses with bipolar cells (axons), ganglion cells (dendrites/soma), interplexiform neurons, and other amacrine cells.
  - 30 to 40 different types, described as stratified or diffuse.
  - Four groups: narrow field, small field, medium field, and large field (extent of coverage by branching processes).
  - Most contain inhibitory neurotransmitters (GABA, glycine).
  - Combine information from rod and cone pathways prior to innervating ganglion cells.
- **Ganglion Cells**: 3rd order neuron

- Can be bipolar or multipolar, and variable in size.
- Three types:
  - **W cells** project to the midbrain, carry information on pupillary response and reflexive movements.
  - **Y cells** project to lateral geniculate body, collateral branches to the midbrain, with pupillary information.
  - **X cells** project to lateral geniculate body, carry information on visual discrimination.

- **Receptive Fields**: the area of the retina in which the stimulation leads to a response in a given cell
  - Response may be depolarizing or hyperpolarizing, depending on the spatial configuration of the stimulus.
- Spatial antagonism – the center of the area of stimulus produces an opposite effect to the surround
  - On-center with off-surround
  - Off-center with on-surround
- Pathway of visual information processing:
  - Coupling of receptive fields → outer plexiform layer → LGN
- Factors that affect neuronal response:
  - **Type of cell:** Horizontal cell have larger, slower hyperpolarization than photoreceptors
  - **Shape:** Ring of light gives greater response than with a spot
  - **Location:** Contrast in the inner plexiform layer is temporal **and** outer plexiform layer is spatial
- Visual information travels from bipolar and amacrine cells → ganglion cells → LGN via action potentials
  - Possible receptive fields of the ganglion cell:
    - On-center with off-surround
    - **X type:** Sustained tonic from bipolar cell input
    - **Y type:** Phasic from amacrine
  - In the macula
    - receptive field is small
    - X type detects motion.

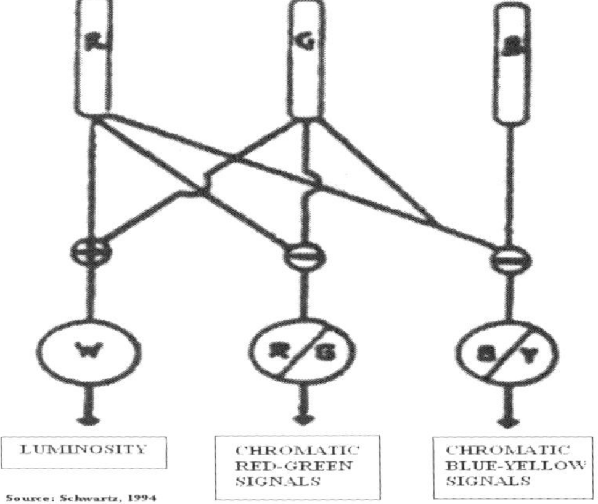

9. Retinal Neural Mechanisms of Color Vision (Spatial, Temporal, and Chromatic)

- Hering's Opponent color theory (1872)
  - Neural mechanisms display spatially antagonistic achromatic and chromatic behavior in the retina and cortex.
  - Color is processed by bipolar hue channels referred to as the R-G and B-Y channels.
    - Red and green are not seen simultaneously, either red or green. Same with blue and yellow →At any point in time, only one color in each channel is signaled.
    - A chromatic stimulus causes an afterimage of a complementary color.
    - "Bipolar" channel indicates the channel can only signal one of the two colors it is capable of coding.
- Trichromatic theory(Young-Helmholtz Theory -1802)
  - Color is coded by relative amounts of 3+ cone types that have preferential sensitivity to blue, green, and red.
- Modern opponent color theory
  - Combines Hering's opponent color theory & the trichromatic theory.
  - Opponent Theory is supported by hue cancellation experiments, Trichromatic theory is supported by color-matching experiments.

10. Physiological Relationships in the Choroid and the Retina, Including Retinal Metabolism

Relationship between the Choroid and the Retina

- The photoreceptors are nourished by choroid vessels (long & short posterior ciliary and anterior ciliary arteries).
- Hydrostatic pressure in the retina and choroid are about the same.
- Oncotic pressure of the choroid tissue causes a gradient of fluid absorption from the retina into the choroid of about 12mmHg.
    - May be a mechanism to help keep the retina attached to the choroid.
- The vessel walls of the choriocapillaris are fenestrated:
    - Permeable to particles up to 200 angstroms in diameter.
    - Allows Vitamin A to reach the RPE.

Relationship between the RPE and Photoreceptor Outer Segment

- The RPE provides nutrients for the photoreceptors:
    - Vitamin A (precursor for photosensitive pigments rhodopsin and iodopsin)
    - Oxygen
    - Glucose
- The RPE cells contain lysosomes that digest phagocytized outer segments discs.
    - There are melanin granules in the apical projections of the RPE that surround the photoreceptors outer segments. These absorb excess light that passes through the retina to minimize scatter between adjacent photoreceptors.

Age related changes

- Retina:
    - Decreased rod density
    - Decreased glial cells
- RPE:
    - Atrophy
    - Hyper and hypo pigment changes
    - Lipofuscin accumulation
- Vasculature:
    - Decreased blood supply
    - Vessel attenuation
    - Cystoid and Pavingstone degeneration

11. Unique Environment of the eye (High Extravascular Pressure)

- Metabolism in the outer retina (photoreceptors and RPE) has high metabolic activity, receives most blood supply from the choroid.
- Metabolism of the inner retina is less demanding, and supplied by retinal circulation.
- Glucose metabolism:
    - Retina has the highest rate of aerobic glucose consumption of any tissue.
    - 80% of glucose if used by photoreceptors.
    - Insulin-independent tissue (glucose enters directly by extracellular concentration regulation), uses GLUT 1 and GLUT 3 transporter proteins.
- Protein metabolism
- Lipid metabolism:
    - Varied and complex
    - Renders retina susceptible to oxidative damage

12. Retinal Blood Flow (Unique Characteristics, Dual Supply, Functions)

- Retinal blood flow is autoregulated – blood flow is varied according to nutritional demands of tissue and cardiac output.

- Blood Retinal Barrier
  - Tight junctions between endothelial cells of retinal vessels and RPE.
  - Impermeable to passage of molecules greater than 20-30,000 Da.
  - Small molecules (glucose, ascorbate) are actively transported.
- Outer retina
  - Receive blood from the choroidal capillary bed (through Bruch's membrane→ RPE→Neural retina.
  - Retina outer to outer plexiform layer is avascular and receives dual blood supply from retinal and choroidal vessels.
- Inner retina
  - Receives blood from **Central Retinal Artery** (enters the retina through the optic disc).
  - Two capillary networks:
    - **Deep** – between inner nuclear layer and outer plexiform layer.
    - **Superficial** – in the nerve fiber layer or ganglion cell layer.
- Retinal Vessels = "End" Vessels → do not anastomose with other blood vessels.
  - Terminate 1mm from the ora serrata.
- **Cilioretinal Artery** nourishes the macula, found in only 15-20% of population.

RETINA (PATHOLOGY)

- **Age-related macular degeneration (ARMD)**
  - Epidemiology:
    - Disease of the RPE, Bruch's, and choriocapillaris
    - Leading cause of blindness in US for patients over 65 years old
    - Risk factors:
      - Age
      - Family history
      - Smoking
      - Malnutrition
      - Hypertension
      - High cholesterol
      - Hyperopia
  - Nonexudative (Dry):
    - Drusen
      - Mucopolysaccharides, lipids, hyaline, and other basement membrane material deposits under RPE
      - Result of improper RPE cell function
    - Calcific drusen
    - Geographical atrophy of the RPE
    - 10% will develop wet AMD in 5 years
  - Exudative (Wet) :
    - Choroidal neovascularization in the macula
    - 12% per year risk of developing in fellow eye
  - Symptoms :
    - Dry:
      - Asymptomatic in early stage
      - Gradual VA loss
    - Wet:
      - Metamorphopsia
      - Central scotoma
      - Rapid VA loss
  - Signs:
    - Dry:
      - Drusen

            - RPE clumping and atrophy
        - Wet:
            - Choroidal neovascularization
            - Exudates
            - Retinal hemorrhage
            - RPE tears or detachment
    - Observation, inspection, techniques:
        - Amsler grid
        - Non-contact fundoscopy
        - Fluorescein angiography
        - Optical coherence tomography
- **Diabetic retinopathy (DR)**
    - Diabetes mellitus:
        - Insulin-dependent (Type I):
            - Juvenile onset
            - After 15 years, almost all patients with have DR
        - Non-insulin-dependent (Type II):
            - Adult onset
            - DR usually present at time of diagnosis
            - Risk factors
                - Hypertension
                - Pregnancy
                - Renal disease
                - Chronic hyperglycemia
    - Symptoms:
        - Early stages – asymptomatic
        - Reduced vision with macular edema or proliferative stages
    - Signs:
        - Non-proliferative (NPDR):
            - Microaneurysms (first sign)
            - Dot blot and flame hemorrhages
            - Venous beading
            - Intraretinal microvascular abnormalities
            - Hard exudates
            - Cotton wool spots
        - Proliferative (PDR):
            - neovascularization of the disc (NVD) or elsewhere (NVE)
            - Pre-retinal or vitreal hemorrhage → fibrosis → tractional retinal detachment
        - Macular edema
    - Observation, inspection, techniques:
        - DFE
        - Lab tests
            - fasting blood glucose
            - Hb A1C
            - blood urea nitrogen
            - creatinine
        - Fluorescein angiography
        - Optical coherence tomography
- **Retinal Detachment**
    - Risk factors:
        - PVD
        - Horseshoe retinal tear (30% risk)
        - Trauma
        - Lattice (<1% risk)

        - Atrophic holes (7% risk)
        - Cystic retinal tufts (10% risk)
        - High myopia (2% risk)
        - Ocular surgery
        - Aphakia
        - Retinal detachment in other eye (10% risk)
    - Must be treated immediately unless chronic
    - Rhegmatogenous:
        - Full-thickness retinal break that allows fluid from the vitreous to enter the subretinal space
        - Cause
            - Vitreoretinal traction (most common)
            - Traumatic
    - Non-rhegmatogenous:
        - Subretinal fluid beneath retina without retinal break
        - Cause
            - Exudative
            - Hemorrhagic
            - Tractional (caused by fibrosis)
    - Symptoms:
        - Acute onset of flashes or floaters
        - Dark curtain across field of view
        - May be asymptomatic
    - Signs:
        - Tobacco dust
        - Vitreal hemorrhage
        - Lower IOP in affected eye
        - Mild APD
        - Tear is red, flap is white (degenerated tissue)
        - Acute RD
            - Undulating
            - Hazy
            - Elevated
        - Chronic RD
            - Immobile
            - Transparent
            - Bullous
            - Pigment demarcation lines present at least 3 months

	Chronic RD	Acquired retinoschisis
Layer of retina split	Sensory retina and RPE	OPL and INL
Visual field	Relative defect	Absolute defect
Laterality	Unilateral	Bilateral
Tobacco dust	Present	Absent
Pigment lines	Present	Absent
Symptoms	Usually present in history	Rare

    - Observation, inspection, techniques
        - Slit lamp evaluation for tobacco dust
        - DFE with scleral indentation
        - Pupils
        - B scan ultrasonography (if unable to see fundus)
        - Fluorescein angiography for serous type to look for subretinal fluid
    - Complications: Macula off RD → severe visual loss

- **Acquired Retinoschisis**
    - Splitting of the inner nuclear and outer plexiform layer
    - Usually asymptomatic
    - Signs:
        - Most common location: inferotemporal
        - Bilateral
        - Snowflakes (persistent Muller fibers on inner wall of schisis)
        - No associated pigment

        - Not mobile
    - Observation, inspection, techniques:
        - Check for tobacco dust
        - DFE with scleral indentation
        - OCT to asses layer of splitting
        - Visual field
    - Complications: If break forms in outer retinal layer, fluid may travel through and cause a RD

- **Trauma to retina**
    - Epidemiology: Usually young males
    - Commotio Retinae (aka Berlin's Edema)
        - disruption of the photoreceptor outer segment following a traumatic eye injury
        - Usually asymptomatic unless near macula
        - Signs:
            - grey/white discoloration of the retina
            - can be associated with retinal hemorrhages or choroidal rupture
    - Dialysis:
        - Tearing of peripheral retina near ora serrata
        - Usually inferior temporal with <90 degree involvement
        - Usually asymptomatic
        - Signs: possibly vitreal hemorrhage
        - Complications: slow progression toward RD

Retinal Holes

- **Atrophic hole**
    - Pathophysiology:
        - Avascular area of sensory retina → focal retinal degeneration → Progressive thinning → Full thickness break in peripheral retina
        - Leads to a hole if there is traction or trauma
    - Epidemiology: 2-7% of population
    - Signs:
        - Round red lesion
        - Peripheral
        - Pinpoint to 2DD in size
        - Often multiple
        - 25% bilateral
        - Usually associated with lattice
    - Observation, inspection, techniques:
        - Scleral indentation
            - Whitish cuff surrounding hole indicates small RD or edema
            - Pigment indicates chronicity
    - Complications: 7% risk of RD
- **Operculated hole**
    - Small, focal area of retinal tissue separated by vitreoretinal adhesion and liquefaction
    - Signs:
        - White operculum in the vitreous overlying red hole
        - Pigment due to vitreal traction
    - Complications: High risk for RD
- **Macular hole**
    - Pathophysiology: Circular depression usually caused by macular edema or retinal breaks
    - Epidemiology:
        - >60 years old
        - white females
        - <10% chance of developing hole
    - Lamellar holes: Ruptured macular cyst

- Symptoms:
  - Metamorphopsia
  - Decreased VA (20/200 for full thickness holes)
  - Central scotoma
- Signs:
  - Round, red lesion
  - Surrounding fluid cuff - gray edema appearance
  - Watzke Allen sign

- **Retinal venous occlusions**
  - Pathophysiology:
    - Arteriosclerosis
    - Thickened arterioles compress vein
  - Risk factors:
    - Age
    - Hypertension
    - Hyperlipidemia
    - Diabetes
    - Elevated IOP (risk of CRVO)
  - **Branch retinal venous occlusion (BRVO):** Occurs at major retinal branch or minor macular branch
  - **Hemiretinal:** Least common, Involves superior or inferior branch of central retinal vein
  - **Central retinal venous occlusion (CRVO)**
    - Non-ischemic
    - Ischemic – much more severe
  - Symptoms:
    - Metamorphopsia or blurred vision if macular edema
    - Sudden, severe vision loss with CRVO
  - Signs:
    - Venous engorgement
    - Dot blot and flame hemorrhages
    - Cotton wool spots
    - All 4 quadrants in CRVO affected
    - APD in CRVO
  - Observation, inspection, techniques:
    - Pupils
    - DFE
    - Gonioscopy for CRVO→Iris or angle neovascularization
    - Fluorescein angiography
  - Complications: Neovascularization in retina and iris if large area of ischemia (CRVO)

Benign Peripheral Retinal Findings

- **Lattice degeneration**
  - Thinning of retina due to loss of inner retinal layers down to ONL (loss of retinal neurons) with strong vitreoretinal adhesion
  - Associations:
    - Myopia
    - Marfan's syndrome
  - Symptoms: Asymptomatic
  - Signs:
    - Whitish gray circumferentially oriented cigar-shaped lesion
    - Vitreal liquefaction
    - Usually found at 11, 1, 5, and 7 o'clock
    - 82% pigmented
    - 18% have atrophic holes
    - 12% have white lines (sclerosed retinal blood vessels)

- Other presentations: Snail track degeneration
- Complications: 0.3% risk of RD

- **Cystic retinal tuft**
  - Small focal vitreoretinal adhesion
  - Present at birth
  - Signs:
    - Discrete white gray lesion
    - Pigment if traction
    - Around retinal equator
    - 95% Bilateral
  - Causes 10% of all RDs
- **Snowflake degeneration**
  - Signs:
    - Small, yellow white spots
    - Circumferential
    - Superior/temporal quadrant
- **Central serous retinopathy (CSR)**
  - Fluid in macular area
  - Epidemiology:
    - Age 30-40
    - Type A personality and stress
  - Symptoms:
    - Decreased VA
    - Metamorphopsia
    - Dyschromatopsia
    - ma:y present with central scotoma
  - Signs:
    - Hyperopic shift
    - Unilateral
    - Loss of foveal reflex (due to elevation in macula)
  - Prognosis:
    - Spontaneous recovery 1 to 6 months later
    - High recurrence rate
- **Cystoid macular edema**
  - Pathophysiology: Fluid accumulation in retinal OPL and INL
  - Causes:
    - Vaso-occlusive disease
    - Cataract surgery
    - Pars planitis
    - Retinitis pigmentosa
    - Progressive pigmentary degeneration
    - Ocular inflammation
  - Signs:
    - Subtle elevation
    - Loss of foveal reflex
  - Observation, inspection, techniques:
    - Fluorescein angiography →Petal-like pattern
  - Prognosis: Usually spontaneous recovery

Retinitis

- **Histoplasmosis**
  - Pathophysiology: infection of the choroidal tissue by histo capsulatum
  - Epidemiology:
    - 1% prevalence
    - Age 20-50 years

        - Endemic to Ohio Mississippi River Valley
    - Symptoms:
        - Asymptomatic until macular involvement
        - Decreased VA
        - Metamorphopsia
    - Signs:
        - Peripapillary atrophy
        - Atrophic histo-spots (choriodal scarring)
        - Maculopathy
- **Toxoplasmosis**
    - Retinochoroiditis caused by infection by Toxoplasma Gondii protozoan
    - Pathophysiology:
        - May stay dormant in NFL for years
        - Reactivation may occur in immunocompromised patients
    - Epidemiology:
        - #1 cause of posterior uveitis
        - Caucasian
        - Adolescent
    - Symptoms:
        - Hazy vision
        - Floaters
        - Visual field loss
    - Signs:
        - Focal retinitis with overlying vitritis
        - Whitish yellow lesions with surrounding pigmented scar
        - Papillitis & papilledema are sometimes present
        - Size usually 1 DD

White Dot Syndromes

- **Multiple evanescent white-dot syndrome (MEWDS)**
    - Epidemiology:
        - More common in females
        - Age 20-40 years
    - Symptoms:
        - Unilateral 80%
        - Photopsia
    - Signs:
        - Reddish granular changes
        - Foveal/macular area
        - Small punctuate white lesions at RPE level
- **Acute posterior multifocal placoid pigment epitheliopathy (APMPPE)**
    - Epidemiology:
        - Equally common in male and females
        - Age 20-50
        - History of flu
    - Symptoms:
        - Bilateral
        - Paracentral vision loss
    - Signs:
        - RPE inflammation
        - Diffuse area of white, plate like lesions
        - Well defined edges
    - 95% resolve without treatment

Chapter 16 – Optic Nerve/Neuro-Ophthalmic Pathways

OCULAR AND ORBITAL NERVES (GROSS ANATOMY)

1. Cranial Nerves I, III, IV, V, VI, VII

- **Cranial Nerve I: Olfactory Nerve**
  - Olfactory nerves arise from olfactory receptor cells in the olfactory epithelium of the nasal cavity, which bundle together and pass through the cribriform plate of the ethmoid bone to synapse with the olfactory bulb, which extends as the olfactory tract under the frontal lobe to the olfactory cortex.
  - It functions for the sense of smell only.
- **Cranial Nerve III: Oculomotor Nerve**
  - 3rd n. innervates SR, MR, IR, IO, Levator and also provide route for autonomic fibers travel to innervate iris sphincter muscle, ciliary muscle, and smooth muscles of the eyelid.
  - 3rd n. nucleus is located in the midbrain at the level of the superior colliculus, right above the trochlear nucleus.
  - There is a cluster of subnuclei within the oculomotor nucleus. Each of these subnuclei controls each muscle. There are 2 subnuclei for muscles, except for levator.
  - Fibers extend from the nucleus in the ventral midbrain near the superior junction of the pons, pierces through roof the cavernous sinus, runs along the cavernous sinus's lateral wall, right above the trochlear nerve, and enters the orbit through superior orbital fissure, *within* the oculomotor foramen. Then, this nerve divides right before entering the muscle cone into the superior and inferior muscular branches.
    - The superior branch runs medially above the optic nerve and innervates the *levator* and *superior rectus*. These fibers enter along the underside of the superior rectus, additional fibers either pierce through the muscle or pass around it to innervate the levator.
    - The inferior branch runs below the optic nerve, innervates the *medial* and *inferior recti* and the *inferior oblique*. First branch enters medial rectus, second enters inferior rectus, the third branch sends parasympathetic root to the ciliary ganglion, then innervates inferior oblique.

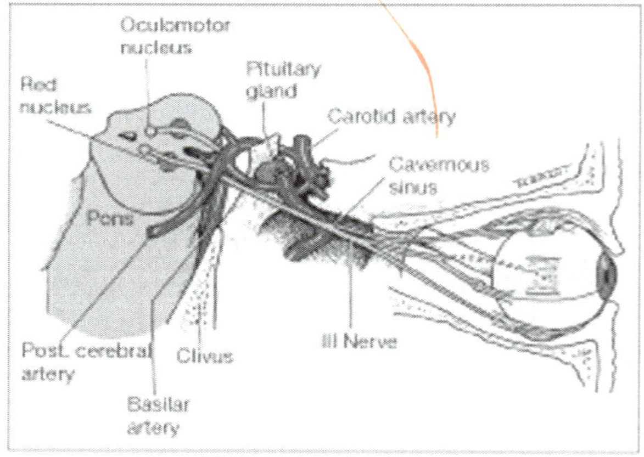

- **Cranial Nerve IV: The Trochlear Nerve**
  - It is the thinnest nerve originates from nuclei right below the oculomotor nuclei at the level of the inferior colliculus in the midbrain. It is the only nerve that runs dorsal, decussates then curves around the cerebral peduncle right above the pons. It enters the cavernous sinus, moves to the superior orbital fissure, and enters the orbit outside of the muscle cone above the common tendinous ring. It goes above the levator to innervate the superior oblique 1/3 of the way along the muscle. This nerve runs the longest course and is most prone to traumatic damage.
  - The superior obliques are innervated by trochlear nerves that originated from the contralateral side of the brain.
- **Cranial Nerve V: The Trigeminal Nerve**

- These nerves arise from the gasserian ganglion outside the brainstem, which is composed of the sensory and motor roots.
- The ganglion splits into three branches: the ophthalmic division, the mandibular division, and the maxillary division.
  - The ophthalmic division splits into 3 subdivisions: the nasociliary nerve, the frontal nerve that innervates the skin of the brow and forehead, and the lacrimal nerve that innervates the lacrimal gland and the skin of the face.
    - Nasociliary nerve consists of infratrochlear nerve, anterior and posterior ethmoid nerves, 2 long ciliary nerves and sensory roots of the ciliary ganglion. The nasociliary nerve exits the orbit by passing through the common tendinous ring and the superior orbital fissure into the cranial cavity.
    - Frontal nerve consists of supratrochlear nerve and supraorbital nerve. It travels between levator muscle and the periorbita, exiting the orbit through the SOF, above the common tendinous ring. Both of these nerves innervate the skin, muscle of the forehead, and upper lid.
    - Lacrimal nerve innervates the lateral aspect of the upper lid, temple area and lacrimal gland.
- The mandibular division gives sensory innervation to the teeth, gums, and skin of the lower jaw.
- The maxillary division includes infraorbital n. which sends sensory fibers from the cheek, upper lip and lower eyelid through infraorbital foramen and infraorbital groove in the maxillary bone. Some branches from the upper teeth joined this nerve in the maxillary sinus. Over stimulation to upper teeth can be sent to the infraorbital nerve leading to orbital pain sensation.
  - The zygomatic nerve is the second nerve that makes up the maxillary division of 5th N. It contains 2 smaller nerves known as zygomaticotemporal n. which innervates the lateral aspect of the forehead and zygomaticofacial n. which innervates the lateral aspect of the cheek, and lower eyelid.

- **Cranial Nerve VI: The Abducens Nerve**
  - The nuclei of the abducens nerve are located near the midline of the pons beside the floor of the 4th ventricle. It exits the brainstem in the groove between the pons and the medulla oblongata. It runs along the occipital bone, then takes a sharp bend over the petrous portion of the temporal bone before entering the cavernous sinus. Within the sinus, it sits next to the internal carotid artery. It then enters the orbit through the SOF within the common tendinous ring and innervates the lateral rectus muscle. 6th nerve damage is very common as trauma occurs to the side of the head and 6th n. runs most laterally and innervates the eye on the ipsilateral side.
  - 6th nerve nucleus also contains internuclear neurons that communicate with the nucleus for the contralateral medial rectus muscle in the oculomotor complex via the medial longitudinal fasciculus. This is the pathway for conjugate horizontal eye movement. It received its signal from higher CNS centers such as: paramedial pontine reticular formation (PPRF), cerebellum, and the vestibular nucleus. Coordinated movement of the ipsilateral LR and the contralateral MR results in conjugate horizontal eye movement.

- **Cranial Nerve VII: The Facial Nerve**
  - The nuclei are near the abducens and the nerves emerge from the brainstem near the lower border of the pons running laterally to the internal auditory meatus, where one branch innervates the middle ear and the other exits the skull by the stylomastoid foramen to branch to supply the muscles of the face and jaw, the submandibular and sublingual salivary glands, the lacrimal glands, and sensation to the soft palate and anterior 1/3 of the tongue.
  - The upper and lower zygomatic branches supply the orbicularis oculi.

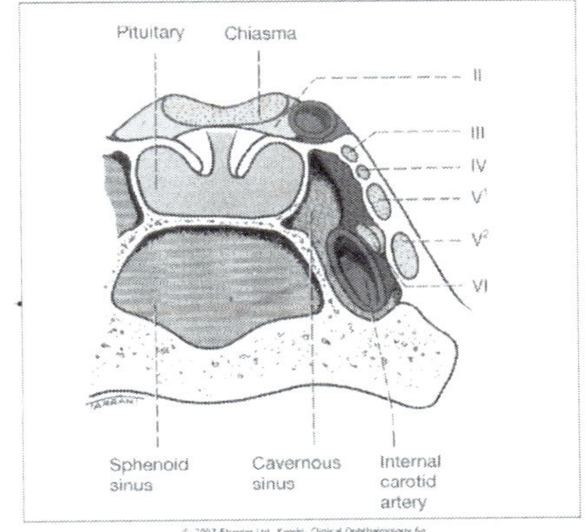

Note: *It is important to know which nerves travel through the cavernous sinus and their relative location to each other.*

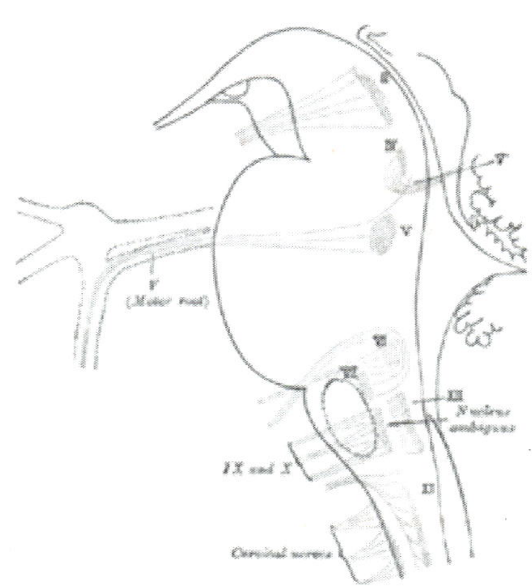

Sagittal section through brain stem showing trigeminal, oculomotor, trochlear, abducens and facial nuclei.

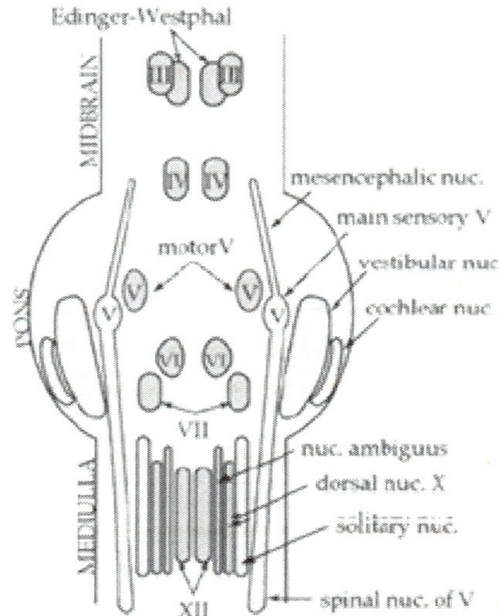

Dorsal view of the brainstem nuclei of the cranial nerve

Note: *You will need to know the positions of the nuclei within the brainstem, so that you can localize central lesion.*

2. Parasympathetic Nerves (Course, Branches, Tissue Innervated)

- Originate in the ciliary or pterygopalatine ganglion and travel from the **Edinger-Westphal nucleus** to the **ciliary ganglion** by the **oculomotor nerve**, and then to the eye with the **short ciliary nerve**, where the fibers innervate the sphincter of the iris, the ciliary muscle and the choroidal vasculature.
- The lacrimal gland receives parasympathetic innervation from the pterygopalatine ganglion in the pterygopalatine fossa of the sphenoid bone which passes through the maxillary nerve to the zygomatic nerve to the zygomatic-temporal branch.

3. Sympathetic Nerves (Course, Branches, Tissue Innervated)

- Sympathetic fibers controlled by the hypothalamus travel through the cervical spinal cord. The **preganglionic** fibers leave the spinal cord via the ventral root and enter the sympathetic ganglion chain located adjacent to the vertebrae. These fibers travel up the sympathetic chain and synapse in the **superior cervical ganglion**. They then become **postganglionic** fibers that leave the ganglion and form the **carotid plexus** around the internal carotid artery. These fibers separate from the plexus in the cavernous sinus (CS) and travel different routes to reach their target structures.
    - Some fibers travel with the ophthalmic division of 5th n. from the CS into the orbit. Once in the orbit, the sympathetic fibers follow the nasociliary nerve and travel with the long ciliary nerves to innervate the iris dilator and ciliary muscle.
    - Other fibers from the carotid plexus take the same route as the nasociliary nerve and branch to the ciliary ganglion as the sympathetic root. These fibers pass through the ganglion without synapsing. They enter the globe as the short ciliary nerves to innervate the choroidal blood vessels.
    - The rest of the fibers from the carotid plexus join the oculomotor nerve and travel with it into the orbit to innervate the smooth muscle of the upper eyelid.

Note: *Sympathetic innervations to iris dilator, Muller's muscle, blood vessels, and lacrimal gland.*

OPTIC NERVE (GROSS ANATOMY)

- The optic nerve contains about 1 million visual fibers, 90% of which will end at the LGN and 10% will travels to that area responsible for pupil response and the circadian rhythm.
- The ONH is 5-6cm long and can be divided into 4 sections: intraocular, intraorbital, intracanalicular, and intracranial. They can be further divided into smaller portion: intraocular (prelaminar, laminar, and retrolaminar).

1. Surface Features

- RPE crescent: Pigmented crescent is caused by exposed pigment epithelium of the retina (dark crescent).
- Choroidal crescent: If the retinal pigment epithelium does not reach the edge of the optic nerve, a choroidal crescent becomes visible at the optic nerve (grayish crescent).
- Scleral crescent: Is due to having an exposed lip of the sclera (whitish crescent).

2. Prelaminar Portion (Composition, Blood Supply)

- The prelaminar portion is in front of the lamina cribrosa behind which the nerve fibers become myelinated.
- Many **central retinal arteries** and veins emerge in this portion.
- The small capillaries lose their internal elastic lamina supplying this portion of the nerve with blood.
- Myelin may appear in the papillary region.
- Astrocytes in the optic nerve surround, line and protect it:
    - Intermediary tissue of Kuhnt and the marginal border of Elschnig are specialized regions of glial tissue where the retina and choroid terminate at the optic nerve.
    - The glial mantle of Fuchs or Graefe, which is the name for the pia mater of the optic nerve in this portion.
    - The border tissue of Jacoby, glial tissue where the sclera terminates at the optic nerve head and is continuous with the intermediary tissue of Kuhnt.
- The inner limiting membrane of Elschnig is where the glial layer thickens over the optic nerve head.
- The meniscus of Kuhnt is where the inner limiting membrane of Elschnig thickens and fills in the optic cup.
- The Muller cells disappear when the axons curve sharply to form the optic nerve in this portion.

3. Laminar Portion (Composition, Blood Supply)

- The lamina cribrosa or cribriform plate is perforated to allow ganglion cell axons and vascular passage.
- Firm attachment for the optic nerve to the back of the eye.
- Blood vessels have an internal elastic lamina.
- Axons begin to be myelinated.
- Capillaries from the Circle of Zinn and choroidal vasculature supply the blood.

4. Retrolaminar Portion (Composition, Blood Supply)

- The optic nerve proper.
- The axons are all myelinated in this region behind the lamina cribrosa.
- The septal connective tissue appears and continues laterally with the pial connective tissue and the lamina cribrosa internally.
- Blood is supplied by the pial arteries, central retinal and pial system of vessels.

5. Central Retinal Artery and Vein (Location)

- The central artery branches off from the ophthalmic artery just as it enters the orbit. It travels beneath the optic nerve and then inserts into the optic nerve 12-13 mm behind the eye. It emerges inside the eye in the optic disc.

- The central retinal vein travels along with the central retinal artery, also leaving the sheath of the optic nerve 12-13mm behind the eye.

6. Optic Disc/Cup

- The optic disc/cup is where the nerve fiber layer dips down into the optic nerve – it is where ganglion cell axons accumulate and exit the eye.
- Slightly elongated vertically (1.7mm horizontal, 1.9mm vertical)
- Number of nerve fibers are positively correlated with the size of the optic nerve head
- Optic disc lacks all retinal elements except the nerve fiber layer and internal limiting membrane. No RPE or photoreceptors
- Internal limiting membrane of Elschnig covers it.

VISUAL PATHWAY (GROSS ANATOMY)

1. Localization of Retinal Fibers Along Visual Pathway

- **Optic nerve:** groups of nerve axons from the retina form into approximately 1000 fascicles to pass through the lamina cribrosa. The fibers are in a regular array.
- **Optic chiasm:** fibers from the nasal retina cross over to the other side. Nasal macular fibers cross at the center of the optic chiasm. Temporal fibers stay on the same side.
- **Optic tract:** As the fibers leave the chiasm in the optic tract, the crossed and uncrossed fibers mix together. The superior fiber (from the ipsilateral superior nasal retina) moves to the medial side of the tract. The fibers from the inferior retina (ipsilateral inferior temporal retinal fibers and contralateral inferior nasal retinal fibers) occupy the lateral area of the tract.
  - Nerve fibers in the optic tract make first contact with the brain by wrapping around the cerebral peduncles. The optic tract divides into two roots:
  - The lateral root, which goes to the lateral geniculate nucleus and is concerned with conscious vision
  - The medial part goes to the superior colliculus and the pretectum, carrying 10% of the fibers, which are not involved in conscious vision.
- **Lateral Geniculate Nucleus (LGN):**
  - The fibers from the superior retinal quadrants end in the medial aspect of the LGN and the fibers from the inferior retinal quadrant terminate in the lateral aspect.
  - The primary synaptic point of the optic axons. A single LGN cell may receive signals from a single optic axon but usually are contacted by several (3-4) optic axons. One optic axon can connect to six LGN cells in the same layer.
  - These cells project to the pulvinar, superior colliculus, pretectum and other nuclei.
  - The macula is mapped onto the body of the LGN, axons of the superior retina go to the medial part, the inferior retina to the lateral part of the LGN, the temporal crescent is mapped onto the contralateral spur at the anterior section of the LGN.
  - Each layer of the LGN has a retinotopic map which is a "point-to-point localization" of the retina. Many of these maps are stacked on each other such that if a line were passed through all six layers, perpendicular to the surface, the intercepted cells all would be carrying information about the same point in the visual field. Therfefore, fibers that carry information from the same site in the visual field of each eye terminate in adjacent layers of the LGN, right next to each other
- **Optic radiations** are fibers that fan out from the LGN, and the *retinotopic map* is maintained.
  - It is important to know that the lateral fibers of LGN which representing inferior retina will travel into the temporal lobe and loop around the tip of the temporal horn of the lateral ventricle, known as Meyer's loop, then continue to travel to the parietal lobe to from the inferior radiation.
  - *Remember:*
    - *Lateral LGN fibers- inferior radiation*
    - *Medial LGN fibers- superior radiation*

- **Visual cortex** is located at the posterior pole of the brain. 1/3 of the cortex is taken up by macular representation.
    - The cuneus or upper calcarine fissure maps the lower visual field, i.e., the superior retina.
    - The linguinal gyrus (below the calcarine fissure) maps the upper visual field, i.e., the inferior retina.
    - The parieto-occipital fissure maps the monocular segment of the peripheral visual field.
    - Fibers from the macular area terminate in the most posterior part of the striate cortex.

2. Layers of Lateral Geniculate Body (Afferents, Efferents)

- The input from the 2 eyes is kept separate until the striated cortex. Therefore, the LGN is separated into 6 layers.
    - Layers 1, 4, 6 are contralateral, nasal hemiretina, temporal crescent
    - Layers 2, 3, 5 are ipsilateral, temporal hemiretina
- Three types of Axons:
    - Optic axons or retinogeniculate axons travel from the retina to the striate cortex
    - Geniclo-cortico axons travel from the principal cells in the LGN to the striate cortex
    - Cortico-geniculate axons go from the cortex to the LGN
- Two Main Pathways:
    - Optic nerve to principal cell to the cortex
    - Optic nerve to intrinsic cell to principal cell to the visual cortex

3. Layers of Visual Cortex (Areas)

- **Supragranular layers (I,II,III):**
    - I is the superficial layer that lies against the pia mater (almost no cells, mostly fibers)
    - II and III are densely cellular, composed of many stellate and pyramidal cells
- **Layer IV (A, B, C):** receives main input from the LGN. Granular layer due to loss of stellate cells.
    - IV A has almost exclusively stellate cells.
    - IV B has some stellate and some pyramidal cells. The Stripe of Gennari is due to this layer.
    - IV C alpha has densely packed stellate cells and is characterized by structures called ocular dominance columns.
    - IV C beta also has densely packed stellate cells.
- **Infragranular layers (V, VI):**
    - Layer V or the inner line of Baillarger is a relatively sparse cell layer with very big pyramidal cells.
    - Layer VI is very dense with cells containing both stellate and pyramidal cells.
- **Broadmann Area 18 (V2)** is a mirror of area 17, the primary visual cortex
- **Broadmann Area 19 (V3)** is a mirror of area 18, making 17 and 19 similar

4. Blood Supply

- **Intracranial optic nerve:** ophthalmic, internal carotid, anterior cerebral, anterior communicating arteries, and a small amount by the anterior hypophyseal artery
- **Optic chiasm:** ophthalmic, anterior cerebral, anterior and posterior communicating arteries, internal carotid artery, anterior and superior hypophyseal, middle cerebral, and anterior choroidal arteries
- **Optic tract:** middle and posterior cerebral, anterior choroidal, and the posterior communicating arteries
- **LGN:** anterior and posterior choroidal arteries and a branch of the posterior cerebral artery
- **Optic radiations** (3 sections)
    - **Anterior**: the anterior choroidal artery
    - **Middle**: deep optic branch of the middle cerebral artery
    - **Posterior**: the posterior cerebral artery near the striate cortex
- **Visual cortex:** middle cerebral and posterior cerebral artery, may have macular sparing because of this dual supply which anastomoses

5. Anatomy Related to Visual Pathology

- The macular area of the visual cortex sits out at the back of the occipital lobe; some of it is folded into the occipital bone. This places it in a very vulnerable position, and loss of vision can be very precise with sharp and distinct borders, usually binocular.
- The temporal loop of the optic radiations is the more vulnerable pathway, lesions to this pathway effects the upper quarter of the visual field. A bilateral quadratic defect. "Pie In The Sky".
    - *Tips: Know the abbreviation of PITS stands for Parietal lesion resulted in Inferior VF defect, and Temporal lesion resulted in Superior VF defect.*
- All lesions posterior to the chiasm will affect visual fields on the opposite side. If you have a lesion on the right side of the brain, then you will be a bilateral superior left quadranopsia.
- Remember all the left side of the visual field is seen by the right striate cortex. These are contralateral fields.
- Pituitary tumors which press on the posterior part of the optic chiasm will cause the superior nasal field to be affected resulting in a bilateral temporal-inferior visual defect, i.e., a quadranopsia. If it pushes on the center of the chiasm, then you will get a bilateral temporal hemianopsia because fibers from the nasal maculas of both eyes are affected.
- Lesions to the optic nerve and retina will result in monocular losses in the visual field directly corresponding to those areas which the affected neurons had served.
    - **Remember the more posterior a lesion is the more congruous the VF defect pattern will be.*

Chart 1: Summary of different types of VF defect patterns and location of lesion.

VF defects	Sites of interruption of nerve fiber
Monocular complete VF loss	Before chiasm in same eye.
Bitemporal hemianopia	In midline of optic chiasm
Complete VF loss in OD, and superior temporal loss for OS	Lesion at right anterior knees + lesion at right ON at junction w/ chiasm
Incongruent right homonymous hemianopia	OS optic tract
Total OS homonymous hemianopia	Complete interruption in right optic tract, LGN, or optic radiation
Incongruent right homonymous hemianopia	Left optic radiation involving Meyer's loop
Incongruent right homonymous hemianopia	Optic radiation in left parietal lobe
Complete right homonymous hemianopia	All left optic radiations
Right homonymous hemianopia w/ macular sparing	Left anterior striate cortex
Left homonymous hemianopia with macular and temporal crescent sparing	Right striate cortex
Left macular homonymous hemianopia	Right posterior striate cortex
Left temporal crescent loss	Right anterior striate cortex

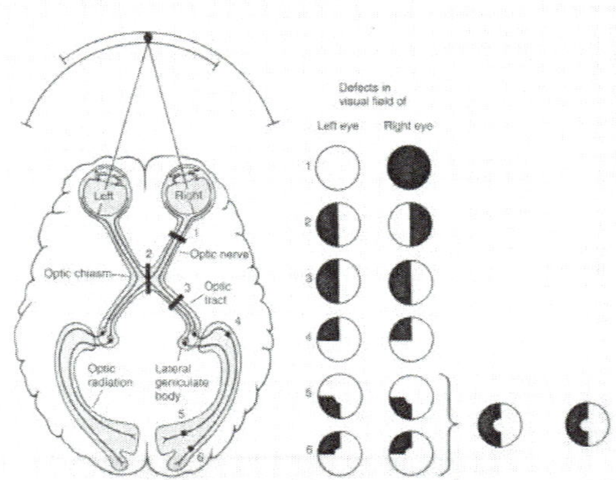

OPTIC NERVE & VISUAL PATHWAY (DEVELOPMENTAL ANATOMY)

1. Developmental Stages of Lower Visual Pathway, Before Lateral Geniculate Body

- **Optic nerve:**
  - Developed from the optic stalk or pedicle.
  - As the optic stalk develops, it consists of two parts; a distal, primitive portion associated with the fetal fissure, and a proximal portion.
  - Nerve fibers from the ganglion cell layer grow into the stalk, towards the brain and form the optic nerve. ← Inner neuroblastic layer
  - The optic nerve then grows thicker.
  - Cells in the optic nerve vacuolate and disappear.
  - Outer epithelial cells develop into supporting glial cells. ← neural ectoderm?
  - Glial cells also develop around the hyaloid artery at its entrance into the vitreous. This mass of glial cells is known as Bergmeister's Papilla. The optic nerve fibers must pass through the papilla as they come from the ganglion cells to the optic stalk.
- Developmentally, the optic nerve resembles a tract of the brain, because like the brain, the fibers do not possess a neurilemma sheath.
- **Meninges:** the optic nerve is surrounded by sheath made from all three layers of meninges of the brain. Between the layers are spaces continuous with the subdural and subarachnoid space, bathing the optic nerve in cerebrospinal fluid. At the 5th month the dura, arachnoid and pia can be distinguished from each other.
- During the 6th month a network of scleral tissue penetrates the optic nerve to form the lamina cribrosa.
- Differences between crossed and uncrossed fibers:
  - Fibers from the lateral half of the retina grow into the optic tract on the same (ipsilateral) side.
  - Fibers from the medial half of the retina pass through the optic chiasm into the optic tract on the opposite (contralateral) side.
  - One-third of the optic nerve fibers represent the macula (which is only 10% of retinal space).
  - Macular fibers are split such that temporal fibers stay near the temporal portion of the optic nerve.
  - Nasal macular fibers cross over in the center of the chiasm.

2. Myelination of the Visual Pathway (Lower visual pathway vs. upper visual pathway)

- Optic nerve fibers become medullated late in fetal life.
  - Many double layers of myelin are wrapped around optic nerve fibers by oligodendroglial cells.
  - Nodes of Ranvier and mesaxons form as myelin sheaths grow.
- Developmental sequence of myelin sheath
  - The process begins in the chiasm around the 24th week of fetal life.
  - Medullation of the optic nerve proceeds from the brain to the eye, unlike optic nerve fiber growth which goes from the eye to the brain. Medullation opposite to growth
  - By birth the myelination has reached the lamina cribrosa.
- The pathway is divided into two parts:
  - Non-medullated part consisting of bare axons continuous with the nerve fibers of the retina. The loss of the medullary sheath allows the diameter of the nerve to be diminished as it enters the scleral foramen.
  - Medullated part runs from the lamina cribrosa to the brain.
- The layers of the retina usually cease before the optic nerve is reached; in which case, a mass of tissue continuous with the neuroglia of the optic nerve is interposed called the intermediary tissue of Kuhnt.

3. Relationship Between Development of Upper Visual Pathway and Central Vision

- A point-to point relationship develops between the origin of the optic nerve fibers in the retina and their termination in the LGN.
- Neurons develop in the lateral geniculate body whose axons form the geniculocalcarine tract.
  - Neurons in the geniculocalcarine tract develop a point-to-point relationship between the LGN and cortex.
  - The geniculocalcarine tract grows into the visual cortex which is located on either side of the calcarine fissure. (Calcarine fissure: During the 6th month of fetal life the visual area of the cerebral cortex becomes folded along its axis.)

4. Physiological Cupping

- The **physiological cup** is a **congenital** depression in the center surface of the disc and varies greatly in size and depth. It is the absence of neural tissue and glial elements.
- The size is determined by heredity (multofactorial/polygenic) and race:
  - African Descent have larger cups than Caucasians.
- Physiological cupping should be symmetrical between the two eyes.
- Congenital neuroretinal rim is thick uniformly, full, with a distinct border.

NEUROPHYSIOLOGY (PHYSIOLOGY)

1. Integration of Nerve Signals

- **Synaptic processes**
  - There are two types of synapses in the nervous system, electrical synapses and chemical synapses. An electrical synapse consists of gap junctions that permits the direct passage of ions and other small molecules from one cell to another. Electrical synapses transmit information in both directions. In chemical synapses, on the other hand, there is a space, called a synaptic cleft, between one cell and the other that prevents the direct passage of ions. In order for ions to flow into the second cell, chemical transmitters must be released from the first cell into the synaptic cleft, where they bind specifically with chemically activated ion channels in the second cell.
  - The structure of the electrical synapse is similar to the gap junctions seen in other cells. Studies have shown that the pre- and postsynaptic cells are connected by a protein channel called a connexon that spans the gap between them. The connexon is made of six protein subunits called connexin that are arranged into a hexagonal assembly. Electrical synapses are found between axons and soma, axons and dendrites, dendrites and dendrites, and soma and soma. These "electrical" synapses serve as channels for both electrical and metabolic communication. These synapses synchronize the activity of many adjoining cells as well as provide a pathway for a rapid communication between cells.
  - Although electrical synapses are found in many areas of the nervous system, the predominant type of synapse is the chemical synapse. In chemical synapses at least two cells participate: the cell producing the chemical signal, called the presynaptic neuron, and the target cell that receives the signal, called the postsynaptic neuron. The terminal ending is part of the presynaptic neuron, and it contains vesicles. These vesicles, filled with chemicals referred to as neurotransmitters, fuse with the presynaptic membrane. The fusion of the vesicle with the presynaptic cell membrane causes the release of the chemical neurotransmitters into the synaptic cleft. The transmitters in turn act upon the receptors located on postsynaptic cell membranes. When transmitters bind the receptors, one of two things can happen: there is either depolarization of the membrane or hyperpolarization of the membrane. Finally, the termination of synaptic transmission occurs when the transmitter is removed from the synaptic cleft. This process is accomplished in most neurotransmitter systems by the transport of the transmitters back into the presynaptic terminal. Other transmitters are removed from the

synaptic cleft by degrading enzymes, and the metabolic products are then transported back into the presynaptic terminal. Spinal cord reflexes represent the most basic of motor responses. These reflexes are carried out entirely within the spinal cord and are modified by inputs from higher centers to generate complex movements. They are also used to help diagnose disorders of the motor system. The following is a list of spinal reflexes that are explained in further detail in another section.

- **Reflexes:** automatic body movements, which do not require conscious thought. Examples include:
  - Stretch reflex: commonly called the knee jerk reflex.
  - Inverse myotic reflex: involves the Golgi tendon organ.
  - Flexor withdrawal reflex: involves cutaneous receptors.
- **Feedback:** the return of some of the output of a system as input allowing for some control over the process. Feedback controls are a type of self-regulating mechanism by which certain activities are sustained within prescribed ranges. There are two types of feedback, one is positive and the other is negative. In a positive feedback system there tends to be an increase of activity or product to get back to the normal set point. It reinforces and accelerates certain factors within a given system. In negative feedback, the controlling mechanism responds in a manner that decreases activity or product to get back to the normal set point level. It is, therefore, a corrective action that returns a factor within the specific system to a normal range.
- **Adaptation:**
  - Often, when a stimulus is continuously applied, the brain at some point no longer consciously perceives it. This adjustment happens, for example, with background noise such as the ticking of a clock. After a period of time it is unnoticed. This phenomenon is called sensory adaptation. The adaptation to a sensory stimulus can be caused by mechanisms either within the brain or at the receptor site. Adaptation mechanisms that work at receptor sites are the most clearly understood and best illustrated by the Pacinian corpuscle.
  - When pressure applied to the Pacinian corpuscle is continuously maintained, the free nerve ending eventually reverts back to its original shape even though the layers of connective tissue remained deformed. Since the Na+ channels embedded within the nerve membrane are opened only when the nerve fiber is deformed, they close only when the form of the nerve fiber is again circular. Consequently, even though pressure on the Pacinian corpuscle is still maintained, it ceases to produce a generator potential when it resumes its normal shape and thus no longer transmits information about the pressure of the stimulus.
  - Mechanisms of adaptation are also found at the molecular level. Chemical receptors on membranes, for example, are internalized and removed from the surface of the membrane after continued exposure to drugs. With the removal of these chemical receptors, higher levels of the drug are necessary to achieve the same effect. This may be why, after repeated use, the body develops a tolerance to drugs.
- **Habituation:** Habituation, or the decrease in a behavioral response to a repeated stimulus, can be explained at the cellular level in terms of a decrease in synaptic transmission, as a result of the inactivation of Ca^{2+} channels in the presynaptic terminal. The reduction of Ca^{2+} influx in turn decreases the amount of neurotransmitter that is released into the synaptic cleft. In addition, the number of synapses that contain active zones for the release of vesicles decreases, as does the area of the active zones. Together, these mechanisms diminish the functional capacity of the synapse.

2. Sensory Coding (e.g. receptive field concept)

- Sensory organs are highly specialized extensions of the nervous system in that they contain sensory neurons adapted to respond to specific stimuli and conduct nerve impulses to the brain for interpretation. A sensation is the arrival of a sensory impulse to the brain. The interpretation of a sensation is referred to as perception. In order to perceive a sensation, the following four conditions are necessary:
  - A stimulus sufficient enough to initiate a response in the nervous system must be present.
  - A receptor must convert the stimulus to a nerve impulse. A receptor is a specialized, peripheral dendritic ending of a sensory fiber or the specialized receptor cell associated with it.
  - The conduction of the nerve impulse must occur from the receptor to the brain along a nervous pathway.

- The interpretation of the impulse in the form of a perception must occur within a specific portion of the brain. Only impulses reaching the cerebral cortex are consciously interpreted as sensation. If impulses reach the spinal cord or brain stem, they initiate a reflex motor response rather than a conscious sensation.

- **Receptor potentials:**
  - Sensory receptors are activated when they detect a specific stimulus. This specific stimulus is called an adequate stimulus and is unique to each type of sensory receptor. In the visual system, for example, the photoreceptors detect light but are insensitive to frequencies of sound. Likewise, the auditory receptors of the ear respond only to sound and are insensitive to light.
  - An adequate stimulus will produce a change in the membrane potential of the sensory receptor cell. This change in the membrane potential is called a generator potential. In some sensory receptors, such as somatic sensory receptors, the generator potential is a depolarization of the membrane. In others, such as the photoreceptors of the eye, it is a hyperpolarization of the membrane. The generator potential, in turn, produces an action potential or a series of action potentials. The action potentials can be generated by the receptor cell itself or by a neuron connected to the receptor cell. These action potentials transmit information about the nature of the stimulus to the central nervous system.
- **Receptive field concept:**
  - For any neuron in a sensory pathway, the receptive field consists of all the sensory receptors that can influence its activity. Thus, cell A in the figure below has a receptive field consisting of the two receptors (2 and 3) which connect to it. Cell B, at the second level in this system, has a receptive field consisting of receptors 1, 2, and 3. The connections to a cell may be excitatory or inhibitory, and they may be mediated by interneurons at a given level as well as relay neurons between connecting levels. The properties of receptive fields generally reflect the increasing degree of information processing and feature extraction that occurs in neurons at successively higher levels in sensory pathways.

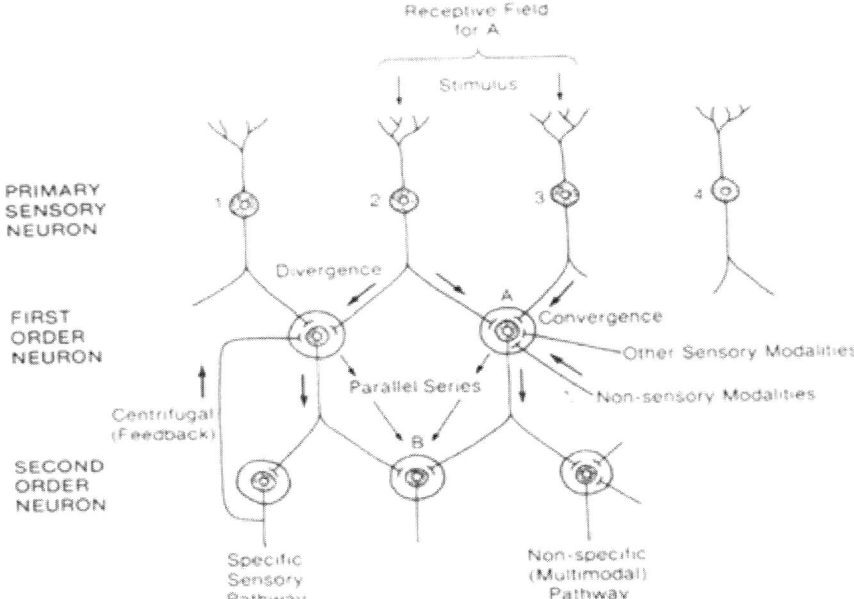

3. Somatosensory System

- Transmission of tactile, proprioceptive, temperature, and pain sensations: This is the system concerned with bodily sensations. The "somasthetic area" in the brain is a region in the postcentral gyrus of each parietal lobe that receives nerve impulses carrying somasthetic information.
- **Tactile:** The receptors that respond to touch, or tactile, stimuli are called Pacinian corpuscles. This type of receptor is located beneath the skin and consists of a free nerve ending that is encapsulated by layers of connective tissue. The nerve ending is wrapped with myelin along the length of the fiber.

The fiber itself extends into the spinal cord, where it forms synapses with other nerve cells. The adequate stimulus for the Pacinian corpuscle is pressure applied to the skin. This pressure causes the layers of connective tissue and free nerve ending to compress. The compression of the free nerve ending causes an opening of Na+ channels in the nerve membrane. The resulting influx of Na+ ions depolarizes the membrane and produces a generator potential. If the generator potential is of sufficient amplitude, it will then depolarize the membrane in the region of the first node of Ranvier to threshold and initiate an action potential.

- **Proprioceptive:**
    - The position of the body's limbs is detected by proprioceptors. One type of proprioceptor detects the stationary position of the limbs in space with respect to the other parts of the body. Other proprioceptors transmit dynamic information about limb movement to convey the sense of movement, or kinesthesia. The brain needs this information to determine where the arms and legs are located in order to calculate how much further they need to go to complete a certain movement.
    - The sense of stationary or static position is transmitted to the brain by mechanoreceptors located in joint capsules, cutaneous mechanoreceptors, and mechanoreceptors in muscles that are specialized to transduce the stretching of the muscle. Extremes of joint angles are transduced by the muscle spindle receptor.
    - The static proprioceptors produce a continuous frequency of action potentials in response to different joint positions. If the joint is left in one particular position, the receptor will generate action potentials at one specific frequency. This type of action potential response is called a tonic discharge. The dynamic proprioceptor generates action potentials only with a change in direction of movement. The burst of action potentials that they produce is very brief. This type of action potential response is called a phasic discharge.
    - The information from somatic sensory receptors is transmitted to the central nervous system by several different pathways organized according to four general principles:
        - (1) Each type of somatic sensation has its own pathway.
        - (2) Most pathways cross over from one side of the brain to the other.
        - (3) Each pathway is made of connections between clusters of cell groups called nuclei.
        - (4) The nerve cells within each nucleus are topographically organized according to the location of their sensory receptor on the surface of the body. These four principles also apply to the organization of other sensory systems.
- **Temperature:**
    - Sensory receptors that respond to temperature are called thermal receptors. There are two types of thermal receptors: one type responds to temperatures below 30°C, while the other type responds to temperatures above 30°C. These thermoreceptors are capable of adapting to the external environment. When exposed to cold weather, for example, the cold thermoreceptors do not become activated until temperatures lower than 30°C are reached, while the warm thermoreceptors become activated well before 30°C.
    - Temperature receptors that measure skin and shell temperature are located just beneath the skin. Peripheral temperature receptors are naked nerve endings that are very sensitive to temperature and are classified as cold receptors or warm receptors. Cold receptors are characterized by increasing steady-state discharge rates as the skin is cooled. Warm receptors, in contrast, are those whose steady-state discharge rates increase in response to warming of the skin. While both types of temperature receptors are found throughout the body surface, cold receptors are about 10 times more numerous than warm receptors. Nerve impulses from peripheral receptors enter the spinal cord at all levels and ascend to the brain.
- **Pain Sensations** (nociceptors): The receptors that detect painful stimuli are called nociceptors. In general, there are two types of nociceptors: mechanical nociceptors that are activated by intense mechanical stimulation such as a knife cut on the arm or a slap to the head, and heat nociceptors that respond to temperatures above 45 C. The transduction of pain is activated by a chemical process that also involves the immune system.

4. Auditory System

- The nerve fibers of the auditory and vestibular systems arise in the 8th cranial nerve (vestibulocochlear nerve). This nerve has two well-defined parts: the cochlear nerve for hearing and the vestibular nerve for equilibrium.
- **Functions of the middle ear and cochlea**: Sound is the adequate stimulus of the auditory system and is transmitted through the air by the compression and expansion of air molecules in the form of air pressure waves. The sense organ for the transduction of sound is the ear. The ear consists of the outer ear, middle ear, and inner ear. The outer ear channels the sound waves to the eardrum, located at the interface between the outer and middle ear. The sound waves cause the eardrum to vibrate much like the vibration of the speakers of a stereo system. The vibration of the eardrum, in turn, causes the small bones or ossicles within the middle ear to move. These bones are called the malleus, incus, and stapes (also known as the hammer, anvil, and stirrup). Vibrations at the tympanic membrane cause the ear ossicles to move and transmit sound waves across the tympanic cavity to the oval window. Vibration of the oval window moves a fluid within the inner ear and stimulates the receptors for hearing.
- The stapes, the last in the series of ossicles, is connected to the inner ear at the oval window, a membranous structure that vibrates with the movement of the ossicles. The inner ear consists of a fluid-filled chamber called the cochlea. The cochlea is a cone-shaped structure that is wrapped in a coil much like the shape of a snail's shell. Along the length of the cochlea is a membrane called the basilar membrane. This membrane is a flexible structure that vibrates when sound impinges upon the ear drum. The vibrations of the basilar membrane are in the form of traveling waves that deform the shape of the membrane. As the traveling wave progresses down the length of the membrane, the amplitude of the deformation become greater and greater until it reaches a peak. As the traveling wave progresses further, its amplitude diminishes. The location of the peak amplitude of the traveling wave along the basilar membrane depends upon the frequency of the sound. High frequency sounds cause the traveling wave to reach its peak amplitude near the base of the cochlea. Low frequency sounds cause the traveling wave to reach its peak near the apex of the cochlea. Intermediate frequencies of sound causes peak amplitudes to occur at locations along the membrane between the base and apex of the cochlea. Thus, the basilar membrane is designed mechanically to respond to different frequencies of sound by changing its form.
- The deformations of the basilar membrane are transduced into action potentials by hair cells. The hair cells sit upon the basilar membrane and have 20 – 50 fiber-like microvilli and one cilium called kinocilium that protrude from the cell. These microvilli are embedded in another membranous structure called the tectorial membrane. When the basilar membrane vibrates and reaches a peak amplitude, the hair cells are bent in the direction of the kinocilium. This bending of the hair cells causes the ion channels of the hair cells to open, leading to a depolarization of the membrane potential. When a hair cell is depolarized, Ca^{+2} ions flow into the cell and release transmitters that in turn depolarize auditory nerve fibers. It is the auditory nerve fiber that then generates action potentials that are transmitted to the brain to convey information relating to frequencies of sound. When the hair cells are bent in the opposite direction to the kinocilium the basilar membrane is hyperpolarized and the sensory neuron is inhibited.
- **Central auditory mechanisms**
    - The peripheral fibers of the auditory nerve make contact with the cochlear nucleus in the brain stem. Information from the cochlear nucleus is transmitted to both sides of the brain and eventually reaches the medial geniculate nucleus of the thalamus. From the medial geniculate nucleus, information is transmitted to the primary auditory cortex.
    - The receptive field characteristics of neurons along the auditory pathway are characterized by using tones of sound with different frequencies and intensities. A tone is a sound wave of one frequency. If the frequency of the tone is varied, one frequency will be found that most effectively activates a particular auditory nerve fiber. Different auditory nerves have different characteristic frequencies. These auditory nerve fibers have a tono-topic organization such that those with a high characteristic frequency innervate hair cells near the base of the cochlea, while those with a low characteristic frequency innervate hair cells near the apex of the cochlea.

- Neurons of the auditory system respond in a variety of different ways to a particular tone. Some neurons initiate action potentials only when the tone is on; other neurons are prevented from generating action potentials with the onset of the tone. Some neurons generate action potentials when the frequency of the tone is suddenly changed whereas others generate action potentials only when the amplitude changes.

- **Afferent system:** The cochlear nerve originates in the spiral organ of Corti, in the cochlea in the inner ear. Its cell bodies lie in the spiral ganglion from which its central fibers pass through the internal acoustic meatus to terminate in the dorsal and ventral cochlear nuclei in the medulla. The secondary auditory fibers arising from the cochlear nuclei form three acoustic striae:
  - The dorsal and intermediate acoustic striae ascend as the lateral lemniscus to synapse in the contralateral nucleus of the inferior colliculus. From the inferior colliculus tertiary auditory fibers arise and travel to the medial geniculate nucleus of the thalamus. These fibers are then sent laterally to the hearing center in the temporal cortex.
  - Part of the auditory relay in the medulla is uncrossed and terminates in the reticular formation, the superior olivary nuclei and others.
  - The ventral acoustic striae synapse in the ipsilateral nucleus of the superior colliculus.
- **Efferent system:** There is an efferent cochlear bundle which projects from the olivocochlear bundle in the brain stem back to the cochlea. This is a pathway by which the central nervous system may influence itself and represents an inhibitory feedback system.

5. Vestibular System

- The primary vestibular fibers arise from the superior and inferior vestibular ganglia with peripheral receptors in the semicircular canals of the inner ear. The secondary vestibular fibers arise from the vestibular nuclei in the medulla and send axons to many structures such as:
  - Nuclei of the extraocular muscles- via the vestibuloencephalic pathway for coordination of eye movements.
  - Spinal cord- via crossed and uncrossed fibers that descend in the medial longitudinal fasciculus in a pathway called the vestibulospinal tract for coordination of head and body movements.
  - Thalamus- sends fibers to cortex area 2.
  - Cerebellum and reticular formation- to facilitate posture and equilibrium. Fibers from the vestibular nuclei pass through the juxtarestiform body (medial portion of the inferior cerebellar peduncle) and terminate in the archicerebellum (flocculonodular lobe) and in the fastigial nuclei of the cerebellum. The fastigial nuclei project efferent fibers to the vestibular nuclei, which passes through the vestibular nerve and terminate on the hair cells of the membranous labyrinth. These efferent neurons probably exert inhibitory effects to ameliorate the effects of motion sickness and nystagmus.
- Functions of the vestibular apparatus:
  - The vestibular apparatus, the semicircular canals in the inner ear and the utricle and saccule, serves three functions:
    - (1) Maintaining balance of equilibrium during posture and movement by reflex alterations in muscle activity
    - (2) Stabilizing the visual world by reflex eye movements that compensate for changes in head position
    - (3) Conscious awareness of position in space, or “which way is up.”
  - All of these functions are accomplished by a close coordination of vestibular, visual, and proprioceptive sensory systems. Any two of these are able to compensate for the loss of one, as in the person who is blind.

- Brain stem mechanisms of vestibulocochlear and postural reflexes: When a person changes his direction of movement rapidly, or even leans his head sideways, forward, or backward, it would be impossible for him to maintain a stable image on the retina of his eyes unless he had some automatic control mechanism to stabilize the direction of gaze of the eyes. In addition, the eyes would be of little use in detecting an image, unless they remained "fixed" on each object long enough to gain a clear image. Fortunately, each time the head is suddenly rotated, signals from the semicircular canals cause the eyes to rotate in an equal and opposite direction in relation to the head. This rotation comes from reflexes transmitted from the canals through the vestibular nuclei and the medial longitudinal fasciculus to the ocular nuclei.
- Postural reflexes are usually divided into static reflexes and statokinetic reflexes. The static reflexes are those present when a person is at rest. They are also called position reflexes since they serve to maintain the body in a given position, such as standing, lying or sitting. The statokinetic reflexes are also known as righting reflexes; they include reflexes aimed at restoring the normal orientation of the head and body in space. The static reflexes are mainly elicited from the labyrinth and from the proprioceptors in the neck muscles. The statokinetic reflexes depend not only on the labyrinth organs and the proprioceptors of the neck muscles but also on visual input and the input from muscle and skin receptors in the trunk and limbs.

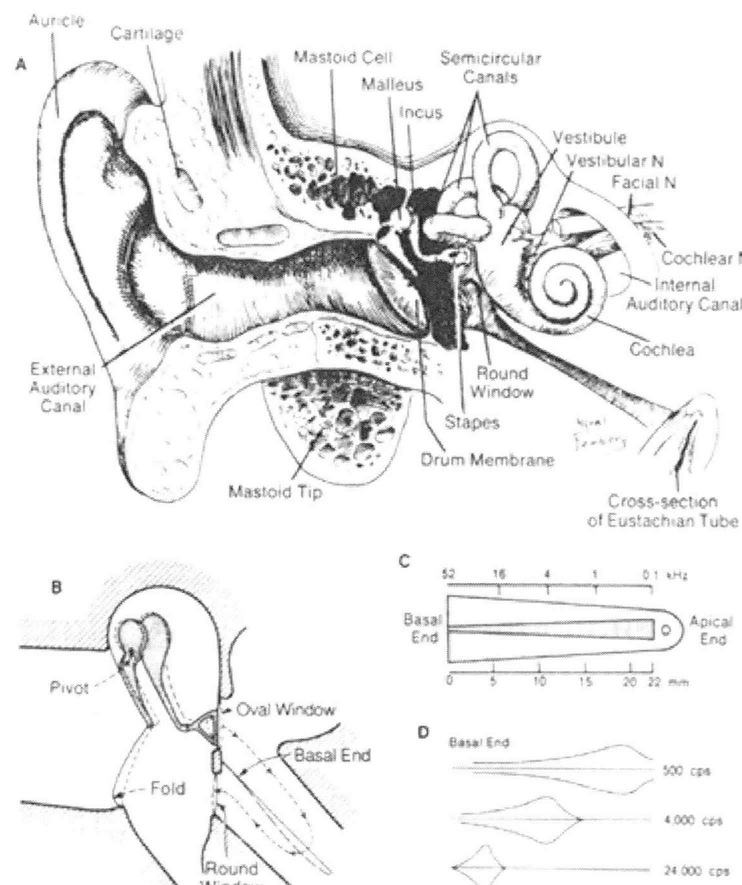

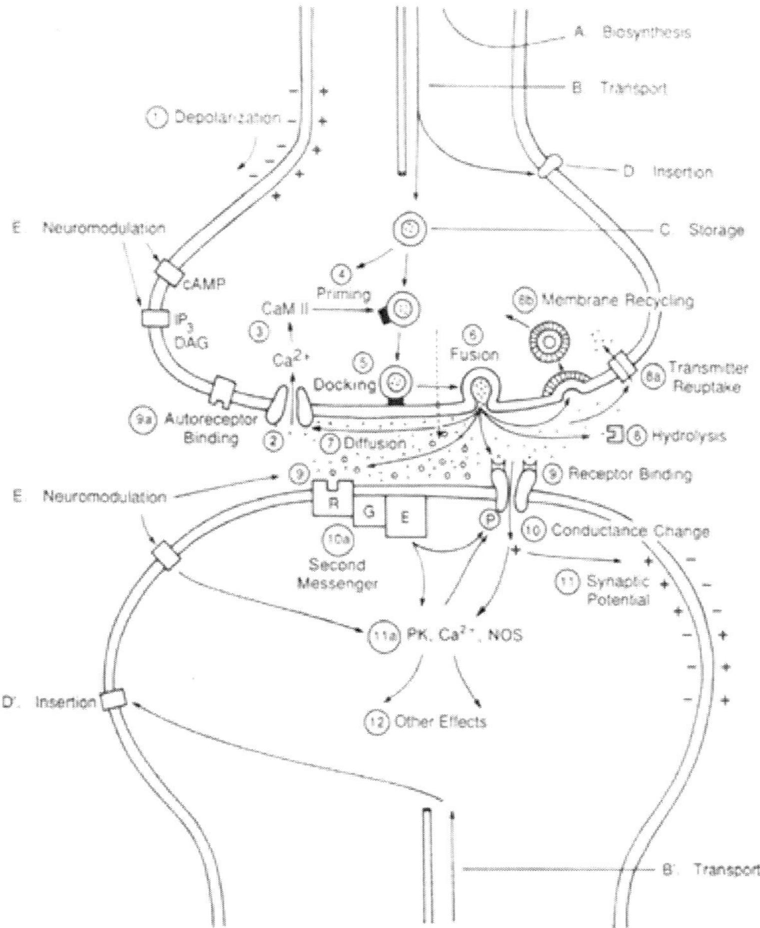

Fig. 6.14 A summary of some of the main biochemical mechanisms that have been identified at chemical synapses. A–E. Long-term steps in synthesis, transport, and storage of neurotransmitters and neuromodulators; insertion of membrane channel proteins and receptors; and neuromodulatory effects. ①–⑫. These summarize the more rapid steps involved in immediate signaling at the synapse. These steps are described in the text, and are further discussed for different types of synapses in Chapter 8. Abbreviations: IP_3, inositol triphosphate; CaM II, Ca/calmodulin-dependent protein kinase II; DAG, diacylglycerol; PK, protein kinase; R, receptor; G, G protein; E, effector.

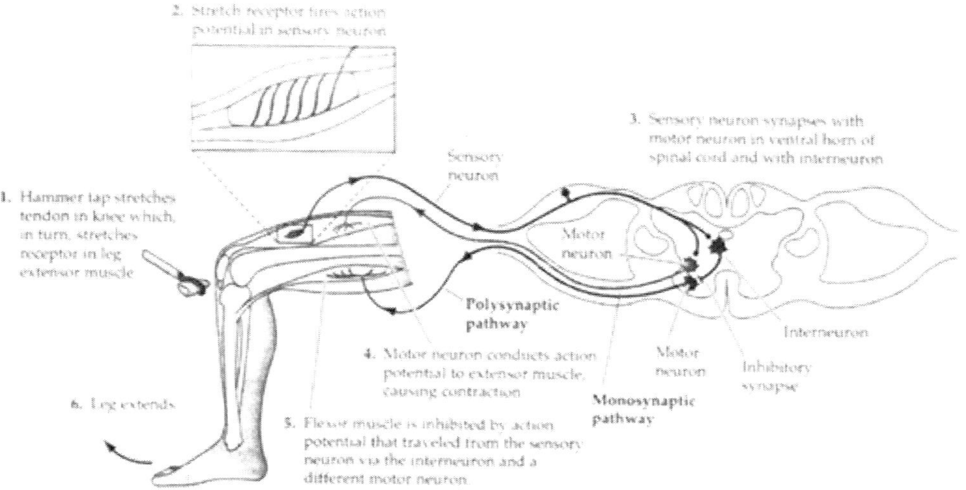

6. Motor Pathways

- **Spinal reflexes:**
  - Spinal cord reflexes represent the most basic of motor responses. These reflexes are carried out entirely within the spinal cord and are modified by inputs from higher centers to generate complex movements. They are also used to help diagnose disorders of the motor system.
  - The stretch reflex is commonly called the knee jerk reflex. An example of a stretch reflex is that activated by tapping the patellar tendon below the knee to stretch the muscle spindles. Action potentials conducted along the muscle spindle sensory neurons enter the spinal cord via the dorsal roots. The fiber from the muscle spindle branches after entering the spinal cord, with the ascending branch joining the dorsal column pathway. The other branch forms synaptic connections with motor neurons in the ventral horn. These motor neurons activate muscle fibers, causing the leg to extend quickly or kick out. In order for the leg to extend, however, the antagonistic muscles that would cause the leg to flex must be inhibited. This inhibition comes about by the activation of inhibitory interneurons within the ventral horn. These interneurons receive information from muscle spindle sensory neurons and in turn inhibit synaptic connections with motor neurons of flexor muscles. The activation of these interneurons thus prevents the contraction of the flexors. By inhibiting flexors and activating extensors, the interconnections of nerve cells within the spinal cord produce well-coordinated motor responses.
  - The inverse myotatic reflex is a reflex that involves the Golgi tendon organ. This reflex is seen when a person attempts to lift more weight than he/she can actually carry. The inhibition of the biceps occurs because the Golgi tendon organ detects excessive force, which might damage the muscle. With increasing force, the Golgi tendon organ begins to discharge action potentials. As with the muscle spindles, these action potentials are transmitted to the dorsal column nuclei and subsequently to the somatic sensory cortex. In the spinal cord, however, information about excessive muscle tension is transmitted to inhibitory interneurons that turn off the motor neurons innervating the biceps. At the same time, interneurons turn off any muscles (flexors) synergistic to the biceps and turn on any muscles (extensors) that are antagonistic to the biceps, so that the arm will extend and drop the weight. This reflex thus protects the muscle from damage that might occur when a person attempts to lift too heavy a weight.
  - A reflex that involves cutaneous receptors is the flexor withdrawal reflex. An example of this reflex is activated by pain receptors on the bottom of the foot. When you step on a tack, for instance, pain information is transmitted to the spinal cord and causes a contraction of the flexors to remove the foot from the tack. At the same time, extensors of the leg that would normally keep the foot on the tack are inhibited. In order to support the rest of the body, however, the extensor muscles in the other leg are activated while its flexors are inhibited.
- **Muscle Spindles**
  - The sensory receptors that detect the length of the muscle and its velocity of contraction are called muscle spindles. These structures are formed by sensory neurons that entwine intrafusal muscle fibers. The muscle spindle is composed of two types of intrafusal fibers: nuclear bag fiber and nuclear chain fibers. The nuclear bag fiber is innervated by Type Ia nerve fibers, which transmit information about muscle length and velocity of contraction to the CNS. Nuclear chain fibers are innervated by Type II nerve fibers, which transmit information about muscle length.
  - The muscle spindle acts as a stretch receptor and it increases its discharge of action potentials when the intrafusal fibers stretch. As a muscle contracts, both the extrafusal and intrafusal fibers shorten. The shortening of the intrafusal muscle fiber causes a decrease in the action potential discharge of the Ia nerve fibers. As the extrafusal muscle fiber continues to shorten, the muscle spindle further reduces its discharge of action potentials.
  - Muscle spindle sensitivity is maintained even at short muscle lengths by gamma motor neurons. The gamma motor neurons specifically innervate contractile elements at the poles of the muscle spindles. The activation of these contractile elements causes the central region of the muscle spindle to stretch as a rubber band would. In this manner, the gamma motor neurons can regulate the sensitivity of the Type Ia sensory nerves of the muscle spindles.
- **Control of movement by the motor cortex**

- The fine control of voluntary movement is due to instructions transmitted via descending pathways to the spinal cord from the motor cortex. The motor cortex occupies a cortical region rostral to the somatic sensory cortex. The cells in the motor cortex are organized in a topographic manner similar to that of the somatic sensory cortex. Cells in the medial region of the motor cortex cause the contraction of muscles in the leg. Nerve cells located in more lateral regions of the motor cortex activate the muscles of the torso, arm, and face. The parts of the body that are involved with fine movements, such as fingers, occupy more space in the motor cortex than parts of the body involved in gross movement, such as the torso. This relationship is in keeping with the general principle that the amount of cortical space that is devoted to different parts of the body is in proportion to its sensory sensitivity or degree of fine motor control.
- Information from the motor cortex is transmitted to the spinal cord and brain stem by the corticospinal pathway and corticobulbar pathway, respectively. Inputs to the brain stem control axial muscles near the midline for the maintenance of posture, while inputs to the spinal cord control the distal limb muscles. As these axons descend from the motor cortex, they form the pyramidal tract. When the pyramidal tract reaches the level of the brain stem, the majority of the fibers that continue to the spinal cord cross the midline of the body and continue their descent along the lateral corticospinal tract. Nerve fibers exit from the lateral corticospinal tract at various levels of the spinal cord. Fibers from neurons in the motor cortex innervate motor neuron pools that control distal limb muscles. The direct connections from motor cortex to spinal cord permit the independent control of individual muscles.
- In addition to the lateral corticospinal tract, a minority of the fibers from the motor cortex descend to the spinal cord without crossing the midline of the body. These fibers from the ventral corticospinal tract and primarily innervate motor neurons in the medial region of the ventral horn associated with axial muscles of the body.

- **Cerebellum**
  - The cerebellum and the basal ganglia are the major subcortical components of the motor system. They both receive inputs from the neocortex and transmit information back to the cortex by way of the thalamus. The inputs to the basal ganglia are from the entire cortex, while those to the cerebellum are primarily from sensory and motor areas. The basal ganglia do not receive direct sensory information from somatic receptors, nor do they transmit descending information directly back to the spinal cord as does the cerebellum. These differences suggest that the basal ganglia are involved with the control of movement that requires constant monitoring by sensory feedback.
  - The cerebellum has three basic functions: (1) the planning of a movement, (2) the control of posture and equilibrium, and (3) the control of limb movement. The cerebellum accomplishes the latter two functions by comparing information with sensory feedback about the actual movement and adjusting its output to compensate for differences between the two. It participates in the planning of a movement by receiving information from motor and parietal cortices and then uses these inputs to initiate a planned movement.
- **Basal ganglia**
  - The basal ganglia are involved in the programming of motor patterns. The basal ganglia include the caudate nucleus and the lentiform nucleus which include the putamen, which is the lateral portion, and globus pallidus, the medial portion. The caudate nucleus and putamen receive inputs to the basal ganglia, while the globus pallidus provides the output. The caudate nucleus and putamen control unconscious contractions of certain skeletal muscles such as those involved in involuntary arm movements during walking. The globus pallidus regulates the muscle tone necessary for specific intentional body movement. Inputs to the basal ganglia are from the entire neocortex, thalamus, and substantia nigra of the brain stem. The primary input, however, is from the neocortex. The extensiveness of this suggests that the basal ganglia are involved in other functions besides motor activities. In fact, diseases of the basal ganglia often produce cognitive abnormalities, motor movement dysfunction including rigidity, tremor, and rapid and aimless movements.
  - The major output of the basal ganglia is to the prefrontal and premotor cortices by way of the thalamus. Through this pathway, the basal ganglia can modulate the descending components of the motor system. The basal ganglia also have outputs to the substantia nigra. The nerve

fibers from the substantia nigra that terminate in the basal ganglia release dopamine as the neurotransmitter. The degeneration of these dopamine fibers is responsible for the motor disorder called Parkinson's disease.

- **Brain stem structures:**
  - One of the primary roles of the brainstem is to maintain the body's posture and balance. Nerve cells within different clusters in the brain stem send axons that terminate in the spinal cord. Three pathways from the brain stem provide input to the motor neurons of the spinal cord:
  - The ventromedial pathway impinges on motor neurons that control axial muscles. This pathway has three major components, all of which descend along the ventral and medial region of the spinal cord. The first component is the vestibulospinal tract, which originates in the vestibular nucleus and carries information for the reflex control of equilibrium and conducts impulses that regulate tone in response to head movements. The second component of the ventromedial pathway is the tectospinal tract, which originates in the tectum, a structure involved in the coordinated control of head and eye movements in response to visual, auditory and cutaneous stimuli. The third component is the medial reticulospinal tract, which originates in the reticular formation, a structure involved in maintaining posture by the activation of extensor muscles and control of sweat gland activity.
  - The lateral reticulospinal tract is the second major descending pathway from the brain stem to the spinal cord. Nerve fibers in this pathway are derived from the lateral reticular nucleus and descend the spinal cord in the lateral region of the cord. These fibers innervate flexors in the control of posture.
  - The rubrospinal tracts have fibers that originate in the red nucleus of the brain stem. These fibers descend along the dorsal and lateral border of the cord to innervate motor neurons that control distal flexor muscles

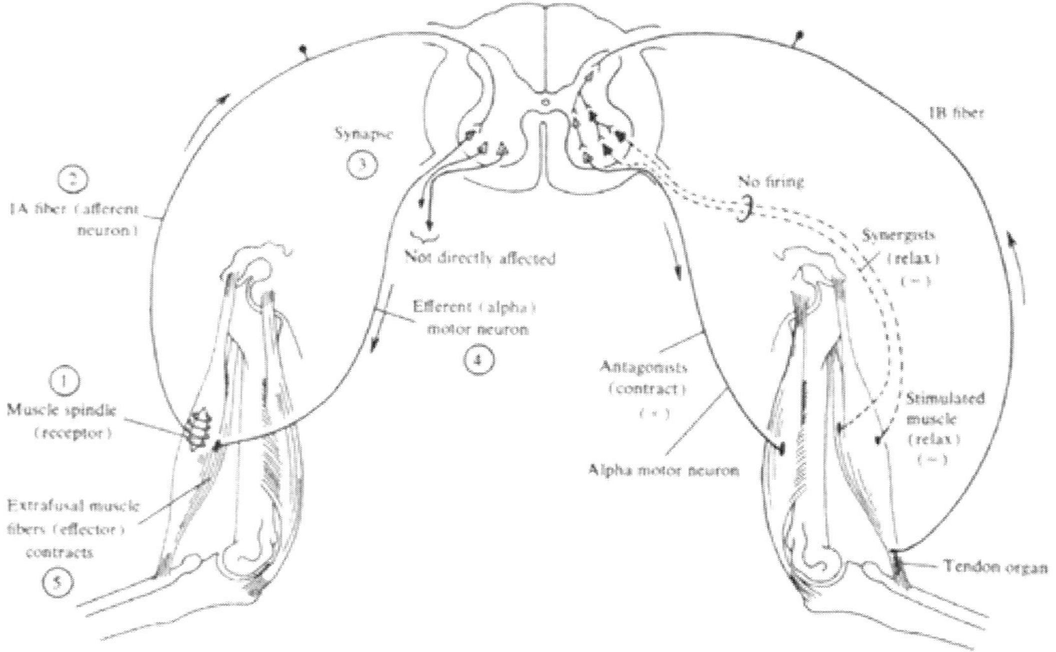

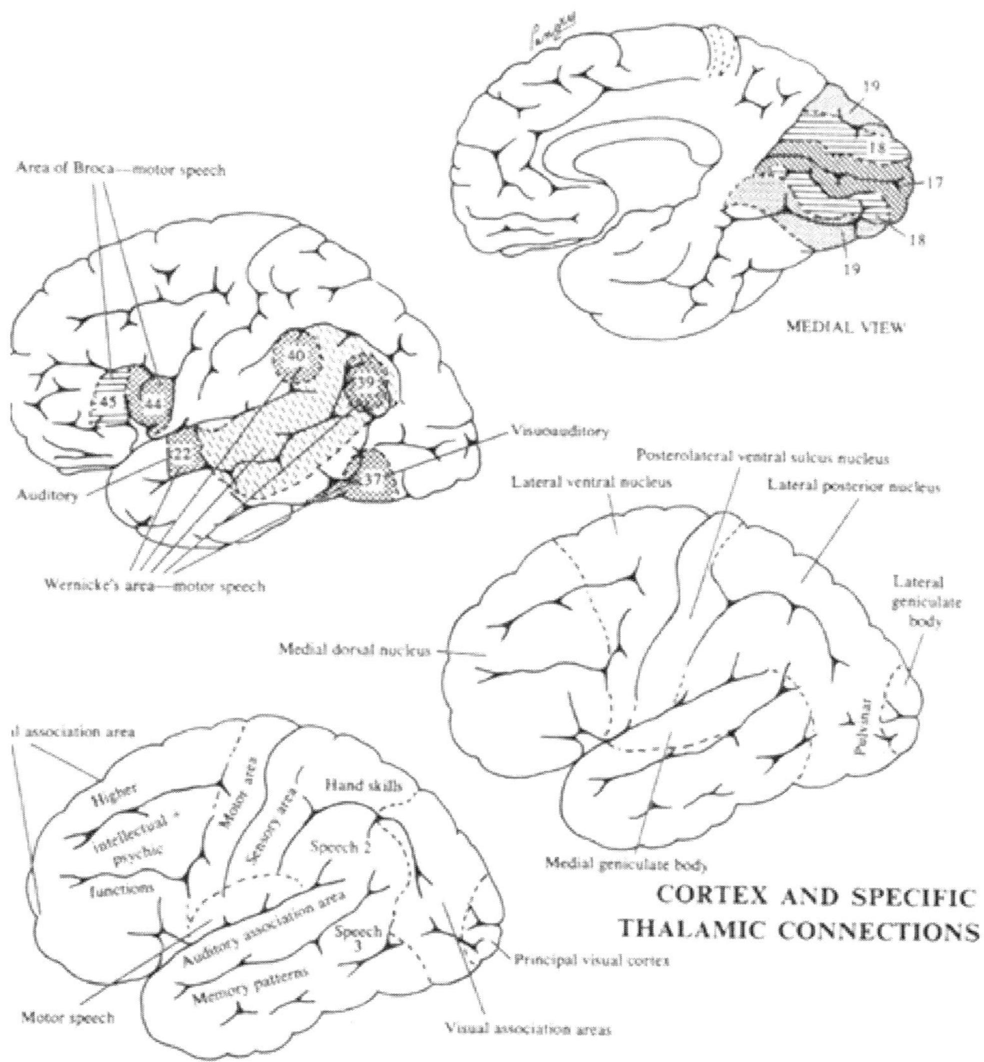

GENERALIZED FUNCTIONAL AREAS OF LEFT CORTEX

7. Autonomic Nervous System

- The ANS coordinates bodily functions that are needed for survival. It is also a regulatory system that maintains an environment necessary for the cells in the body to function properly. The actions of the ANS are all subconscious and not under direct voluntary control. Autonomic processes transmit sensory information from "visceral" organs to the central ANS, which in turn send instructions to the smooth muscles and other cells of those organs, producing an appropriate autonomic response.
- **Function of the adrenal medulla:**
    - The adrenal medulla is an important component of the sympathetic nervous system. The sympathetic nervous system and the adrenal medulla are often referred to together as the sympatho-adrenal system. The adrenal medulla secretes the catecholamines epinephrine and norepinephrine.
    - The primary product secreted by the adrenal medulla is epinephrine. Note that norepinephrine is an intermediate in the synthesis of epinephrine. However, the adrenal medulla secretes only small amounts of norepinephrine. Input of sympathetic stimulation to the medulla increases epinephrine synthesis and causes the release of large amounts of epinephrine and smaller amounts of norepinephrine into the blood. These hormones are then carried in the blood to all

tissues of the body, where they produce the same effects as those resulting from direct sympathetic stimulation of the tissue, except for one important difference. Because epinephrine and norepinephrine are removed from the blood more slowly than from the area of the sympathetic nerve terminal, the effects of the circulating hormones are more prolonged than the effects of direct sympathetic stimulation.

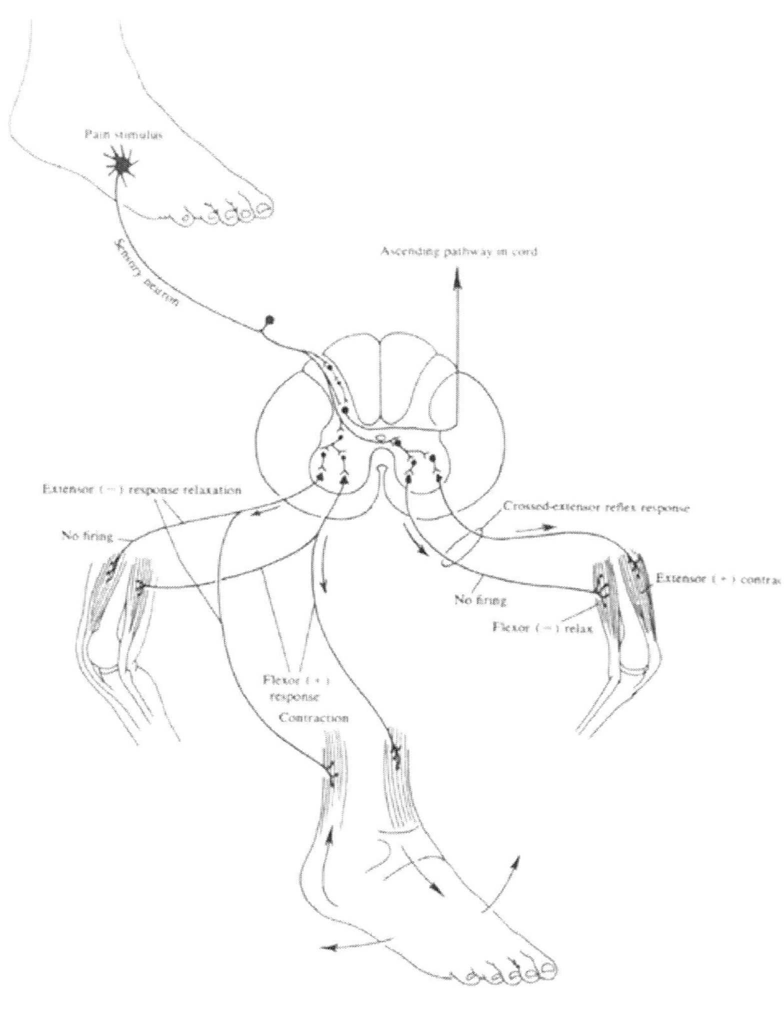

    - The adrenal medulla is part of a general alarm system in the body that triggers a sequence of events appropriate to "fight-or-flight" situations. The net result of this response is to increase the capability of the body to perform vigorous muscle activity. Thus, if faced with a life-threatening situation, the body can respond more effectively, therefore bettering its chances of survival.

- **Central regulation of visceral function:**
    - The actions of the sympathetic and parasympathetic inputs to an organ have opposite effects. These actions operate to control various parameters in the body. The sympathetic and parasympathetic nerve endings secrete one of the two synaptic transmitter substances, acetylcholine and norepinephrine. Those fibers that secrete acetylcholine are cholinergic and those that secrete norepinephrine are adrenergic. All preganglionic neurons are cholinergic in both the sympathetic and parasympathetic nervous systems. Thus, acetycholine will excite both sympathetic and parasympathetic postganglionic neurons. The postganglionic neurons of the parasympathetic system are also all cholinergic. On the other hand, most of the postganglionic sympathetic neurons are adrenergic.
    - Acetylcholine activates two different types of receptors. These are called muscarinic and nicotinic receptors. The muscarinic receptors are found in all the effector cells stimulated by the postganglionic neurons of the parasympathetic nervous system, as well as those stimulated by the postganglionic cholinergic neurons of the sympathetic system. The nicotinic receptors are found in the synapses between the pre- and postganglionic neurons of both the sympathetic and parasympathetic systems and also in the membranes of skeletal muscle fibers at the neuromuscular junction.
    - There are two major types of adrenergic receptors, called alpha receptors and beta receptors (beta 1 and beta 2). Norepinephrine excites mainly alpha receptors but excites beta receptors to a very slight extent as well. On the other hand, epinephrine excites both types of receptors approximately equally. Therefore, the relative effects of norepinephrine and epinephrine on

different effector organs is determined by the types of receptors in the organs. Sympathetic stimulation causes excitatory effects in some organs but inhibitory effects in others. Likewise, parasympathetic stimulation causes excitation in some organs but inhibition in others. There is no generalization one can use to explain whether sympathetic or parasympathetic stimulation will cause excitation or inhibition of a particular organ. Therefore, to understand sympathetic and parasympathetic function, one must learn the functions of these two nervous systems.

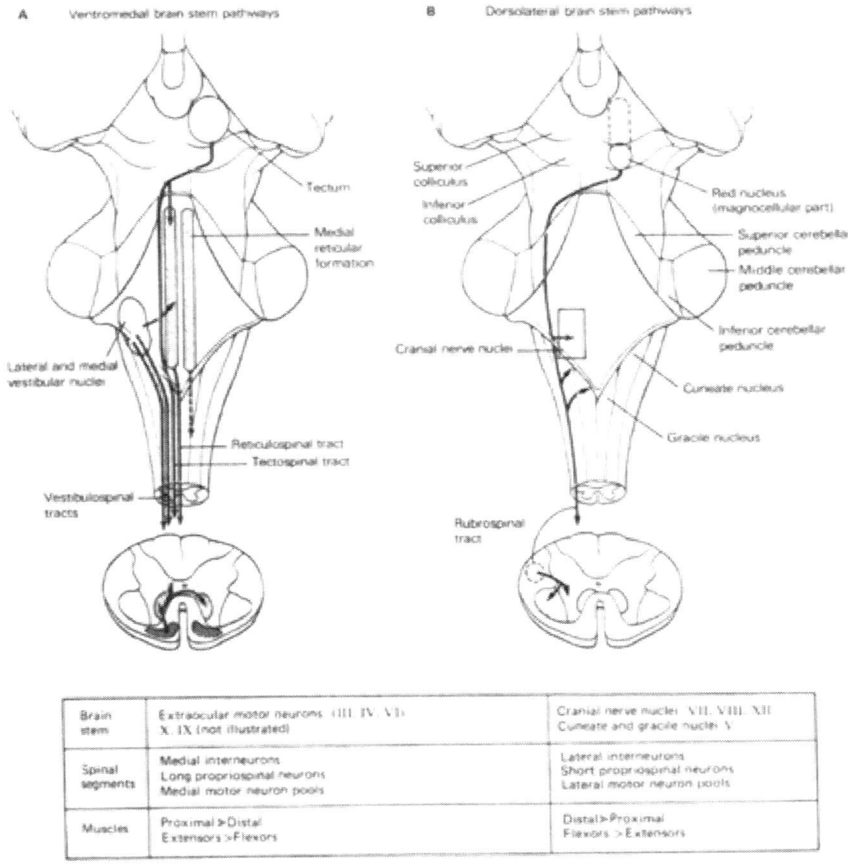

Brain stem	Extraocular motor neurons (III, IV, VI) X, IX (not illustrated)	Cranial nerve nuclei (VII, VIII, XII) Cuneate and gracile nuclei (V)
Spinal segments	Medial interneurons Long propriospinal neurons Medial motor neuron pools	Lateral interneurons Short propriospinal neurons Lateral motor neuron pools
Muscles	Proximal > Distal Extensors > Flexors	Distal > Proximal Flexors > Extensors

8. Significance of Evoked Potentials, CT and PET Scanning, and MRI

- The significance of evoked potentials, CT & PET scanning, and MRI is that these are all neurologic diagnostic tests. Thus, these are procedures that allow assessment of possible neurologic pathology.
- **Evoked potentials**: Visual, auditory, and tactile stimuli that activate their corresponding neuro-anatomic tracts and result in a cortical potential. The latency, duration, and amplitude of the evoked responses reflect the physiologic integrity at various levels of the tested sensory pathway. This approach is useful for detecting cryptic lesions in demyelinating disease, appraising sensory systems in uncooperative infants, quantifying deficits in histrionic patients, and following the subclinical course of disease.
- **CT scanning:** Computed tomographic X-ray (CT scan) provides rapid, noninvasive imaging of cerebral sulci, the ventricles, gray and white matter, and bony and calcified structures. The technique passes a series of collimated x-ray beams through the region of interest and measures their attenuation by the various tissue densities within a transverse plane. A computer transforms these measurements into a 2-dimensional image of high resolution that resembles an anatomic "slice."
- **Pet scanning**: Positron emission tomography (PET) is a research tool using the uptake of trace amounts of radioisotopes to measure blood flow, glucose, and oxygen metabolism in the living brain. Although it can provide important information about epilepsy, brain tumors, and stroke, currently it has little practical utility in clinical diagnosis.

- **Magnetic resonance imaging (**MRI): Magnetic resonance imaging yields extraordinary resolution in imaging neural structures without known risk to the patient. The head or body is placed in a confined space with a strong magnetic field that aligns the hydrogen protons in the direction of the field. An additional, specific radiofrequency pulse then "flips" the aligned intra- and extracellular protons into a higher energy state. When the radio pulse is turned off, the protons "relax" back to their original alignment, and the energy emitted gives information about the chemical makeup of the tissue. The regional relaxation times are used to compute an anatomic image in virtually any plane desired. MRI helps particularly to identify brain stem lesions and other abnormalities of the posterior fossa. It is also useful for detecting demyelinating plaques, subclinical brain edema, cerebral contusions, abnormalities of the craniocervical junction, and syringomyelia. MRI is contraindicated in patients who are dependent on respirators, prone to severe claustrophobia, or have a cardiac pacemaker, a ferromagnetic aneurysm clip, or any moveable metallic prostheses.

9. Plasticity

- Three types of plasticity have been studied in the visual cortex:
  1) Ocular Dominance Plasticity:
     - This is a shift in whether the cells are dominated by the left eye, right eye, or both. These changes are found in cases of monocular deprivation, strabismus, anisometropia, and other conditions. This is thought to be mediated through glutamate synapses, where the cells become hyperpolarized. GABA may also play a role as suppression of input from deprived eyes suggests a role for increased inhibitory interactions in the neurons. The critical period for this plasticity is thought to be from when the eyes open to close to puberty, though mostly animal studies have been done on this subject. We also know that rearing animals in the dark extends the period for ocular dominance plasticity. It delays the start of plasticity, so that the ocular dominance shift occurs more slowly.
  2) Orientation and Direction Plasticity:
     - A cell is selective for a specific orientation if the response along one axis is greater than the response on a perpendicular axis. It is thought that visual cortex cells receive input from LGN cells that have receptive fields lined up along the preferred axis of orientation. There are also lateral inhibitory connections that contribute to orientation selectivity. Direction selectivity is thought to be mainly due to inhibitory connections, but this is according to the rabbit model. The critical period for changes here is up to the first 7 weeks of life. Thus orientation selectivity is fully developed when ocular dominance is not.
  3) Long Term Potentiation (LTP) and Long Term Depression (LTD):
     - LTP is the increase in the size of the excitatory postsynaptic potential and LTD is a decrease in the size of that potential lasting for more than 30 minutes. LTP is produced by high frequency stimulation and LTD is produced by low frequency stimulation. Both depend on the firing of the cells nearest neighbors. The magnitude of LTP and LTD declines with age.
     - The effects of visual deprivation depend on the type of deprivation. So the eye could be totally deprived of light or only look at stimuli with a single orientation, but the results would be different and depend on the pattern of electrical activity that reaches the brain.

VISUAL PATHWAY (PHYSIOLOGY)

Receptors → Ganglion cells → optic nerve → LGN → Visual cortex

1. Function of Lateral Geniculate Body

- The LGN represents the first level in the visual pathway at which the modification of the information by the CNS may occur. The LGN functions as a relay for information from the outer retina to the higher visual centers. The parvocellular cell layers 3,4,5, and 6 relay the ganglion cells to the visual cortex. The magnocellular cells in layers 1 and 2 relay information from the primary visual cortex to the secondary visual cortex and on to the MT and MST region.

- The LGN is responsible for segregation of motor input. Contralateral (crossed) ganglion cell axons end in layers 1, 4, 6, ipsilateral (uncrossed) fibers in layers 2, 3, 5. The LGN in the human has 6 layers. The superficial layers 3, 4, 5, and 6 have small cells (parvocellular laminae), while the deep layers 1 and 2 have large cells (magnocellular laminae). Each layer receives input from either one eye or the other eye.
- The LGN has 2 classes of cells, the principal cells and the interneurons. The principal cells are the major relay to the visual cortex and the interneurons mediate interactions within the LGN. Transformation of the visual information occurs through the physiological processes in the glomerulus involving inhibitory input from the interneurons (a.k.a. the intrinsic cells) onto principal cells. This retroactive inhibition by the intrinsic cell on the principal cell serves to sharpen the signal once the signal has passed.
- All 6 layers of the LGN have a retinotopic map of the retina; macula to the posterior, lateral retina to the anterior. Input from the two eyes is kept separate. The visual world is unified in the visual cortex.

2. Receptive Fields of Cells in Lateral Geniculate Body (Relationship to Color Vision, Binocularity, Space Perception, etc)

- Receptive fields of cells in the lateral geniculate body closely resemble ganglion cells; the majority has center surround receptive field mechanisms. Although the LGN surround is stronger, the LGN response is weaker relative to the ganglion cell. Input to one LGN cell arrives from a few ganglion cells with offset receptive fields. An on-center ganglion cell connects to an on-center LGN cell, and vice versa. The LGN neurons can be categorized according to the way they respond. In the cat, Y type (large) rapidly conducting axons, with large receptive fields and phasic response, are differentiated from medium size X type, which conduct with medium velocity and have smaller receptive fields and tonic responses. Both relay to the visual cortex. W-type ganglion cells (sluggish cells) have small axons and slow conductance. These cells are a heterogeneous class with a variety of different properties, including responding to brightness. They project to the pretectum, superior colliculus, and suprachiasmatic nucleus.
- **Color opponency:** color specific receptive fields give only one polarity of response for one color, and a response of opposite polarity for another color. ie: "on" response to red, and "off" response to green, with no response to white light. Double opponent cells respond on to one color in the center, and off to the other color in the surround. There is no response to uniform illumination. Double opponent cells are concerned with simultaneous color contrast. Regarding binocularity and space perception in the LGN: there is limited information on this in the LGN, although there is evidence of a weak inhibitory input from the corresponding part of the retina in the other eye.
- **Color detection** depends on the location on the retina: red and green cones have about the same density of distribution at the fovea. Blue cones make up less than 10% of the cone photoreceptors and have a peak density 1° from the fovea. The cone density drops sharply with eccentricity.
- **Color formation** processing has been studied in the monkey retina and has shown that red and green photoreceptors antagonistically share the same pathway. These signals sum to yellow and antagonize the blue cone signals in the blue/yellow pathway, and also sum to contribute to the luminosity signal.
- **Critical Flicker Fusion (CFF)**. CFF is when the temporal frequency is increased to a point when flicker can no longer be resolved. CFF varies with eccentricity on the retina, and depends on the number of rods and cones stimulated. Cones have a higher CFF, and the CFF decreases with an increase in rod population. In an area of both rods and cones, a bipartite CFF function will be observed in respect to receptive fields. Horizontal cells have a large receptive field presumable because horizontal cells connect with neighboring horizontal cells. Bipolar cells respond to spots of light. Again, they have a center/ surround antagonism orientation that processes visual information by discriminating between light falling on it versus light falling next to it. Amacrine cell receptive fields respond to the onset of spots of light. They give a transient response when they see light and thus process the temporal contrast

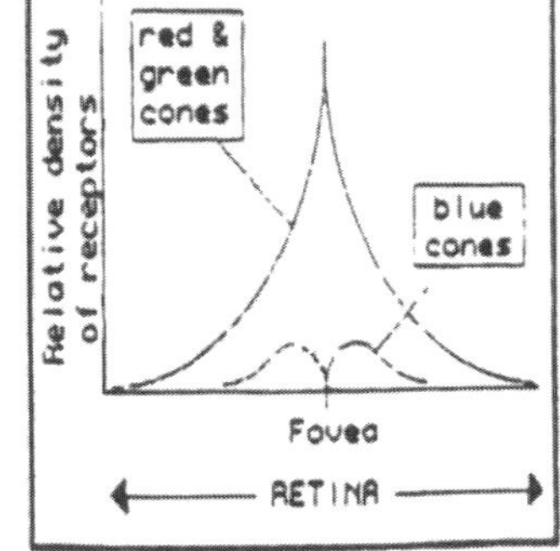

aspect of visual processing. The ganglion cells have on center off surround and receive information from the bipolar cells and the amacrine cells and feed the information back to the LGN. Their response can be transient like the amacrine cells or sustained like the bipolar cells. As the receptive fields are processed along the visual pathway, they become more complex. There is a hierarchy involved in signal processing.

3. Function of Visual Cortex

- Integration and transformation of visual information. The visual world is mapped out and organized, represented by binocularity, orientation, and position in visual space. The two major functions are:
    - Elaboration of angular properties in visual space.
    - Binocular integration. The most widely used region in the visual cortex receiving information from the LGN is area 17

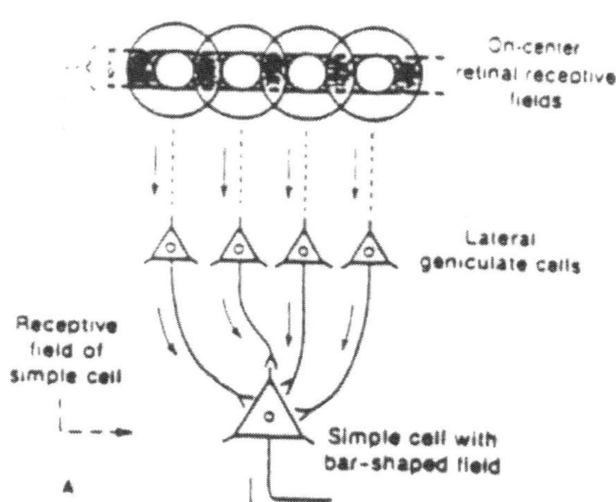

4. Receptive Field Properties (single cell properties)

- Simple cells have elongated center surround receptors that respond to extended stimulus of light. Simple cell receptors are found primarily where LGN input occurs, layers 4, 6, and lower 3. Input comes from the X-cells. The elongated receptive field has parallel bands of on and off regions that are usually equal in size and mutually antagonistic. The stimulus must have proper orientation at the border of the on-off region, diffuse illumination is not effective, and the illumination must be on axis. There is one other type of simple cell, the special simple cell. The main difference is that the response depends on the length of the stimulus.
- Complex cells prefer stimulus of correct orientation and size (up to a degree). Position of a stimulus on the receptive fields is not important, since on/off regions in the receptive field are mixed. As long as the orientation is correct, stimulus anywhere in the receptive field produces a response. However, illumination of the whole field gives no response. Complex cells are sensitive to length variations, and also directionally selective to movement of the stimulus. A subcategory of complex cells includes hypercomplex cells, which respond to short bands. Complex cells are said to receive input from both eyes and are therefore termed binocular.

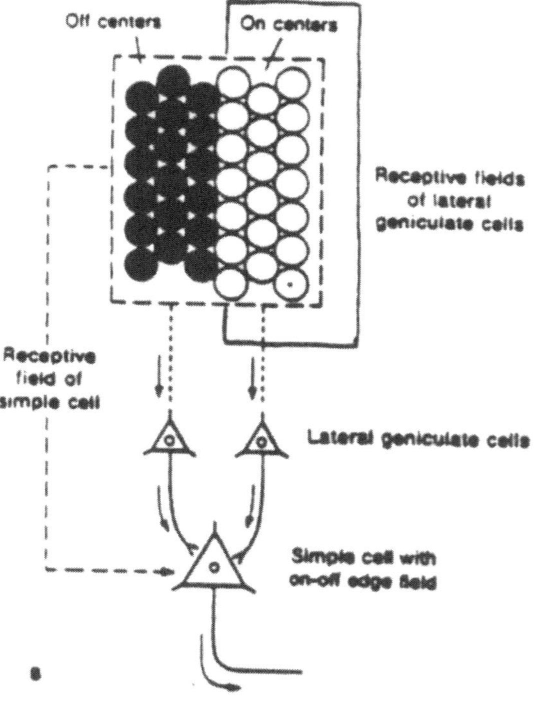

- There are two theories of processing in the visual cortex: the hierarchical and the parallel processing principle. In the hierarchical principle, it is believed that the receptive field properties of cells in the visual cortex may be built up from receptive fields of peripheral cells, such as LGN cells feeding to simple cells, which then feed to complex cells. In parallel processing, streams of information go from the retina to the LGN to the cortex in separate channels. Instead of everything being processed sequentially, information is being processed in parallel. It is believed that hierarchical processing occurs within the pathways of parallel processing.

5. Functional Organization

- There are six layers of the visual cortex. The primary input from the LGN goes to layer four. Collaterals of both M and P cells terminate in layer six and intralaminar cells terminate in layers two and three. (There is reciprocal interconnection between the striate cortex and the other cortical and subcortical regions.) There are two primary cell types: pyramidal cells have large, long axons and spiny type processes. Stellate cells have short axons and both smooth and spiny type processes. Spiny stellate and pyramidal cells are excitatory; smooth stellate cells are inhibitory. Pyramidal cells project out of the cortex, whereas stellate cells are local.
- The major unit of organization in the visual cortex is a column going down through the six layers of the cortex. The columns have neurons that are specific to one orientation and have the same ocular dominance. If a probe is inserted into the visual cortex at a right angle to the surface, cells with similar orientation preference will be found. If the microelectrode is not inserted at a right angle, a systematic change in the orientation preference is found. Therefore, the columns are arranged in sequence such that the column next to it has a slight change in orientation preference. Ocular dominance is the classification of the binocularity of a particular cell. Those cells completely stimulated by only the contralateral eye are classified as group 1. Group 2 and 3 are cells that are codominant to both eyes, but respond more to the contralateral eye. Group 4 has equal binocular response to both eyes. In group 5 and 6, codominance with more response to the ipsilateral eye is found. Group 7 has only response to the ipsilateral eye. A hypercolumn is defined by the orientation preference (of the stimulus) and the ocular dominance, which has a consistent dimension throughout the central visual field.

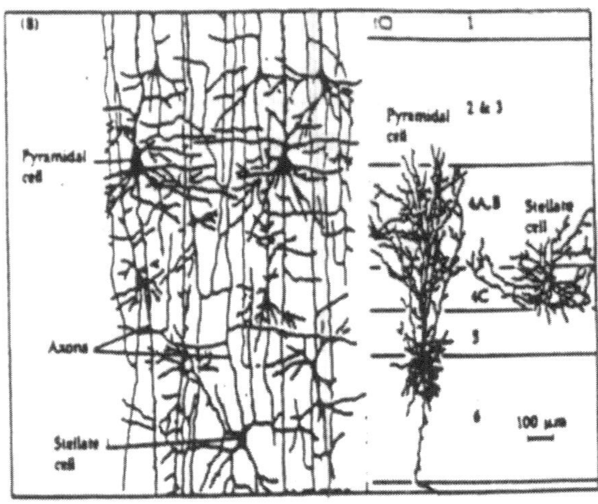

6. Physiology of Binocular Vision

- Discoveries by Hubel and Wiesel have shown that the receptive fields from the binocular cortical cells that are on corresponding regions of the retinal have similar organization. Stimuli either summate or cancel, with some cells responding only with binocular stimulation. 84% of visual cortex cells respond to either eye (binocular responsiveness), while most cells have some degree of contralateral dominance.
- Disparity sensitive cells respond to a stimulus presented to corresponding areas of the retina. Tuned excitatory cells respond when stimulus is presented on or near the fixation point, but are inhibitory on either side. The inhibition only occurs over a limited region in space, known as Panum's Fusional Area, which is determined by the size of the inhibitory sideband. Tuned inhibitory cell responses are inhibited when the stimulus is on or near the fixation point.
- Near cells/ far cells respond when the stimulus is nearer/further than the fixation point. These near/ far cells are usually monocular (dominated by one eye). Simple cells (binocular organization) show phase specific binocular interaction similar to simple cells. 40% are non-phase specific, and result in suppression or facilitation. A small number appear monocular but show binocular inhibition from the silent eye. The receptive fields of the eyes are matched for orientation tuning, spatial frequency tuning, dimension, etc. There is an exquisitely tuned binocular interaction, a linear summation of the signals from each eye. These cells are disparity selective and are therefore involved directly in depth perception.

7. Mechanism of Feature Detection

- The feature detectors are cortical neurons that respond only to features with specific orientations and patterns. The feature detectors abstract particular aspects of a pattern stimulus and dismiss all irrelevant information coming from the retina. For example the visual cortex might respond to a triangle using both complex and simple cells.
- The feature detectors detect the edges of the triangle such as the apex, corners, and sides. The apex is detected by hypercomplex cells, which respond best to exact position and orientation. The inside of the triangle may stimulate the retina and send impulses to the brain, but will not trigger feature detection because the inside of the triangle gives diffuse illumination which is not effective on feature detection neurons. Feature detection is possible due to the tuning of the cell neurons to stimuli with specific spatial frequencies and orientations. This is possible because the cell does a 2-dimensional Fourier analysis on the pattern. To do this, the cell breaks down a complex sine wave to smaller, simpler sine wave components that have specific spatial frequency and orientation.
- The cortical cells responding to the individual sine wave gratings can detect features in complex images.

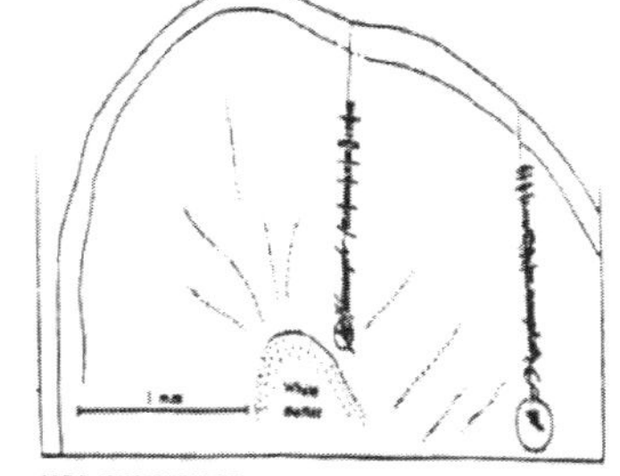

AXIS ORIENTATION of receptive fields in the cortex

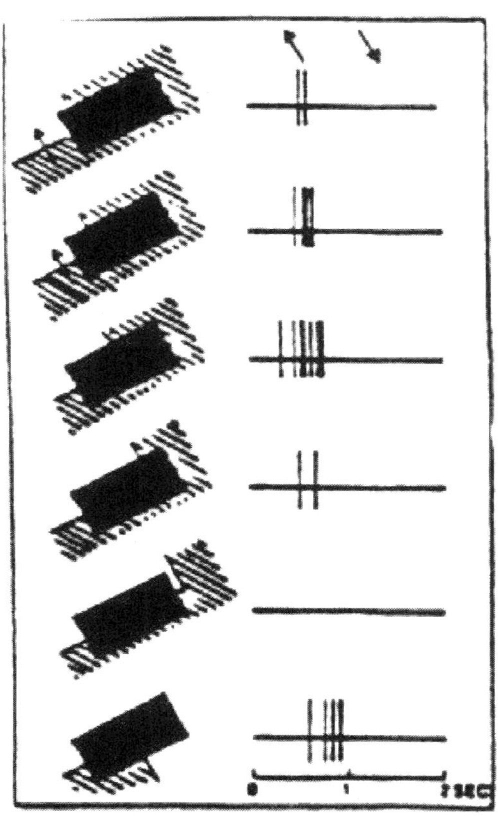

END INHIBITION OF A COMPLEX CELL

In V2 (area 18) of the cat cortex. The best stimulus for this cell (third from top) is a moving, oriented edge, that does not encroach on the antagonistic right-handed portion of the receptive field. The records also show selective sensitivity of the cell to upward movement.

Summary of Receptive Fields in the Visual System

Type of Cell	Shape of Field	Best Stimulus	How good is diffuse light as a stimulus	Is orientation of stimulus important?	Are there distinct "on" or "off" areas within receptor fields?	Are cells driven by both eyes	Can cells respond selectively to movement in one direction?
Photoreceptor		Light	Good	No	No	No	No
Ganglion		Small spot or narrow bar over corner	Moderate	No	Yes	No	No
Geniculate		Small spot or narrow bar over corner	Poor	No	Yes	No	No
Simple (layers 4 and 6)		Narrow bar or edge	Ineffective	Yes	Yes	Yes (except layer 4)	Some can
Complex (not layer 4)		Bar or edge	Ineffective	Yes	No	Yes	Some can
End-inhibited complex (not layer 4)		Line or edge that stops, corner or angle	Ineffective	Yes	No	Yes	Some can

8. Gross Electrical Potentials

- Gross electrical potentials are the summed electrical activity of a large number of neurons. There are three noninvasive methods of measuring them:

Electrooculogram (EOG):

- The basis is that the front of the eye has a positive charge relative to the back of the eye, generating a resting potential.
- Electrodes are at the patient's inner and outer canthi and the patient is instructed to look back and forth between two points, which move the eyes from extreme right to extreme left gaze.
- EOG is larger in light adapted than dark adapted conditions.
- The minimum is the dark trough, reached at 8 minutes of dark adaptation, and the maximum is the light rise, reached after 10-15 minutes of light adaptation.
- The **Arden ratio** is the ratio of the light rise to the dark trough. A normal ratio is 165-180% and anything below is abnormal.
- The dark adapted EOG comes from the RPE and the light is mainly due to rod activity.
- Four conditions that reduce EOG, but not ERG are:
    - Butterfly shaped dystrophy of the macula,
    - Flavimaculatus,
    - Advanced drusen,
    - Best's Disease.

Electroretinogram (ERG):

- Full-field ERG is the retinal potential elicited by a brief flash of light that evenly illuminates the entire retina. ERG is smaller than EOG.
- The ERG is first biphasic (the early receptor potential), then a negative a-wave, the positive b-wave, then the after-potential and the c-wave. ERP comes from the outer segments of photoreceptors, mostly cones. The a-wave from the photoreceptors, the b-wave from Muller/bipolar cells, and the c-wave possibly from the RPE. Each a- and b-wave consists of photopic and scotopic components, but in clinic the stimulus is presented at 30 Hz that is too high for the scotopic, but resolvable by the photopic system.
- **Focal ERG:** The light flash is confined to the area of interest, so only the stimulated tissue contributes and damage becomes obvious.
- **Multifocal ERG:** ERGs are recorded for many different locations in a short time. The patient is presented with a stimulus array of 240 hexagons, half of which are illuminated at one time. mfERG is useful for diagnosis of localized retinal abnormalities and may allow early recognition of more generalized disease like retinitis pigmentosa and glaucoma.
- **Pattern ERG:** Obtained with a temporally modulated stimulus whose average spatial luminance remains constant. Retinal ganglion cells play a large role in generating a PERG.
- The ERG is recorded with a rigid contact lens containing an electrode connected to an amplifier.
- Full field ERG is helpful for diagnosing retinitis pigmentosa, where both photopic and scotopic ERGs are reduced.

Visually Evoked Potentials (VEP):

- VEPs are very small cortical potentials elicited by visual stimuli and are imbedded in the randomly fluctuating electroencephalogram (EEG). Electrodes are positioned on the scalp and measured with an averaging computer. Transient VEPs are collected with flash stimuli and Steady-state VEPs are collected with patterned or non-patterned stimuli presented at moderate frequency.
- VEPs allow an objective determination of threshold contrast as well as visual acuity when using high contrast targets. Thus VEPs are useful to determine visual acuity in the mentally retarded, infants, hysterics, and other nonresponsive patients. Though, VEPs overestimate infant acuity and mostly tests central vision function.
- VEPs may be reduced in macular, optic nerve, and cortical lesions. VEPs also have increased latency in the affected eye of patients with multiple sclerosis and optic neuritis. This helps in making the initial diagnosis of MS.

PUPILLARY PATHWAYS (PHYSIOLOGY)

1. Sympathetic Pathway to Iris

- Figure 1. The pathway of the pupil control system begins in the cortex with a diffuse pathway to sympathetic centers in the hypothalamus and reticular tract that synapse within the cord in the ciliospinal center of Budge.
- Sympathetic fibers emerge from the cord with the first, second, and third thoracic roots and form the sympathetic trunk, which ascends the vertebral column. In the neck the fibers synapse at the superior cervical ganglion. The post-ganglionic fibers are called the internal carotid nerve, which follows the course of the internal carotid artery into the skull. The fibers eventually reach the orbit, where they form the long ciliary nerve. This nerve follows the course of the optic nerve to the eyeball, where it penetrates the sclera and travels to the iris to innervate the dilator muscle. The fibers may also travel through the ciliary ganglion without synapsing and enter the eye with the short ciliary nerves.

Pupillary dilation

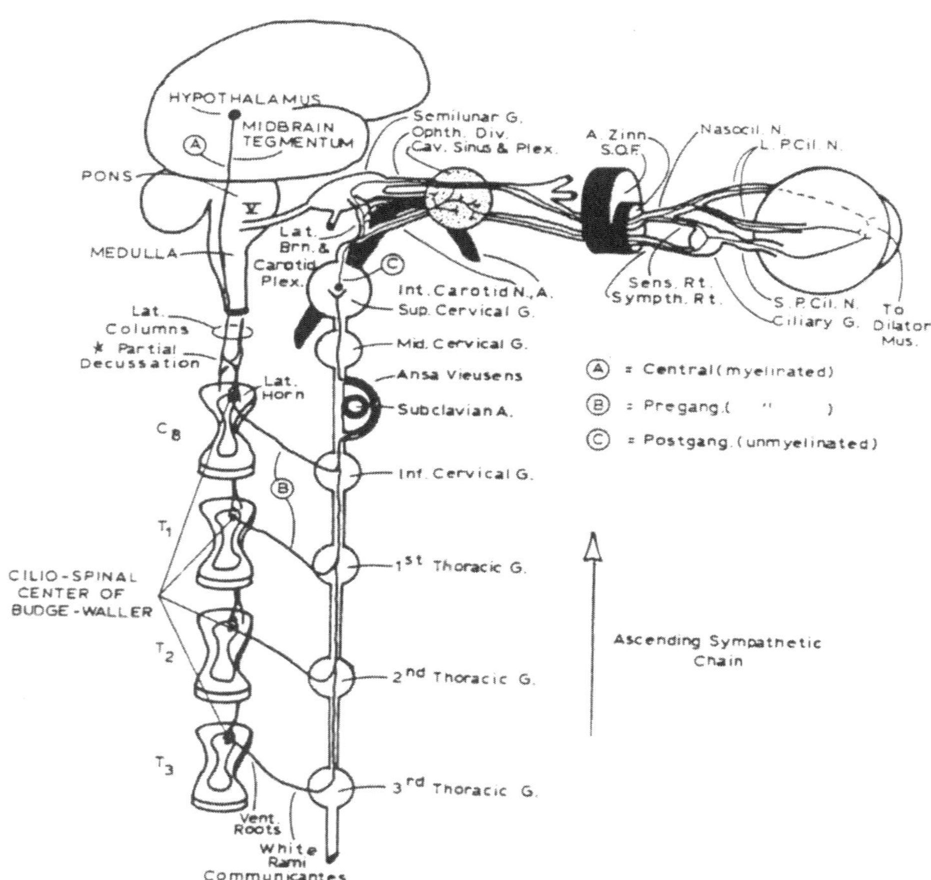

2. Parasympathetic Pathway to Iris

- Figure 2. The parasympathetic pathway begins at the lateral geniculate body, where branches of retinal ganglion cells which synapse in the LGB descend to the midbrain and synapse at the pretectal nucleus. Post-synaptic fibers travel to the Edinger-Westphal (EW) nucleus on both the same and contra lateral side. Postsynaptic EW fibers join with nerve fibers from the oculomotor nuclei and travel along the surface of CN III.

Pupillary constriction

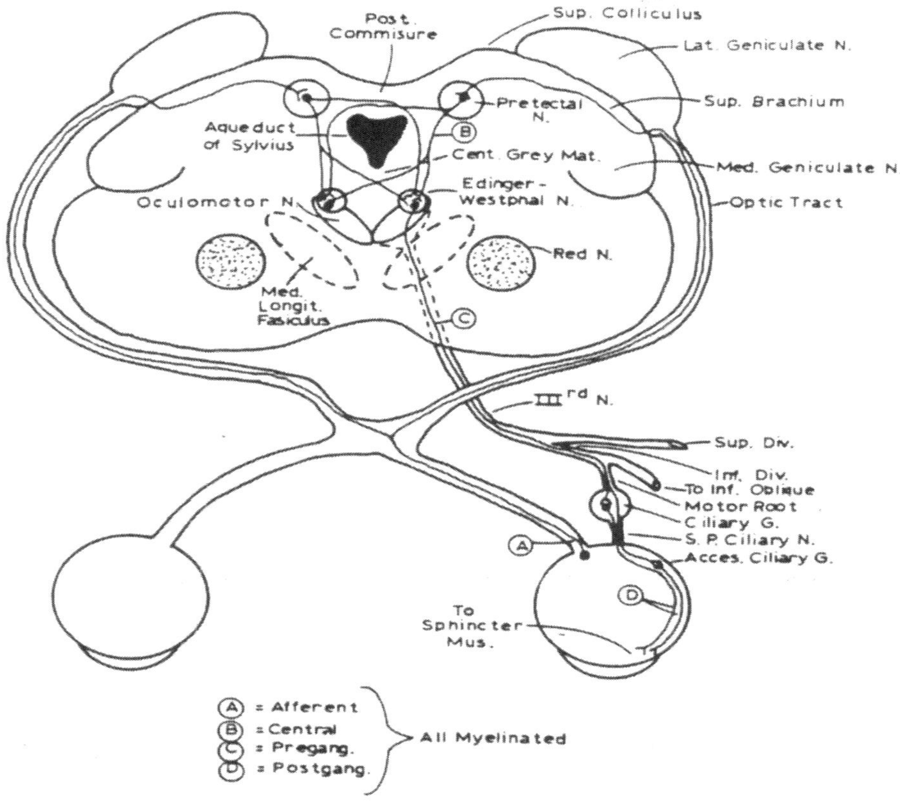

3. Functional Relationships between Pupillary Pathways and Central Nervous System

- The central synapse of the pupillomotor reflex arc in the EW nucleus is subject to sensory or emotional stimuli provided by the environment, spontaneous thoughts or emotions; they travel by the brain stem, cervical cord, and peripheral sympathetic chain to the dilator muscle of the iris. Under the influence of these mechanisms the pupil in healthy alert subjects is relatively large and quiet in darkness. But when the subject becomes tired, the pupils gradually become smaller and begin to oscillate.

NEURO-OPHTHALMIC DISORDERS (PATHOLOGY)

---

1. Optic Nerve Pathology

- **Papillitis (Optic Neuritis):**
  - Observations: Swelling of disc; accompanied by decreased VA (over hours to days), color vision loss, venous pulsation possible, pain upon eye movement; disc elevation <2D, (+) Marcus Gunn pupil, red desaturation; blurred disc, hemorrhages, disc hyperemia.
  - Epidemiology: Suspect optic neuritis if patient > 40 y/o, optic atrophy presents with short history, VF defects respect the vertical meridian, no recovery. Obliteration of physiological cup and vitreous cells; most common type on children (also occurs in adults).
- **Retrobulbar Neuritis:**

- Observations: Inflammation behind orbit; decreased VA. Pain on eye movement. 25-40% of these patients develop Multiple Sclerosis. Normal optic nerve head and fiber layer.
    - Epidemiology: Most common in adults; frequently associated with demyelination diseases.
- **Papilledema:**
    - Observations: Normal VA; bilateral transient loss of vision (usually last a few seconds), nausea, vomiting, diplopia, blurred disc margins, enlarged blind spot. No SVP, even if pressure is put on globe. No pain on eye movement; disc elevation >2D. Bilateral. Transitory obscuration of vision, for about 5-10 sec. Usually resolves itself if underlying condition is treated.
- **Ischemic Optic Neuropathy**
    - Observations: Infarct of prelaminar or laminar anterior optic nerve due to blockage of two main posterior ciliary arteries supplying optic nerve and choroid.
    - Main types are giant cell arteritis (temporal arteritis), non-arteritic arteriosclerosis, and autoimmune. Also involved: abrupt decrease in VA, pallor (not hyperemic like papilledema) and swelling of optic nerve head, no pain, transient monocular visual loss (2-5 min), afferent pupil defect in eye with severe ischemic papillitis or CRA occlusion. Also systemic symptoms: temporal pain/ headache, tenderness of temporal artery, fatigue, neck pain.
    - Epidemiology: Mostly Caucasian males of Northern European descent. Mean age is 70s.
- **Optic Atrophy**
    - Observations: Patient must have decreased VA's or a visual field defect.
- **Consecutive Optic Atrophy:**
    - Observations: Most frequent form. Includes all diseases causing retinal ganglion injury (Tay Sachs, Menke's Kinky Hair Syndrome). Also follows more common conditions as tobacco alcohol amblyopia, ethambutol, and other drug induced neuropathies; follows trauma, ischemia, demyelination, compressive lesions. Signs are pale disc, decreased VA, field defects.
- **Secondary Optic Atrophy**
    - Observations: Follows papillitis and chronic papilledema; yellow cup, possible association with glaucoma.
- **Pseudotumor Cerebri:**
    - (Benign Intracranial Hypertension)
    - Suspect this when see an obese, middle aged female with bilateral papilledema with high CSF (>250mm in adult, normal is <210mm in adult, and , 90mm in children), but has normal MRI.
    - Symptoms of HA in the morning, can be generalized or localized, can be intensify with head movement. Might reports hearing “whooshing” sound, transient blurred of vision. Management: lose weight.
- **Marcus Gunn Pupil (Relative Afferent Pupillary Defect)**
    - Sensory or afferent limb of reflex arc can provide evidence for impaired function of retina or optic nerve; can roughly quantify with neutral density filters in front of normal eye to "balance" visual loss.
- **Horner’s Pupil (Pupilodilator Dysfunction)**
    - May be pre/postganglionic lesion along the sympathetic pathway.
    - Associated with lung cancer, but seen in <5% of lung cancer patients. Pupil dilator fibers governed by SANS (3 neuron arc); SANS damage decreases norepinephrine output.
    - Signs: (unilateral) ptosis, miosis, facial anhydrosis (absence of sweat secretions
    - Tests:
        - Cocaine: If Horner's, pupil dilates poorly (NE reuptake blocked, so pupil will dilate if not Horner's).
        - Paredrine (hydroxyamphetamine) 1%. Indirect acting sympathomometic. Causes release of NE into synaptic cleft; postganglionic lesion leads to degeneration of adrenergic nerve endings, so will see a loss of catecholamines in the iris. Pupil will not dilate with indirect acting sympathomimetic (Paredrine), but does react to Phenylephrine which acts directly on alpha receptors. Preganglionic lesion shows normal response to both drugs, as preganglionic fibers are intact. If no reaction (dilates) to Paredrine then suggests a postganglionic lesion.
        - Dilation lag-lag of affected pupil in dilation.
- **Melanocytoma**

- Benign tumor of melanocytes that looks like a large mass on the disc.
- **Sarcoid Nodule of Optic Disc**
  - A white mass, with no associated hemorrhage and the rest of the disc margin is distinct.
- **Optic Pit**
  - A large hole, often in the area of the fetal fissure. There is a visual field defect if the pit interferes with nerve fibers. It may be associated with macular edema since subretinal fluid at the optic nerve can spread to the macula.
- **Optic Nerve Head Drusen**
  - Obervations: Disc has blurred margin and large "blobs" are sometimes visible on the disc. No visible optic cup and CRA branches in front of the optic disc.
  - Typically drusen begin buried in the substance of the nerve and then move forward with age and can have visual field defects.
  - Epidemiology: Hereditary condition, typically people of Northern European descent.
- **Argyll Robertson Pupil**
  - Light-near dissociation: pupils are very small and poor in response to light, but have a (+) result on alternating light from eye to eye, when enlargement of the pupil is seen when light is shone into the affected eye and constriction is seen when light is shone into the unaffected eye. Miosis is a component of the AR syndrome and is more prominent in the dark. The affected pupil is smaller than would be seen in the normal individual. This syndrome is bilateral is 90% of the cases but two sides would be affected unequally. The affected pupil does not directly response to light very well but does constrict with near response.
  - Seen in patients with neurosyphilis, diabetes neuropathy, and alcoholic neuropathy and lesions tend to be in the midbrain.
- **Adies Tonic Pupil**
  - Tends to be women 20-40 y.o, 90% of these patients have diniminished tendon reflexes. Unknown etiology.Tonic pupil seen, usually after damage to the ciliary ganglion or postganglionic fibers of the short posterior ciliary nerves. Tonic pupil characterized by poor pupillary light response and loss of accommodation. In some cases, decreasing in corneal sensitivity also occurs before some afferent sensory fibers from cornea passed through SCN and the ganglion also being affected.
  - Administration of 0.125% pilocarpine leads to an intense constriction of pupil if there is denervation supersensitivity resulting from injury to the fibers directly innervating muscles. Remember you are using a extremely diluted amount of pilocarpine which should not induced an huge reaction on normal pupil.
- **Nerve Toxicology**
  - *Optic Neuritis:* chloramphenicol, sulfa drugs, ethambutol, nicotinic acid, salicylates, streptomycin, isoniazid, chlorpropamide, tryparsamide, MAO inhibitors.
  - *Optic Atrophy*: barbiturates, quinine.
  - *Papilledema:* tetracycline, vitamin A, corticosteroids (associated w/pseudotumor).
  - *Papillitis:* birth control pills.
  - *Color Vision Disturbances:* ibuprofen, MAO inhibitors, digilatis (yellow vision).
- **Color Vision Testing in ON Disorders**
  - Expect red/greed defects, check with Ishihara or D15.
- **Visual Field Testing**
  - Amsler Grid: Qualitative evaluation that can detect edge of glaucomatous Bierrrum scotoma, and peripheral field defects secondary to CNS disorder.
  - Confrontation Tests: Rough estimate of VF, can pick up gross alteration in VF due to advanced glaucoma, brain tumor, or hemorrhage.
  - Perimetry (i.e. Goldmann. Kinetic vs static).
  - Tangent Screen: Examine 30 degrees.
- **Testing for Objective and Subjective Marcus Gunn Pupils**
  - (+) result on alternating light from eye to eye, see enlargement of pupil when light shone into affected eye and constriction when light shined in unaffected eye. Quantify by using neutral density filters to eliminate relative afferent defect by balancing the visual loss in the two eyes.
- **Pupil Cycle Times**

- Possibly how quickly the pupil responds to light, which should be almost instantaneous with bright light and a healthy system.
- Hippus: physiologic pupillary unrest. In a normal, healthy, awake person, the size of pupil changes constantly reflects the balance between parasympathetic and sympathetic systems.

- **Pulfrich Phenomenon**
    - Apparent motion in depth of a moving object viewed with a neutral density filter before one eye. Eye with filter in front of it sees a lag in target location with respect to that seen by the other eye.
- **Interpretation of Electrodiagnostic Tests, Contrast Sensitivity, Etc**
    - Reflects the presynaptic function of the retina.
    - Electroretinogram (ERG) reflects the chain of graded electrical responses from each layer of the retina: human response is biphasic. ERG is normal in diseases of visual pathway i.e. optic atrophy.

Observation of ONH and Peripapillary Retina with Ophthalmoscope, Fundus Lenses, and Stereography

- **Optic Nerve Head**
    - Circular to oval shape; pink color; temporal edge lighter than nasal, center depressed aka cup
    - In glaucoma, ON will have extensive cupping.
    - Changes in these characteristics can be indication of ON pathology. For example, ONH color: if pale = optic atrophy. Indistinct margin of ONH, or no present of cupping can indicate swollen papilledema/ papillitis. Size of ONH or pattern of insertions can varies with refractive error of person (hyperopes smaller, myopes tends of have oblique insertion).
- **Peripapillary Retina**
    - Arteries red, smaller than veins (2/3); shiny central reflex strip due to thicker walls. Arteries never cross arteries, veins never cross veins. Arteries only cross veins.
    - Hemorrhage:
        - Flame shaped: intraretinal, hypertension
        - Round pre-retinal: diabetes mellitus
    - Spontaneous venous pulsations are normal.
    - Foveal reflex may be present, seen mostly in children. Whitish sheen throughout retina indicates presence of healthy NFL.

Carotid Assessment

- **Ophthalmodynamometry**
    - Approximate measure of relative pressures in the CRA and indirect assessment of carotid artery flow on either side. Press a probe on the sclera while observing blood vessels emerging from the optic disc with an ophthalmoscope. Increase the pressure on the sclera until the CRA pulsates where it leaves the disc. This is the diastolic pressure in the ophthalmic artery on that side. Keep the pressure until the CRA stops pulsating. This is the systolic pressure. Repeat on the other eye a 25% difference between eyes indicates carotid insufficiency on side with lower reading.
- **Doppler Ultrasound:** Scans carotids when conducted up and down the neck.
- **Indirect Ophthalmoscopy:** Touch dilated eye. If fundus arterioles collapse, there is a low volume of blood present, indicating carotid insufficiency.
- **Plain X Ray:** Bones make it difficult to see ocular details well
- **Tomograms:** Good at localizing small fractures and presence of orbital tumors; this blurs out surrounding structures and clearly visualizes a given spot at a given depth
- **CAT scan**: Creates a picture of the structure based on density of the tissue involved. Non-invasive. Good at locating tumors, lesions.
- **Ultrasound**: Propagation of high frequency sound waves through tissue. Waves are deflected, create echoes which produce a picture.
- **Intravenous fluorescein**: Diagnosis of retinal disorders affecting retinal vascular system, choriocapillaris, Bruch's membrane, and pigmented epithelium.
-
- Signs and Symptoms of related Systemic Diseases

- Optic Neuritis: Reiter's Syndrome, temporal arteritis, chickenpox, measles, smallpox, herpes zoster, mumps, influenza, TB, malaria, alcoholism, emphysema, hypothyroidism, Stevens/Johnsons Syndrome (Erythema multiforme).
- Papilledema: Systemic lupus erythematosus., TB, Addison's disease, emphysema, multiple myeloma, sickle cell, hyperthyroidism.
- Optic Atrophy: German measles, hyperthyroidism, Addison's disease, hypothyroidism.
- Papillitis: Infectious mono, leukemias.
- Optic Nerve Glioma: Von Recklinghausen's disease (neurofibromatosis).
- Optic Nerve Neovascularization: Diabetes Mellitus.

2. Sensory Neuro-Visual Pathology

- **Multiple Sclerosis**
  - This is a chronic demyelinating idiopathic disorder of the CNS. It rarely presents before age 15 or after 55 (mean onset age is 30) and tends to affect women more than men. There is a tendency to involve the optic nerves, chiasm, brain stem, cerebella peduncles and spinal cord.
  - Multiple focal demyelinating lesions are caused by degeneration of the myelin sheaths of nerve fibers with a relative sparing of the axon. The specific signs and symptoms depend on the location of the lesion.
  - Symptoms present as ocular disturbances (seeing phosphenes- tiny white or colored flashes or sparkles), muscle weakness, ataxia, urinary disturbances, parasthesia, and sensory disturbances. Temporary visual loss that last for a few days during attack. Mild pain and discomfort with eye movement.
  - Often patients complain of blurred vision. This is most likely due to a retrobulbar optic neuritis characterized by acute unilateral loss of vision with a tendency for recovery. With each attack there may be some residual permanent loss of VA or color vision and optic nerve appearance (pale).
  - Diplopia is frequently an early symptom of extraocular muscle involvement due to internuclear ophthalmoplegia. The lesion is in the medial longitudinal fasciculus. Typically there is a paralysis of one or both medial rectus muscles.
  - Nystagmus is a common early sign and is often permanent.
  - The visual evoked response (potential) may confirm the diagnosis since it is abnormal in 80% of MS patients.
- **Pituitary Tumors**
  - The anterior lobe of the pituitary gland is the site of pituitary tumors. The pituitary lies over the optic chiasm and pressure due to the tumor results in bitemporal heminaopsia. The pituitary dysfunction may also result in extraocular muscle palsies. Confirmation of the diagnosis can be made with CT scan.
- **Ischemic Optic Neuropathy**
  - This is caused by thrombosis or embolism of the posterior ciliary artery. The onset is abrupt and usually in the elderly men. Vision may be abolished completely, or there may be a segmental defect. Both eyes may be affected and prognosis for recovery is poor. If vision loss is preceded by headache, pain on chewing, the diagnosis is usually temporal arteritis. Fluorescein angiography can confirm the retinal vascular abnormality.
- **Transient Neuro-Visual Episodes**
  - See part about strokes and transient ischemic attacks).
- **Visual Field Defects**
  - Scotomas -are small areas of impaired vision within the visual field. They can be related to toxic reactions to drugs or alcohol, nutritional disorders, systemic and/or vascular disease (see next section for detailed visual field losses).
  - Different pattern of visual fields defect:
    - Optic Nerve Lesions:
      - Chief characteristic is that vision is lost in one eye whereas the other eye is usually normal. If field defects occur in both eyes it must be determined whether there are bilateral optic nerve lesions or a single lesion at the optic chiasm.
    - Optic chiasm lesions:

    - Tumors arising in the pituitary or in the adjacent dura mater can compress the chiasm and produce a characteristic bitemporal hemianopia. If the chiasm is involved anteriorly, there may be total vision loss in one eye and a temporal hemianopia in the other eye.
- Optic tract lesions:
    - Post chiasmic lesions typically present as homonymous hemianopias where the field defect is in the opposite hemifield of the two eyes. Details of the hemianopic defect as well of signs generated from the involvement of adjacent brain areas, will aid in the localization of the lesion. The field defects can be congruous, where the fields from each eye are affected identically, or incongruous.
- Lateral geniculate lesions:
    - Lesions in the terminal optic tract, the lateral geniculate body or the initial part of the optic radiations all produce similar homonymous hemianopias. Fibers from the upper retinal quadrants terminate medially whereas fibers from the inferior quadrants terminate laterally within the geniculate. The macular fibers project to the posterior portions of the geniculate.
- Lesions in the optic radiations:
    - Fibers pass through the posterior part of the internal capsule and then appear to spread out forming a large fan that passes around the lateral wall and posterior horn of the lateral ventricle. The fibers originating from cells in the medial portions of the lateral geniculate (superior retina) pass almost directly posteriorly to the visual cortex. Those fibers from the lateral aspect of the geniculate (inferior retina) form an anterior loop (Meyer's loop) before turning posteriorly to terminate in the visual cortex. Meyer's loop passes through the temporal lobe, so lesions causing homonymous superior visual field loss can indicate a lesion there. Alternatively, parietal lobe lesions may interrupt the fibers that do not loop forward and may produce inferior homonymous hemianopia. Lesions in the left temporal and parietal lobes often produce various types of aphasia which may aid in the diagnosis of the lesion.
- Primary visual cortex lesions:
    - The striate (primary) cortical visual area is located on the medial aspect of the posterior cerebral hemisphere (occipital pole) within the calcarine sulcus. Fibers carrying information from superior retinal quadrants terminate on the superior lip of the sulcus whereas the inferior retinal quadrant information is projected inferiorly. The macular area is represented in a large area extending onto the posterolateral aspect of the occipital pole. Lesions within a single hemisphere will almost always result in a congruous homonymous hemianopia; as opposed to lesions of the optic chiasm or tract which are usually incongruous.
- Macular sparing refers to homonymous hemianopias in which there is a zone of preserved vision (up to 5 degrees) around the fixation point. An occipital cortical lesion is expected, however the mechanism for this phenomenon is unknown.
- Bilateral destruction of the occipital poles usually results in total blindness even though pupillary reflexes and the retinas are normal. Bilateral damage (due to trauma) to the visual cortices typically occurs due to their close proximity within the skull. Also, both occipital poles share a blood supply from branches of the basilar artery which may be occluded by thrombosis or embolization.
- Secondary Visual Cortex Lesions:
    - These cortical areas lie within the temporal and parietal lobes. The ability to recognize objects and words depends on the integrity of these areas and the pathways running through them. The loss of these abilities is termed visual agnosia (objects) and alexia (words).
- Effects of unilateral disease of the dominant temporal lobe: (left hemisphere, right handed patients) homonymous quadrantopia, Wernike's aphasia
- Effects of unilateral disease on nondominant temporal lobe: homonymous quadrantopia, impairment of mental function, visual alexia and agnosia (although these may also be attributed to contralateral lesions as well), dressing and constructional apraxia, bland or indifferent moods.

- Effects of bilateral temporal lobe disease: Korsakoff's amnesic defect, apathy and placidity loss of sexual capacity, Kluver- Bucy syndrome.
- Effects of unilateral parietal lobe disease (right or left): cortical sensory syndrome (total or partial hemianesthesia), mild hemiparesis, homonymous hemianopia or visual inattention, abolition of optokinetic nystagmus to one side.
- Effects of unilateral disease of the dominant parietal lobe: alexia, tactile agnosia, bilateral apraxia of the ideomotor type.

Detailed Headache (HA) Workup

- **HA History**
  - Location of HA, aggravating factors of pain duration and character of HA age of HA onset -this is critical to diagnosis. Migraines usually begin between the ages of 15 and 40. If Has begin before age 10 a tumor should be suspected. Has beginning after the 5th decade may indicate temporal arteritis, stroke, cerebral orsubarachnoid hemorrhage, brain tumor or glaucoma.
- **Type of HA**
  - Vascular – migraine, cluster, symptomatic vascular
  - Tension
  - Increased cranial pressure -tumor, subarachnoid hemorrhage
  - Inflammatory – Temporal arteritis
  - Traumatic – HAs following injury to the head and/or neck
  - Others – HAs related to medical disorders such as: hyperthyroidism, Cushing's disease, withdrawal of corticosteroid med, ldosterone producing tumors, occasionally Addison's disease, use of the "pill", acute anemia with low hemoglobin count.
- Most commonly ordered tests and their diagnostic usefulness:
  - CT Brain Scan is the best test for mass lesions. Used for tumors, infarcts, hemorrhages, subdural hematoma.
  - X-Rays are useful for any bony abnormalities such as, metastasis, fracture, primary tumor, osteo-myelitis or arthritis, sinusitis.
  - EEG is useful for seizures and encephalopathies.
  - Lumbar Puncture can help rule out CNS infection, bleeding, tumor and increased pressure.
  - Blood Tests: Sedimentation rate is used to rule out temporal arteritis. Other useful tests are, complete blood count, antinuclear antibodies, measurement of platelets, glucose, calcium, blood urea nitrogen (BUN) or serum glutamic oxaloacetic transaminase (SGOT).
  - * Consultation with ophthalmologist, neurologist, dentist, arteriography may determine, subarachnoid hemorrhage, aneurysm, cerebral vasculitis, venous occlusion, or atherosclerotic lesions.

3. Oculomotor Neuropathology

- Infranuclear pathology is indicated by the isolated paralysis of any one or more of the extraocular muscles. The lesion could affect neurons within the CNIII, IV, and VI nuclei; the course of the nerve from the nucleus to the muscle it supplies; or the muscle itself.
- Supranuclear pathology is indicated by the presence of a lesion either in the pathways connecting the various oculomotor nuclei or in the higher brain centers.
- Factors to consider about deviations of the eye:
  - Magnitude, direction, and laterality
  - Commitancy (deviation is the same in all visual directions) vs Non-commitancy
  - Constancy
  - Time of onset
  - Paralytic vs. non-paralytic
    - Which muscle are affected (external vs internal ophthalmoplegia)
    - Where is lesion (supranuclear, nuclear or myopathic)
- Paralysis of individual ocular muscles produces the following:
  - Loss or limitations of certain movements of the eyeball.
  - Secondary contraction of the antagonist(s).
  - Deviation of the eyeball, producing non-correspondanceof the visual axes (i.e. strabismus).

The acquired deviation undergoes 3 major changes known as the "spread of comitance"

- Weakness of the paretic muscle +overaction of its direct antagonist.
- Contracture of antagonist deviation "spreads" into all fields of gaze.
- Diplopia
- Ocular torticollis

Causes of Paralysis of Nerve Palsies (%)			
Cause	CN III	CN IV	CN VI
Undetermined	23	36	27
Head trauma	16	32	17
Neoplasm	12	4	15
Vascular	21	19	18
Aneurism	14	2	4
Other	14	7	19

- Differential diagnosis of paralytic vs. non-paralytic strabismus:
  - Paralytic- often sudden onset with history of head trauma, may occur at any age, primary finding is the difference between primary and secondary deviations, diplopia, typically non-comitant
  - Non-paralytic- gradual onset during childhood or congenital, presence of ARC or amblyopia or both, comitance

4. Infranuclear Neuropathology

- Objective and Subjective Testing for Non-comitance:
  - **Objective:** Cover tests in all fields of gaze; amblyoscope; corneal light reflection tests; Bielschowsky head tilt test.
  - Subjective: Red filter or Maddox rod (diplopia tests); Hallden and Lancaster (projector tests).
- Strength and Fatigue Testing in Myopathies:
  - **Forced duction test:** Diagnostic for the presence of a mechanical restriction of ocular motility. Eye is moved with a forceps in a direction opposite that in which mechanical restriction is suspected. If resistance is encountered, mechanical restrictions exist.
  - Determination of generated muscle force: Can estimate the force generated by a contracting muscle by stabilizing the eye with forceps while the patient tries to move the eye against this obstacle.
- Eye movement velocity:
  - Record eye movements via electro-oculography. Used as an auxiliary diagnostic tool in evaluating paralytic conditions. However, an astute clinician can detect differences in eye movement velocities with his/her own clinical expertise.
- Recognition and examination for orbital signs:
  - N. III Paralysis:
    - S. Rectus – Isolated paralysis is rare and most commonly congenital. Paretic eye is hypotropic in primary position and Bell's phenomenon is absent. Frequently-associated with weakness of the ipsilateral levator palpebrae.
    - M. Rectus – Isolated paralysis without involvement of other muscles supplied by the third nerve is rare. Exotropia in primary position. Must be differentiated from internuclear ophthalmoplegia.
    - Inf. Rectus – Isolated paralysis is also rare and usually congenital. Incyclotropia and hypertropia are seen in primary position.
    - Inf. Oblique – Least likely to become paralyzed. Greatest deviation seen upon elevation in the adducted position. Overaction of the unopposed superior oblique causes incyclotropia. The forced duction test is necessary to differentiate this paralysis from Brown's syndrome.
  - Complete N. III Paralysis:
    - Typically the eye will be abducted, depressed and intorted. Ptosis and slight proptosis are also observed. The intrinsic muscles of the eye are involved only in acquired conditions, causing the pupil to be dilated and nonreactive and accommodation paralyzed. During recovery of acquired third nerve paralysis, aberrant regeneration of nerve fibers results in a pseudo-Graefe sign.
  - N. IV Paralysis:
    - The overaction of the inferior oblique will produce hypertropia in the primary position with a characteristic head tilt towards the noninvolved side. The palsies are bilateral in about 1/5 of the cases of traumatic trochlear nerve damage. The acquired paralysis due to trauma is the most common cause.

- N. VI Paralysis:
  - Esotropia is seen in primary gaze due to the unopposed action of the antagonist medial rectus. The head is tilted towards the involved side. It must be differentiated from Duane's retraction syndrome, and from the nystagmus blocking syndrome causing congenital esotropia.
- Understanding Indications for Intravenous Tension:
  - The tension test consists of 2 mg of edrophonium (an anti- cholinesterase) given IV over 15 seconds. A relief of ptosis constitutes a positive response and confirms the diagnosis of myasthenia gravis. If no response occurs in 30 seconds, an additional 8 mg are given.

Signs and Symptoms of Related Systemic Diseases

- Graves' Disease:
  - Signs are limitation of elevation of one or both eyes, exophthalmos and lid retraction, myopathy of edematous nature of extraocular muscles. The myopathy is more frequent in women and usually affects middle aged individuals. Diplopia is reported with an insidious onset usually correlating to an onset of exophthalmos. Involvement frequently remains unilateral or is asymmetric if involvement is of both eyes. CT scan of the extraocular muscles is used to confirm diagnosis.
  - Non-metabolic bone disease of unknown etiology. Causes excessive bone degeneration and repair with associated deformities since the repair takes place in an unorganized fashion. Up to 3% of persons over age 50 will show isolated lesions, but many are clinically insignificant. There is a strong familial incidence. Deep bone pain is reported and X-rays show the involved bone to be expanded and denser than normal. The head becomes larger and restrictions of the extraocular muscles may result.
- Möbius Syndrome:
  - A congenital disorder of autosomal recessive inheritance and unknown etiology. There is bilateral paralysis of lateral gaze, esotropia is common, bilateral facial palsy and malformation with lower lid ectropion, tongue weakness, and mental retardation.
- Myasthenia Gravis:
  - Diplopia and ptosis are the presenting symptoms in over 75% of the patients. Any extraocular muscle can be affected. A positive Tensilon test is diagnostic.
- Multiple Sclerosis:
  - (covered in part B.)
  - Muscles most affected are the medial and lateral recti and the levator palpebrae.
- Orbital Blowout Fractures:
  - Usually caused by a traumatic force, the fracture typically occurs within the anterionasal section of the orbital floor, where the bone is thinnest. The following signs and symptoms are present: periorbital swelling and ecchymosis; anesthesia of nose and lower lid; vertical diplopia with restrictions of up or down gaze; enophthalmos.
- Duane's Retraction Syndrome:
  - Characterized by the following signs: severe limitation of abduction; slight limitation of adduction; globe retraction and narrowing of the palpebral fissure on adduction. A strabismus may or may not be present with the eyes in the primary position. When present, the strabismus is esotropic. Many patients adopt a head turn to maintain binocular fixation. Complaints of diplopia are rare, but cosmesis is a major concern.
- Brown's Superior Oblique Tendon Sheath Syndrome:
  - Characterized by the following signs: absence of elevation in adduction; positive forced duction test; divergence (V-pattern) in upward gaze. Symptoms include diplopia on adduction, and anomalous head positions. The positive forced duction test differentiates this from paralysis of inf. oblique m.

5. <u>Supragranular Oculomotor Neuropathology</u>

- Observation, inspection and testing stability of eyes in fixation:
  - Testing relies on subjective and objective signs and symptoms of eye stability:
    - Oscillopsia – An illusionary movement of the environment in which stationary

objects seem to move. May be associated with coarse nystagmus due to a brain stem lesion. The movement or positional distortion of single visualized objects may be a part of metamorphopsia from cerebral lesions.

        - Opsoclonus – Sustained, irregular, conjugate “dancing” movements usually associated with cerebellar disease due to a viral infection or neuroblastoma
        - Ocular dysmetria – An overshoot of the eyes on attempted fixation, followed by several cycles of oscillations of diminishing amplitude about the fixation point. Usually due to a disease of the cerebellum or its pathways

- Parinaud’s Syndrome
    - Refers to lesions within the midbrain tegmentum, ventral to the superior colliculi which interfere with voluntary upward gaze, and convergence movements and abolish the pupillary light reflex.a lesion in the pontine center for conjugate lateral gaze, near the abducens nucleus, causes ipsilateral gaze palsy, with the eyes turning to the opposite side.

TESTING

- Testing for adequacy of pursuits:
    - Have the patient follow some target.
    - Aberrant movements include a constant lag, overshoots, undertracking, or a midline hesitation (common with disabled or dyslexic kids).
    - Smooth pursuits can break down due to conditions listed in the above sections. An acute lesion, such as an infarct, in one frontal lobe may cause paralysis of contralateral gaze, and the eyes will turn toward the side of the lesion. This type of disorder is usually temporary (several days).
    - Gaze paralysis of cerebral origin is not attended by stabismus or diplopia
    - Smooth ocular pursuits may be lost with lesions in the occipital lobe.
- Testing for adequacy of saccades:
    - Use two objects held apart and have the patient look from one to the other in rapid succession. Look for movement asymmetry, left to right vs. right to left. Check in all fields of gaze.
- Testing extraocular muscle reflexes:
    - Optokinetic Nystagmus
    - Vestibular Ocular Reflex
    - Nystagmus
    - Vestibular Nystagmus
    - Congenital Nystagmus
- Assessment of “dizzy” patient:
    - A careful case history is always important. Inspection of the eardrums, x-rays of the mastoids middle and inner ears, as well as auditory and caloric testing are all useful in differentiating labyrinth from nerve disease. The association of vertigo with auditory signs and symptoms always signifies a disease process of the end organ or eighth nerve. Labyrinth and auditory tests and the presence of neurologic signs referable to structures adjacent to the eighth cranial nerve nuclei are useful as a means of differentiation. Pure vertigo as a manifestation of brainstem disease is rare.

Chapter 17 – Ocular Pharmacology

GENERAL PRINCIPLES

1. Factors Affecting Drug Bioavailability

- **Bioavailability** is the amount of drug present at the desired receptor site.
- **Active Ingredients:** therapeutic and diagnostic drugs given topically or systemically can have major effects on uptake of other drugs as a result of their own actions on tissue permeability, blood flow, and fluid secretion.
- **Stability:** low concentration of buffer in the drug vehicle is often used to prevent a change in tear pH; which can cause irritation and stimulation of lacrimation and decrease in drug penetration.
- **Osmolarity:** Increasing tonicity above that of the tears causes immediate dilution by osmotic water movement from the eyelids and eye. Simple or complex salts, buffering agents, or certain sugars are often added to adjust osmolarity of the solution to the desired value.
- **Preservatives:** used at high concentrations can irritate and damage the ocular surface.
- **Vehicles:** agents other than the active drug or preservative added to a formulation to provide proper tonicity, buffering, and viscosity to complement drug action.
- **Drug Release Systems:** soft contact lenses and collagen shields absorb drugs from solution and then slowly release them when placed on the eye. This form of drug therapy can be valuable when continuous treatment is desired.

2. Routes of Administration

- **Solutions and Suspensions**: Solutions are the most commonly used mode of delivery for topical ocular medications. Suspensions must be resuspended by shaking. Solutions or suspensions are usually preferred over ointments, because the former are more easily instilled, interfere less with vision, and have fewer potential complications.
- **Sprays:** topical sprays represent an alternative method of administering ophthalmic solutions that may be less irritating and less objectionable.
- **Ointments:** When applied to the inferior conjunctival sac, ophthalmic ointments melt quickly, and the excess spreads out onto the lid margins, lashes, and skin of the lids. Ointment at the lid margins acts as a reservoir and enhances drug contact time.
- **Lid Scrubs:** application of solutions or ointments directly to the lid margin is especially helpful in treating seborrheic or infectious blepharitis.
- **Gels:** advantage of this sustained delivery system is the once-daily dosage regimen, with the drug usually administered at bedtime. Minor side effects include superficial corneal haze and superficial punctuate keratitis.
- **Solid Delivery Devices**: used to provide continuous drug delivery; soft contact lenses, collagen shields, filter paper strips, cotton pledgets.
- **Continuous Flow Devices**: used to delivery large volumes of fluids; conventional irrigating system, continuous irrigating system.
- **Periocular Administration:** used when higher concentrations of drugs are required in the eye than can be delivered by topical administration; subconjunctival injection, sub-Tenon's injection, retrobulbar injection, peribulbar injection.
- **Intracameral Administration**: used to deliver drug directly into the anterior chamber of the eye.
- **Intravitreal Administration**: used to inject drug directly into the vitreous.

3. Pharmacokinetics of Ocular Tissues

- **Pharmacokinetics** is the study of the time course of absorption, distribution, metabolism, and elimination of an administered drug.
  - Drug absorption depends on:
    - Molecular properties of the drug

        - Viscosity of its vehicle
        - Functional status of the tissue forming the barrier to penetration
    - Distribution depends on bioavailability.
    - Metabolism plays a part in drug elimination, prodrug activation, and toxic byproduct production and removal.
- **Tear Film**
    - Normal tear volume is 8-10mcl with a total volume up to 30mcl held in eyelids if not squeezed after dosing. Single drop of medication is typically 50mcl, leading to some medication being nasolacrimally drained and some spilling over the lid margin.
    - Concentration of drug absorption in the anterior segment depends on tear flow rate and tear volume.
    - To increase corneal absorption block nasolacrimal drugs and administer ophthalmic solutions at 10 minute intervals.
- **Cornea**
    - Major site of absorption of topically applied drugs.
    - Epithelium and stroma have major effects on pharmacodynamics acting as depots and reservoirs for lipophilic and hydrophilic drugs.
    - Epithelium:
        - Resists penetration of hydrophilic drugs:
            - Hydrophilic drug penetration can be increased with epithelial erosion or cationic preservatives.
        - Lipophilic drugs can readily penetrate.
    - Stroma:
        - Major ocular depot for topically applied hydrophilic drugs.
        - Keratocytes are the major reservoir for lipophilic compounds.
    - To penetrate cornea effectively, drug must have hydrophilic and lipophilic properties.
- **Sclera/Conjunctiva**
    - Vascularized, results in removal of drugs.
    - Can account for up to 1/5 of drug absorption to iris and ciliary body.
- **Iris**
    - Contains pigment that absorbs light and lipophilic drugs. Usually drug-binding is reversible, and causes a slow release of the drug over time.
    - Iris serves as a reservoir for some drugs.
    - Effective dosing can only be achieved by reaching a saturation equilibrium where the amount of drug being bound is the same as the being released from the reservoir.
- **Aqueous Humor**
    - Formed by ciliary body, drains through Schlemm's canal (conventional pathway) or through walls or iris or other tissues that form margins of anterior chamber through the uveoscleral (nonconventional) pathway.
- **Ciliary Body**
    - Systemic drugs enter anterior and posterior chamber by passing through the ciliary body vasculature and diffusing into the iris.
    - Major source of drug metabolizing enzymes- begins process of drug detoxification and removal from the eye.
    - Melanin in pigmented ciliary epithelium absorbs polycyclic compounds.
- **Crystalline Lens**
    - Anterior lens epithelium most metabolically active and most prone to damage from drugs or toxic substances.
    - Lipid-soluble drugs can pass through the lens cortex slowly.
- **Vitreous**
    - Free diffusion of small molecules.
    - Acts as both a reservoir and temporary depot for metabolites.
- **Retina and Optic Nerve**
    - Tight junctional complexes (zonula occludens) in RPE prevent ready movement of antibiotics and other drugs from the blood to the retina and vitreous (blood-retinal barrier).

- Lipophilic drugs can cross BRB easily.

- **Ocular Blood Supply** – Removal of Drugs and Metabolites
  - Two circulatory pathways in the eye that drugs exit through:
    - Retinal vessels- use active transport to remove many drugs, metabolites, and agents like prostaglandins from the vitreous and retina.
    - Uveal vessels – (choroid, ciliary body, iris) – use bulk transport to remove drugs from the iris and ciliary body.
  - Drugs can also exit via aqueous drainage into the general circulation.

AUTNOMIC AND/OR NEUROMUSCULAR JUNCTION DRUGS

1. Drugs Affecting Neurohumoral Transmission: Autonomic and Somatic Motor Nervous Systems

- The autonomic nervous system controls unconscious motor control and is divided into two parts:
  - **Parasympathetic System**: "Rest and digest" – discrete output:
    - Originates in cranial nerves from medulla.
    - Preganglia are very long and myelinated.
    - Maintains normal function in the body.
    - Aka Cholinergic/Muscarinic System.
  - **Sympathetic System:** "Fight or Flight" – diffuse output :
    - Sympathetic preganglia originate in spinal cord.
    - Preganglia are very short and myelinated → fast conduction.
    - Directly innervates adrenal glands, causes epinephrine and norepinephrine release.
    - Aka Adrenergic System.

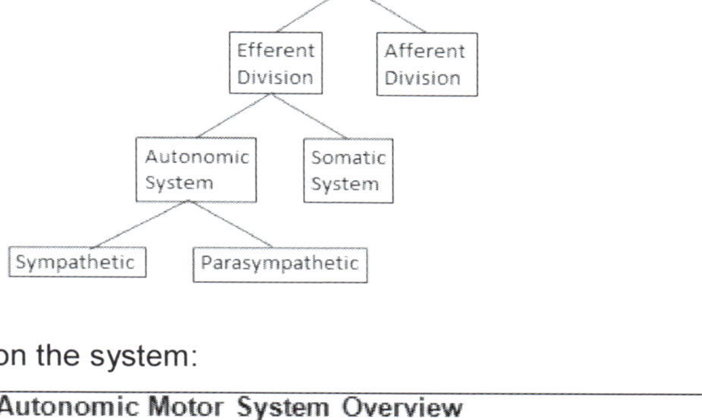

  - Autonomic Neurotransmitters vary depending upon the system:
    - Acetylcholine is the common ganglionic neurotransmitter to activate both sympathetic and parasympathetic systems.
    - The parasympathetic nerves release acetylcholine to regulate nerve terminals and trigger muscarinic receptors.

Autonomic Motor System Overview		
Body Part	**Parasympathetic**	**Sympathetic**
Pupil	Constricts (Miosis)	Dilates (Mydriasis)
Exocrine Glands (Salvation)	Stimulates	Inhibits
Heart	Slows	Accelerates
Bronchi	Constricts	Relaxes
Stomach/pancreas	Stimulates	Inhibits
Gallbladder	Stimulates	
Liver		Stimulates glucose release
Bladder	Constricts	Stimulates
Gonads	Causes erection	Promotes ejaculation

    - The sympathetic nerves release norepinephrine to trigger adrenergic (α,β) receptors:
      - Exceptions to sympathetic nerve secretion of norepinephrine:
        - Sympathetic nerves acetylcholine actively triggers Norepinephrine/Epinephrine release in the adrenal gland and to stimulate sweat glands.
        - Renal vasculature is stimulated by dopamine instead of norepinephrine.

- **Cholinergic (Muscarinic) Neuron**
  - All aspects of the cholinergic neuron are possible target sites for drug action.
  - *Acetylcholine synthesis:*
    1. **ChAT** (choline acetyltransferase) makes acetylcholine from Acetyl-CoA (Krebs cycle in mitochondria) and choline (recycled).

2. Acetylcholine is actively transported (ATP and Substance P co-transporters) into vesicles by vesicle-associated transporter pumps.
3. Neuron depolarizes, Ca2+ channels open, Ca2+ rushes in, causing the vessel to fuse with the membrane. Specific anchoring proteins on the vesicles (VAMPs) and on the membrane (SNAPs) interact, fuse, and anchor the vesicle to the membrane that allows the membrane fusion and neurotransmitter release into the synapse.
4. Acetylcholine is released into the synapse and will work on cholinergic (muscarinic receptors).

- *Acetylcholine Metabolism:*
  1. **Acetylcholinesterase** and **pseudocholine esterase** rapidly metabolize acetylcholine into choline and acetate. The choline gets recycled into the neuron and other cells use the acetate.
  2. Acetylcholine receptors are present on the presynaptic neuron for negative feedback → acetylcholine can activate the inhibition of additional acetylcholine.

- **Adrenergic Neuron**
  - *Catecholamine Synthesis:*
    1. Tyrosine is converted to L-DOPA by **tyrosine hydroxinase** (rate limiting step).
    2. L-DOPA is converted to dopamine by **DOPA decarboxylase.**
    3. Dopamine is converted into norepinephrine by **Dopamine hydroxylase.**
    4. Norepinephrine is converted into epinephrine by **N-methyl transferase.**
  - *Storage:*
    - Dopamine and Norepinephrine are complexed with ATP (co-transmitter) and chromogranin A (stabilization)
  - *Norepinephrine Release:*
    - Three mechanisms:
      1. Exocytosis (Ca2+ dependent and driven release) – activated nicotinic receptors cause depolarization and ion channel opening.
      2. Inhibitory feedback via α2 and DA2, AcH (muscarinic) receptors – slows down further release of norepinephrine (**heterotypic inhibition**).
      3. Stimulatory feedback via β2, AII (Angiotensin II) Receptors – increases further release indirectly via cAMP.
  - *Norepinephrine Reuptake:*
    - Either neuronal or extraneuronal reuptake.
  - *Metabolic Termination of Norepinephrine:*
    - **Monoamine Oxidase (MAO)** located in neurons and effector cells. Two Types, MAO-A oxidizes norepinephrine and serotonin. MAO-B oxidizes dopamine.
    - **Catechol-O-methyl-transferase (COMT)** is located at effector sites and may act in series with MAO.
- The **Somatic Motor Nervous System** controls conscious motor control (skeletal muscle)
  - Somatic nerves use acetylcholine to activate nicotinic receptors (ion channels) at the neural/muscular junction.
- **Drug Agonists (-mimetics)** increase activity of the receptor it binds to.
  - Direct: turns on receptor.
  - Indirect: increases acetylcholine at nerve junction to activate receptor.
- **Drug Antagonist (-lytic)** decreases receptor activity.
  - Direct: binds to receptor but does not activate signal.
  - Indirect: indirectly decreases agonist (acetylcholine).
  - Reversible: adding more agonist can overcome antagonist.
  - Irreversible: inhibition remains no much how much agonist is added.

Sympathetic Receptors		
Receptor	**Location**	**Normal Receptor Action**
α-1	Peripheral blood vessels	Vasoconstriction
	Blood lipids	Increased blood lipids
	Heart (limited)	Not much change
	Bladder neck	Vasoconstriction
	Seminal tract	Vasoconstriction
	Eye- Dilator Muscle	Mydriasis
	Eye- Blood vessels	Vasoconstriction
α-2	Medullary vasomotor control center	CNS depression
	Peripheral nerves at pre-synapse	Decreases NE Release
	Peripheral blood vessels	Vasodilation
	Pancreas	Decrease Insulin
	Eyes-Ciliary Epithelium	Increases Aqueous Outflow
β-1	Kidneys	Increase renin release
	Heart	Increase cardiac output
	CNS	Increase tone
	Pre-synaptic nerves	Increases NE release
β-2	Peripheral blood vessels to muscle	Vasodilation
	Lungs	Bronchodilation
	Blood glucose	Increased blood glucose
	Eyes-Ciliary Epithelium	Decreases Aqueous Outflow
β-3	Adipose tissue	Lipolysis (increases VLDL)

2. Adrenergic Agonists

- Adrenergic agonists (**sympathomimetics**) increase adrenergic receptor activity. Can be selective for an α or β receptor or both (nonselective).
- **Mechanism of Action:** Stimulate both α and β receptor sites.
  - α1 Receptors located on blood vessel smooth muscle, GI tract, and genitourinary tract→ vasoconstriction.
  - β1 Receptors located in heart muscle → increased contractility and heart rate.
  - β2 Receptors located in bronchial muscle→ bronchodilation.
- **Indications**
  - α-agonists are used to relieve hypotension, hemostasis, nasal congestion, reduces bleeding in conjunction with local anesthetics, and causes **mydriasis.**
  - β-agonists used to treat asthma and bronchitis.
  - Many are potent ocular hypotensive agents used for treating glaucoma. **α2 Agonists:** Decrease cAMP. Can decrease aqueous humor production by epithelial cells and thus decrease IOP.
- **Adverse Effects**
  - α-agonist effects due to vasoconstriction → hypertension, decreased heart rate.
  - β-agonist effects →headache, tremors, mild leg cramps, nervousness, fatigue, hypertension, palpitation, nausea, vomiting, shortness of breath.
  - General side effects of adrenergic agonists:
    - Cardiac arrhythmias
    - Headache
    - Hyperacuity
    - Insomnia
    - Nausea

- Tremors

- **Contraindications**:
  - Patients with known hypersensitivity
  - Elderly – more sensitive to adverse effects
  - Patients with blurred vision, seizures, chest pain, palpitations
  - Children <2 years (α-agonists)
  - Cardiac arrhythmias associated with tachycardia, hyperthyroidism, pregnancy, lactation (β-agonists)
  - Used with caution in patients that have hypertension, cardiovascular disease, hyperthyroidism, and diabetes
- **Direct acting agonists** – act directly on α or β receptors, producing effects similar to those of stimulation from adrenal gland epinephrine release. Activated receptor initiates synthesis of second messengers and subsequent intracellular signals.
- **Indirect acting agonists** –block the uptake of norepinephrine or are taken up into the presynaptic neuron and cause the release of norepinephrine.
  - **Amphetamine** – displaces norepinephrine
  - **Cocaine** – inhibits reuptake of norepinephrine at the junction
  - Tyramine
- **Mixed action agonists** – capacity to stimulate adrenergic receptors directly and to release norepinephrine from the adrenergic neuron.
  - Ephedrine
  - Pseudo-ephedrine
  - Metaraminol

Examples of Adrenergic Agonists					
α1 Agonists	**α2 Agonists**	**α1/α2 Agonists**	**β1 Agonists**	**β2 Agonists**	**β1/β2 Agonists**
Phenylephrine Methoxamine Naphazoline Oxymetazoline Tetrahydrozoline	Clonidine Aproclonidine Bromonidine Guanfacine α-methyldopa	Methoxamine	Dopamine Dobutamine	Salbutamol Terbutaline Salmeterol Dopezmine	Isoprenaline Ephedrine

3. Adrenergic Antagonists

- Adrenergic antagonists (**sympatholytics**) decreases receptor activity. Can be selective for an α or β receptor or both (nonselective). These drugs are the most commonly prescribed class of autonomic drugs.
- **Mechanism of Action**
  - Reduce the delivery of catecholamines to the adrenergic receptors by inhibiting catecholamine synthesis, storage, or release.
- **Indications**
  - Hypertension
  - Dysrhythmias, angina, heart failure
  - Glaucoma
  - Migraines
- **Adverse Effects**
  - Orthostatic hypotension, edema, headache, dizziness, vertigo, somnolence, fatigue, nervousness, anxiety.
  - Abdominal pain, nausea, vomiting, diarrhea, peptic ulcer exacerbation.
  - β-Blockers – respiratory disturbances, bradycardia, peripheral vascular insufficiency, palpitations, postural hypotension, behavioral changes, **blurred vision, dry eye.**

Examples of Adrenergic Antagonists					
α1 Antagonists	**α2 Antagonists**	**α1/α2 Antagonists**	**β1 Antagonists**	**β2 Antagonists**	**β1/β2 Antagonists**
Prazosin Doxazosin Tetrazosin	Yohimbine	Phentolamine Thymosamine Dapiprazole	Practolol Betaxolol Atenolol Metoprolol Carteolol	Butoxamine	Propranolol Metipranolol Timolol Levobunolol

4. Cholinergic Agonists = Parasympathomimetics = Muscarinic Agonists

- **Acetylcholine**
  - Quaternary ammonium compound that cannot penetrate membranes. It is the Neurotransmitter of the parasympathetic and somatic nerves as well as ganglion nerves.
  - There is no therapeutic importance because of multiplicity of action and rapid inactivation by cholinesterases.
  - Has both muscarinic and cholinergic activity:
    - Decreases heart rate and cardiac output.
    - Decreases blood pressure - cholinergic receptors on blood vessels lead to vasodilation due to acetylcholine-induced rise in intracellular Ca2+, which results in the formation of nitric oxide (NO) from arginine in endothelial cells.
    - Increases salivary secretion, intestinal secretions, and motility.
    - Stimulates ciliary muscle contraction for near vision (**accommodation**) and constriction of the sphincter muscle (**miosis**).
- **Mechanism of Action**
  - Cholinergic agonists either directly mimic the effects of acetylcholine by binding to the receptors or indirectly by inhibiting acetylcholinesterase, thus prolonging the duration of acetylcholine in the synapse.
- **Adverse Effects**
  - Central: Light-headedness, dizziness, motor disturbances (tremor, rigidity).
  - Other: Diarrhea, Diaphoresis, Nausea, Urinary urgency, **Miosis.**
- **Direct Cholinergic Agonists**: mimic the effects of acetylcholine by binding to cholinergic receptors. They all have longer durations of action than acetylcholine. As a group of drugs, most direct-acting agonists show little specificity in their actions, which limits their clinical usefulness.
  - Synthetic esters of choline:
    - **Bethanechol** – major actions on smooth musculature of bladder and GI tract, muscarinic only.
    - **Carbachol**- hard to metabolize, has both muscarinic and nicotinic actions. Can decrease IOP. Has many side effects. Used to cause miosis during ocular surgery or to reduce IOP in open or closed-angle glaucoma patients that are intolerant to pilocarpine.
  - Naturally occurring alkaloid:
    - **Pilocarpine** – far less potent than acetylcholine and its derivatives. Exhibits muscarinic activity and is used primarily in ophthalmology. It is able to penetrate the CNS.
      - Used in open- and closed-angle glaucoma to decrease IOP.
- **Indirect Cholinergic Agonists (anti-cholinesterases) – reversible:** Acetylcholinesterases specifically cleave acetylcholine to acetate and choline, terminating acetylcholine's actions in the synapse. These enzymes are located both pre- and post-synaptically in the nerve terminal. Inhibitors of acetylcholinesterase indirectly provide cholinergic action by prolonging the lifetime of acetylcholine produced endogenously at the cholinergic nerve endings.
  - **Donepezil, Tacrine, Rivastigmine** – used in Alzheimer's treatment
  - **Edrophonium**
    - Therapeutic Uses:
      - Diagnosis of myasthenia gravis
      - Antidote for tubocurarine
      - Short duration of action
  - **Neostigmine** – a synthetic compound that is also a carbamic acid ester

- Its quaternary nitrogen makes the molecule more polar so it cannot penetrate into the CNS
- Has a greater effect on skeletal muscle than physostigmine and can stimulate contractility before it paralyzes.
- Therapeutic effects:
  - Used to stimulate the bladder and GI tract – prevents postoperative abdominal distention and urinary retention
  - Antidote to tubocurarine and other competitive neuromuscular blocking agents
  - Symptomatic treatment of myasthenia gravis
- **Physostigmine –** alkaloid and tertiary amine
  - Carbamic acid ester = substrate for acetylcholinesterase. Forms a stable carbamoylated intermediate with enzyme.
  - Therapeutic uses:
    - Increased intestinal and bladder motility
    - Reduce IOP in glaucoma
    - Reverse CNS and cardiac effects of tricyclic antidepressants
    - Reverse CNS effects of atropine
    - Penetrates CNS
- **Indirect Cholinergic Agonist - irreversible:** synthetic organic phosphate compounds that covalently bind to acetylcholinesterase. This results in long lasting increases in acetylcholine at all sites where it is released. These drugs are extremely toxic and have been developed by the military as nerve agents.
  - Ecothiopate – irreversibly inhibits acetylcholinesterase
  - Isofluorphate
    - Therapeutic effects:
      - Treatment of open-angle glaucoma
      - Long duration of action (1 week)
  - **Sarin (Nerve gas), Parathion/Malthione (insecticides)**

5. Cholinergic Antagonists

- Cholinergic antagonists (**parasympatholytics**) bind to cholinergic receptors but do not trigger the usual receptor-mediated intracellular effects. Most useful agents selectively block muscarinic synapses of the parasympathetic nerves, allowing for sympathetic stimulation to be left unopposed
- **Mechanism of Action**
  - Selectively block all muscarinic responses to acetylcholine.
- **Indications**
  - Adjunct treatment of GI disorders (peptic ulcer, pylorospasm, GI hypermotility, irritable bowel syndrome, spastic disorder of biliary tract).
  - **Cycloplegia**
  - **Anterior Uveitis**
  - **Iritis**
  - General anesthesia, bradycardia, asystole during CPR
- **Adverse Effects**
  - Headache, ataxia, dizziness, excitement, irritability, convulsions, drowsiness, fatigue, weakness, mental depression, confusion, disorientation, hallucinations, hypertension or hypotension, ventricular fibrillation, inability to swallow, cycloplegia.
  - Central:
    - Sedation at therapeutic doses
    - Excitement at higher doses
    - Atropine fever (peripheral effect) – pronounced in children, leads to shutting down of sweat glands causing systemic over heating
  - Other:
    - **Blurred vision**
    - Confusion
    - **Mydriasis**

    - Constipation
- **Contraindications**
  - Hypersensitivity to belladonna alkaloids
  - Synechiae, angle0closure glaucoma
  - Parotitis, obstructure uropathy, intestinal atony, paralytic ilius, obstructive GI tract diseases, severe ulcerative colitis, toxic megacolon
  - Tachycardia, acute hemorrhage
  - Myasthenia Gravis
  - Use with caution in patients with:
    - Myocardial infarction, hypertension, hypotension, coronary artery disease, congestive heart failure and irregular heart rhythms
    - Gastric ulcer, GI infections, hiatal hernia, reflux esophagitis, hyperthyroidism, chronic lung disease, renal disease, hepatic disease
    - Elderly, debilitated patients, children <6
    - Down Syndrome, autonomic neuropathy, spastic paralysis, brain damage
- **Drug Interactions**
  - Amantadine
  - Antihistamines
  - Tricyclic antidepressants
  - Quinidine
  - Procainamide
  - Methotrimeprazine (precipitate extrapyramidal effects)
  - Phenothiazines (decreased absorption)
- **Indirect Cholinergic Antagonists:** block the synthesis of acetylcholine
  - **Hemicholinium** – inhibit choline recycling by competing with choline in uptake, decreasing the synthesis of acetylcholine
  - **Triethylcholine –** false transmitters that inhibit synthesis
  - **Vesamicol –** inhibit transport of acetylcholine into storage vessels
  - **Botulinum toxin** – inhibits acetylcholine release by inhibiting the fusion of vesicle to the membrane
  - **Magnesium** – inhibits acetylcholine release as a Ca2+ blocker, inhibiting the cascade
  - **Aminoglycoside antibiotics (streptomycin, neomycin), Local Anesthetics –** inhibits the release of acetylcholine
- **Cholinergic Blocker Examples**
  - Atropine
  - Scopolamine
  - Tropicamide
  - Cyclopentolate
  - Homatropine
  - Ipratropium

6. Ganglionic Agonists and Antagonists

- Both sympathetic and parasympathetic nervous system ganglia are effected by acetylcholine, so most ganglionic agonists and antagonists are non selective and effect both autonomic nervous systems creating undesirable side effects.
- **Ganglionic Agonists** are of no therapeutic use. They are used to analyze the mechanism of ganglionic function. They enhance action at nicotinic acetylcholine receptors. The classic ganglionic agonist is Nicotine.
    - Nicotine causes arousal at low doses.
    - Nicotine causes calming at high doses as it essentially acts as a ganglionic and neuromuscular antagonist.
    - Very addicting drug.
    - Symptoms of poisoning:
      - Sweating, hypertension, decreased GI activity, arrhythmia, tachycardia, flaccid paralysis, convulsions, vomiting.

- **Ganglionic Antagonists**: show a preference for nicotinic receptors (N_N) of sympathetic and parasympathetic ganglia.
    - **Mechanism of action**
        - Drugs compete, mimic, or interfere with acetylcholine metabolism at the autonomic nervous system ganglia indirectly inhibiting postganglionic transmission.
    - **Therapeutic Uses**
        - Hypertension (first effective therapy but had many side effects)
        - Aortic dissection
        - Limited therapeutic uses are due to this drug groups tendency to produce vasodilation causing extreme hypotension, rapid onset tachyphylaxis.
    - **Adverse Effects**
        - Venous pooling, postural hypotension, dry mouth, constipation, sexual dysfunction
        - Tachycardia, dry mouth, urinary retention.
        - **Mydriasis,** blurred vision
    - **Examples**
        - Hexamethonium
        - Mecamylamine
        - Trimethaphan
            - All three produce a selective non-depolarizing blockage of neurotransmission without producing neuromuscular blockage indicating their selectivity for N_N versus N_M receptors.

8. Neuromuscular Transmission Agonists and Antagonists

- Neuromuscular junctions are between skeletal muscle effectors sites in the somatic nervous system. Acetylcholine is released from motor nerve endings and binds to nicotinic receptors (N_M) on the postsynaptic membrane of endplates of the skeletal muscle, leading to a muscle fiber action potential.
- The action potential is caused by the opening of ion channels in the muscle membrane altering the sodium and potassium concentrations across the membrane, depolarizing the membrane from -80mV to 0mV.
- **Neuromuscular Agonists**
    - Agonists cause skeletal muscle contraction by either directly binding to the N_M receptor subunit, or by increasing the concentration of acetylcholine in the synapse increasing acetylcholine bound N_M receptors, causing conformational change and ion channel opening.
    - Examples include acetylcholinesterase inhibitors and acetylcholine analogs.
- **Neuromuscular Antagonists**
    - Aka muscle relaxants
    - Neuromuscular blockers are divided into two groups depending upon their mechanism of action. They are either non-depolarizing or depolarizing blockers. Both groups interfere with transmission of efferent impulses to skeletal muscles and cause varying levels of paralysis.
    - **Mechanism of Action-** Non-depolarizing.
        - Competitive antagonists that reversibly bind to N_M receptors, physically preventing the binding of acetylcholine, inhibiting receptor activation and ion channel opening.
        - These agents can be reversed by high concentrations of acetylcholine (anticholinesterases).
    - **Mechanism of Action** – Depolarizing
        - Long acting agonists
        - These antagonists maintain depolarization at the end-plate (chemically active region of skeletal muscle) which initially opens channels causing a large muscle contraction. Breakdown of these agents is slower than acetylcholine causing a prolonged state of depolarization. This receptor state renders the muscle unexcitable until the drug is broken down. This causes a transmission inhibition by preventing re-initiation and action potential propagation.
        - The receptors eventually desensitize, making the receptor less responsive to acetylcholine itself.
        - This type of blockade can be caused by large doses of agonists.

- Contrary to non-depolarizing antagonists, this blockage is enhanced by anticholinesterases which can lead to pain and muscle damage.

- **Therapeutic use**
  - Complete skeletal muscle relaxation during surgery.
  - Can allow for avoidance of deep anesthesia and its side effects.
- **Side Effects**
  - Myalgias
  - **Increases IOP**
  - Increases intracranial pressure
  - Masseter muscle spasm
  - Cardiovascular effects
  - Prolonged block
  - Anaphylaxis
  - Malignant hyperthermia → high morbidity and mortality

Neuromuscular Antagonist Examples	
Non-Depolarizing	**Depolarizing**
Tubocurarine Atracurium Pancuronium Vecuronium Rocuronium Cisatracurium Mivacurium	Suxamethonium Devamethonium

- **Pharmacological Inhibition of Neuromuscular Antagonists**
  - Recovery from non-depolarizing relaxants occurs spontaneously, but can take a long time and be unpredictable.
  - Administration of anti-cholinesterase drugs (**neostigmine, pyridostigmine, edrophonium**) increases the concentration of acetylcholine in the synapse to compete with non-depolarizing neuromuscular antagonists.

ANTI-INFECTIVE AGENTS

1. Antimicrobials

- Ocular infections involve bacteria, viruses, fungi, protozoa, or helminthes (worms).
- Ocular tissue damage is caused by both microbial factors and host immune responses:
  - Microbial factors: mechanical (penetration, invasion, adhesion), causes cell death
  - Virulence factors: exotoxins, endotoxins, polysaccharide capsules
  - Host response: complement, phagocytosis, inflammation, neovascularization
- Ocular tissues susceptible to infection:
  - **Conjunctiva**: is the most commonly infected tissue.
  - **Cornea**: is less commonly infected, but infection of the cornea is more threatening to vision.
  - **Lids/Adnexa**: endophthalmitis, orbital/preseptal cellulitis.
  - **Retina**: more common than corneal infections, very vision threatening.
  - Scratches are the most common pathway for pathogens to get into the eye.
- Treatment of ocular infections must be rapid, appropriate and of sufficient duration to resolve the infectious process.
- Antimicrobials help the immune system overcome bacterial resistance and decrease bacterial load.
- Antimicrobials are specific towards the microbe with minimum cross over between groups (anti-bacterials, anti-virals, anti-fungals).
- Agents are divided into narrow and broad spectrums, indicating the range of organisms that are affected. Antibacterial spectrum refers to the range of activity of the compound:
  - A **narrow spectrum** antibiotic is effective against either gram-positive of gram-negative organisms and may be either bactericidal or bacteriostatic.
  - A **broad spectrum** antibiotic is effective against gram-positive and gram-negative organisms, and also inhibits the *Rickettsia* (causes spotted fever and typhus) and *Chlamydia*.

Ocular Pathogens		
Gram-Positive Bacteria	**Ocular Effects**	**Special Characteristics**
Staphylococcus Aureus	Keratitis, Conjunctivitis, Blepharitis Endophthalmitis, Orbital Cellulitis	Most Strains B-lactamase producers
Staphylococcus epidermidis	Keratitis, Conjunctivitis, Blepharitis	Broad drug resistance
Streptococcal pneumonia	Keratitis, Conjunctivitis	Drug resistance increasing) -No B-lactamase
Bacillus cereus & Enteroccucs faecalis	Endophthalmitis	Broad drug resistance
Gram-Negative Bacteria	**Ocular Effects**	**Special Characteristics**
Haemophilus influenza	Conjunctivitis, Orbital Cellulitis	Many strains B-lactamase producers Most common cause of ocular disease
Pseudomonas aeruginosa	Keratitis, Endophthalmitis	Many strains B-lactamase producers Common cause of corneal infections
Chlamydia trachomatis	Inclusion Conjunctivitis, Trachoma	
Neisseria gonorrhoeae	Keratoconjunctivitis	Increasing drug resistance to penicillins
Viruses	**Ocular Effects**	**Special Characteristics**
Herpes Simplex (HSV)	Keratitis, Conjunctivitis	
Varicella Zoster (VZV)	Keratitis, Conjunctivitis	
Cytomegalovirus (CMV)	Retinitis	Lots of drug resistance
Adenovirus	Keratitis, Conjunctivitis	
Vaccinia virus	Keratitis, Conjunctivitis	
Fungal	**Ocular Effects**	**Special Characteristics**
Candida albicans	Endophthalmitis	
Fusarium spp	Keratitis, Conjunctivitis	
Protozoa	**Ocular Effects**	**Special Characteristics**
Acanthamoeba	Keratitis	
Toxoplasmosis gondii	Chorioretinitis	
Helminths	**Ocular Effects**	**Special Characteristics**
Tamea solium	Ocular cysticerosis	Pork tapeworm
Onchocerca volvulus	River blindness	
Loa loa	Eye worm	

Antimicrobial Drug Targets			
Microbe	**Drug Target**	**Mechanism**	**Drug Classes**
Bacteria	Peptidoglycan Cell Wall	Selectivity due to absence in mammalian cells	Penicillins Cephalosporins Bacitracin Vancomycin
	Protein Synthesis	Selectivity due to 70s vs. host 80s ribosomes	Aminoglycosides Macrolides Tetracyclines
	DNA Synthesis	Folic acid synthesis	Sulfonamides Trimethoprim
		DNA gyrase inhibition	Fluoroquinolones
	Cell/Outer Membrane	Little selectivity leads to toxicity	Polymyxin B

Fungi	Cell Membranes	Ergosterol selectivity	Amphotericin B Nystatin Azole Antifungals
Protozoa	DNA Synthesis	Folic acid biosynthesis	Sulfonamides Trimethoprim
Viruses	DNA synthesis	Viral protein specific	Trifluridine Ganciclovir Acyclovir
Helminthes	Metabolic System/ Nervous System	Fragmentation of parasite – potential exacerbation of ocular disease	

2. Antibiotics

- Antibiotics are substances that destroy or inhibit the growth, reproduction, or pathogenic activity of microorganisms. Bacterial agents destroy microorganisms and are more effective during periods of rapid growth of the microorganisms.
  - **Note:** Gram-Negative bacteria have a cell wall structure that is LESS permeable to antibiotics.
- Antibacterial drugs are classified according to their principal site of action including the bacterial cell wall, bacterial cell membrane, protein synthesis, and intermediary metabolism.
  - **Cell Wall**: good target because mammalian cells don't have a cell wall or peptidoglycan.
    - Drugs in this group are useful and good for safety and efficacy.
    - Disadvantage: **very allergenic**, a lot of hypersensitivity to these drug groups. Also, tend to disturb normal flora causing numerous side effects.
  - **Cell Membrane:** similar in mammalian and bacterial cells leads to high toxicity.
    - Gram-negative bacteria have additional outside membranes anchored to peptidoglycans that contain lipopolysaccharides. Certain drugs can selectively interfere with the outer membrane, disburse it, and then destroy the inner cytoplasmic membrane.
    - Disadvantage: **very cytotoxic,** must apply topically. No systemic applications.
  - **Protein Synthesis:** while processes are similar in mammalian and bacterial cells, but different ribosomal subunits (70s-bacteria, 80s-mammalian) allow for selectivity.
  - **DNA synthesis:** to selectively inhibit DNA synthesis, drugs can either inhibit the folic acid synthetic pathway (specific to bacteria) or directly inhibit DNA gyrase.
    - The dihydrofolate reductase enzyme is different in mammalian and bacterial cells allowing for selectivity.
    - DNA gyrase allows bacterial DNA to uncoil and supercoil to fit the large genome in the small cell. Uncoiling is necessitated for DNA synthesis, thus inhibition of this enzyme inhibits bacterial replication.

Eyelid Infections	**Antibacterial Drug**	**Administration**
Blepharitis (Staphylococcal, Angular, Seborrheic)	Bacitracin or Erythromycin	Topical
Acne Rosacea	Doxycycline or Erythromycin	Oral
Meibomianitis	Doxycycline or Tetracycline	Oral
External Hordeolum	Bacitracin or Erythromycin	Topical
Internal Hordeolum (nonresolving)	Dicloxacillin or Cephalexin	Oral
Conjunctivitis	**Antibacterial Drug**	**Administration**
Acute mucopurulent	Gentamicin, Tobramycin, Trimethoprim/Polymyxin B, Ciprofloxacin, Norfloxacin, Ofloxacin, Levofloxacin	Topical
Gonoccal	Ceftriaxone	Parenteral
Chlamydial (adult)	Doxycycline or Azithromycin	Oral
Dacryocystitis	**Antibacterial Drug**	**Administration**
Acute	Amoxicillin/clavulanate, Cefaclor, Cefuroxime, Cefazolin, Erythromycin	Oral Parenteral
Neonatal	Trimethoprim/Polymyxin B	Topical

Cellulitis	Antibacterial Drug	Administration
Mild Preseptal	Amoxicillin/clavulanate, Dicloxallin, Cephalexin, Cefaclor	Oral
Moderate to Severe Preseptal	Ceftriaxone and Vancomycin, or Cefuroxime and Ampicillin/sulbactam	Parenteral
Orbital	Nafcillin and Ceftazidime or Ampicillin/sulbactam	Parenteral
Keratitis	**Antibacterial Drug**	**Administration**
Local	Ciprofloxacin or Ofloxacin	Topical
Expansive	Fortified cefazolin and Gentamicin or Tobramycin	Topical
Other Ocular Infections	**Antibacterial Drug**	**Administration**
Endophthalmitis	Vancomycin and amikacin or Vancomycin and Ceftazidime	Intravitreal
	Vancomycin and Amikacin or Vancymycin and Ceftazidime	Topical
Neurosyphilis	Penicillin G or Procaine penicillin and Probenecid	Parenteral

3. Ocular B-Lactams (Cephalosprins & Penicillins)

- **B-lactams** are chemical structure rings characteristic of cephalosporins and penicillins that conveys the activity of the drugs.
- **Mechanism of Action:** irreversibly inhibits **transpeptidase enzyme** in cell wall, inhibiting the cross linking of peptidoglycan weakening the cell wall. The cytoplasm is highly concentrated with solutes (strong osmotic pressure into the cell), with decreased structural integrity, the cell autolysis due to osmotic pressure. Some drugs can stimulate **autolysins** which further blocks crosslinking and stimulates cell wall breakdown.
  - Activity: **Bactericidal**
    - **Penicillins** mostly effective against **gram-positive bacteria**
    - **Cephalosporins** and **cephamycins** are effective against both **gram-positive microorganisms** as well as **penicillin-resistant staphylococci**
      - Not effective against *Enterobacter, Pseudomonas aeruginosa, Serratia*, and some *Proteus*
- **Resistance Factors:** Limited due to B-lactamase expression and Penicillin-binding proteins (PBPs)
  - **B-lactamase** is a bacterial produced enzyme that can destroy penicillin and cephalosporins. It is one of the main causes of increasing drug resistance as it is encoded on chromosomes (stably expressed) and plasmids (transferable). The presence of this enzyme allows for drug-resistant strains of B-lactamase bacteria (*Bacillus, Pseudomonas*, etc).
  - **B-lactamase inhibitors**- not necessarily anti-microbial, but prevents resistance of bacterial strain to the co-administered antibiotic. Examples: **Clavulonic acid, Silvactin**
    - **Augmentin**= amoxicillin + clavulonic acid = effective antibiotic for B-lactamase expressing strains.
    - Disadvantage: expands antimicrobial activity and can increase normal flora death.
    - **Methicillin** – a penicillin derivative that is designed so that B-lactamase cant destroy it.
  - **Penicillin-Binding Proteins** are proteins on the bacterial cell wall that binds the penicillin drug. By altering PBPs, bacteria are expanding their resistance by making it harder for drugs to bind to them.
- **Therapeutic Use**
  - Topical use limited to blepharitis and conjunctivitis due to poor ocular penetration.
  - Many administered orally.
  - Preseptal or orbital cellulitis (soft tissue infections) cannot be cured with topical drug use; they necessitate oral administration for systemic circulation absorption.
    - The infectious bacteria is often a B-lactamase producing *S. aureus*, soothe first choice tends to dicloxacillin/cloxacillin
- **Adverse Effects**
  - Hypersensitivity – VERY allergenic, can produce any type of hypersensitivity reaction (1-4). Can lead to hemolytic anemia.
  - Cross-sensitivity between penicillins and cephalosporins is 20%.

- Interfere with GI tract normal flora leading to antibiotic associated diarrhea (oral administration).

Penicillins	Special Characteristics	Ocular Use
Penicillin G	Injection Only. Widespread resistance Effective against *Neisseria* and *Streptococcus*	Keratitis
Amoxicillin	Broader spectrum than penicillin, little resistance, high clinical use	
Carbenicillin	Not the 1st choice. Effective against *P. aeruginosa*	Keratitis
Dicolaxillin	Oral. Particularly effective against B-lactamase producing staphylococci	Preseptal Cellulitis Internal hordeolum
Augmentin (Amoxycillin +Clavulonic Acid)	Oral. Particularly effective against B-lactamase producing staphylococci	Preseptal Cellulitis Orbital cellulitis Dacrocystitis

Cephalosporins	Special Characteristics	Ocular Use
Cefazolin	1st generation, good against gram-positive, including B-lactamase producing *S. aureus* Solubility allows fortified preparations→ good for topical use for acute corneal infections	Corneal ulcers
Cefaclor	Oral. 2nd generation. Not usually a 1st choice drug. Commonly used in upper respiratory infections	Preseptal Cellulitis Internal Hordeolum
Ceftazidime	Injection. 3rd generation. Not stable in stomach. Can penetrate BBB, so good for CNS infections. Broad spectrum, often used in hospitals for drug resistant strains	Endophthalmitis
Ceftriaxone	Injection. Effective against *neisseria gonorrhoeae* and penicillin resistant *S. pneumonia* and *H. influenza*	Ophthalmia neonatorum Keratoconjunctivitis Keratitis

4. Bacitracin

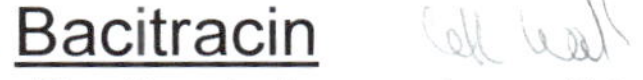

- Bacitracin is a polypeptide mixture from *Bacillus subtilis.*
- **Mechanism of Action:** inhibits bacterial cell wall formation by interfering with the transfer of peptidoglycan polymer units to growing cell walls.
  - Activity: **Bactericidal**
    - Primarily effective against **gram-positive organisms** including B-lactamase producing Staphylococci .
    - Not effective against gram-negative organisms due to impermeability of the outer membrane of gram-negative bacteria to these drugs.
  - Spectrum: relatively narrow.
  - Availability: commercially only available as an **ointment** due to instability in solution and in combination with other antimicrobial drugs.
- **Therapeutic Use**
  - **Blepharitis**
  - Combination drugs reduces the chance of resistance occurring in bacteria.
- **Adverse effects**
  - Currently restricted to topical dermatologic and ocular application because of serious **nephrotoxic effects associated with its parenteral administration**.

5. Vancomycin

- Vancomycin is a glycopeptide antibiotic.
- **Mechanism of Action:** inhibits cell wall synthesis by preventing the incorporation of N-acetylmuramic acid (NAM)- and N-acetylglucosamine (NAG)-peptide subunits into the peptidoglycan matrix which

forms the major structural component of Gram-positive cell walls. Thus, it inhibits the peptidoglycan chains themselves from growing. It also damages cell membrane function.

- Activity: **Bactericidal** ONLY against **gram-positive organisms**
- Spectrum: Wide. Can kill B-lactamase *Staphylococcus* and MRSA, and *Enterrococcus* (except Vancomycin-resistant enterrococcus –VRE)
- Availability: Topical and injection. Not active orally.

- **Therapeutic Use**
  - Topically for MRSA-related conjunctivitis and keratitis.
  - Injection for MRSA and *Enterrococcus* related endophthalmitis.
  - Often in combination with aminoglycosides.
  - It has traditionally been reserved as a **drug of "last resort",** used only after treatment with other antibiotics had failed, although the emergence of vancomycin-resistant organisms means that it is increasingly being displaced from this role by linezolid and daptomycin.
- **Adverse Effects**
  - Systemically toxic: fever, chills, rash
  - Neurotoxicity
  - Nephrotoxicity (with aminoglycosides)
  - Ototoxicity

6. Aminoglycosides

- **Mechanism of Action:** Selectively inhibits 30s subunit of ribosomes, inhibiting bacterial protein synthesis.
  - Activity: **Bactericidal** against both **gram-positive** and **gram-negative bacteria**.
    - Primarily used against *P. aeruginosa & S. aureus*
    - Activity is enhanced by cell-wall destructive drugs.
    - Not effective against anaerobic bacteria.
  - Availability: Topical and injection, not orally active. Solutions, ointments, fortified preparations.
    - **Gentamicin/tobramycin** are the ocular aminoglycosides. Come in standard concentrations of 3mg/mL.
- **Therapeutic Uses**
  - Bacterial keratitis
  - Corneal ulcers (standard treatment)
  - Endophthalmitis
- **Adverse Systemic Effects**
  - Nephrotoxicity (5-25%)
  - Ototoxicity (0.5-3%)
  - Blood dyscrasia
  - Pain
  - *Generally occur with systemic use. Systemic absorption with topical use is minimal*
- **Adverse Ocular Effects**
  - Hypersensitivity reactions:
    - Lid pruritus (itch) /edema,
    - Conjunctival erythema, conjunctival paresthesia,
    - Punctuate keratitis
    - Mydriasis
  - Optic neuritis, peripheral neuritis (Streptomycin)

Aminoglycosides	Special Characteristics	Use
Gentamicin	Broad Spectrum of Activity. -It is effective against Streptococcus pneumoniae, *Streptococcus pyogenes, Aerobacter aerogenes, Escherichia coli, Klebsiella pseamoniae, Pseudomonas aeruginosa*, and most strains of Staphylococcus. -It is frequently used **alone or in combination** with other antibiotics in the treatment of serious gram-negative infections.	Ocular Use

	- Its **antibacterial activity is reduced when gentamicin is administered together with chloramphenicol**. Gentamicin is widely used in the topical antibiotic therapy of **conjunctivitis, blepharitis, and keratitis**, and is commercially available in both ointment and solution preparations.	
Tobramycin	**-Safe in children** - Superior activity against *Pseudomonas aeruginosa*. Bacterial resistance can develop, and cross-resistance between tobramycin and the other aminoglycosides has been observed. -For topical ocular use, tobramycin is available as a 0.3% **solution and ointment.**	Ocular Use
Streptomycin	-Bactericidal in high concentrations and bacteriostatic in low concentrations	Tuberculosis
Neomycin	-Broad spectrum of activity and is bactericidal - Neomycin is rarely administered parentally because of severe nephrotoxicity and ototoxicity. Because of its systemic toxicity, neomycin is best reserved for topical administration to the eye -However, there has been an increasing number of hypersensitivity reactions associated with topical use of this drug; approximately **6-8%** of treated patients develop **contact dermatitis of the lids and conjunctiva**. -Neomycin is available in many ointments and solutions, both alone or combined with **bacitracin, gramicidin**, other antibiotics, and with various corticosteroids.	Ocular use

7. Tetracyclines

- **Mechanism of Action:** Inhibits bacterial protein synthesis by blocking the access of aminoacyl transfer RNA to the acceptor site on the messenger RNA 70s ribosome complex.
  - Activity: **Bacteriostatic** broad spectrum.
    - Effective against a wide variety of gram-positive and gram-negative organisms as well as being highly **effective against Chlamydia.**
  - Ocular Preparations: ointment or suspension 10mg/mL.
- **Therapeutic Use**
  - Topical:, prophylaxis of **ophthalmia neonatorum**
  - Oral: **trachoma, injection conjunctivitis**, acne rosacea, **blepharitis, meibomianitis, chalazia**
  - Tetracyclines are the drugs of choice in infections caused by *Francisella tularensis, Pseudomonas pseudomallei, Vibrio cholerae, ribrio fetus, Hemphilus ducreyi, Mycoplasma pseumoniae*, rickettsial infections, and Chlamydia infections.
  - Their absorption is inhibited by food.
- **Adverse Effects**
  - Gastrointestinal irritation, nausea, vomiting, abdominal distress, epigastric burning and distress.
  - Phototoxic reactions are usually manifested as an exaggerated sunburn.
  - Cause teeth discoloration and hypoplasia ofenamel in children < 8 years old.
- **Contraindications**
  - Not for conjunctivitis or keratitis unless pathogen is known to be susceptible.
- **Examples**
  - Tetracycline
  - Oxytetracycline
  - Chlortetracycline
  - Minocycline
  - Doxycycline

8. Macrolides

- **Mechanism of Action:** inhibits bacterial protein synthesis
  - Activity: **Bacteriostatic**, narrow spectrum.
    - Effective against **most gram-positive** cocci, including *Staphylococcus aureus, Streptococcus pyogenes, S. pneumoniae, S. viridans,* and many strains of *S. faecalis.* It is also effective against gram-positive bacilli including Clostridiumtetani, Cornyebacterium diptheriae, and Actinomyces israelii.
    - Not active against most aerobic gram-negative bacteria; however, Haemophilus *influenzae, Neisseria meningitidis,* and *N. gonorrhoeae* are sensitive.
- **Therapeutic Uses**
  - Topical administration is highly effective in the treatment of staphylococcal **blepharitis** and most cases of **hordeolum** respond to **oral dosages of erythromycin** Erythromycin is indicated in the treatment of **mild infections** caused by sensitive strains.
  - It is the drug of choice in the treatment of pneumonia caused by the legionnaires bacillus, and is used primarily as an alternative to treat infections in patients who are allergic to penicillin.
  - Erythromycin is an alternate choice to penicillin for the treatment of syphilis, and is used for the treatment of uncomplicated gonorrhea in pregnant women. It is also used in cases of primary pneumonia and chlamydia.
- **Adverse Effects**
  - When administered orally, erythromycin may produce nausea, vomiting, epigastric irritation, and urticaria, but serious adverse effects are rare.

Macrolide Example	Preparation	Ocular Use
Erythromycin	Ointment 5mg/g	Prophylaxis of *ophthalmia neonatorum*
Azithromycin	Oral	Prophylaxis and treatment of inclusion conjunctivitis and trachoma

9. Chloramphenicol

- **Mechanism of Action:** inhibits bacterial protein synthesis
  - Activity: **Bacteriostatic**, broad spectrum. Effective against many strains of both **gram-positive and gram-negative bacteria**, Rickettsiae, Chlamydiae, and Mycoplasma.
  - Resistance to chloramphenicol occurs when bacteria have CAT (chloramphenicol acetyl transferase) which inactivates the drug.
  - Chloramphenicol is used as an **ointment and solution** and is available in combination with polymyxin B, hydrocortisone, or prednisolone.
- **Therapeutic Uses:** not used ocularly or systemically in the United states due to unpredictable and irreversible potential for bone marrow toxicity.
  - Used for conjunctivitis (3rd line) in other regions of the world.
  - Chloramphenicol is the drug of choice in the treatment of **typhoid fever** and other types of **Salmonella** infections. Because of its **ability to penetrate the blood-aqueous barrier**, it is a preferred drug in the initial treatment of **endophthalmitis**.
    - When topically applied, its therapeutic use should be limited to those infections in which the beneficial effects outweigh the potential toxic effects.
- **Adverse Effects**
  - Severe anemia
  - Bone marrow toxicity
  - Nausea, vomiting, diarrhea, anterocolitis, stomatitis, mild fever,
  - Delirium, depression, and confusion

10. Fluoroquinolones

- **Mechanism of Action:** inhibits bacterial DNA gyrase, which is responsible for the uncoiling and supercoiling of bacterial DNA, thus inhibiting DNA replication.
  - Activity: **Bactericidal**, broad spectrum

        - Effective against many **gram-positive** and **gram-negative** bacteria including *P.aeruginosa, S. aureus,* and *H. influenza.*
        - Due to its recent emergence on the market, the resistance is low and efficacy is high.
- **Therapeutic Use**
    - Topical: Bacterial corneal ulcers, severe conjunctivitis
    - Pseudomonas keratitis
- **Adverse Reactions**
    - GI upset, antibiotic associated diarrhea
    - Superinfection
    - Renal excretion
    - Hypersensitivity
- **Drug Interactions**
    - **Theophylline** – elevates levels to toxic, causing cardiac arrhythmias and possibly fatal.
    - **Warfarin** – increased levels enhance anticoagulant action leading patient more prone to bleeding. Can occur with systemic absorption of topical administration of fluoroquinolones.
- **Contraindications**
    - Ciprofloxacin contraindicated in children <18 years old due to the interference in proper joint formation in the knees and hips.
    - Norfloxacin/ofloxacin contraindicated in infants < 1 year.
- **Examples**
    - Ciprofloxacin
    - Norfloxacin
    - Ofloxacin
    - Levofloxacin

11. Trimethoprim

- **Mechanism of Action:** inhibits bacterial dihydrofolate reductase (DHFR) preventing the supply of tetrahydrofolate needed in purine synthesis, thus interfering with the synthesis of DNA.
    - Activity: **Bacteriostatic**, broad spectrum
        - Effective against many **gram-positive** and **gram-negative** bacteria EXCEPT *P.aeruginosa, and Bacteroides fragilis.*
- **Therapeutic Use**
    - Used in combination with polymyxin B (**Polytrim**) in ointment form for **bacterial conjunctivitis.**
    - Used in combination with sulfamethoxazole (**Bactrim**) in oral form for **Toxoplasmosis.**

12. Sulfonamides

- **Mechanism of Action:** Sulfonamide structure is similar to **PABA**, and acts as **competitive antagonists,** inhibiting folic acid synthesis and thus DNA synthesis.
    - Activity: **Bacteriostatic**, broad spectrum
        - Effective against a wide range of activity against many **gram-positive** and **gram-negative** organisms.
    - Preparations: sulfacetamide sodium 10%, 15%, 30% solution or ointment
- **Indications**
    - Not the drugs of choice for major infections because of high resistance and allergic reactions.
        - However for the topical treatment of minor ocular infections, the sulfonamides are valuable agents when used both alone and in combination with corticosteroids for steroid-responsive inflammatory ocular conditions with risk of bacterial infections.
        - Ex: Sulfacetamide sodium 10% + fluoromethalone 0.1% or prednisolone 0.5%
    - Sulfonamides are the drugs of choice for the treatment of acute, non-complicated urinary tract infections due to sensitive bacterial strains. They are also useful in the treatment of diseases cause by *Toxoplasma gondii* and *Plasmodium falciparum* as well as *Chlamydia* (Trachoma).
    - **Conjunctivitis or corneal ulcers**
- **Systemic Adverse Reactions**
    - **Hypoallergenic** – many people are allergic to sulfonamides as a class of drug

- Fever, headache, GI upset, nausea, maculopapular rash, contact dermatitis, anorexia photosensitivity, liver damage, bone marrow suppression, anemia, type III hypersensitivity, **Stevens-Johnson Syndrome exacerbation**

- **Ocular Adverse Reactions**
  - Headache, brow ache
  - Transient myopia (blurred vision)
  - Local irritation: pruritus, edema, burning, stinging
  - Transient epithelial keratitis
  - Conjunctival edema
- **Drug Interactions**
  - **Warfarin** – increases levels enhance anticoagulant action leading patient more prone to bleeding. Can occur with systemic absorption of topical administration of fluoroquinolones
- **Contraindications**
  - Children< 2 months
  - Pregnant or lactating women
- **Examples**
  - Sulfamethoxazole
  - Sulfacetamide sodium
  - Sulfacetamide solution = sulfamethoxazole + sulfacetamide sodium
  - Sulfonamide

13. Polymyxin B

- **Mechanism of Action:** a cationic polypeptide, polymyxin B interferes with bacterial cell and outer membrane function. The polymyxin antibiotics interact with the **phospholipid** component of the cell membrane, thereby disrupting the membrane structure and changing its **permeability** characteristic.
  - Activity: **Bactericidal**, broad spectrum
    - Effective against **gram-negative bacteria**
    - The activity of the polymyxin antibiotics is related to the phospholipid content of the cell membrane, such that **the higher the phospholipids content, the greater the activity.**
    - Resistance is high in *Proteus, Serratia,* and *Neisseria*
- **Therapeutic Use**
  - Mostly used in combination preparations with other drugs
  - **Pseudomonas Keratitis** (gram-negative)
  - Polymyxin B does not penetrate the intact cornea when applied topically. However, **after epithelial damage, the drug achieves effective stromal penetration** when administered topically or by subconjunctival injection.
  - Topical applications of concentrations of **0.25% are well tolerated** by the eye, however concentrations **1.0% can cause ocular irritation**. Polymyxin B is a popular antibiotic for use in treatment of common **bacterial infections of the conjunctiva and lid**.
- **Adverse Reactions**
  - Nephrotoxicity, and neurotoxicity with systemic use.

14. Antiviral Drugs

- Viruses are obligate, intracellular parasites and can infect the cells of humans, animals, plants, and bacteria. They contain a molecule of DNA or RNA as their genome which is encased in a protein shell called a **capsid**.
- Antiviral drugs target:
  - 1. Absorption and Penetration of Virus
    - **Amantadine, Rimantidine**
      - **Mechanism of Action:** interacts with M2 protein on virus coat and inhibits virus uncoating, thus blocking viral replication and release. Effective against *H. influenza* A, rubella.
      - **Therapeutic Uses:** Chemoprophylaxis of influenza A for high risk professionals (health care practitioners).
    - **Gammaglobulins** and moderate to high pH.

- 2. Inhibit Nucleic Acid (DNA/RNA) Synthesis
    - Most are anti-metabolites. Structural analogs of endogenous purine or pyrimidine nucleosides used in DNA or RNA.
    - Require bioactivation by viral and/or host kinase enzymes to active triphosphate form.
    - Often toxic to host cells.
    - Various mechanisms of action:
        - Incorporates into viral DNA producing faulty DNA or early termination of DNA chain elongation.
        - Inhibits viral DNA polymerase.
        - Inhibits the synthesis of nucleoside precursors.
- 3. Inhibit Protein Synthesis and Viral Release
    - **Rifampin:** : topical for vaccinia lesions
    - **Interferons:** herpes zoster, suppression of viremia in hepatitis B, cancer treatment; adverse effects include GI irritation, fatigue, and anemia
    - **Methisazone:** vaccine for small pox (variola) virus

15. Anti-Herpetic (Simplex, Zoster) and Anti-CMV Drugs

- **Idoxuridine**: inhibits nucleic acid synthesis. Can be used topically for herpes simplex keratitis; but, very toxic to the cornea, and more effective drugs are available.
- **Trifluridine**
    - **Mechanism of Action:** Effective inhibitor of thymidine synthetase, thus inhibiting DNA synthesis in both virally infected cells and host cells.
    - **Therapeutic Use**
        - Current drug of choice for topical treatment of primary and recurrent HSV keratitis (1 and 2)
        - Dendritic and geographic corneal ulcers.
        - Thygeson's superficial punctate keratitis
    - **Adverse Effects**
        - Less toxic than idoxuridine
        - Transient burning, stinging
        - Contact dermatitis
        - Corneal punctate keratopathy and edema
        - Conjunctival hyperemia, chemosis, impaired stromal wound healing
        - Keratitis sicca, punctual narrowing
        - Increased IOP
        - Long term use can cause conjunctival scarring and cicatrization
- **Acyclovir**
    - **Mechanism of Action:** A purine analogue to guanine that is specific for virus-infected cells of HSV-1, HSV-2, and VZV. It is preferentially bioactivated to triphosphate form by using virus encodes enzyme, **thymodine kinase**. As an analogue it causes DNA chain termination
    - **Therapeutic Use**
        - Not available as a topical ointment in the US
        - Orally FDA approved for Herpes Zoster Ophthalmicus (VZV)
        - Orally off-label (not FDA approved) for HSV epithelial keratitis
    - **Adverse Effects**
        - Very safe drug
        - Nausea, vomiting, diarrhea, abdominal pain
        - Skin rash, photosensitivity, headaches, dizziness, hallucinations, lethargy, confusion, seizures coma
        - Side effects more frequently in patients with renal impairment
        - Cautious dosing in elderly and immunocompromised
- **Valacyclovir, Famciclovir**
    - **Mechanism of Action:** Prodrug of acyclovir that is hydrolyzed in the GI tract and liver by esterases.
    - **Therapeutic Use**
        - Better bioavailability than acyclovir

- HSV keratitis
- Adverse Effects
  - Same as acyclovir

- **Ganciclovir** Zirgan
  - **Mechanism of Action:** inhibits CMV DNA polymerase and incorporates into viral DNA results in termination of DNA chain elongation.
  - **Therapeutic Use**
    - Very toxic to host cells, limits use
    - Prevents/treats sight or life-threatening CMV infection of AIDS and other immunocompromised individuals
    - CMV retinitis, pneumonia, GI lesions (IV injections, intraocular inserts, oral)
    - Viral suppressive agent
  - **Adverse Effects**
    - Bone Marrow Depression
    - Renal Dysfunction
    - Seizures
    - Carcinogenic
- **Foscarnet** Foscavir
  - **Mechanism of Action:** phosphonoformate antiviral. Active without phosphorylation. Inhibits viral DNA polymerase at doses that do not affect host DNA polymerase and also inhibits reverse transcriptase (HIV)
  - **Therapeutic Use**
    - CMV retinitis in AIDS
    - Suppressive therapy only
    - Continual treatment
  - **Adverse Effects**
    - Renal Damage
    - Seizures
- **Cidofovir**
  - **Mechanism of Action:** nucleoside analogue that inhibits DNA synthesis
  - **Therapeutic Use**
    - CMV, herpes virus and other herpes groups (adenovirus, pox virus)
  - **Adverse Effects**
    - Nephrotoxicity
    - Neutropenia
    - Neuropathy
- **Ribavirin** Rebetol
  - **Mechanism of Action:** interferes with guanosine monophosphate formation and nucleic acid synthesis. Effective against DNA and RNA viruses (Influenza, RSV).
  - **Therapeutic Use**
    - Aerosol inhalation for RSV in infants
    - Reduces severity and duration of illness
  - **Adverse Effects**
    - Anemia

16. Anti-Retroviral Drugs

- **HIV** is an RNA retrovirus that infects lymphocytes, macrophages and dendritic cells.
- **HAART** is a treatment strategy that lowers the likelihood of resistance by combining several types of antiretroviral drugs. there are four categories of antiretroviral drugs for HIV therapy.
- **Nucleoside Reverse Transcriptase Inhibitors**
  - Nucleoside analogs converted into nucleotide analogs. Taking nucleotide analog reverse transcriptase inhibitors (NtARTIs or NtRTIs) allows conversion steps to be skipped.
  - **Examples**
    - Nucleotide: Tenofovir, Adefovir

- Nucleoside: Zidovudine, Didanosine, Zalcitabine, Stavudine, Lamivudine, Abacavir, Emtricitabine, Entecavir, Apricitabine

- **Non-nucleoside Reverse Transcriptase Inhibitors**
  - **Examples:** Efavirenz, nevirapine, delavirdine, etravirine, rilpivirine
- **Protease Inhibitors**
  - **Examples:** Saquinavir, ritonavir, adinavir, nelfinavir, amprenavir
- **Fusion Inhibitors**
  - **Examples:** Maraviroc, enfuvirtide

17. AZOL Antifungals

- **Mechanism of Action:** interferes with the biosynthesis of ergosterols, thus interfering with the growth and replication of fungi. **Ergosterols** are cholesterol-like membrane components of fungi.
  - Activity: **Fungistatic,** broad spectrum
  - Preparations: creams, ointments, OTC, capsules, tablets, infections
  - Systemically absorbed
- **Therapeutic Use**
  - Candidiasis
- **Drug Interactions**: Metabolized in liver so can interfere with various drugs
- **Examples**
  - Ketaconzole
  - Fluconazole
  - Itraconazole
  - Miconazole

18. Polyene Antifungals

- **Mechanism of Action:** binds to ergosterol in fungal cell membranes
  - Activity: **Fungicidal,** broad spectrum
  - Preparations: creams, ointments, OTC, capsules, tablets, infections
- **Adverse Effects**
  - From systemic use, drug can follow host cholesterol pathways and cause liver damage
  - Neurotoxicity
  - Nephrotoxocity
  - Cardiotoxicity, hypotension, electrolyte imbalance

Polyene Antifungals	**Special Characteristics**	**Therapeutic Use**
Amphotericin B	Major antifungal drug -VERY Toxic	Treatment of life-threatening fungal infections – Cryptococcus (yeast), candida albicans, aspergillus, coccidioides, infections
Nystatin	Slightly soluble in water, does not cross skin or mucous membranes -VERY Toxic	Oral suspensions are used for infections of the GI tract in infants and the immune compromised
Natamycin	Only topical ophthalmic antifungal available -Limited Toxicity	Fungal blepharitis, conjunctivitis, Keratitis (*Fusarium)* Filamentous fungi and yeasts (candida, cephalosporum, aspergillis)

Other Antifungals

- **Flucytosine:** is a nucleic acid analog that acts by altering the function of fungal RNA into which it has been incorporated.

- Its action is limited to Cryptococcus and Candida albicans. (All classes of antifungals act on Candida.) Flucytosine causes reversible inhibition of bone marrow.
- **Griseofulvin:** is the major systemic drug for **superficial fungal infections. Decreases fungal mitosis** by an unknown mechanism can cause headaches, GI irritation, and neural dysfunction.

ANTI-INFLAMMATORY AGENTS (PHARMACOLOGY)

- **Eicosanoids** are potent bioactive lipid signals that are generated from the essential polyunsaturated fatty acid (w-6 PUFA). Virtually every cell in the body can generate these potent lipid signals.
    - Cell membranes contain phospholipids and polyunsaturated fatty acids (arachidonic acid) that are absolutely essential to normal function.
- Inflammatory pathway:
    - Stimulus to cell activates **phospholipase A2** which cleaves off **arachidonic acid** from the phospholipid membrane.
    - Arachidonic acid is a substrate for numerous enzymes:
        - **Cyclooxygenase** converts arachidonic acid to prostaglandin G2 (PGG2), which then becomes Prostaglandin H2 (PGH2). PGH2 can differentiate into:
            - **Prostacyclin (PGI2)**: causes vasodilation and inhibits platelet aggregation.
            - **Prostaglandin E2, F2, D2 (PGE2, PGF2, PGD2):** causes vasodilation and potentiates edema.
            - **Thromboxane A2 (TXA2):** causes vasoconstriction, promotes platelet aggregation.
        - **Lipoxygenase** converts arachidonic acid to 5-HPETE which convert to various leukotrienes (LT) and other lipid mediators:
            - **LTB4**: causes chemotaxis
            - **LTC4, LTD4, LTE4**: causes vasoconstriction, bronchospasm, and increased permeability
            - **Lipoxin A4 and B4 (LXA4, LXB4)**: causes vasodilation, inhibits neutrophil chemotaxis, and stimulates monocyte adhesion
- NSAIDs and corticosteroids target the eicosanoid process, inhibiting the formation of prostaglandin and leukotriene mediators of inflammation.
    - **Corticosteroids** inhibit phospholipases
    - **NSAIDs** inhibit cyclooxygenase

1. Steroids

- In response to ACTH, the adrenal cortex produces several kinds of steroid molecules known as adrenocorticosteroids. One of these, the glucocorticoids has powerful anti-inflammatory effects. In humans, the major glucocorticoid is cortisol (hydrocortisone). Cortisol is synthesized from cholesterol, metabolized in the liver, and excreted by the kidney. Steroids act by binding to receptors in the cytoplasm of the target cell. The steroid-receptor complex then enters the nucleus, where it regulates the formation of mRNA.
- The commonly used anti-inflammatory steroids (hydrocortisone, cortisone, prednisone, prednisolone, and dexamethasone) act by essentially shutting down the immune response.
- **Mechanisms of Action**
    - Alters transcription and protein synthesis at the level of the nucleus
    - Upregulates anti-inflammatory peptides
    - Represses master regulator of most inflammatory response
    - Blocks transcription of phospholipase At
    - Inhibits expression of COX-II, iNOS, collagenase→ inhibits synthesis of all eicosanoids
    - Inhibits expression of cytokines, chemokines, and growth factors
    - All actions are mediated by **nuclear receptors**
    - These actions lead to physiological anti-inflammatory effects:
        - Inhibition of migration of inflammatory cells (Decreased capillary permeability to neutrophils prevents them from leaving the bloodstream and reaching the site of inflammation
        - Interferes with lymphocyte activation

        - Inhibits fibroblast proliferation and activity (important for wound healing)
        - Decreases collagen and GAG synthesis
        - Vasoconstriction, reduced capillary permeability and proliferation (angiogenesis)
        - Suppresses the production of antibodies (in high doses).
- **Therapeutic Actions**
    - **Very potent** anti-inflammatory and immunosuppressant
    - Inhibits mediator synthesis (cytokines)
    - Decreases healing rates
    - Potency: base-dependence = acetate>alcohol>phosphate
- **Ocular Indications**
    - Inflammation:
        - Uveitis
        - Scleritis
        - Keratitis
        - Neuritis
    - Diabetic macular edema
    - Cystoids macular edema
    - Age-related macular degeneration
    - Infection (herpes, bacterial keratitis → corneal ulcer formation prevention)
    - Allergic conjunctivitis
    - Auto-immune ocular disease:
        - Mooren's ulcer
        - Cicatrical penphigoid
        - Rheumatoid arthritis - scleritis
    - Anti-graph rejection (corneal transplant surgery)

Ophthalmic Corticosteroids			
Drug	**Vehicle**	**Formulation/concentration**	**Indications**
Prednisolone	Acetate Phosphate	Suspension- 0.125, 1% Solution -0.125, 1%	Anterior Segment Inflammation
Dexamethasone **Highest risk for IOP increase*	Alcohol Phosphate	Suspension -0.1% Solution -0.1% Ointment – 0.05%	Ocular Inflammation
Fluorometholone	Alcohol Acetate	Suspension -0.1, 0.25% Suspension – 0.1% Ointment -0.1%	Anterior Segment inflammation Allergies
Rimexolone		Suspension – 1%	Post-op inflammation Anterior Segment Inflammation Allergies
Loteprednol **Lowest risk for IOP increase*	Etabonate	Suspension -0.2, 0.5%	Ocular inflammation Allergies
Medrysone	Alcohol	Suspension- 1%	Superficial Ocular Inflammation
Triamcinolone			Posterior segment inflammation (CME, DME)

- **Systemic Indications**
    - Auto-immune Diseases (Rheumatoid Arthritis, Psoriasis, Lupus erythematosus, Crohn's)
    - Asthma
    - Allergies
    - Infection
    - Gout
    - Inflammatory bowel disease
    - Certain kinds of leukemia and anemia
    - Sarcoidosis

Systemic Corticosteroid Examples
- Dexamethasone
- Hydrocortisone
- Prednisolone
- Triamcinolone
- Fluticasone
- Mometasone
- Bethamethasone
- Budesonide
- Fluocinolone
- Desonide

- Certain skin disorders.

- Steroids are the most frequently used agents for the control of ocular inflammatory disease. They are effective in protecting the delicate tissue of the eye from many deleterious effects of the inflammatory response, in particular, scarring and neovascularization. In general, ocular allergic reactions and uveal tract inflammations respond satisfactorily. Steroids appear to be more effective in acute than in chronic conditions. Degenerative diseases are usually refractory to steroid therapy.
- Steroids are notorious for relieving inflammation while allowing the underlying disease to progress unchecked, so patients receiving them must be carefully monitored.
- Intermittent, rather than daily doses, often give useful therapeutic results with fewer side effects.
- Systemic effects of topically applied steroids are minimal, but they can cause adverse local effects including skin atrophy, erythema, increased IOP, and hypersensitivity.

- **Adverse Ocular Effects:**
  - Posterior subcapsular cataract
  - Elevated IOP/Glaucoma
  - Retardation of Corneal Epithelial Healing
  - Infections
  - Steroid Uveitis
  - Mydriasis
  - Ptosis
  - Transient ocular discomfort
  - Refractive changes, blurred vision
  - Increased corneal thickness
  - Dry eye syndrome

- **Adverse Systemic Effects**
  - Metabolism
    - Osteoporosis, growth retardation
    - Muscle/skin wastage
    - Increased blood glucose/diabetes exacerbation
    - Obesity, acne
  - Immune system (increased susceptibility to infection)
  - Altered Water/salt balance – hypertension, edema, hypokalemia, hypernatremia
  - Adrenal suppression
  - Hirsutism (excessive hair)
  - Depression/psychosis/behavioral disturbances
  - Peptic ulcer

2. Non-Steroids

- **Mechanism of Action:** Non-steroidal anti-inflammatory drugs (NSAIDs) act by inhibiting the action of cyclooxygenase, the enzyme that converts arachidonic acid into the precursors of prostaglandin and thromboxane. There are three major classes based on different mechanisms of action.
  - **1. Irreversible Inhibition of Cyclooxygenase**: by salicylic acid (aspirin) produces anti-inflammatory, analgesic, and antipyretic effects. GI discomfort and bleeding (due to platelet inactivation) are possible at low doses. Higher doses may result in tinnitus and vertigo. Overdoses can cause hyperventilation, fever, dehydration, coma, respiratory collapse, and renal failure. Some evidence supports the conclusion that aspirin can cause Reye's syndrome in children.
  - **2. Reversible Inhibition of Cyclooxygenase:** Ibuprofen (Motrin, Advil, Nuprin), a simple derivative of phenylproprionic acid, is metabolized in the liver, and may decrease the anti-inflammatory effect of aspirin if the two are used together. Possible adverse effects include GI bleeding and irritation (less than with aspirin), rash, pruritus, tinnitus, dizziness, headache, and anxiety.
  - **3. Slow Acting Anti-inflammatory Agents:** of uncertain mechanism of action are used to control rheumatoid inflammation. These include several anti-malarial drugs (i.e. Hydroxychloroquine) which may interfere with T-lymphocyte function, and gold salts, which appear to alter the function of macrophages.
- **Ophthalmic Therapeutic Uses**
  - Analgesic for inflammatory related pain
  - Prevent intraoperative miosis (often co-administered with mydriatic)
  - Prevent/treat cystoids macular edema

- Control post-operative inflammation and/or pain
- Prevent breakdown/re-establishing blood-aqueous barrier
  - Prostaglandins regulate barrier functions

Ophthalmic NSAIDs		
NSAID	**Concentration**	**Therapeutic Use**
Diclofenac	0.1%	-Intraoperative miosis -Inflammation (post-op) – *off label* -Allergic conjunctivitis – *off label* -Pain/photophobia control
Ketorolac	0.4-0.5%	-Inflammation (post op) – *off label* -Allergies -Chronic CME -Pain control – *off label* **Relative COX-1 Selectivity*
Flurbiprofen	0.03%	-Intraoperative miosis -Inflammation (post-op) – *off label* -Uveitis
Nepafenac	0.1%	-Inflammation (post-operative)- ECCE **Relative COX-2 Selectivity*
Bromfenac	0.09%	-Inflammation (post-operative)- ECCE

- **Systemic Therapeutic Uses**
  - Symptomatic/anti-inflammatory
    - Analgesia (headache, dental, dysmenorrheal)
    - Fever
    - Corns, muscle sprains
    - Auto-immune diseases (rheumatoid arthritis)
    - Gout
    - Post-surgical pain control
    - Ulcerative colitis
    - Colon cancer prophylaxis
    - Cardiovascular protection (aspirin)

Systemic NSAID Examples	
Group	**Examples**
Aspirin and Salicylate derivatives	Methyl/copper salicylate Diflunisal Sulfasalazine
Proprionic acid derivatives	Ibuprofen Naproxen Ketoprofen Flurbiprofen
Fenamates	Diclofenac Meclofenamate
Oxicams	Piroxicam Meloxicam
COX-2 Inhibitors	Celecoxib Meloxicam (less selective)
Pyrazoles	Phenylbutazone

- **Ophthalmic Side Effects**
  - Transient ocular inflammation (stinging, burning, conjunctival hyperemia)
  - Delayed wound healing → corneal melts
    - Macrophages release PGE2, which is an integral part of wound healing and drives angiogenesis

        - Higher incidence with Diclofenac and Bromfenac
    - Allergic hypersensitivity, possible cross-reactions with aspirin (aspirin sensitive asthmatic)
    - Ocular effects (less common)
        - Corneal deposits, keratitis, epithelial breakdown
        - Nystagmus, retinopathy, retinal hemorrhage, optic neuritis
- **Systemic Side Effects**
    - GI distress/bleeding
        - PGE2 regulates proton production, inhibition of PGE2 increases stomach acidity
    - Prolongation of bleeding (inhibits thromboxane)
    - Hypersensitivity
    - Reye's Syndrome (children with viral infections
    - CNS effects
- **Contraindications for NSAIDs**
    - Soft contact lenses (irritation, preservative issues) → Ophthalmic NSAIDs
    - Children (Reye's Syndrome risk)
    - Pregnant women
- **Drug interactions with NSAIDs**
    - Brimonidine, carbachol ← Cholinergic agonist
    - PG analogs
    - Problematic for most drug clearance due to prostaglandins role in kidney function

---

OCULAR (LOCAL) ANESTHETICS

- Neural Transmission Review
    - There is a sodium/potassium gradient in which there is a higher concentration of sodium outside and potassium inside a cell (resting potential) such that the inside of the cell is relatively negative to the outside. When stimulated, calcium binds to the receptor, which changes the membranes' permeability. An influx of sodium ions occurs (depolarization), the membrane loses its increased permeability to sodium and potassium outflow along its concentration gradient (repolarization),and the ion influx/outflow creates an electrical current that is self-propagating down the nerve.
- **Mechanism of Action:**
    - Main action: Block sodium channels. They directly inhibit permeability of the nerve to sodium
    - Some newer drugs block substance P release
    - Prevents depolarization/action potentials in neural tissues.
        - Small nerves more vulnerable
        - Myelinated fibers generally more sensitive for matched fiber sizes
        - Active/recently inactivated fibers more sensitive (activity-dependent)
    - Most anesthetic effects last 10-30 minutes.
- **Ophthalmic Diagnostic Uses**
    - Tonometry
    - Gonioscopy/fundus contact lens biomicroscopy
    - Foreign body removal
    - Modified Schirmer test
    - Improved topical drug absorption (e.g. mydriasis)
- **Ophthalmic Therapeutic Uses**
    - Corneal epithelial debridement
    - Anterior segment (minor conjunctival, cataract, refractive) surgery
    - Enhanced mydriasis
    - Forced duction
    - Electrophysiology
    - Herpes (shingles: Lidoderm)

Common Ophthalmic Local Anesthetics	
Topical use (esters)	**Injection**
Cocaine Proparacaine Benoxinate Tetracaine	Procaine Chloroprocaine Bupivacaine Mepivacaine Lidocaine

- **Ocular Adverse Effects**
    - Mild to severe corneal epithelial desquamation, superficial punctate keratitis

- Slowed corneal healing
- Disrupted tear layer
- Mytotoxicity
- Allergic reactions (ester drugs) – conjunctival edema, hyperemia, edematous lids
- Lacrimation
- Less common but potential side effects also include marked epithelial cell loss, iritis, blepharitis, corneal ulceration, and filamentary keratitis

- **Systemic Adverse Effects**
  - Urticaria
  - Angioneurotic edema
  - Bronchospasm
  - hypotension
- **Drug Interactions**
  - Allergic cross-reactivity
  - PABA derivatives/metabolites and sulfonamides (decreases activity)
  - Interactions with drugs sharing secondary actions:
    - Cocaine and adrenergic agonists (MAOIs, TCAs, methyldopa, phenylephrine)
    - LAs and Beta-blockers with MSA
    - Type I antiarrhythmic drugs
  - Interactions with enzyme inhibitors:
    - Ester drugs
    - Anticholinesterases (physostigmine, echothiophate)

ANTIHISTAMINES

- Antihistamines are useful for the symptomatic relief of Type I allergic reactions as sedatives, anti-emetics, and occasionally as local anesthetics. They are used mainly for seasonal and perennial allergies. **Allergic conjunctivitis** is an immediate response triggered by histamine.
- Histamine and Allergies
  - When an allergen enters the body, the immune system produces specific antibodies to the allergen. When the antibody is of the IgE variety, the potential for mast cell sensitization is established. The IgE antibodies attach to mast cells.
  - Upon re-exposure to the same antigen, the antigen reacts with the IgE antibody on the sensitized mast cell or basophil membranes. This binding results in mast cell degranulation and the release of pharmacologic mediators (Histamine, SRS – slow reacting substance of anaphylaxis, ECF-A – eosinophil chemotactic factor of anaphylaxis, prostaglandins, serotonins, and kinins.
  - **Histamine** can drive the triple response of allergies
    - Capillary dilation (heat and flare)
    - Vasodilation (pre-capillary beds)
    - Venule vasoconstriction
    - Edema/chemosis
    - Pruritis

H1 Receptors	H2 Receptors
Blood vessels	Blood vessels
Bronchi	Heart
GI	GI parietal cells
CNS/nerves	Mast cells
Mucous membranes	CNS

- **Mechanism of Action:** Antihistamines work by reversibly binding to the histamine receptor, and thus preventing histamine-receptor interaction. There are two types of histamine receptors.
  - **H1 Antagonists** inhibit the allergic reactions (reduce itch, pain, capillary dilation, edema) and have a local anesthetic effect (antipruritic effect)
    - 1st **Generation** drugs cause **CNS depression/sedation** because they penetrate the CNS easily. These drugs act on **muscarinic, serotonin, and/or α1 receptors.** These drugs are very lipophilic
    - 2nd **Generation** drugs are less hypophilic and do not penetrate CNS nor have any anti-muscarinic activity. Thus these drugs are more selective and avoid sedation and other side effects.
- **Therapeutic Uses**:

- Ocular Allergies (itchy, watery eyes, congestion, swelling, mucus discharge, papillary hypertrophy
- Allergic Conjunctivitis
- Allergic Rhinitis

Topical Antihistamine Examples		
Generic Name	**Brand Name**	**Adjunct Featuers**
Olopatadine 0.1% 0.2%	Pataday Patanol	Mast cell stabilizer, inhibits TNF-α
Azelastine 0.05%	Optivar	Mast cell stabilizer, inhibits PAF and leukotrienes
Emedastine 0.05%	Emadine	Potent
Epinastine 0.05%	Elastat	Mast cell stabilizer, inhibits ME (α1, α2), Serotonin
Ketotifen 0.025%	Alaway Refresh Zaditor	Mast cell stabilizer, Potent

- **Adverse Effects of 1st Generation Antihistamines**
  - H1-Receptor Mediated
    - Decreased neurotransmission in CNS
    - Increased sedation
    - Decreased cognitive and psychomotor performance
    - Increased appetite
  - Muscarinic Receptor Mediated
    - Increased dry mouth
    - Increased urinary retention
    - Sinus tachycardia
  - α-Adrenergic Receptor Mediated
    - Hypotension
    - Dizziness
    - Reflex tachycardia
  - Serotonin Receptor Mediated
    - Increased appetite
  - Cardiac Ion Channel Mediated
    - Ventricular Arryhythmias

Adverse Effects of 2nd Generation Antihistamines

- H1 Receptor Mediated
  - Decreased neurotransmission in CNS - Headaches
  - Decreased cognitive and psychomotor performance
  - Increased/decreased appetite

Oral Antihistamine Examples		
Generic Name	**Brand Name**	**Adjunct Features**
FIRST GENERATION		
Dimenhydrinate	Dramamine	
Diphenylhydramine	Benadryl	Strongly Sedating
Hydroxyzine	Atarax	
Promethazine	Phenergen	Strongly Sedating
Chlorpheniramine	Chlor-Trimeton	Weakly Sedating
SECOND GENERATION		
Fexofenadine	Allergra	Non-Sedating
Loratadine	Claritin	Non-Sedating
Cetirizine	Zyrtex	Non-Sedating
Desloratadine		Non-Sedating

LUBRICANTS AND TEAR SUBSTITUTES

- Dry eyes could be present in all ages. However, it is more common in the elderly than the young. Dry eyes have variable presentations and symptomatology. Patients often complain of burning, itching, and foreign body sensation. The symptoms are often reported as worsening as the day progresses. Based on the knowledge of the tear film physiology and clinical observations, we can classify dry eye conditions into five groups.

Aqueous Tear Deficiency	Mucin Deficiency	Lipid Abnormality	Impaired Lid Function	Epitheliopathy
Acetylcysteine Artificial Tears Sodium hyaluronate Lacrisert Punctual plug	Artificial Tears Lacrisert	Artificial Tears Ointments	Artificial Tears Ointments	Artificial Tears Ointments Vitamin A

- Ideally the ingredients of artificial tear formulations should fulfill the physiochemical role of a normal tear film. An effective tear substitute should:
  - Lower surface tension of the tear film
  - Aid in the formation of a hydrophilic layer
  - Enhance tear volume
  - Not alter the functions of the lipid layer of the pre-corneal tear film.
- Lubricants currently available include preparations formulated as solutions, ointments, or artificial tear inserts.
- For mild or occasional dry eye symptoms, preserved artificial tears instilled up to four times daily is usually adequate.

Artificial Tear Solutions

- Lubricants formulated as solutions consist of inorganic electrolytes to achieve tonicity and maintain pH, preservatives to prevent bacterial growth, and water soluble polymeric systems.
- **Substituted Cellulose Ethers:**
  - Methylcellulose (MC) and other substituted cellulose ethers such as hydroxyethylcellulose (HEC), hydroxypropylcellulose (HPC), hydroxypropylmethylcellulose (HPMC), and carboxymethylcellulose (CMC) have been used as artificial tear formulations.
  - These cellulose ethers dissolve in water to produce colorless solutions of varying viscosity. They have the proper optical clarity and a refractive index similar to the cornea, and they are nearly inert chemically.
  - They are not only useful for artificial tear preparations, but also useful for moistening contact lenses. More viscous solutions are used for application of gonioscopic and fundus contact lenses to the eye.
- **Polyvinyl Polymers:**
  - Polyvinyl alcohol (PVA) is a suspending agent and an emulsifier. PVA is transparent and colorless in solution. PVA solutions can withstand high temperatures so they can be easily autoclaved or filter sterilized through a millipore filtering system. They enhance ocular contact time of ophthalmic medications and the stability of the pre-corneal tear film.
  - Although PVA is compatible with many commonly used drugs and preservatives, certain agents (such as sodium bicarbonate, sodium borate, and the sulfates of sodium, potassium, and zinc) can thicken or gel solutions containing PVA. Therefore, we should be cautious in the clinical use of PVA solutions and the solutions containing any of these agents to avoid incompatibility.
- **Other Polymeric Systems:**
  - Polyvinylpyrrolidone (povidone, PvP) has less ability to lower the interfacial tension at a water oil interface than cellulose ethers. However, it appears capable of forming hydrophilic coatings

in the form of adsorbed layers. Therefore, it is a benefit for both mucin and aqueous deficient dry eyes.

Trade Name (manufacturer)	Active Ingredient	Preservative
Adsorbotear (Alcon)	HEC, povidone	Thimerisol 0.004%, EDTA 0.1%
Akwa Tears (Akom)	PVA, NaCL	Benzalkonium chloride 0.01%, EDTA
Artificial Tears Solution (Rugby)	PVA 1.4%	Chlorobutanol, EDTA
Hypotears (Iolab)	PVA 1%, PEG-80 dextrose	Benzalkonium chloride, EDTA
Isopto Tears (Alcon)	HPMC	Benzalkonium chloride 0.01%
Lacril (A Uersan)	HPMC, gelatin A	Chlorobutanol 0.5%
Lacrisert (Merck)	HPC (solid)	None
Liquifilm Fotne (Allergan)	PVA 3%	Thimerosal 0.002%, EDTA
Liquifilm Tears (Allergan)	PVA 1.4%	Chlorobutanol 0.5%
Lyteers (Bausch & Lomb)	HEC	Benzalkonium chloride 0.01%, EDTA
Moisture Drops (Bausch & Lomb)	HPMC, dextran 0.1%	Benzalkonium chloride 0.01%, EDTA
Mum Tears (Bausch & Lomb)	HPMC, dearran 40	Benzalkonium chloride 0.01%, EDTA
Murocel (Bausch & Lomb)	MC, propylene glycol	Parcbens
Neo-Tears (Barnes-Hind)	PVA, ttEC, PEG-3UO	Thimerosal 0.04%, EDTA 0.02%
Refresh (Allergan)	PVA 1.4%, povidone 0.6%	None
Tear Gard (Mediech)	HEC, locithin	Sorbic acid, edetate disodium
Tearisol (Lolab)	HPMC	Benzalkonium chloride 0.01%, EDTA
Tears Naturale (Alcon)	HPMC, dextran 70	Benzalkonium chloride 0.01%, EDTA
Tears Naturale II (Alcon)	HPMC, dextran 70	Polyquatemium 0.001%, EDTA
Tears Plus (Allergan)	PVA 1.4%, povidone	Chlorobutanol 0.5%
Tears Renewal (Akom)	HPMC, dextran 70	Benzalkonium chloride 0.01%, EDTA
Ultra Tears (Alcon)	HPMC	Benzalkonium chloride 0.01%
Viv-A-Drop (Vision Pharmaceuticals)	5000 IU Vitamin A, polysorbate 80	None
CMC: carboxymethylcellulose, HEC: hydroxyethylcellulose, HPMC: hydroxypropylmethylcellulose, HPC: hydroxypropylcellulose, MC: methylcellulose, PVA: polyvinyl alcohol, EDTA: ethylenediaminetetraacetic acid.		
* Available only by prescription.		

- Vitamin A Derivatives:
  - Epidermal keratinization and squamous metaplasia of the mucus membranes, including the cornea and conjunctiva, respond to both oral and topical vitamin A therapy. Recent evidence suggests that retinol is secreted by the lacrimal gland and is metabolized in the cornea to retinoic acid. Topical use of both tretinoin and retinol, the alcohol form of vitamin A, has been advocated for treatment of various dry eye disorders. However, the benefits of vitamin A solution in the dry eye remain unknown. Retinol is available over the counter in solution form as Viv-A-Drops.
- Viscoelastic Agents:
  - Sodium Hyaluronate: a polysacchride polymer, is a structural component of vertebrate connective tissue matrices.
  - It has been used with success in intraocular surgical procedures such as cataract extraction, intraocular lens implantation, corneal transplantation, glaucoma filtration, and procedures to repair retinal detachment. It has also been used to treat patients with severe dry eye syndromes, and shows to have beneficial effects including decreased itching and burning, reduced foreign body sensation, and reduction of mucus strands. When used topically on the eye at the 0.1% concentration, it appears to be free of adverse ocular or systemic effects.
  - Chondroitin Sulfate: is 350,000 times as viscous as saline and shows to alleviate symptoms of itching, burning, and foreign body sensation in patients with keratoconjunctivitis sicca. However, its benefits compared with other viscous agents need to be further studied.
- Mucolytic Agents:
  - Acetylcysteine has been clinically useful as a mucolytic agent in acute and chronic bronchopulmonary conditions. It is available as Mucomyst in a 10% or 20% solution. It is not commercially available for ocular use, but it can be prepared by diluting the commercial preparation to 2% to 5% in artificial tear or saline solution. When used on the eye, Mucomyst can dissolve mucus threads and decrease tear viscosity.
- Lipid-containing Formulations:
  - Tear-Gard, one of several lipid containing products, is formulated by incorporating a phospholipid into an aqueous solution of hydroxyethylcellulose (HEC) and inorganic buffers. Although the manufacturer claims that this product replaces all 3 layers of the tear film, no clinical study has been done to support this claim.
- Non-preserved Tear Preparations:
  - For patients with moderate to severe dry eye, where the ocular surface is already compromised, or for patients who are sensitive to preservatives such as benzalkonium chloride and thimerosal, using preservatives is not a good idea. The clinical disadvantages of these formulations are that they are more expensive and easily contaminated by the patients during use. Following are the preservative-free artificial tears that should be prescribed to these patients.
- Similasan Eye Drops #1 is an herbal-based, "homeopathic" product. Homeopathy is the concept of treating diseases with minute amounts of antigenic substances. These two products appear to be popular among clinicians. However, there are no well-controlled clinical studies to guide the use of these products.
- Bland Ointment Formulations:
  - Bland ointment is a non-medicated, semisolid preparation of petrolatum and mineral oil. It melts at the temperature of the ocular tissue and disperses with the tear fluid, but retains longer on the eye than other ophthalmic vehicles. Bedtime instillation of ointments is often helpful in the treatment of exposure to keratopathy secondary to nocturnal lagophthalmos. They should be avoided in eyes with impending corneal perforations because of the possibility of ointment entrapment.
- Artificial Tear Inserts:
  - Artificial tear inserts (Lacrisert, Merck) have been used for the treatment of moderate to severe dry eye syndromes. When placed in the inferior cul de sac, these solid inserts dissolve over a

period of hours while releasing their polymeric contents. They are well accepted by many patients, but some patients complain of blurred vision associated with the intense release of polymer after the first 4 to 6 hours following instillation. Artificial tear can be added to reduce the viscosity and minimize the visual complaints.

- Active ingredients: hydroxypropyl methylcellulose, polyvinyl alcohol, carboxymethylcellulose, glycerin, polycarbophil.

OPHTHALMIC DYES

---

1. Topical Diagnostic Agents

- **Fluorescein sodium**
  - A water-soluble compound that easily dissolves in the aqueous portion of the tears.
  - **Mechanism of Action:** vital dye stains epithelial defects, and is excited by wavelengths of 465-490nm.Repelled by intact corneal and conjunctival epithelium. Attracted to corneal stroma.
  - **Diagnostic Uses**
    - Testing for intact corneal epithelium
    - Aqueous flow rate determination
      - Detection of aqueous leaks (post-surgery, post-trauma)
    - Reverse staining in the area of cornea.
    - Evaluation of Lacrimal duct patency (Jones' test)
    - Labeling/evaluation of tear film (TBUT, applanation tonometry, contact lens fits)
    - Evaluation of Meibomian gland function (Marx line).
  - **Formulations**
    - Solutions (favor pseudomonas growth) – 0.5-2% unpreserved for topical use
    - Sterile impregnated strips
    - Combinations with local anesthetic:
      - **Fluress** – 0.25% with benoxinate. Self-sterilizing.
    - **Fluorexon** – large molecular weight form
      - "limited" penetration of soft contact lenses
      - Stains devitalized tissue
      - Increased vulnerability to bacterial contamination
  - **Contraindications**: Fluorescence is quenched by local anesthetics
  - **Adverse Effects:** "ingested" doses most problematic
    - Mild reaction (1-10%) – nausea, vomiting, headaches, tissue necrosis associated with extravasation
    - Less problem with lower concentration, faster injection
    - Serious reactions possible – anaphylactic shock, myocardial infarction, death
- **Rose-Bengal**
  - **Mechanism of Action**: a photoreactive dye that causes erythrocyte hemolysis, significant anti-viral activity, with intrinsic cytotoxicity. Stains mucus and all "exposed" conjunctival and corneal cells a brilliant purple color. It will not stain stroma or healthy cells.
    - Doesn't stain "covered" breaches in epithelium
    - Not a vital stain
  - **Therapeutic Uses**
    - Dry eye diagnosis
    - Differential diagnosis of dendritic ulcer
  - **Formulations** – 1% unpreserved solutions and sterile impregnated strips
  - **Adverse Effects:** Irritation and discomfort on instillation (more than fluorescein)
- **Lissamine Green**
  - **Mechanism of Action:** Stains dead, degenerating, membrane damaged epithelial cells, mucus, and exposed corneal stroma. It has very weak intrinsic activity and antiviral activity
  - **Therapeutic Uses**
    - Dry eye/squamous cell metaplasia (highlights mucus deficiency)
    - Herpetic keratitis (stains deduced stroma)

        - Superior limbic keratitis
    - **Formulation** – sterile strips
    - **Adverse Effects**: stings on instillation, hypersensitivity reactions rare

2. Oral and Intravenous Agents

- **Fluorescein Sodium**
    - **Mechanism of Action**: Fluorescein solution is injected in the anticubital space (brachial vein); serial fundus photographs taken with cobalt blue filter – retinal vascular circulation followed through various phases.
        - Many disease entities alter the characteristics of the retinal circulation. Retinal vessels normally impermeable to water soluble products.
        - Many diseases alter the permeability of the vessel wall (e.g. diabetes, sickle cell anemia, various leukemias) – leaks show up as hyperfluorescent "hot spots."
        - Devascularized area (arteriosclerotic occlusive disease, diabetes, etc.) are delineated by hypofluorescence. Vascular anomalies are clearly outlined as well as neovascularization and "feeding" vessels or neoplasms.
        - Subtle early changes can be detected by skilled observers – oral fluorescein useful only for endstage phase slow leaks – not useful for dynamic vascular evaluation. Somewhat useful in evaluation of macular edema, but not useful for determination in the etiology of the edema.
    - **Therapeutic Uses**
        - Evaluation of integrity of retinal blood vessels and RPE (fluorescein angiography)
        - Visualization of vitreous for vitrectomy (oral administration)antidote for aniline dye poisoning
    - **Formulations**
        - 20-25% for angiography
        - 5mL of 10%/ 3mL of 25% injected rapidly via IV. Circulation time: 13 sec, persists 20 sec
        - 1g in 200mL, oral use (peak blood concentration in 30 min)
    - **Fluorescein sodium**
        - Intravenous injection
        - Used for fluorescein angiography in detecting i) retinal abnormalities, ii) neovascularization, iii) increased capillary permeabilities (i.e. CME)
- **Rose Bengal**
    - Can be used for laser photothrombosis (Argon laser after IV injection, 8mg/kg)
    - Avoid IV injection if liver disease/dysfunction
- **Indocyanine Green**
    - **Mechanism of Action:** A green water-soluble dye that stains diseased/dead endothelial cells. It has a peak absorption and fluorescence above 800nm.
        - Highly protein bound to α1-lipoproteins allowing for minimal leakage and trapping of ICG in the choroid
        - RPE is transparent to IR wavelengths, so can get through the RPE to the choroid
    - **Therapeutic Uses**
        - Visualizing choroidal vasculature/defects using infrared excitation
        - Aid in retinal surgery – highlight the removal of epiretinal membranes and macular holes
    - **Formulations**: Powder + diluents to a final concentration of 25 mg/mL
    - **Adverse Effects**
        - Dose-dependent retinal/RPE toxicity
        - Mild reactions (nausea, vomiting, sneezing)
    - **Contraindications**
        - Patients with allergies to iodine and shellfish could have a related anaphylactic allergic reaction
        - Uremia and liver disease
        - Pregnant/lactating women
- **Verteprofin (Visudyne)**

- **Mechanism of Action:** Verteprofin is a photosensitizing dye (liposomal formulation), that can be intravenously infused, and binds to lipoprotein receptors and aggregates on certain blood vessels (usually abnormal blood vessels have more lipoprotein receptors). The dye is then non-heat laser activated to produce and release cytotoxic oxygen species that accumulate in regions of abnormal blood vessels. This causes endothelial cell damage, platelet activation, and thrombosis leading to vascular occlusion
- **Therapeutic Uses:** Clinical treatment of choroidal neovascularization
- **Adverse Effects:** Photosensitivity reactions, injection site/back pain

HYPEROSMOTIC AGENTS

- Hyperosmotic agents are topically used to treat corneal edema, especially when it is caused by endothelial damage.
- The endothelium maintains normal corneal hydration levels through active transport of water and electrolytes from and to the aqueous humor. The endothelial layer can fail in this function if the transport system becomes defected or elevated intraocular pressure causes stromal compression.
  - Corneal swelling leads to loss of transparency and subsequent vision loss.

Causes of Corneal Edema	
Endothelial	**Increased IOP**
Birth Trauma Congenital Hereditary Corneal Dystrophy Fuch's Dystrophy Keratoconus and Hydrops Mechanical/Surgical Trauma Inflammation	Acute-Angle Closure Glaucoma Chronic Glaucoma

- **Mechanism of Action**: By increasing the tonicity of the tear film these agents (which are hyperosmolar to the ocular tissue) enhance the rate of movement of fluid from the cornea into the tear film, which is then eliminated through normal tear mechanisms.
- **Therapeutic Uses:** These drugs are most efficacious in minimal to moderate epithelial corneal edema.

Topical Hyperosmotic Agents			
	Sodium Chloride	**Glycerin**	**Glucose**
Formulations	2%, 5% solution 5% ointment	50-100% solutions	30-50% solutions
Time to maximum Reduction in corneal thickness	3-4 hours	1-2 minutes	3-4 hours
Adverse Effects	Mild discomfort on instillation	Painful upon application to the eye	Transient discomfort

- **Hyperosmotic Agents**
  - **Sodium Chloride** – has limited effectivity in traumatized corneal epithelium.
  - **Glycerin** – necessitates prior instillation of topical anesthetic due to pain upon administration, limiting its therapeutic use. Glycerin is primarily used for diagnostic purposes like the ophthalmoscopic and gonioscopic examination of the eye in acute-angle closure glaucoma, bullous keratopathy, and Fuch's endothelial dystrophy.
  - **Glucose** – necessitates preservatives to maintain sterility of the solution.

MAST CELL STABILIZERS

- **Mast Cell** activation is an essential and healthy response. They have important functions in:
  - Cardiovascular disease
  - Tumor biology
  - Host defense
  - Limitation of inflammation
  - Tissue pathology

- Some actions are protective

- **Mechanism of Action**
  - Mast cell stabilizers prevent the release of mediators (like histamine) from mast cells. There is also a possible anti-allergy effect which has proposed mechanisms through inhibition of sensory nerve firing (chloride channels), eosinophil accumulation, and IgE production (lymphocytes).
  - As a group they generally do not have intrinsic antihistamine, vasoconstrictive, or anti-inflammatory reactions.
- **Therapeutic Uses**
  - Usually recommended for prophylaxis because they are slow in onset and take 1 week before an effect is seen.
  - Seasonal allergies (including asthma)
  - Vernal allergic keratitis
  - Keratoconjunctivitis
  - Conjunctivitis
  - GPC (Giant papillary conjunctivitis)
  - More useful in generally allergic patients
  - Helps to reduce/terminate corticosteroid therapy
  - Newer drugs are more potent than cromolyn
- **Adverse Effects**
  - Ocular reactions generally mild
  - Burning and stinging (15% lodoxamide)
  - Less common:
    - Itching, pruritis, hyperemia, tearing/discharge/dry eyes
    - Crystalline deposits (lodoxamide)
    - Styes (cromolyn)
  - Systemic effects from ophthalmic formulations (up to 40%, mostly mild):
    - Nasal congestion, headaches (nedocromil)
    - Flu-like symptoms (pemirolast)
- **Contraindications**
  - Pregnant/lactating women
  - Young children:
    - <2 yo (lodoxamide)
    - <3 yo (nedocromil, pemirolast)
    - <4 yo (cromolyn)
  - Patients sensitized to one/more ingredients
- **Ophthalmic Mast Cell Stabilizers**
  - Cromolyn sodium 4%
  - Lodoxamide tromethamine 0.1%
  - Nedocromicl sodium 2%
    - Also has direct antagonism of histamine and LTB2 and a more rapid onset
  - Pemirolast 0.1%
    - Inhibits eosinophils too (chemotaxis, mediator release)

VASOCONSTRICTORS

- Ocular decongestants or **vasoconstrictors** are α1-adrenergic (sympathomimetic) agonists.
- **Mechanisms of Action**
  - Topical application leads to vasoconstriction of superficial conjunctival vessels as the agonists bind to α1 receptors on the conjunctival vessels. This counter regulates edema and swelling, reducing hyperemia and congestion. They have no effect on deeper episcleral vessels.
- **Therapeutic Uses**
  - Allergic conjunctivitis
  - Decreasing the redness and irritation of mild allergies

- Provide only palliative (symptomatic) therapy because have no effect on conjunctival response to antigen that is causing the allergic reaction .
  - Often combined with antihistamines, corticosteroids, and antimicrobial agents.
  - They are usually used as quick and acute relief in emergencies and as a last resort.
- **Adverse effects**
  - Relatively safe
  - Major ocular effect is transient stinging
  - Mild pupillary dilation
  - Blurred vision
  - Epithelial erosions
  - Rebound conjunctival congestion
  - Slight increase in IOP

Vasoconstrictors
Phenylephrine 0.12%
Imidazole Derivatives
Naphazoline 0.1%, 0.012%, 0.03%
Oxymetazoline 0.025%
Tetrahydrozoline 0.05%

- **Rebound Conjunctival Congestion**
  - Long term use of ocular decongestants can cause rebound congestion, resulting in conjunctivitis medicamentosa. i.e. When the drug use is discontinued, the symptoms often come back worse than before .
  - This occurs most commonly with phenylephrine. The imidazole derivatives are less likely to induce rebound congestion.
  - Body releases norepinephrine and acetylcholine all of the time, if you flood a tissue with adrenergic receptor agonists, the through off the homeostatic balance and the tissue will stop producing enough norepinephrine. Imidazoles are more α-selective, and cause less rebound vasoconstriction.
- **Contraindications**
  - Patients with angle-closure glaucoma or potentially occludable angles
  - Diseased or traumatized corneas (can result in sufficient absorption to cause systemic vasopressor response)
  - Cardiovascular disease
  - Hyperthyroidism
  - Diabetes
  - Children

IMMUNE MODULATORS

- **Immunological Mechanisms**
  - When a foreign antigen invades a tissue, it causes an acute response. Physical injury to the eye and damage of the epithelium releases pro-inflammatory cytokines, which upregulate vascular endothelial adhesion molecules causing the movement of immune cells from the blood vessels to the damaged/invaded tissue.
  - At the end of the acute response, antigen-presenting cells like macrophages infiltrate the inflamed tissue and engulf the foreign antigen, processing it into peptides. These peptides are presented on outer cell membrane MHC Class II molecules.
  - Lymphocytic T cells recognize and interact with the antigen bound MHC class II molecule, causing T cell activation, forming memory T cells and Helper T cells.
    - The differentiation of helper T cells into Th1 and Th2 cells is dependent upon the cytokine expression at the site of injury.
      - Th1 cells produce interferon (IFN)-γ and TNF-α
      - Th2 cells produce interleukin (IL)-4, IL-5, and IL-13
- **Dry Eye** disease or Keratoconjunctivitis Sicca is a disease of ocular surface inflammation that is mediated by CD4+ T-cell activation and Th1 differentiation.
  - Dry eye results from an unstable tear film or tear evaporation which results in physical damage to the ocular surface, causing an acute response.
  - In susceptible individuals, a chronic response will develop if the antigen causing the acute response is not eliminated and inflammatory cytokines remain at the site of injury.

- **Immunomodulators** are drugs that weaken or modify the inflammatory system which decreases the inflammatory response. More specifically they work by modifying the specific immune sensitization of lymphoid cells. There are four types of immunomodulators effective for ocular inflammation:
    1. **Alkylating Agents**: interfere with DNA replication and transcription which leads to a depression of T- and/or B-cell populations. Examples: **Cyclophosphamide, chlorambucil**
    2. **Antimetabolites**: selectively compete for intermediary metabolites that are critical to immune cell function causing a cytotoxic effect. Examples: **Methotrexate** inhibits folic acid, **Azathioprine** and **Mycophenolate mofetil** interfere with purine metabolism
    3. **Antibiotics**: Inhibit T-cell proliferation and block production of inflammatory mediators. Examples: **Cyclosporine, Tacrolimus**
    4. **Biologic agents**:
        - **Interferon-α** managed the refractory disease-associated uveitis in Behcet's disease.
        - **Infliximab** may be beneficial to unresponsive uveitis my being a monoclonal antibody directed against TNF-α.
        - **Etanercept** binds to extracellular TNF-α, truncating the autoimmune cascade and is approved by the FDA to treat rheumatoid arthritis, JLA, psoriasis and psoriatic arthritis.
- Ophthalmic diseases that may necessitate immunosuppressants/immunomodulators:
    - Cicatricial pemphigoid
    - Sjogren's syndrome
    - Behcet's disease
    - Mooren's and other sterile corneal ulcers
    - Ocular manifestations of rheumatoid arthritis (scleritis, keratitis, dry eye, retinopathy)
    - Corneal grafts
    - Severe atopic/vernal keratoconjunctivitis
    - Uveitis
    - Sympathetic ophthalmia
- **Cyclosporine A**
    - Derived from a soil fungus *Tolypocladium inflatum*
    - **Mechanism of Action:** binds to cyclophilin and inhibits its action. Cyclophilin normally inhibits and regulates calcineuron, a phosphatase that removes phosphate from the transcription factor NFAT (nuclear factor of activated T cells). NFAT is inactivated when phosphate-bound, and is unable to bind to the promoter region for IL2. Thus, cyclosporine indirectly inhibits the synthesis of interleukin 2 (IL2) by T helper cells.
    - **Therapeutic Uses**
        - Immune-mediated conjunctival diseases
        - Keratoconjunctivitis Sicca
        - Chronic tear film dysfunction
        - Transplant patients (oral administration)
        - Behcet's disease
        - Bird-shot retinochoroiditis
        - Uveitis
    - **Topical Adverse Effects**
        - Burning/stinging
        - Hyperemia
        - Itch
    - **Systemic Adverse Effects**
        - Renal dysfunction
        - Hypertension
        - High serum creatine

MYDRIATICS AND CYCLOPLEGICS

- **Adrenergic Innervation of the Eye**
    - Sympathetic innervations from the posterior and lateral nuclei of the hypothalamus descend the lateral aspects of the brainstem into the intermediolateral columns in the cervical cord.

Myelinated preganglionic neurons emerge from the thoracic section and synapse onto the superior cervical ganglion. Then unmyelinated postganglionic fibers travel through the cavernous sinus alongside the carotid plexus, and join the ophthalmic division of CN V. These fibers then accompany the long ciliary nerves to the iris dilator and Muller's muscle.
  - Sympathetic nerves reach the ciliary muscles to cause **accommodation** through uveal blood vessels.
- **Cholinergic Innervation of the Eye**
  - Parasympathetic preganglionic fibers from the Edinger-Westphal nucleus travel through the oculomotor nerve (CN III) to synapse in the ciliary ganglion. Postganglionic fibers than enter the globe through the short ciliary nerves and terminate on muscarinic receptors on the iris sphincter muscle and ciliary body.
- Both adrenergic (α, β) and muscarinic (M) receptors on ocular tissues are responsible for pupillary size changes and accommodation.
  - α1-Receptor – Iris Radial Muscle – stimulation causes mydriasis
  - M3-Receptor – Iris Sphincter Muscle – stimulation causes miosis
  - β2-Receptor – Ciliary Muscle – stimulation causes relaxation of accommodation
  - M3-Receptor on Ciliary Muscle – stimulation causes accommodation
- **Mydriatics** are adrenergic (α-1) agonists or antimuscarinics.
- **Cycloplegics** are adrenergic (β-2) agonists or antimuscarinics.

1. Mydriatics (Phenylephrine)

- **Mechanism of Action:** synthetic sympathomimetic amine of epinephrine that acts on α1 receptors causing the contraction of the iris dilator and smooth muscle of the conjunctival arterioles. This leads to pupillary dilation and conjunctival blanching. It also stimulates Muller's muscle and widens the palpebral fissure and may decrease IOP.
- **Therapeutic Uses**
  - Mydriasis- 2.5%, 10% solution
  - Breaking posterior synechiae
  - Peripheral corneal vessel vasoconstriction during LASIK
  - Ptosis resulting from sympathetic denervation (Horner's Syndrome)
  - Diagnostic test for Horner's Syndrome:
    - 1% phenylephrine can markedly dilate the pupil with postganglionic sympathetic denervation but causes minimal or no dilation in the normal eye or in an eye with a lesion that is central or preganglionic.
- **Ocular Adverse Effects**
  - Transient pain
  - Lacrimation
  - Keratitis
  - Allergic dermatoconjunctivitis
  - Pigmented aqueous floaters
  - Rebound miosis
  - Rebound conjunctival congestion
  - Conjunctival hypoxia
- **Systemic Adverse Effects**
  - Systemic hypertension
  - Occipital headache
  - Subarachnoid hemorrhage
  - Ventricular arrhythmia
  - Tachycardia
  - Reflex bradycardia
  - Blanching of skin
- **Contraindications**
  - Use 10% solution with caution in patients with cardiac disease, idiopathic orthostatic hypotension, hypertension, aneurysms, insulin-dependent diabetes, advanced arteriosclerosis
  - Only use 2.5% in infants and elderly

- **Drug Interactions**
    - MAOIs
    - Tricyclic antidepressants
    - Reserpine
    - Guanethiodine
    - Methyldopa
    - Atropine

2. Cycloplegics

- Cycloplegics are cholinergic (muscarinic) antagonists that can be nonspecific (Atropine, Scopolamine) or receptor type selective (Tropicamide – M4).
- They cause both reduced accommodation and mydriasis
- All agents are influenced by iris pigmentation due to depot effects
- **Atropine**
    - Naturally occurring alkaloid isolated from *Atropa belladonna*.
    - **Mechanism of Action**: non-selectively inhibits muscarinic receptors. It is the most potent mydriatic and cycloplegic agent presently available.
    - **Therapeutic Action**:
        - Cycloplegic refraction in young children with suspected latent hyperopia or accommodative esotropia
        - Anterior uveitis – relieves pain by relaxing ciliary muscle spasm. Decreases excessive permeability of inflamed vessels (decreasing cells and flare)
        - Slowing myopia progression
        - Penalization occlusion in amblyopia
    - **Ocular Adverse Effects**
        - Direct irritation
        - Allergic contact dermatitis (eyelid erythema with pruritus and edema)
        - Risk of angle-closure glaucoma/IOP elevation
    - **Systemic Adverse Effects**
        - Depression of salivation and dry mouth
        - Facial flushing
        - Sweat inhabitation
        - Cognitive impairment and delirium in elderly
        - Convulsions (children)
    - **Contraindications**
        - Open-angle/closed-angle glaucoma
        - Children, especially those with Down's syndrome (vasovagal hypersensitivity)
- **Homatropine**
    - 1/10th as potent as atropine. Amount of cycloplegia is less than cyclopentolate but longer in duration
    - **Therapeutic Use**
        - Anterior Uveitis treatment
        - Cycloplegia for patients with darkly pigmented irides
    - Adverse Effects and Contraindications the same as atropine
- **Scopolamine**
    - Found in shrub *hyoscyamus niger* and *Scopalia carniolica*
    - Therapeutic uses
        - Drowsiness/confusion (can penetrate blood-brain barrier)
        - Motion sickness
    - Adverse Effects: CNS toxicity more common
- **Cyclopentolate**
    - **Therapeutic Uses**
        - Cycloplegic agent of choice for routine cycloplegic refractive procedures, especially infants and young children

- Anterior uveitis treatment
  - **Ocular Adverse Effects**
    - Irritation, lacrimation, transient stinging upon initial instillation
    - Conjunctival hyperemia
    - Allergic blepharoconjunctivitis
    - Elevated IOP in patients with glaucoma
  - **Systemic Adverse Effects**
    - More CNS effects than atropine: drowsiness, ataxia, disorientation, incoherent speech, restlessness, visual hallucinations
- **Tropicamide**
  - **Mechanism of Action**: selective M4 receptor antagonist.
  - **Therapeutic Uses**
    - Drug of choice for ophthalmoscopy → fast onset, short duration, and sufficient intensity of action
      - Pupillary dilation with tropicamide is less dependent on iris pigmentation as t is with atropine, homatropine, and cyclopentolate
  - Adverse effects and contraindications similar to cyclopentolate and atropine

	Time to Maximum Dilation (min)	Dilation Recovery (days)	Time to Maximum Cycloplegia (min)	Cycloplegia Duration (days)
Phenylephrine	45-60	0.25	n/a	n/a
Atropine	30-40	7-10	60-180	7-12
Homatropine	40-60	1-3	30-60	1-6
Scopolamine	20-30	3-7	30-60	3-7
Cyclopentolate	20-45	1	20-45	0.25-1
Tropicamide	20-35	0.25	20-45	0.25

MIOTICS

- **Miotics** are cholinergic agonists or parasympathetic antagonists.
  - Direct-acting cholinomimetics activate cholinergic receptors directly at the iris sphincter muscle and ciliary body. Examples: Acetylcholine, Methacholine, Pilocarpine, Carbachol
  - Indirect acting cholinomimetics inhibit cholinesterase, increasing acetylcholine concentrations at the synapse. Examples: Physostigmine, Neostigmine, Edrophonium, Demecarium (Reversible), Echothiophate, Diisopropylfluorophosphate (irreversible)
- **Pilocarpine**
  - Alkaloid of natural plant
  - **Mechanism of Action:** directly agonize cholinergic receptors in the central and peripheral nervous sstems. Ocularly, pilocarpine causes miosis, accommodative spasm, and IOP reduction
    - **IOP** is believed to be decreased by causing ciliary body contraction which widens the scleral spur and trabecular meshwork spaces allowing for increased aqueous outflow
    - This effect is dose and ocular pigmentation dependent
  - **Therapeutic Use**
    - Primary open-angle glaucoma
    - Acute angle-closure glaucoma
    - Secondary glaucomas
  - **Ocular Adverse Effects**
    - Accommodative spasm
    - Miosis
    - Follicular conjunctivitis
    - Pupillary block with secondary angle-closure glaucoma

- Band keratopathy
- Allergic blepharoconjunctivitis
- Retinal detachment
- Conjunctival injection
- Lid myokymia
- Anterior subcapsular cataract
- Iris cyst formation

- **Systemic Adverse Effects**
  - Headache, brow ache
  - Marked salivation
  - Profuse perspiration
  - Nausea
  - Vomiting
  - Bronchospasm
  - Pulmonary edema
  - Systemic hypotension
  - Bradycardia
  - Generalized muscular weakness
  - Increased tone and motility of gastrointestinal tract (abdominal pain, diarrhea)
  - Respiratory paralysis
- **Contraindications**
  - Presence of cataract
  - Patients younger than 40 years of age
  - Neovascular and uveitic glaucoma
  - History of retinal detachment
  - Asthma
  - Phakic eyes
  - Surgical procedures using succinylcholine

NUTRITIONAL SUPPLEMENTS

- **Age-Related Macular Degeneration**
  - ARMD is a disease where the RPE and photoreceptors (rods and blue-light sensitive cones most sensitive to damage) in the macular area atrophy and loss of rods and cones
  - Risk factors include:
    - Family history of macular disease
    - Cigarette smoking
    - Light (UV) exposure
    - Light iris pigmentation
    - Chemical exposure
    - History of cardiovascular disease
    - Hyperopia
  - The etiology is somewhat unknown but there is substantial evidence suggesting free radical damage from sunlight exposure and lipid peroxidation of the photoreceptor membranes
  - Normally there are high concentrations of antioxidants like Vitamin C, Vitamin E, and Carotenoids (lutein and zeaxanthin), especially in the macula.
    - Lutein and zeaxanthin are two major components of macular pigment which decreases the amount of blue wavelength and UV light from reaching the RPE, Bruch's membrane and photoreceptors.
  - Patients with ARMD tend to have lower density of macular pigment. And smoking cigarettes may also contribute to decreased macular pigment density.
  - Supplementation with antioxidants **Vitamin A, Vitamin E, Ginkgo Biloba** and carotenoids **Lutein** and **Zeaxanthin** can increase pigment density and decrease oxidative stress in the retina that leads to ARMD.

- AREDS (Age-Related Disease Study) formulation has been shown to slow the risk of progression of AMD in patients 55 years of age and older who had some macular changes consistent with early age-related maculopathy.
  - Above medium intake of **beta-carotene,** Vitamin C, Vitamin E, and zinc are associated with reduced risk of AMD
  - Zinc deficiency has been found to cause deterioration of the macula.
    - **Zinc** is present normally in high concentrations in ocular tissues, especially the retina and choroid.
      - Interacts with taurine and Vitamin A
      - Modifies photoreceptor plasma membranes
      - Regulates the light-rhodopsin reaction (required to convert retinol to retinal)
      - Modulates synaptic transmission
      - Antioxidant
  - AREDS is a major clinical trial run by the NEI and NIH.
  - AREDS II is evaluating the potential benefits of antioxidants lutein/zeaxanthin and omega-3 acids in delaying progression of vision loss in AMD.

- **Diabetic Retinopathy**
  - High blood glucose leads to glycosylated proteins that generate free radicals which leads to tissue damage and glutathione depletion. These glycosylated proteins can deposit in the blood vessels of the retina and contribute to neovascularization.
  - Decreased blood plasma levels of selenium also lead to increased blood viscosity which contributes to blood vessel blockage, decreased oxygenation of the retina and neovascularization.
  - There are numerous nutrients and botanicals that are used to prevent and treat diabetic retinopathy:
    - Antioxidants (**Vitamin C, Vitamin E, Ginkgo biloba, Acetyl-L-carnitine**) prevent protein glycosylation, free radical scavenging
    - Some botanicals decrease capillary fragility (**Bilberry**)
    - Other agents correct for deficiencies that may lead to retinopathy:
      - **Magnesium**
      - **Pyridoxine (B6)**

- **Retrolental Fibroplasia (Retinopathy of Prematurity)**
  - ROP is characterized by bilateral neovascularization of temporal regions of retina caused by infantile's immature retinal vascular bed exposure to high postnatal incubator oxygen concentrations.
  - Spindle cells (embryonic precursors of inner retinal capillaries) are in the immature retina and are separated by gap junctions. If the gap junctions increase between spindle cells, neovascularization, dilation, and tortuous retinal vessels are triggered.
  - **Vitamin E** has been found to preserve the embryonic state of spindle cells and retard gap junction increases in premature infants younger than 27 weeks. Vitamin E cannot affect frequency of ROP but can significantly reduce its severity and subsequent eye damage.

- **Retinitis Pigmentosa (RP)**
  - RP is a slowly progressive, bilateral degeneration of the retina that can be autosomal-recessive, autosomal-dominant, or X-linked.
  - Retinal rods are affected most prominently leading to a serious deterioration of night vision as early as childhood, and then a progressive vision loss from the periphery to the center.
  - Some proposed etiologies include:
    - Taurine deficiency
      - **Taurine** is released from the retina in response to light exposure in normal vision.
    - **Vitamin A and E** deficiency in RPE and photoreceptors
      - Possible disturbed utilization or Vitamin A or abnormalities in retinal binding protein.
    - Dopamine system impairment

        - Decrease in cGMP phosphodiesterase can lead to accumulation of cGMP in photoreceptor outer segments.
    - Vitamin A and E supplementation may be helpful in slowing the rate of decline in retinal function.

- **Cataract**
    - Cataracts are characterized by electrolyte disturbances which lead to osmotic imbalances and aggregates of insoluble proteins.
    - Normal lens proteins are in reduced forms by glutathione. Deficient glutathione levels contribute to an inadequate antioxidant defense system in cataractous lenses.
    - Some nutrients can increase glutathione levels (**Vitamin E, Vitamin C, Selenium).**
    - Antioxidants may prevent the formation of cataracts especially in patients deficient in these nutrients (**Vitamin A, Lutein, Zeaxanthin**).

- **Glaucoma**
    - In some cases, faulty glycosaminoglycan synthesis or breakdown in the trabecular meshwork has been associated with impeding aqueous outflow and increased IOP.
        - **Vitamin C** can decrease IOP as a potent osmotic agent and stimulates synthesis of hyaluronic acid in trabecular meshwork (glaucoma may be due in part to a hyaluronic acid deficiency).
    - Some patients have deficiencies of specific nutrients, and supplementation may play a role in treatment:
        - **Thiamin (Vitamin B1)** deficiency associated with degeneration of ganglionic cells of the brain and spinal cord, could also cause optic nerve degeneration.
        - **Chromium** Deficiency – implicated in increased IOP.
        - **Vitamin B12** Deficiency – may cause optic atrophy and visual field defects which mimic glaucoma.
    - **Ginkgo biloba** and other antioxidants are also predicted to have a role in increasing circulation to the optic nerve.

- **Dry Eye Disease (Keratoconjunctivitis Sicca)**
    - Disease of ocular surface inflammation characterized by dryness of the conjunctiva and cornea.
    - Prostaglandin E1 is an anti-inflammatory prostanglanin that is composed of linoleic acids (essential fatty acids).
    - Supplementation of **Omega-3 fatty acids** can decrease chronic inflammation and lead to improved symptoms.

- Adverse Effects and Contraindications of Nutritional Supplements
    - Rare
    - Many can interact with over the counter or prescription drugs:
        - Of particular interest are supplements that interfere with clotting mechanisms.
        - Vitamin C, vitamin E and ginkgo biloba is thus contraindicated to use with NSAIDs and warfarin.

Ocular Effects of Vitamin Deficiencies and Overdoses		
Vitamin	**Deficiency**	**Overdose**
A	Nyctalopia Xerophthalmia	Papilledema
E	Ophthalmoplegia	Vitamin K deficiency
B1	Toxic optic neuropathy	
B2	Light sensitivity Keratoconjunctivitis sicca	
B12	Toxic optic neuropathy	Optic nerve Atrophy

Chapter 18 – Glaucoma

ANTERIOR CHAMBER AND ANGLE

1. Gross Anatomy

- The anterior and posterior chambers are divided by the iris-lens diaphragm.
- The **anterior chamber** is bound anteriorly by the posterior surface of the corneal endothelium, posteriorly by the anterior surface of the iris and pupillary portion of the lens capsule, and peripherally by the anterior chamber angle.
    - It continues through the trabecular meshwork and ends posteriorly at the anterior face of the ciliary muscle (ciliary body).
- The shape of the anterior chamber is ellipsoidal, with the posterior surface of the ellipsoid flattened by the iris. It has an average diameter of 11-12mm, an average axial depth of 3-3.7mm and a volume of 0.25mL.
    - It is shallowest at the iridocorneal junction and deepest in the pupillary area.
    - The depth can increase due to aphakia, buphthalmos, myopia, and vitreal degeneration.
    - The depth can decrease due to lens intumescence, closed angle glaucoma, hyperopia, and involutional changes.
- Anterior chamber angle appearance from anterior to posterior:
    - **Schwalbe's line** – the peripheral boundary of the cornea where Descemet's membrane ends, is the point of base of corneal light edge, and appears as a white line or ridge.
    - **Trabecular Meshwork (TM)** – occupies most of the internal scleral sulcus. Is lightly pigmented anteriorly and darker gray/brown pigmented posteriorly. The greater posterior deposition of pigment is due to the higher aqueous flow rate as the posterior TM lies over **Schlemm's Canal.** There are 3 sections of the trabeculum:
        1) **Corneoscleral meshwork:**
            - Consists of flat, fenestrated, sheets of tissue that have filtering holes called "intratrabecular spaces". The larger filtering holes, (6 to 12 microns in diameter), are called the "spaces of Fontana." These holes are largest near the anterior chamber angle and decrease towards the canal of Schlemm.
        2) **Uveal meshwork:**
            - The most internal component of the TM.
            - Derived from the iris and ciliary body.
            - The most anterior extension of the uvea.
            - Muscular extensions from the ciliary body attach to uveal meshwork and open up trabecular spaces, which increases aqueous outflow.
        3) Pectinate fibers or **iris processes:**
            - Extend from the iris root to the uveal meshwork.
            - There are about 100 per eye.
            - They usually insert at the scleral spur region and extend as far forward as the middle of the trabecular meshwork.
    - **Scleral spur** – found at the posterior insertion of the TM. Consists of a projection of circumferential collagen fibers from the inner sclera forming an external rim of scleral tissue that runs around the internal surface of the sclera. It appears as a white/gray band and is a functionally important insertion point for the longitudinal muscle fibers of the ciliary body and corneoscleral chords. This is also where Schlemm's Canal rests.
    - **Schlemm's canal** – a circular venous channel that lies in the outer portion of the internal scleral sulcus within the limbus. It is a juxtacanalicular tissue, with its inner wall lined with endothelium. **Internal collector channels of Sondermann** are internal collecting channels that

increase surface area. The external collector channels are the main route for aqueous humor outflow from Schlemm's canal into the episcleral veins.

- **Ciliary body** – anterior aspect of the ciliary muscle that appears as dark gray, brown, or bluish purple (depending on irides pigment) in the base of the angle.
  1) Angle recess does not completely form until 5 years of age, so the absence of ciliary body in children under 5 years old is not abnormal.

2. Developmental Anatomy

- Understanding the development of the anterior chamber and angle is critical to understanding the etiology of glaucoma that occurs in childhood.
- **Creation of the anatomical space:**
  - During the 5th-6th week of gestation, the lens vesicle separates from the surface ectoderm and develops as an invagination, while simultaneously a mass of undifferentiated mesenchymal progenitor cells (neural crest origin) form the periphery of the lens.
  - During the 6th-8th weeks of gestation the corneal endothelium, stroma, and iris stroma form from anteriorly migrating mesenchymal progenitor cells from the lens.
    - This marks the beginning of the anterior chamber formation. It begins as a slit and progressively widens with a development.
    - The anterior chamber is characterized as a well marked cleft between the corneal endothelium and the mesodermal portion of the iris. Growth of the chamber is believed to be due to the disappearance of the mesothelium and to the growth of the anterior segment.
- **Factors that promote growth of the anterior chamber:**
  - The differentiation and morphogenesis of mesenchymal progenitor cells is dependent upon signaling from the lens.
  - Secreted signaling molecules like **TGF-β** and ***Foxc1*** and ***Pitx2*** gene transcription factors are believed to be critical for anterior segment development.
  - Studies have noted that if the corneal endothelium does not properly form, the anterior chamber will not form to separate the cornea and lens.
- **Creation of the anterior chamber angle:**
  - When the anterior chamber is small, its periphery is occupied by mesodermal tissue lying between the rim of the optic cup and the surface ectoderm.
  - During the 3rd -4th month of gestation the peripheral corneal endothelium joins the anterior surface of the iris forming the anterior chamber angle.
    - Trabecular meshwork begins to develop from mesenchymal cells and increases in size and cellularity over the next two months.
  - By the 5th months, the angle recess lies at Schlemm's canal and it progressively moves posteriorly for a period time (post birth).
  - At birth the iris inserts at the level of the scleral spur and recesses posteriorly to create adult angle recess. As the angle recess deepens, the open spaces of the trabecular meshwork come into contact with the anterior chamber
- **Theories of the formation of the angle:**
  - Atrophy Theory: Mesodermal absorption over time in the periphery of the anterior chamber (mesenchyme fills the angle recess).
    - Failure of the mesodermal tissue to separate and atrophy leads to congenital glaucoma.
  - Cleavage Theory: The separation of two dissimilar layers of mesodermal tissue grow unequally. The cleavage occurs along the line of the inner layer of the TM. The displacement caused by the growth of the ciliary muscle aids this process.
  - Reorganization Theory: Deepening of the angle occurs due to the gradual rearrangement, expansion and dilation of spaces between existing cells
- **Differentiation of Schlemm's canal, scleral spur, trabecular meshwork:**
  - During the latter part of the 3rd month of gestation, the Canal of Schlemm (COS) appears as a small plexus of venous channels within fibers of the corneo-scleral junction. By the 8th month, an outflow path exists connecting the COS with the scleral veins.
    - Sondermann considers the development of COS as depending on the alterations of IOP, which occur as the fetal eye differentiates.

- During the 5th month, a triangular wedge of dense scleral condensation appears immediately behind the COS. It is continuous with the meridional fibers of the ciliary muscle and gradually consolidates to form the scleral spur.
- The ciliary muscle is slow to reach is full development which is not achieved until shortly after birth.
- During the 5th to 6th month the angle deepens and the loose mesodermal tissue lying between the COS and the root of the iris differentiates into a fan-like bundle of widely spaced anastomosing strands which ultimately constitutes the scleral and uveal portion of the trabeculae.

- **Endothelial membrane**
  - During early development the anterior chamber angle has a continuous endothelial lining.
  - During the 3rd trimester, the endothelial membrane progressively disappears from the pupillary membrane, iris, and anterior chamber. The corneal endothelium still covers a part of the trabecular meshwork.
  - Discontinuity of the endothelial membrane covering of the anterior chamber angle increases outflow of the aqueous humor.
  - Studies have found that the retention of primordial-like endothelium on the iris and iridocorneal angle may occur due to developmental arrest in the 3rd trimester, which can lead to anterior segment dysgenesis and congenital glaucoma.
- **Angle pigmentation**
  - Normal infant/child should not have pigment in the angle.
  - Normal adults will have pigment most prominently inferiorly and nasally with the ciliary body and trabecular meshwork more pigmented than Schwalbe's line.
  - Increased angle pigmentation can be normal or due to:
    - Pigment dispersion syndrome
    - Pseudoexfoliation syndrome
    - Diabetes Mellitus
    - Oculodermal melanocytosis
    - Previous trauma, hemorrhage, inflammation

CILIARY BODY

---

1. Gross Anatomy

- The **ciliary body** is divided into two parts:
  - **Pars plicata** (aka Corona ciliaris or ciliary processes) is the **anterior** portion of the ciliary body.
    - Aqueous humor formation takes place specifically in the **ciliary processes** where there is **fenestrated capillaries**, loose connective stromal tissue, and a metabolically active double-layered epithelium.
      - The **non-pigmented epithelium** is the most internal layer and is continuous anteriorly with the pigmented epithelium of the iris and posteriorly with the nervous retina at the ora serrata. Its heavily folded basement membrane on the internal surface creates the corrugated appearance of the pars plicata, maximizing the surface to produce and secrete aqueous humor.
      - The **pigmented epithelium** is external to the non-pigmented epithelium and is continuous anteriorly with the external non-pigmented epithelium of the iris and posteriorly with the RPE at the ora serrata. It tends to thicken with age.
  - **Pars plana** – (aka Orbicularis ciliaris) is the **posterior** portion of the ciliary body that runs from the ora serrata to the ciliary processes. It is smooth.
    - Avascular; sight for intravitreal injections
    - Produces mucopolysaccharides for vitreous humor
- The ciliary body is the most posterior structure of the anterior chamber and its anterior border forms part of the posterior chamber. It is lateral to and connected to the lens by the zonules.
- The **ciliary muscle** has three types of fibers:
  - Longitudinal (Brucke's muscle or Meridional fibers):

        - Origin at the scleral spur; inserts into choroid and moves it anteriorly.
    - Radial (oblique fibers):
        - Origin at the scleral spur; inserts at the ciliary processes and the pars plana; moves pars plana anteriorly.
    - Circular (Sphincter muscle):
        - Origin at scleral spur; inserts into anterior part of ciliary processes; constricts lens aperture
- The ciliary body is **innervated** by the parasympathetic system at muscarinic receptors on the ciliary body that leads to constriction of the ciliary muscle, which pulls forward relieves tension on the lens zonules, allowing the lens to bow forward during accommodation.
    - **Sensory innervation:** Via the ophthalmic division of CN V (Trigeminal). Leaves the eye with the long posterior ciliary nerves.
    - **Motor innervation:**
        - Sympathetic – Superior cervical ganglion
        - Parasympathetic – Oculomotor (III)

2. Developmental Anatomy

- The **ciliary body** originates from **neuroectoderm** of the optic cup (ciliary body epithelium) and the **mesoderm** (ciliary muscle, ciliary processes, ciliary vessels).
- **Development of pars ciliaris retinae (epithelial layers):**
    - During the 3rd month of gestation, the double-layered neuroectodermal optic cup grows to extend in front of the lens. The tip of the optic cup differentiates into the ciliary body pars ciliaris retinae and iris.
    - The eversion of the inner wall of the optic cup at 10 weeks allows for the double-layered epithelium of the ciliary body.
- **Development of the ciliary processes, ciliary muscles, and ciliary vessels:**
    - The outer pigmented layer of the pars ciliaris retinae forms a number of radial fords around the circumference of the cup, precursors to the ciliary processes. As the eye increases in size, the ciliary processes move farther forward, leaving behind the pars plana.
    - During the 4th month of gestation the ciliary muscle forms from the mesoderm. By the 5th month the meridional portion is formed and continuous with the scleral fibers of the scleral spur. By the 6th month the circular fibers appear and continue to develop after birth.
    - At the beginning of the 6th month, the major circle of the anterior choroidal vasculature is complete and passes forward and runs beneath the ciliary folds. Recognizable branches include:
        - Large superficial vessels of the pupillary membrane
        - Small vessels to the iris stroma
        - Recurrent vessels to the ciliary region
- An anterior insertion of the ciliary body and iris root is present late fetal development and should progress posteriorly during angle recess.
    - If there is arrest of angular development, the anterior insertion may overlap the trabecular meshwork, compressing it, preventing proper development and decreasing aqueous outflow.

CORNEA, LENS, IRIS, PUPIL

---

1. Relevant Gross Anatomy of Cornea, Iris, and Lens to Glaucoma

- The **cornea** forms the roof of the anterior chamber. Anatomically it is normally separated from the iris by the aqueous humor in the anterior chamber.
    - During pupillary block glaucoma, the peripheral iris can bow forward and come into contact with the cornea, closing the angle and blocking aqueous flow.
- The **central corneal thickness (CCT)** is an important measurement and risk factor for ocular hypertensive and normotensive glaucoma cases.
    - The OHTS (Ocular Hypertension Treatment Study) found that :
        - Ocular hypertensives with thinner CCT measurement (<555um) were at a higher risk to progress to primary open angle glaucoma and had more severe glaucomatous field loss.

        - Racial differences are present in CCT measurements with African Americans (who are at high risk for glaucoma) having thinner CCTs than Caucasians and Asians.
    - The risk of developing primary open angle glaucoma is inversely linked with CCT
    - Normal tension glaucoma patients tend to have thinner corneas than the normal population.
    - CCT can affect the IOP measurement:
        - Thicker CCTs can cause an overestimated IOP, while thinner CCTs can cause an underestimated IOP.
- The size of the **crystalline lens** increases throughout life, decreasing the anterior chamber depth, predisposing the elderly to primary glaucoma. Shallow anterior chambers further predispose patients specifically to pupillary block glaucoma.
    - Intumescent lenses (mature cataracts) have increased anteroposterior lengths.
    - Ectopia Lentis and loss of zonular support can lead to spherical lens shape and anterior displacement further decreasing the anterior chamber depth.
    - Senile hypermature (Morgagnian) cataracts can cause leakage of lenticular material (proteins, debris) into the anterior chamber which can block the trabecular meshwork, decrease aqueous outflow and increase IOP.
- Normal **iris processes** appear fine, threadlike, and cross from the iris base to the scleral spur or posterior trabecular meshwork. They are most commonly seen in the nasal and inferior quadrants.
    - Abnormal iris processes extend from the iris base and are thicker and wider than normal. They can be seen in **Axenfold-Rieger Syndrome**.
- **Peripheral anterior synechiae:** ccurs in angle closure from pupillary block and plateau iris.

2. Developmental Anatomy of the Iris/Pupil

- **Development of the iris stroma:**
    - The iris stroma is derived from neural crest cells which are mesodermal in origin. During the 4th month, the rim of the optic cup grows forward in front of the lens to form the pupil. The iris stroma is originally continuous with the pupillary membrane.
    - Optic cup neuroectoderm grows centripetally between the mesenchyme that formed the cornea and anterior lens. As it grows it incorporates the pupillary membrane vessels.
- **Development of the pars iridica retinae (epithelial layer):**
    - The ectodermal iris begins development in the 3rd month and can be seen as a small, blunt margin just anterior to the folds of the primitive ciliary processes. It then grows steadily forward over the anterior surface of the lens so that by 8 months it is practically complete and the pupil fully formed.
    - The pars iridica retinas includes the double layer of pigmented epithelium which covers the posterior surface of the adult iris and also includes derivatives of the pigmented epithelium, the sphincter and dilator muscles.
        - The anterior layer of iris epithelium is directly continuous with the outer wall of the optic cup. The posterior layer of the iris is continuous with the wall of the optic cup.
    - Differentiation of the anterior and posterior layers of ectodermal iris continues with the forward growth of the whole margin of optic cup. Columnar cells of anterior layer are pigmented. Those of the posterior layer are not pigmented at this stage.
    - Pigmentation of the posterior layer of the ectodermal iris occurs gradually and extends from the anterior layer around the marginal sinus and backwards along the posterior layer from the pupil border towards the ciliary region.
- **Development of dilator and sphincter muscles:**
    - Smooth muscles of iris (sphincter and dilator) differentiate directly from the neuroectoderm.
    - **Sphincter** appears first, at 4 months gestation:
        - At first, the muscle forms a compact mass of fibers lying in close apposition with the anterior surface of the ectodermal layer. However, at the 6th month capillaries and connective tissue begin to grow into it, dividing it into bundles finally separating it from the parent epithelium except at the pupillary border where the two remain associated.
    - The **dilator** appears at 6th months gestation, but is not fully formed until after birth
        - Fine longitudinal fibrils appear in the anterior layer of the epithelium; while the nuclei and pigment are posteriorly displaced.

        - The contractile muscle thus represents a direct transformation of the cytoplasm of the epithelial cells to from a myoepithelial unit.
- **Pupillary membrane (atrophy):**
    - The mesodermal layer stretches across the opening of the pupil. At an early stage it includes a portion of mesoderm that will eventually be backed by the ectodermal iris as it grows forward and will then form part of the mesodermal iris stroma.
    - **Pupillary atrophy** occurs as its blood supply diminishes and allows communication between the anterior chamber and the posterior chamber by forming the pupil.
        - If atrophy fails, the condition that exists is called **persistent pupillary membrane**.
- **Cilioiridic circulation:**
    - The nasal and temporal long posterior ciliary arteries run forward on either side of the optic nerve, traverse the scleral condensation, and continue between it and the choroid towards the margin of the pupil. Here each divides into 2 terminal branches, which form the **greater Circle of the Iris** in the deeper layer of mesoderm.
    - From this vascular circle two sets of vessels are given off:
        - Superficial branches to the iris, combining with those of the pupillary membrane to supply the vascular arcades.
        - Intermediate branches running deeply into the peripheral portion of the mesoderm to form a network in the deep layer of the iris stroma.
    - These vessels participate with the sphincter via branches invading the muscle itself, carrying with them mesodermal elements so that the muscle is divided into bundles by vascularized connective tissue.
    - At the 7th month, four layers of vessels present in the iris near the papillary margin: (1) arcades of pupillary membrane laying near the pupil margin, (2) radial vessels of the iris stroma, (3) inter-sphinteric and (4) sub-sphinteric recurrent ciliary branches.
    - Normal vessels emerge from the stroma or ciliary body and are large and have a radial or circular orientation.
        - Infants with congenital glaucoma may have vessels on the iris surface because of incomplete regression of the tunica vasculosa lentis.
- **Development of iris pigmentation:**
    - Pigment-bearing melanocytes are not present in the iris stroma until later in development around birth or later.
    - The stromal thickness and degree of pigmentation are determining factors in eye color at birth.
    - Full pigmentation and pattern of the anterior surface are not complete until a few years post-partum.

3. Glaucoma Related Iris Examination

- Pupil margin, iris and lens surface, zonules, ciliary processes:
    - Sphincter tears – can indicate previous trauma
    - Iris atrophy – can indicate a history of acute angle closure glaucoma and herpetic uveitis
    - Extropion uveae with peripheral anterior synechiae – seen in ICE (iridocorneal endothelial syndrome) or NVG (neovascular glaucoma)
    - Pseudoexfoliuative material
    - Pigment (Pigment dispersion syndrome)
- Iris configuration:
    - Plateau iris, pupillary block
- Iris insertion site – Can indicate pathology
- Factors that affect the width of angle recess:
    - Iris insertion site
    - Iris thickness and rigidity
    - Lens thickness (age, medications, blood sugar)
    - Lens position (medication, accommodative state, changes in ciliary body)
    - Pupil size (light, accommodation, medications, sympathetic/parasympathetic tone)

Iris Insertion Site	Indicative Of
Cornea	Iridocorneal Endothelial Syndrome (ICE) Posterior Polymorphous Dystrophy (PPD) Neovascular Glaucoma (NVG) Trauma
Schwalbe's Line	Angle closure
Trabecular Meshwork	Congenital Glaucoma
Anterior Trabecular Meshwork	Angle closure
Posterior Trabecular Meshwork	Angle Closure Trabeculogoniodysgenesis
Scleral Spur	Hyperopia Narrow angle (early creeping angle closure) Plateau iris Trabeculogoniodysgenesis
Ciliary body	Normal, Emmetropia Myopia
Beyond ciliary body band	Angle Recession
Iris Root detached in one region	Iridodialysis
Ciliary muscle detached from scleral spur	Cyclodialysis
Variable insertion site	Peripheral Anterior Synechiae (PAS) Angle Recession

CHOROID

1. Gross Anatomy

- Four choroidal layers:
    - **Bruch's membrane:** Innermost layer of the choroid. Adjacent to the RPE and continuous with the pigmented layer of the ciliary body.
    - **Choriocapillaris:** Consists of capillaries that have large lumen, many fenestrations.
    - **Stroma:** Makes up the bulk of the choroids.
    - **Suprachoroidia:** Lies between the choroid and sclera and merges with the lamina fusca.
- The choroid as a blood supply to outer retina:
    - **Arterial supply:**
        - 2 long posterior ciliary arteries supply the anterior ½ of the choroid.
        - 7 anterior ciliary arteries that are not major suppliers.
        - Many short posterior ciliary arteries that supply the posterior ½ of the choroid make up the circle of Haller-Zinn which supplies part of the optic nerve head.
    - **Venous drainage:**
        - 4 vortex veins are the major drainage route. They come together at the ampulla.
        - Anterior ciliary veins drain the anterior ½ of the choroid via the limbal plexus.
        - Pial veins drain the optic nerve meninges and a small part of posterior choroid.
- Innervation to the choroid:
    - **Autonomic Nervous System:**
        - Sympathetic causes vasoconstriction.
        - Parasympathetic causes vasodilation.
    - **Circulating Hormones:**
        - **EDVFs (Endothelium Derived Vasoactive Factors)** – released by blood vessel endothelium as an integrated response to physical (sheer stress), chemical (oxygen tension), and biological (hormonal) information.
            - **Nitric Oxide (NO)** – basal production level, which is increased by acetylcholine stimulation of endothelial cells.
                - NO diffuses into neighboring cells (pericyte, smooth muscle cells) stimulating guanylate cyclase which leads to increased levels of cGMP which relaxes smooth muscle cells leading to vasodilation.

        - **Endothelin -1 (ET-1)** is the most important vasoconstrictive factor that is secreted into circulating blood and stimulates ET-receptors on smooth muscle cells causing an increase of cytoplasmic Ca2+ leading to smooth muscle constriction.
        - **Prostacyclin (PGI2)**
      - Fenestration of choroidal vasculature allows for diffusion of ET-1 and NO into choroidal vasculature supplied tissues and thus can regulate parts of the optic nerve perfused by the choroid.

2. Choroidal Vasculature and Glaucoma

- The outer layers of the retina and the outer layer of the optic nerve head is nourished by the choriocapillaris with a strong influence from sympathetic nerves (autonomic nervous system) and circulating hormones.
    - The choroidal blood flow lacks the autoregulation seen in retinal blood flow, indicating that when perfusion pressure changes, the choroidal blood vessels do not automatically respond.
- Studies have indicated that low perfusion pressure is a significant risk factor for glaucoma, especially normal-tension glaucoma.
    - **Perfusion pressure** is the pressure gradient that between arterial blood pressure and venous blood pressure that allows the blood to nourish the local tissue.
    - Low perfusion pressure causes a reduced blood flow to the area causing ischemic tissue damage.
    - Due to the tissues the choriocapillaris nourishes, this ischemic tissue damage is localized to the outer layer of the optic nerve head, leading to ONH excavation and progressive visual field deterioration.
    - It is hypothesized that patients with normal-tension glaucoma, have low perfusion pressure (especially at night due to decreased sympathetic tone to choroidal vasculature) that predisposes the optic nerve to ischemic damage as well as mechanical damage from the intraocular pressure.
        - "High" IOP is an individual phenomenon that is relative to the health of the optic nerve.
- **Vascular dysregulation** (not enough blood supplied) can lead to local vasospasm and/or impaired autoregulation, which is essential to maintain stable blood flow in the eye in response to metabolic demand and ocular perfusion pressure changes. The vascular factors diffuse into the eye via the choroidal vasculature.
- **Peripapillary atrophy (PPA)** of the choroid has also been related to glaucomatous progression.

VITREOUS

---

1. Anatomy

- Posterior hyaloid surface of the vitreous overlies the internal limiting membrane of the retina.
- **Unconventional route** of aqueous outflow involves filtration and passage through the vitreous to the retina and optic nerve head.
    - Studies have found changes in the hyaloids membrane, stroma and constitution of the vitreous that leads to diminished filtration in glaucomatous eyes. In patients that are blinded by glaucoma, their vitreous is more distinctly membranous than in healthy eyes.
- Studies have also found increased concentrations of **glutamate** in the vitreous of glaucomatous eyes
    - It is hypothesized that **hypoxic retinal cells** releases glutamate.
    - Glutamate receptors are abundantly found on retinal ganglion cells.
    - An excitatory neurotransmitter, glutamate, can overstimulate ionotropic glutamate receptors which allows for a large influx of Ca2+ which induces cell death process (apoptosis) of ganglion cells during hypoxic/ischemic conditions.

RETINA

1. Anatomy

Retinal Layers (From Outer to Inner)
RPE (Retinal Pigment Epithelium)
Photoreceptor Cell Layer
ELM (External Limiting Membrane)
ONL (Outer Nuclear Layer)
OPL (Outer Plexiform Layer)
INL (Inner Nuclear Layer)
IPL (Inner Plexiform Layer)
GCL (Ganglion Cell Layer)
NFL (Nerve Fiber Layer)
ILM (Internal Limiting Membrane)

- **Retinal Nerve Fiber Layer (NFL)** noticeably thins and decreases in visibility in glaucoma:
  - Innermost layer of the fundus, separated from the vitreous by the Internal Limiting Membrane.
  - Contains retinal ganglion cells imbedded in astrocytes, and processes of Muller cells).
  - Healthy retinal NFL is slightly opaque with radially oriented striations covering small blood vessels:
    - **Arcuate Nerve Fiber Bundles** are supero- or infero-temporal fibers that arch around the macula. They are separated by the **Horizontal Raphe**. Damage to these bundles lead to arcuate visual field loss
    - **Papillomacular bundles** have straight horizontal course from the nerve to the macula
    - **Nasal fibers** proceed radially into the optic disc.
    - Blood vessels appear blurred because they are embedded in NFL→ thinning of NFL (atrophy) causes the vessels to be clearly visible.
    - NFL is more prominent inferiorly → in glaucoma inferior nerve damage causes the superior NFL to appear more prominent.
      - As the NFL approaches the optic disc, the thickness increases. It is thickest in the superior and inferotemporal arcuate regions (300um) and thinnest in the nasal and papillomacular regions (60um).
    - NFL should be symmetrical between the two eyes.
    - Pseudo-NFL defects occur in 10% of the normal population and tend to be wider than pathological NFL defects and do not extend to the optic disc.
  - Ganglion cell fibers from the more peripheral fundus lie deeper in the NFL (closer to the RPE) whereas more proximal ganglion cell fibers course in the superficial NFL (closer to the vitreous).
    - All fibers course to the optic disc, turn posteriorly, forming the neuroretinal rim of the optic nerve head.
    - The superficial nerve fiber bundles reside in the central regions of the optic nerve head while the deeper nerve fiber bundles reside close to the edge of the optic nerve head near the chorioscleral canal.
  - Retinal NFL changes are the first observable sign in glaucoma patients, and precedes visual field defects.
    - **Retinal NFL Pathological Defects** are slit-like/wedge shaped local areas of thinning. The narrowest tip of the wedge is usually superior or inferotemporally at the optic disc margin or in the peripapillary area.
- Retina blood supply
  - The photoreceptor layer gets its blood supply from the choroid via the long and short posterior ciliary arteries.
  - The rest of the retina gets its supply from the central retinal artery, which breaks into 2 main branches within the optic nerve and then doubles again as it enters the eye. These 4 arteries (Superior temporal and nasal, and Inferior nasal and temporal) supply the 4 quadrants.
  - 20% of individuals have cilioretinal arteries from the choroid vessels and supplying the inner retinal layers in a small area between the optic disc and the macula.
  - Retinal blood flow is **autoregulated** which allows the ocular blood flow to adjust to changes in perfusion pressure.

2. Developmental Anatomy

- **Development of the optic cup:** Develops from the forebrain. The sensory area of the optic vesicle pushes in towards the pigmented layer to form the optic cup.

- The outer wall remains as a thick sheet of cells that become the RPE.
- The inner wall (facing the future vitreous chamber) differentiates into several structures:
    - Peripherally, the single cell thick tissue becomes attached to the RPE to form a double epithelial extension of the double walled optic cup.
    - Centrally, it becomes the neural retina.
- The cell membrane of the inner surface of the retina is formed from glial cell processes, and the surface is covered by the inner limiting membrane.

- **Analogies between development of retina and central nervous system:**
    - The retina develops from the CNS, or neural ectoderm.
    - Comparison of membrane barriers in the eye and brain:
        - There is no physical barrier to diffusion of material from the vitreous through the retina into the ocular ventricles. The terminal bars which link photoreceptors and Muller cells at the level of the external limiting membrane lack occluded zones.
    - The morphology of the photoreceptors suggests that they are related to the ciliated epidymal cells that line the brain ventricle.
    - Analogies between surfaces of the optic cup and tissues in the brain:
        - If the invagination of the optic cup had not occurred, the vitreous surface of the retina would have faced the outside of a sphere, and thus would have been homologous to the pial surface of the brain.
    - The outer surface of the retina without invagination would have faced the cavity of a hollow sphere, thus being homologous to the inner or ventricular surface of the brain.
- **Fetal fissure (formation, function, fusion, failure to fuse)**
    - Invagination of the lower surface of the optic stalk and vesicle occur simultaneously creating the fetal fissure or choroidal fissure or embryonic fissure.
    - The hyaloid artery grows into the fetal fissure.
    - Fusion:
        - The fissure fuses from the center towards the brain and rim of the optic cup. It never completely closes, leaving a canal for the hyaloid artery.
        - The cleft, through which the vessels reach the inner surface, progressively heals. These vessels become restricted to a residue of the cleft in the center of the optic nerve head.
        - Eventually the hyaloid artery atrophies to a point from which the retinal arteries have grown. When this process is complete this artery becomes the central artery of the retina.
    - Function: Allows for the shortest passage for the ganglion cell nerve fibers from the optic stalk to the brain.
    - The ganglion cell nerve fibers have anterograde signals to the brain and retrograde flow of neurotrophic factors from the brain.
        - **BDNF (Brain Derived Neurotrophic Factor)** – delivered to the retinal ganglion cells through retrograde axonal transport. Insufficiency of BDNF has been implicated in retinal ganglion cell death in glaucoma.
- **Retinal differentiation:**
    - Retinal development can be divided into three stages:
    - <u>Stage I</u>: Epithelial stage.
        - The retina develops from pseudostratified neuroepithelium.
        - Tall thin cells run the full retinal thickness.
        - The nuclei migrate towards the ventricle (behind the eye); nuclear and cell division occurs at this level.
    - <u>Stage II</u>: Differentiation Stage
        - Some cells stop dividing and differentiate into a wide variety of nerve or glial cells of the mature retina. These cells lose their connections with the retinal surface.
        - The neural retina divides into two zones: the outer primitive zone and the inner marginal zone.
        - The outer primitive zone then divides into an inner and outer neuroblastic layer:
        - The inner neuroblastic layer: Ganglion cells develop from the inner neuroblastic layer. The cells migrate to the inner marginal zone. Each ganglion cell sends out a process which becomes the retinal nerve fiber layer.

    - Amacrine and Muller cells also develop from the inner layer. By the end of the 3rd month the Muller cells extend between the internal and external limiting membrane.
      - The outer neuroblastic layer: Rods and cones that are ciliated are formed from the outer layer. The cilia later disappear. By week 12, cone cells are differentiated; rod cells differentiate later in the 7th month. The sequence of appearance of recognizable synapses does not correspond with the appearance of cell types.
  - Stage III: Growth stage
    - The differentiation of the neural elements of the optic system develops in the opposite direction of the path of the nerve impulses.
  - The retinal ganglion cell axons course towards the optic nerve head in three zones which relate to the **arcuate scotomas**, **nasal steps**, and **respect of the horizontal midline** seen in glaucomatous visual field loss. These bundles include:
    - Papillomacular bundle
    - Nasal radial bundle
    - Arcuate (thick) bundles
  - The first to develop are the ganglion cells, last to develop are the rods and cones.
- **Macular differentiation:**
  - At 5 months the ganglion cell layer thickens into the future macula.
  - At 7 months the macula thins in the region of the fovea.
  - Differentiation of all parts of the retina is rapid in the first three months, yet the future macula lags behind in development.
  - At 8 months the macular development speeds up again, and development is not complete until 3-4 months after birth.
- **Retinal circulation development:**
  - Several small vessels leading from the internal carotid artery develop in the mesoderm around the optic vesicle forming the primitive dorsal ophthalmic artery.
  - Branches of the primitive dorsal ophthalmic artery anastomose along the rim of the optic cup to form the annular vessel.
    - Other branches that develop from the dorsal ophthalmic artery include the temporal long ciliary artery and the anterior ciliary arteries.
    - The long ciliary arteries unite near the annular vessel to form the major arterial circle.
  - Ventral ophthalmic artery:
    - Branches from the internal carotid artery.
    - Anastomoses with the dorsal ophthalmic artery.
    - Part of it develops into the nasal long ciliary artery. The rest of the artery degenerates.
    - When the ventral ophthalmic artery degenerates, the dorsal ophthalmic artery can be considered the definitive ophthalmic artery.
  - Hyaloid system:
    - As the fetal fissure closes, a branch of the primitive dorsal ophthalmic artery is trapped inside of the cup. This branch is the hyaloid artery.
    - The hyaloid artery divides many times, forming a network over the surface of the lens (the tunica vasculosa lentis) and branching throughout the vitreous chamber (3rd month).
  - The **Ophthalmic artery** (internal carotid branch) enters the orbit and becomes the **central retinal artery (CRA)** and 2 **posterior ciliary arteries (PCAs)**

Optic Nerve Portion	Blood Supply
Retinal Nerve Fiber Layer	Central Retinal Artery
Prelamina	Posterior Ciliary Arteries (Circle of Haller Zinn)
Lamina Cribrosa	Posterior Ciliary Arteries (Circle of Haller Zinn)
Retrolamina	Central Retinal Artery Pial Vessels Intraneural Vessels Posterior Ciliary Arteries

    - The CRA enters ventrally on the optic nerve, 5-15mm behind the eye. It supplies the optic nerve head ONLY at the level of the superficial retinal nerve fiber layer. It does not supply blood from the posterior border of the scleral lamina to the retinal nerve fiber layer.
    - The PCAs travel forward with the optic nerve and become 15-20 short posterior ciliary arteries, entering the sclera in a

ring around the optic nerve known as the **Circle of Haller Zinn**, which supplies blood to the scleral lamina, adjacent choroid, pial circulation, and retrolaminar optic nerve.
    - The long PCAs travel in the suprachoroidal space anteriorly on nasal and temporal side to join the anterior ciliary arteries to supply the iris and ciliary body.
    - The short PCAs supply the anterior optic nerve head and peripapillary choroid.
  - The microvasculature in the optic nerve/retina is under **autoregulation** (as is CNS vessels). Autoregulation is the ability of the blood vessels to respond to local stimuli and maintain constant perfusion in response to changing physiological conditions (Retinal metabolic demands, neuronal function variations, IOP fluctuations).
    - It is hypothesized that insufficient blood perfusion to the optic nerve head due to increased IOP is a cause of glaucomatous optic neuropathy.
    - Damage to the endothelium of blood vessels due to ischemia can result in reduced nitric oxide (vasodilating factor) which can reduce the vascular caliber. It has also been noted that endothelin (vasoconstricting factor) increases during hypoxia and stress in ischemic conditions, which can lead to vasospasm seen in primary open angle glaucoma.
- **Post-natal events:**
  - Development of the cones: At birth the cones at the fovea are still immature, having a short, stumpy appearance. Cones are not fully mature for several months after birth.
  - Other developments.
    - In the foveal region, the outer retinal layer thickens.
    - The density of retinal pigment cells increases.

OPTIC NERVE

---

1. Gross Anatomy

- The retinal ganglion axons bend 90° and rearrange to match the topographical organization of the intraorbital portion of the optic nerve at the optic nerve head, which is the major site of axonal damage in glaucoma. The optic nerve head is the exit point for ganglion cells through the scleral canal.
- Surface features:
  - Pigmented crescent is caused by exposed RPE (dark crescent)
  - Scleral crescent is due exposed sclera (whitish)
- **Elschnig's Ring** (scleral rim) forms the boundary of the optic nerve opening.
- The optic nerve are divided into regions based upon their associated with the lamina cribrosa.
- **Prelaminar portion (Choroidal lamina)**: anterior the lamina cribrosa, this section of the nerve is where the unmyelinated ganglion cell axons from the retinal nerve fiber layer segregate into bundles and begin to turn into the optic nerve head. The bundles are separated and supported by **astrocyte processes.**
  - Many central retinal arteries and veins emerge in this area. The small capillaries lose their internal elastic lamina supplying this portion of the nerve with blood.
  - Astrocytes surround the optic nerve and provide protection.
  - The inner limiting membrane of Elschnig is where the glial layer thickens over the optic nerve head. The meniscus of Kuhnt is where Elschnig's fills in the optic cup.
- **Laminar Cribrosa portion (Scleral lamina):** The lamina cribrosa or cribriform plate is a layer of connective tissue sheets that are perforated to allow ganglion cell axons and vascular passage. Astrocyte processes support the axons with intimate contacts within the axonal bundlers.
  - The lamina cribrosa offers a firm attachment of the optic nerve to the back of the eye.
  - Blood vessels have an internal elastic lamina.
  - Capillaries from the Circle of Zinn and choroid vasculature supply the blood.
  - The pores in the lamina cribrosa are larger and fewer and the laminar beams are thinner the superior and inferior poles of the optic nerve, which are the primary areas of glaucomatous optic neuropathy.
    - Blockage of optic nerve anterograde and retrograde transport occurs at the level of the lamina cribrosa preferentially at the superior and inferior poles of the optic disc.

- The composition of the lamina cribrosa governs the physical behavior and affects axonal damage in glaucoma.
    - With age, the number of axons decrease, the size of the pores increase, and the elasticity of the connective tissue decreases due to increased interpore production of collagen in the laminar beams.
    - Disrupted axoplasmic flow can lead to decreased neurotrophic factors that are necessary to preserve retinal ganglion cells. Thus, the block of axonal transport at the lamina cribrosa is a contributory factor to retinal ganglion cell apoptosis.
        - Ischemia, physical compression, increased IOP, and toxins can all affect axonal transport.
- **Retrolaminar portion** (optic nerve proper): the myelination begins at the posterior limit of lamina cribrosa and the blood is supplied by the pial arteries, central retinal and pial system of vessels.
- Central retinal artery and vein:
    - The central artery branches off from the ophthalmic just as it enters the orbit. It travels beneath the optic nerve and then inserts into the optic nerve 12-13 mm behind the eye. It emerges inside the eye in the optic disc.
    - Each optic nerve portion is supplied by distinct arterial supplies.
- Increased IOP in glaucoma can lead to insufficient blood perfusion the optic nerve head. The **perfusion pressure** to the optic nerve head (arterial BP less IOP) is normally counter regulated by autoregulation. But in glaucoma insufficient autoregulation of optic nerve blood flow leads to ischemia and contributes to optic neuropathy and retinal ganglion cell apoptosis.

2. Developmental Anatomy

- **Developmental stages of lower visual pathway** (before lateral geniculate body)
    - **Optic nerve development:** Nerve fibers from the ganglion cell layer grow into the optic stalk, growing towards the brain and forming the optic nerve. Glial cells develop around the hyaloid artery at its entrance into the vitreous. The mass of glial cells is known as **Bergmeister's Papilla**. The optic nerve fibers must pass through the papilla as they come from the ganglion cells to the optic stalk.
    - **Meninges:** the optic nerve is surrounded by a sheath from all three meningeal layers of the brain. Between the layers are spaces continuous with the subdural and subarachnoid space. At the 5th month, the dura, arachnoid and pia can be distinguished from each other.
    - During the 6th month a network of scleral tissue penetrates the optic nerve to form the lamina cribrosa.
    - At birth, there is an excessive number of neurons in the anterior visual pathway that get pruned through apoptosis over time.
- Differences between crossed and uncrossed fibers:
    - **Uncrossed Fibers** from the lateral half of the retina grow into the optic tract on the same (ipsilateral) side.
    - **Crossed Fibers** from the medial half of the retina pass through the optic chiasm into the optic tract on the opposite (contralateral) side.
    - One-third of the optic nerve fibers represent the macula (which is only 10% of retinal space).
    - Macular fibers are split such that temporal fibers stay near the temporal portion of the optic nerve. Nasal macular fibers cross over in the center of the chiasm.
- **Myelination of the visual pathway:**
    - Optic nerve fibers become myelinated late in fetal life and continue to completion 2 years after birth.
    - Many double layers of myelin are wrapped around optic nerve fibers by oligodendroglial cells. **Nodes of Ranvier** form as myelin sheaths grow.
    - Developmental sequence of myelin sheath:
        - The process begins in the chiasm around the 24th week of fetal life.
        - By birth the myelination has reached the lamina cribrosa.
    - The pathway is divided into two parts:

        - Non-myelinated part consisting of bare axons continuous with the nerve fibers of the retina. The loss of the myelinated sheath allows the diameter of the nerve to diminish as it enters the scleral foramen.
        - The layers of the retina usually terminate before the optic nerve is reached. A mass of tissue continuous with the neuroglia of the optic nerve is interposed called the intermediary tissue of Kuhnt.
- **Relationship between development of upper visual pathway and central vision;**
    - A point-to point relationship develops between the origin of the optic nerve fibers in the retina and their termination in the lateral geniculate body.
    - Neurons develop in the lateral geniculate body whose axons form the geniculocalcarine tract.
        - Neurons in the geniculocalcarine tract develop a point-to-point relationship between the LGN and cortex.
        - The geniculocalcarine tract grows into the visual cortex that is located on either side of the calcarine fissure.
- **Physiological cupping:**
    - By the 2nd month of gestation the photoreceptors and the ganglion cells in the central retina have formed. The ganglion cell axons begin to develop and form a growth cone which guides the axon toward the optic stalk. With the help of guidance molecules within the retina, the axons grow down the optic stalk forming the optic nerve.
    - The size of the cup depends on the diameter of the optic stalk. The ganglion cell axons are laid down from the outside in, so the smaller the diameter of the optic stalk the smaller the cup-to-disc ratio will be.
    - It is essential to differentiate between **pathological cupping** and **physiological cupping** in glaucoma. In physiological cupping, large discs often have large cups, which can make this differentiation complicated.
        - Concentrically enlarged cup without focal glaucomatous features (notching, drance hemorrhage, vessel baring, peripapillary atrophy) in a large disc can be physiological or pathological.
        - Caucausians have smaller discs than African Americans.
        - Complete differential is only with time as physiological cupping remains constant with time and pathological cupping will increase in size and/or result in visual field defects.

INTRAOCULAR PRESSURE PHYSIOLOGY

- Elevated IOP is one of the most important risk factors for glaucoma.
    - But, an elevated IOP does not necessarily equate with a diagnosis of glaucoma and a normal IOP does not necessarily exclude the diagnosis of glaucoma.
    - The true diagnosis of glaucoma is based on the examination of optic discs, retinal nerve fiber layer, and visual function.
- Treatments aimed at lowering IOP have shown a slowed progression of glaucoma and reduces the risk of ocular hypertensives converting to glaucoma.

1. Methods of Measurement

- **Goldmann applanation tonometry:**
    - Procedure: Instill anesthetic + fluorescein in the patient's eye. Use bright illumination and the cobalt blue filter on the slit lamp. Making sure the tip is clean, have the patient look straight ahead, and applanate the tonometer tip on the cornea. Move the measuring drum until the two inside edges of the mires align. Record the findings in mmHg.
    - Theory of measurement: Assumes the Imbert-Fick law that the cornea is infinitely thin, round, perfectly elastic, and 500 microns.
- **Electronic indentation tonometry (i.e. Tono-pen):**
    - Procedure: Instill anesthetic in the patient's eyes. Put a tip cover on the end of the Tono-pen and turn on the instrument. Have the patient fixate on a target and applanate the cornea

several times quickly. The reading that shows on the screen will be an average of several measurements.
    - Theory of measurement: Applanation force = IOP. Applanation diameter is 1.5 mm.
- **Non-contact tonometry:**
    - Procedure: Performed non-anesthetized. The patient stares straight ahead while a puff of air flattens the cornea. The machine automatically calculates the IOP.
    - Theory of measurement: Based on the fact that it takes longer for a puff of air to flatten an eye with a higher IOP than a lower IOP. Not considered to be very reliable or reproducible, and commonly overestimates the IOP.
- **Digital tonometry:**
    - Procedure: The patient closes his eyes while the doctor rubs his thumbs over the eyeball.
    - Theory of measurement: To be used only for screening for very high IOPs.

2. Normative Values

- IOP is a function of the aqueous humor production and outflow.
    - F= aqueous humor formation rate (uL/min)
    - C= Facility of outflow (uL/min)
    - P_v= episcleral venous pressure (mmHg)
    - U= rate of outflow via IOP independent channels

$IOP=F/C+P_v-U$

- Average pressure = 15.5 mmHg $\pm$ 6
- Variation:
    - Highest in the morning, lowest in the afternoon with a variation of approximately 4 mmHg. Some normal subjects have a reversed diurnal variation.
    - Major factor causing IOP variation appears to be a variation in the rate of formation of aqueous. Aqueous rate is affected extrinsically by IOP and ciliary muscle contraction and intrinsically by trabecular meshwork cell activity.
    - Glaucomatous patients may have a much higher daily variation (8 - 11 mmHg).

3. Factors Controlling Aqueous Production and Outflow

- **Production:** Aqueous is produced by the **pars plicata** in the **ciliary body**. Specifically, the aqueous humor is formed in the ciliary process epithelium. The rate of aqueous formation is about **2 - 3 ul/min**. The aqueous passes into the posterior chamber through ultrafiltration, active secretion, and diffusion.
- **Aqueous outflow:** The aqueous is produced in the ciliary body, passes into the posterior chamber and flows to the anterior chamber through the pupil. The aqueous than drains from the aqueous chambers by two routes:
    - **Conventional route (canalicular, trabecular meshwork):** Aqueous flows from the trabecular meshwork into Schlemm's canal which drains into the episcleral veins through collector channels in the limbal sclera.
        - The trabecular meshwork drains 1.8 - 2.5 ul/min and is **dependent on IOP** (as IOP increases, aqueous outflow through the trabecular meshwork decreases).
        - The juxtacanalicular meshwork (outermost component) provides the more resistance to outflow. With low IOP, Schlemm's Canal is wide open, but trabecular spaces adjoining the canal are narrow, so resistance to aqueous outflow is decreased. As IOP increases, the inner wall of the canal is bowed outward into the canal, opening the intertrabecular spaces. However, the net effect on resistance to outflow is probably small.
        - Episcleral venous pressure (P_{ev}) : The pressure forcing fluid through the trabecular meshwork is the difference between IOP (P_{IOP}) and the episcleral venous pressure. A change in episcleral venous pressure causes an almost equivalent change in IOP.

$dP_{IOP} = 0.95\ dP_{ev}$
$F = C(P_{IOP} - P_{ev})$

    - **Unconventional route (uveoscleral)**: Aqueous flows through the anterior face of the ciliary body between the ciliary muscle fibers into the supraciliary and suprachoroidal space. It then passes through emissary canals in the ciliary nerves.
        - The uveoscleral outflow drains 0.2 - 0.5 ul/min of aqueous and is **independent of IOP**.

        - Some small quantities of aqueous can also diffuse through the cornea or posteriorly through the retina/optic nerve head.
    - As age increases, aqueous production decreases and the contribution of unconventional outflow to total aqueous humor outflow decreases.

4. Nervous System Regulation of IOP

- **Epinephrine** and **norepinephrine** increase aqueous formation in human eyes.
- Endogenous catecholamines stimulate aqueous flow during the daytime by binding to ocular receptors via sympathetic nerve terminals.
    - The circulation of these catecholamines governs aqueous production regulation to follow a circadian pattern.
- The absence of sympathetic stimuli during night is hypothesized to contribute to the lower IOP noticed in night due to decreased aqueous production.

5. Factors Influencing IOP

- **Corneal thickness:**
    - Decreased central corneal thickness is an independent predictor for development of glaucoma in ocular hypertensives.
    - Thinner corneas have been correlated with visual field loss.
    - Central corneal thickness affects IOP measurement:
        - Thicker corneas (high CCT) overestimate IOP measurement.
        - Thinner corneas (low CCT) underestimate IOP measurement.
- **Diurnal variation:** always note the time of day the IOP measurement was taken.
- **Body position** (applanation tonometry) affects IOP by increasing episcleral venous pressure and choroidal volume.
    - Mean IOP = 15.4 + 2.5 mmHg for sitting positions
    - Mean IOP = 16.5 +2.6 mmHg for reclining positions
- IOP is greatly affected by changes in plasma osmolarity. Water passes easily across the blood aqueous and blood vitreous barriers from the blood into the eye if plasma is hypo osmotic to the ocular fluids or from the vitreous and aqueous into the blood if plasma is hyper osmotic to ocular fluids. The change in volume causes a change in IOP.
- **Blood osmolarity**: Aqueous has a higher concentration of dissolved substances than does blood filtrate. This concentration difference would fall to zero over time due to movement of solute across the blood aqueous barrier. To maintain IOP, work must be done via active transport by the epithelium of the ciliary body and iris. The result is an osmotic flow of water across the blood aqueous barrier.
- **Blood pressure**: A transient rise in BP is followed by a small, transient rise in IOP, usually only about 10% of the rise in BP. This is caused by an increase in the episcleral venous pressure. There is no consistent relationship between chronic hypertension and IOP in the normal eye.
- **Blood pH:** systemic acidosis will lower IOP.

AQUEOUS PHYSIOLOGY

---

1. Functions of Aqueous

- Nutrition for avascular tissues of the eye (posterior cornea, lens, anterior vitreous, trabecular meshwork). Fills anterior and posterior chambers.
    - Supports metabolic functions, provides glucose, oxygen, amino acids, and removes wastes like lactic acid and carbon dioxide.
- Maintains optical properties of the lens:

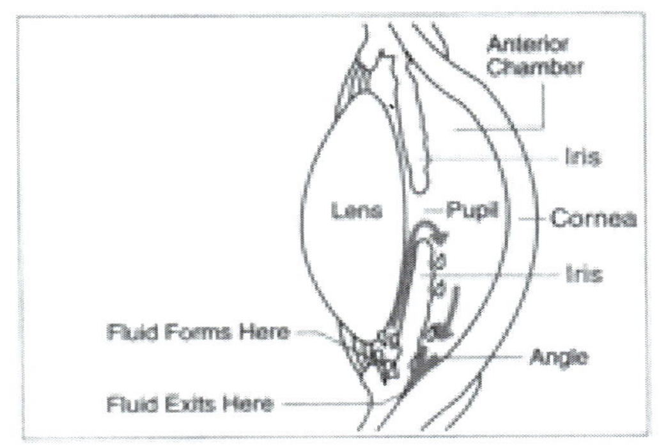

- Index of refraction of aqueous = 1.336. This is slightly lower than that of the cornea, so the corneal-aqueous interface acts as a diverging lens of low power.

- Maintains IOP and preserves the globe in an optical form with the position of the refractive surfaces relative to one another via steady aqueous production and drainage.
- Acts to clear blood, macrophages, and products of inflammation from the anterior segment of the eye.

2. Volume, Osmolarity, Viscosity

- **Volume:**
    - Anterior chamber = 0.25 ml
    - Posterior chamber = 0.06 ml
- **Osmolarity:** slightly hyperosmotic to plasma, about 5 mOsm
- **Viscosity:** 1.025 -1.040 relative to water
- **pH:** 7.6 (pH of plasma = 7.4)

3. Formation

- Both ultra-filtration and active transport contribute to the formation of aqueous. Production rate is approximately 3 ul/min.
- **Ultra-filtration**: Defined as dialysis in the presence of hydrostatic pressure. On the side of membrane containing the protein, a hydrostatic pressure is applied (i.e. blood pressure) and the transfer of salt across the membrane is accelerated.
    - Ultra-filtration is a process in which a finer filter medium is used in comparison to that used in a simple, coarse filtration. Product obtained by ultra-filtration of blood is the plasma without the larger, dissolved proteins.
    - As blood moves through the capillaries, the capillary wall holds back RBC's, plasma proteins, and other blood cells. The plasma, with approximately 10 - 20% of its protein still in solution, fills passages between cells of the epithelium. Some of this plasma enters the ciliary epithelial cells through the epithelial wall membranes. This membrane carries out ultra- filtration by blocking entrance of small to medium sized protein molecules dissolved in the plasma.
- **Active transport:** Accounts for 80-90% of aqueous humor formation, which has a higher concentration of dissolved substances than does blood filtrate. Active transport is done by the non-pigmented epithelium of the ciliary body and iris.
    - The composition of aqueous is different from that produced by just ultra-filtration.
    - Plasma filtrate leaks through space between epithelial cells without any further filtering. The cells take in some of the plasma filtrate, chemically alter it, and return altered material to the filtrate to give a liquid with the composition of aqueous.
    - Solute is transferred or secreted across the blood aqueous barrier as a concentrated solution. Water follows from the concentration gradient established across the barrier.
    - Aqueous formation increases with a drop in plasma osmolarity and decreases with a rise in plasma osmolarity.
    - The primary mechanism for water movement is through Na+ transport with the Na+/K+ ATPase pump, which creates a gradient that allows bicarbonate ions (negatively charged) to follow.

4. Factors Influencing Rate of Flow

- **Neural/neurohumoral mechanism:**
    - Vessels of the ciliary processes have a very dense adrenergic innervation. A vascular receptor could conceivably mediate rate of aqueous formation.
    - Secretory activity of the epithelial cells may be controlled by humoral factor; an adenylate cyclase receptor uses secretory suppression that occurs after administration of adrenergic compounds.
    - Physical characteristics of the membrane barrier separate blood from the aqueous.
- **IOP**: Very high IOP may cause an increase in resistance to outflow through Schlemm's Canal. The outward bulging of the inner wall coming into apposition with the rigid outer wall of the canal may close off access of aqueous to collector channels and aqueous veins.

- **Unconventional outflow (uveoscleral route)**: 20% of outflow may be through outer tunic of eye into the orbit where it is absorbed into the lymphatic system.
  - **Ciliary Muscle Tone**: Contraction of the ciliary muscle stimulated by cholinergic agonists decreases uveoscleral outflow. (Cycloplegics increase outflow through this pathway).
- **ECM**: The extracellular matrix is normally turned over and initiated by the induction of trabecular meshwork metalloproteinases (MMPs). Inhibition of these MMPs can reduce aqueous outflow. Thus ongoing ECM turnover is critical for homeostatic maintenance of normal outflow resistance.

5. Composition

- The concentration of urea and proteins is lower in aqueous than in blood.
- Oxygen and CO_2 are in solution. Oxygen is supplied by blood flow from the ciliary body and iris arterial systems. $C0_2$ is a metabolic product from the cells of the ciliary, iris and lens epithelium, and corneal endothelium. Venous blood flow from the ciliary body and iris carries $C0_2$ away. In the aqueous humor $C0_2$ tension approximates 0_2 tension (50 mmHg).

Component	Plasma	Aqueous
Bicarbonate	27.40	33.60
Lactate	4.30	7.40
Pyruvate	0.22	0.66
Ascorbate	0.02	0.96

6. Blood Aqueous Barriers

- **Location:** A series of variable resistances located between the plasma and the aqueous: Capillary wall, ciliary stroma, basement membrane of the epithelia.
- **Ultrastructure and function:**
  - At the retinal level, tight junctions between the endothelial cells of the retinal capillaries provide a barrier. Tight junctions between the pigment epithelial cells of the retina provide an additional tissue barrier against substances diffusing from the choroid via fenestrated capillaries.
  - 2 types of permeability barriers exist:
    - In the iris vessels, tight junctions between capillary endothelial cells are found which maintain a relatively protein free anterior chamber.
    - The posterior chamber is lined by the inner layer of non-pigmented epithelial cells ringed to each other near their apices with tight junctions. In contrast, ciliary stromal capillaries beneath are fenestrated and large lipid soluble molecules will pass to a moderate degree from fenestrated capillaries into stroma, but are markedly restricted by cells and cell junctions lining the barrier.
  - Barrier to the passage of lipid soluble molecules. Lipid soluble molecules and many ions will pass with relative ease across the blood ocular barrier. If non-ionized compounds have the same lipid solubility the dissociation constant will determine the rate of penetration.
  - Barrier to entry of water. Water penetrates much more rapidly than solutes.
  - Active transport is done by the epithelial cells of the ciliary body and iris. Solute is transferred, or secreted, across the blood aqueous barrier as a concentrated solution.

GLAUCOMA (PATHOLOGY)

---

1 Epidemiology, History, and Symptom Inventory

- Glaucoma is the second leading cause of blindness in the world.
- Epidemiology according to the Beaver Dam Study (a largely Caucasian population):
  - Overall prevalence: 2.1%
  - 0.9% in ages 43 to 54
  - 4.7% over age 75
  - 31.7% of those with glaucoma had IOPs less than 22 mmHg
  - 0.04% had narrow angle glaucoma
  - Prevalence was equal in both males and females
  - According to the Baltimore Eye Study, the prevalence of open angle glaucoma is 4-5 times higher in African Americans than in Caucasian Americans. African American patients also

develop glaucoma 6 to 10 years earlier than Caucasian Americans. African Americans are 3 times more likely to go blind from glaucoma than Caucasians.
    - According to Quigley et al. The prevalence of glaucoma in the Hispanic population is between white Americans and African Americans.
- History:
    - Until late in the last century, glaucoma was considered a blinding disease with no known cause or treatment.
    - The ophthalmoscope was developed by von Helmholtz in 1850, and patients with glaucoma were found to have the characteristic cupped appearance to their optic nerves.
    - The first iridectomy was performed in 1856.
    - It wasn't until the mid-1800s when high IOP was associated with glaucoma, and the first tonometer was developed in 1862.
    - Pilocarpine was the first effective treatment for glaucoma, which doctors began using in the 1870s.
    - In the 1880s, visual field defects were found to be an early sign of glaucoma, and the first perimeter was developed soon afterward.
    - Beta blockers were not used for glaucoma treatment until the 1980s.
    - Xalatan was the first prostaglandin analog, and it came on the market in 1999.
- Symptom inventory:
    - Symptoms for primary open angle glaucoma are rare until the final stages of the disease.
    - Visual acuity can remain 20/20 until right before the patient goes blind.
    - In intermittent angle closure glaucoma, patients can get very severe headaches, see halos around lights, nausea, vomiting, and blurred vision.

2. Pathophysiology

- Pathogenesis:
    - Vascular:
        - Eyes with low perfusion pressure are at higher risk for optic nerve damage.
        - Ischemia/hypoxia to the optic nerve can increase the progression of ganglion nerve cell death.
    - Excitotoxicity:
        - Retinal ganglion cells have neurotoxic reactions to glutamate.
        - Astrocytes are sensitive to mechanical forces and alter their function in response to internal stress. Nitric oxide synthase is upregulated in glaucoma patients and might result in increased levels of neurotoxic nitric oxide.
    - Metabolic:
        - Decreased anterograde and retrograde axoplasmic flow cuts off the ganglion cell's nutritional supply and increases waste build up in the retina. This is believed to enhance the apoptosis of retinal ganglion cells in glaucoma.
    - Mechanical:
        - Elevated IOP causes the plates of the lamina cribrosa to rotate posteriorly, which misaligns the pores and damages the axon bundles running through them either directly (compression) or indirectly (disruption of axoplasmic transport of neurotrophic factors)
        - The regions of greatest damage correspond to the areas of the lamina cribrosa that have the thinnest laminar beams and are thus less resistant to elevated IOP.
    - Genetic
- Glaucoma is a continuum of accelerated retinal ganglion cell death through apoptosis that develops from undetectable disease at the retinal ganglion cell layer to asymptomatic disease, which is detectable by clinicians. With further progression it eventually leads to the functional visial impairment perceived by patients.
- Glaucoma is a **neurodegenerative disease** where excess glutamate becomes toxic to the retina and increases calcium permeability, leading to retinal ganglion cell death.
- Glaucoma is defined by its characteristic optic neuropathy, progressive loss of retinal ganglion cells, topographic optic nerve changes and associated loss of visual function.
- **Risk Factors:**

- IOP elevation:
    - **High IOP** is any IOP (regardless of level) that causes optic neuropathy whereas a normal IOP is one that does not result in glaucomatous optic neuropathy.
    - **Age**: IOP increases with age.
- Family history:
    - Direct relatives most important.
    - Relates to age at diagnosis and severity of disease.
- Ethnicity:
    - African Americans and Hispanics are at higher risk for primary open angle glaucoma.
    - Chinese are at risk for angle closure glaucoma.
    - Japanese are at risk for normal tension glaucoma.
- Corneal thickness:
    - Patients with corneas thinner than 5um are at a 3x greater risk of developing primary open angle glaucoma.
- Large C/D:
    - Pertains to an increased risk for damage due to lamina cribrosa beam strength.
- Myopia (large diameter nerve)
- Systemic health:
    - Disorders that affect the vascular supply to the nerve will predispose the patient to glaucoma.
    - Diabetes
    - Hypertension (decreased perfusion to optic nerve at night time)
    - Hyperviscosity syndromes
    - Hemodynamic crisis (low perfusion pressure)
    - Anemia (less oxygen to the nerve)
    - Vasospastic conditions
    - Cardiac arrhythmias
    - Sleep apnea
- Life style factors
    - Smoking, musical instruments, lifting weights

3. Observation, Investigation and Recognition of Clinical Signs

- The single most important tool in diagnosing glaucoma is observation. Progressive disc cupping and retinal nerve fiber layer defects often precede the onset of glaucomatous visual field loss, so observation is important for diagnosis and detection for early intervention to dampen progression
- Clinical signs of glaucoma:
    - Progressive **neural rim loss:**
        - Nerves that do not follow the ISNT rule (inferior rim should be thickest and temporal rim thinnest). But in glaucoma, rim loss is most prominent in the superior and inferior poles → **vertical cupping.**
        - **Bean pot** appearance of cup is seen in end stage glaucoma where the posterior bowing of the lamina cribrosa and rotation lead to expansion of the cup behind the scleral edge
        - **Vessel bayoneting**: Vessels bend sharply at the disc margin.
    - Deep **focal nothing** of the rim:
        - Acquired optic nerve pit is an extremely deep, localized focal notching that can resemble a congenital pit.
    - **Drance (Disc) hemorrhages** – occur in 40% of glaucoma patients, most common in normal tension glaucoma. They appear as small, flame-shaped (splinter) hemorrhages that lie within the inferotermporal (usually) peripapillary retinal nerve fiber layer and often precede neural rim notching.
    - Nerve fiber layer defects emanating from the optic nerve.
    - **Optic disc asymmetry** between the two eyes normally differs by no more than 0.2, but can be increased due to asymmetric cupping.
    - **Peripapillary atrophy (PPA)**: due to a misalignment of the edges of the retina, RPE, choroid, and sclera.

- **Blood vessel changes**: Vessels may shift due to changes in the neural rim. Collateral disc (shunt) vessels may develop in response to ischemia.
- Signs of pseudoexfoliation: Pseudoexfoliative material on the anterior surface of the lens, pupillary ruff defects, and transillumination defects of the iris.
- Signs of pigmentary dispersion syndrome: Kruckenberg's spindle, pigment on the lens, the iris, or Schwalbe's line.

4. Diagnostic Testing, Techniques and Skills (Applications and Interpretations)

- Anterior Chamber Evaluation:
  - **Gonioscopy:**
    - Function: to visualize and assess the anterior chamber angle to assess if the patient has open-angle or closed-angle glaucoma. The gonioscopy lens allows the clinician to exceed the critical angle of the cornea by altering the corneal air-fluid interface.
    - Technique: must be performed in a dark room to prevent light-induced pupil constriction, which can stretch the iris and open the angle.
    - The direct lens (Koeppe) produces less artifactual distortions in the angle appearance, and the indirect 4 mirror lens is capable of performing indentation gonioscopy.
    - Indicated for glaucoma suspects, grading of angular pigmentation, to determine suitability for pupillary dilation causing acute angle glaucoma.
  - **Indentation gonioscopy**: allows the clinician to distinguish between synechial and appositional angle closure. By pushing onto the central cornea, the aqueous gets displaced to the peripheral anterior chamber and pushes the iris and lens posteriorly.
    - If the angle is closed by apposition, the angle will open on indentation.
    - If the angle is closed by peripheral anterior synechiae or permanent adhesion the angle will remain closed upon indentation.
  - **Anterior angle grading and interpretation:**
    - **Scheie's Grading System** describes the most visible peripheral angle structures from the ciliary body (wide open angle) to no angle structures visible (Grade IV).
    - **Shaffer's Grading System** describes the angle approach and probability of closure based on the angle width in degrees from 35-45° (Grade 4- impossible closure) to 0° (Grade 0- Total angle closure).
    - **Spaeth's Grading System** describes the width of angle recess, peripheral iris configuration (steep, regular, queer), iris root insertion (anterior, behind, in sclera, deep angle recess) and posterior trabecular meshwork pigmentation (graded at 12 o'clock with no pigment (Grade 0) to intense pigment (Grade 4) scaling).
      - Width of angle recess is the angle between the posterior trabecular meshwork and anterior surface of the peripheral iris. Normally the superior and nasal angles are narrower than the inferior and temporal angles.
- Evaluation of IOP:
  - **Tonometry** – IOP >22mmHg warrants additional testing.
  - **Fluorophotometry** – Measures aqueous outflow and trabecular outflow facility.
  - **Tonography** – Measures trabecular outflow facility.
- Evaluation of optic nerve head:
  - **Direct Ophthalmoscopy**
  - **Binocular Indirect Ophthalmoscopy**
  - **Slit Lamp Examination:** Goldman, Zeiss Mirror, 90D, 78D, Hruby lenses
  - Quantitative imaging of the optic disc → **Confocal scanning laser tomography, OCT**
  - **Stereo Photographs:** commonly used to follow glaucoma suspects to better evaluate if there is a change in the optic nerve head over time.
  - Recording:
    - Cup to disc ratio: 10-11% of the population has a C/D of 0.5 or greater. The average C/D is 0.5 horizontal and 0.42 vertical.
    - Vertical C/D is more sensitive in detecting glaucomatous nerve damage.
  - Normal optic nerve head:

        - Neuroretinal rim is thickest Inferior→ Superior → Nasal→ Temporal (ISNT), is intact 360°, and is absent of notching and hemorrhages.
        - The optic disc size is normally symmetrical between the two eyes and proportional to their cups (Large discs: large cups, small discs: small cups).
- Evaluation of retinal nerve fiber layer:
    - **OCT (Optical Coherence Tomography)** assesses the retinal nerve fiber layer thickness by measuring its light reflection properties. It is noninvasive, and noncontact. It can detect diffuse thinning, but has limited potential for localized defects.
        - Common sources of error are tilted nerves, optic nerve head myelination, and nerve heads that are much larger or smaller than average.
    - **Funduscopy**: Retinal nerve fiber layer atrophy makes the fundus appear darker red in white light. Since short wavelength light does not penetrate the nerve fiber layer, the defects can be better seen with red-free filter because in areas where the nerve fiber layer is destroyed, the RPE absorbs light (making areas appear darker).
    - **Wide Angle Red-Free Photographs**: Help in the assessment of retinal nerve fiber layer thickness
    - **Scanning Laser Ophthalmoscopy, HRT** (Heidelberg Retinal Tomograph): Indirectly measures the thickness of the retinal nerve fiber layer at the optic disc margin by assembling multiple tomographic laser scans and compares it to a standard reference plane.
    - **Polarimetry with the Nerve Fiber Analyzer**: A confocal scanning laser ophthalmoscope that measures the chane in the polarization state of polarized laser light induced by the bifringent properties of the retinal nerve fiber layer. It estimates the peripapillary retinal nerve fiber layer thickness.
- Evaluation of corneal thickness:
    - **Pachymetry**: According to the OHTS, patients with central corneal thicknesses less than 550 microns are at a higher risk for glaucoma. A thicker CCT makes the tonometry measurement artificially higher than the true IOP.
    - Goldmann applanation tonometry is calibrated for a CCT of 500 microns.
- Evaluation of visual fields (Perimetry):
    - **Automated Static Perimetry** is the current gold standard for clinical assessment of visual function. Typically, instruments used include Humphrey Field Analyzer, Frequency Doubling Threshold (FDT), or Goldmann perimetry.
    - **Characteristic glaucomatous defects** correlate with physical changes in the optic nerve and retinal nerve fiber layer. The field loss is initially in either the superior or inferior hemifield.
        - **Nasal Step** – The arcuate nerve fibers are more susceptible to the initial glaucomatous damage. This deviation respects the horizontal midline in the nasal visual field
        - **Arcuate Scotoma** – Later in the disease as the nerve loss progresses the nasal step connects to the optic nerve head.
        - **Paracentral Scotoma** – Appears as an extension of the blindspot or an isolated defect in the arcuate fibers close to fixation.
    - Visual field defects are not pathopneumonic for glaucoma, as many other diseases can mimic glaucomatous visual field defects, like:
        - Branch artery occlusions
        - Chorioretinal scars
        - Optic neuritis
        - Optice nerve head drusen

TYPES OF GLAUCOMA

- Glaucoma is classified based upon the etiology (primary vs. secondary) and appearance of the angle (open vs. closed).

1. Ocular Hypertension and Glaucoma Suspects

- A patient who has elevated IOP >21mmHg but no glaucomatous optic nerve damage and visual field loss is classified as having **ocular hypertension.** These patients are at an increased risk of developing optic nerve changes with time and being classified to have glaucoma.
    - These patients are managed by periodic monitoring and medical treatment if IOP raises to >30mmHg, or there is visible optic nerve damage or visual field defects.
- A **Glaucoma suspect** has a normal IOP (<21mmHg) but suspicious optic nerve changes that appear to be glaucomatous.

2. Primary Open-Angle Glaucoma (POAG)

- POAG defined as "chronic, generally bilateral and often asymmetrical disease, which is characterized (in at least one eye) by all of the following:
    1. Evidence of glaucomatous optic nerve damage
        - Thinning or notching of the disc rim, progressive change, nerve fiber layer defects
        - Characteristics visual field abnormalities – arcuate defect, nasal step, paracentral scotoma, generalized depression
    2. Adult onset
    3. Open, normal appearing anterior chamber angles
    4. Absence of secondary causes of open angle glaucoma
- Risk factors:
    - **Elevated IOP:**
        - Increased IOP is correlated with increased prevalence and incidence of glaucoma.
        - Elevated IOP does not necessarily equate with a diagnosis of glaucoma, and normal IOP does not exclude the diagnosis of glaucoma
    - **Age** – Risk increases with age
    - **Ethnicity** – African Americans and Hispanics at higher risk
    - Positive **family history**
        - Strongest risk in siblings, genetic basis of "Glaucoma" genes.
    - Optic nerve head cupping – wide, deep physiological cups are at higher risk of visual field loss
    - Thin central cornea
- Potential clinical risk factors:
    - **Diabetes Mellitus** – tend to have higher IOPs, and ischemic ocular vessels may lead to increased susceptibility of the optic nerve to damage by elevated IOP
    - **Systemic hypertension**
    - Myopia
    - Migraines
- Pathogenesis:
    - Aqueous humor outflow is obstructed due to changes in the trabecular meshwork including endothelial cell loss and collagen abnormalities in the extracellular matrix.
    - The increased IOP causes mechanical compression on the optic nerve leading to posterior bowing of the lamina cribrosa, neuronal blockage of axoplasmic flow, and loss of optic nerve and ganglion cell fibers.
- Symptoms:
    - Most patients are asymptomatic in the early stages of the disease.
    - As IOP elevates, corneal edema (due to aqueous flowing into the corneal stroma) leads to halos around lights and blurry vision.
    - As the disease advances, acquired blue-yellow color vision defects followed by visual scotomas occur.

- As the optic nerve damage advances even further, patients may develop an afferent pupillary defect in eye with the most damage.

- Management – Can only be directed towards decreasing IOP
  - Medical management
  - Laser trabeculoplasty
  - Glaucoma filtration surgery
- **Normal Tension Glaucoma (NTG):**
  - Glaucomatous optic nerve changes in NTG are caused by pressure independent causal factors.
  - The patients might have a heightened sensitivity to "normal" IOP pressures due to anatomical features of their optic nerve head.
  - Patients tend to have conditions that alter blood flow to the optic nerve head like vasospasm or systemic hypertension that leads them to have more ischemic etiologies of glaucomatous damage.
  - Most patients are asymptomatic but might have a history of shock, severe blood loss, and/or Raynaud's phenomenon.

3. Primary Angle-Closure Glaucoma (PACG)

- PACG is defined as "appositional or synechial closure of the anterior chamber angle caused by relative pupillary block in the absence of other causes of angle closure" – AAO, 1996
  - It is the sudden/complete blockage of aqueous outflow that causes a rapid and severe rise in IOP.
- Epidemiology: PACG accounts for 9% of all types of glaucoma
- Diagnosis: depends on gonioscopy
- **Risk factors:**
  - Ethnicity:
    - Eskimos (20-40x higher risk than Caucasians) and Asians (Chinese) at higher risk due to smaller eyes size, more crowded anterior chamber
  - Age:
    - Increased risk with age due to steady growth of crystalline lens and shallowing anterior chamber and angles
    - Most prevalent beyond 5th decade of life
    - Prevalence of pupillary block increases with age, peak incidence during 60s-70s
  - Gender – Women at increased risk (smaller eyes and anterior chambers than men)
  - Refractive error: Hyperopia
  - Positive Family History: Strong risk factor
- **Symptoms:**
  - Severe pain in ocular/maxillary regions – due to CN V
  - Nausea, vomiting
  - Bradycardia, sweating – due to oculocardiac reflex
  - Blurred vision/Halos – due to corneal edema from aqueous humor forced into cornea by high IOP
- **Signs:**
  - Shallow anterior chamber, convex iris insertion (visualized with gonioscopy).
  - Acute iritis (can lead to iris congestion, conjunctival hyperemia, cells and flare in anterior chamber).
    - Excess protein in anterior chamber predisposes patient formation of peripheral anterior synechiae (PAS) and posterior synechiae.
  - Mid-dilated/fixed pupil – Extremely high IOP causes ischemia, temporary paralysis, and/or necrosis of the pupillary sphincter leading to mydriasis and iris stroma atrophy.
  - Glaukomflecken – Gray-white anterior subcapsular lens opacities visible in the pupillary region.
- **Angle closure with pupillary block:**
  - **Pupillary block** is the relative obstruction of aqueous humor movement from the posterior chamber to the anterior chamber due to the apposition of the iris to the anterior surface of the lens.

- **Primary angle closure** with pupillary block involves an anatomically narrow angle and apposition of the iris. As the pressure rises in the posterior chamber, it pushes the iris to bow forward in a condition known as **"iris bombe"** which occludes the angle which was narrow to begin with. This can be acute, intermittent, or chronic (chronic occurring due to progressive increase of apposition – "creeping glaucoma").
    - **Mydriasis** causes the iris to become flaccid and pushed anteriorly into the trabecular meshwork provoking an acute angle-closure (AAC) attack.
    - **Factors favoring AAC attack** include narrow anterior chamber angles, shallow anterior chamber depths, short axial lengths (hyperopia), small corneal diameters, increased thickness, physiologic/pharmacologic mydriasis, and systemic medications that have anticholinergic effects.
- **Secondary Angle Closure** with pupillary block is usually unilateral, and caused by physical blockage of the pupil by things like the lens, inflammation (posterior synechiae), anterior hyaloids face of the vitreous, and can be caused by intravitreal gas, pseudophakia, miotics, and retinopathy of prematurity
- **Treatment** (for primary and secondary) is laser iridotomy or peripheral iridectomy

- **Angle closure without pupillary block:**
    - Angle closure without pupillary block is diagnosed as an acute angle closure that is not resolved by laser iridotomy. Its primary causes include a **plateau iris configuration**, or **ciliary body angular rotation** which pushes the peripheral iris against the angle.
    - Secondary causes of angle closure without pupillary block are caused by forces pushing posteriorly and/or pulling forces anteriorly that force the peripheral iris to appose the trabecular meshwork and peripheral cornea. The secondary causes affect the angle, not the pupil.
        - Anterior forces include peripheral anterior synechiae (PAS), neovascularization of the angle, iridocorneal endothelial syndrome (ICE), aniridia, and iridoschisis
        - Posterior forces include malignant ciliary block, suprachoroidal hemorrhage, intraocular tumors, choroidal effusion, and swelling/anterior rotation of the ciliary body which can be caused by retinal detachment surgery, panretinal photocoagulation, and other ocular diseases that obstruct blood flow.
    - Medical treatment and iridoplasty used for management.

4. Secondary Open-Angle Glaucoma

- **Pigmentary Dispersion Syndrome:**
    - Chronic rubbing of the iris pigmented epithelium against the lens zonules leads to pigment release into the anterior chamber. The pigment deposits onto the cornea, iris, lens and trabecular meshwork, and has characteristic radial iris transillumination defects.
        - Anatomically, these patients have larger eyes, with a posterior bowing of the iris (concave iris insertion) which allows it to rest on the zonules facilitating the mechanical rubbing.
        - The aqueous humor pressure in the anterior chamber exceeds the posterior chamber enhancing the posterior bowing of the iris onto the lens in a **reverse pupillary block.**
    - Usually sporadic in etiology (can be autosomal recessive), most patients are diagnosed in their 30s-40s, and commonly tend to be young myopic males. 25-50% of patients with PDS develop **pigmentary glaucoma.**
        - Pigment deposits in the trabecular meshwork block aqueous outflow, elevating IOP.
    - Triad of signs:
        - Kruckenburg spindles – pigment deposits on the corneal endothelium
        - Dense pigment dusting in the trabecular meshwork
        - Transillumination defects
- **Pseudoexfoliation Syndrome:**
    - A pseudoexfoliative material deposits on the lens, pupillary margin, and anterior segment structures, appearing as white, dandruff-like flakes. The pseudoexfoliation occurs most commonly on the anterior lens capsule with a characteristic central disc, clear intermediate zone, and peripheral granular zone. Some of the material can fill in the trabecular meshwork, and occlude the Schlemm's canal, leading to glaucoma in 50% of afflicted persons.

- The etiology of this pseudoexfoliative material is unknown, but hypothesized to arise from abnormal basement membrane of degenerated elastic fibers.
- This is seen more often in women than men, and has a high genetic incidence in those of Northern European descent.

- **Iridocorneal Endothelium (ICE) Syndrome:**
  - A broad range of ocular diseases that entail abnormal corneal endothelial proliferation and collagenous deposition posterior to Descemet's membrane, which leads to corneal edema and progressive alterations in the iris and anterior chamber angle.
  - 50% of patients with ICE syndrome develop glaucoma when the abnormal endothelial membrane grows posteriorly over the angle structures.
- **Traumatic glaucoma:**
  - **Acute traumatic glaucoma** is secondary to blood, cellular debris, pigment, lens particles, steroids, and trabecular meshwork dysfunction.
  - **Angle recession glaucoma** occurs when significant trauma to the globe causes the angle to recess through the ciliary body, causing acute trabecular meshwork injury, fibrosis of the trabecular meshwork, and endothelialization which increases the patients risk for glaucoma for 2 months to 20 years after the trauma.
- **Neovascular glaucoma:**
  - A severe form of acute open-angle glaucoma associated with posterior segment disease. Ischemia of 50% of the retina releases diffusible growth factors (VEGF) which promote iris neovascularization.
  - The new blood vessels in the anterior segment are fenestrated and leak leading to inflammation. Blood vessels in the trabecular meshwork obstruct aqueous outflow.
  - Predisposing conditions for neovascularization include CRVO, diabetic retinopathy, carotid artery occlusion and uveitis.
  - Early in the disease the symptoms are mild (decreased acuity) and neovascularization of the pupil, iris, and angle (trabecular meshwork) is visible.
  - Later in the disease the symptoms exacerbate (brow ache, nausea) and neovascularization causes angle closure, ectropion uvea, anterior chamber inflammation and increased IOP.
  - Peripheral anterior synechiae can cause angle closure in neovascular glaucoma.
  - Management entails medical management of the glaucoma and treatment of the underlying retinal condition.
- **Inflammatory glaucoma:**
  - Ocular inflammation can directly and indirectly alter aqueous humor dynamics and IOP.
  - Anterior Uveitis (commonly associated with glaucoma) increases the permeability of anterior segment vasculature allowing for inflammatory cells, mediators, and proteins to accumulate in the iris, ciliary body, anterior and posterior chambers.
  - Open-angle glaucoma secondary to inflammation is caused by inflammatory debris obstruction and alteration of the function of the trabecular meshwork.
  - Closed-angle glaucoma secondary to inflammation is caused by peripheral anterior synechiae, scarring, posterior synechiae, pupillary block, fibrous adhesions, anterior rotation of the ciliary body, and ciliary body swelling.

5. Childhood Glaucoma

- Most glaucoma cases in childhood are caused by obstruction to aqueous humor outflow due to abnormal anterior chamber angle development, inflammation, or trauma.
- **Congenital (Infantile) glaucoma** is usually on open-angle glaucoma that presents from birth to 3 years of age with a peak onset at 1 year of age. It is caused by the arrest of angle development leading to anterior placement of the iris root and ciliary body anterior to the scleral spur which either partially or completely covers the trabecular meshwork.
  - Genetic etiology
  - **Symptoms**: photophobia, blepharospasm, and epiphora caused by corneal edema,
  - **Signs:** Buphthalmos (enlargement of the globe), enlargement of the cornea (diameter >12mm), Haab's Striae (breaks in Descemet's membrane due to stretching of immature tissues), axial elongation, and myopia.

- IOP in infants is normally lower than adults, and an IOP >20mmHg in infants is indicative of glaucoma.
  - Glaucomatous nerve changes like asymmetric cupping between the two eyes and a C/D >0.3 may also indicate glaucoma.
  - **Management**: surgical goniotomy/trabeculotomy
- **Juvenile glaucoma** presents in older children and young adults between 10-35 years. There is a higher incidence among African heritage, and has a genetic component tied to defective gene.
- **Axenfold-Rieger Syndrome** a group of bilateral congenital anomalies due to abnormal anterior chamber angle, iris, and trabecular meshwork development. 50% of people with Axenfold-Reiger's syndrome have glaucoma.
  - **Axenfold's Anomaly** – prominent anteriorly displaced Schwalbe's line with attached iris processes
  - **Reiger's Anomaly** – Axenfold's anomaly in addition to iris hypoplasia and altered pupils
  - **Reiger's Syndrome** – Axenfold's anomaly, Reiger's anomaly, in addition to ocular and systemic developmental problems with the teech and facial bones
- **Peter's Anomaly** – bilateral central corneal opacities with adhesions between the central iris and corneal endothelium. 50% of patients with Peter's anomaly have glaucoma. Etiologically stemmed from the embryologic arrest and lack of separation of the lens vesicle from the surface ectoderm
- **Aniridia** – 50-75% of patients with marked iris hypoplasia develop glaucoma due to the anterior rotation of the rudimentary stump of the iris which progressively covers and obstructs the trabecular meshwork

---

ANTI-GLAUCOMA AGENT PHARMACOLOGY

1. General Principles

- The aim of medical treatment of glaucoma is to lower IOP, which does not cure the disease but slows its progression.
- Numerous studies have indicated the advantages of lowering IOP in glaucoma treatment.
  - Decreasing IOP by 20% decreases the incidence of POAG.
  - Each 1mmHg decrease in IOP decreases the risk of progression by 10%.
  - Decreasing IOP decreases the risk of vision loss in normal tension glaucoma.
  - With aggressive therapy aimed at decreased IOP, VF loss in general can be minimized.
- The best treatment is a consistently decreased IOP.
- The **target IOP** is a variable target that is based on the degree of glaucomatous damage:
  - No VF damage and an intact neuroretinal rim → IOP in high teens/low 20s.
  - VF loss on one side of the horizontal meridian → IOP in mid-teens.
  - VF loss on both side of horizontal meridian → IOP <12mmHg.
- Topical anti-glaucoma therapy:
  - Drugs affect either aqueous humor production or outflow.
  - Prodrugs improve transfer and decrease systemic and ocular side effects.
  - Due to asymptomatic nature of POAG, compliance of patients to topical therapy is reduced due to subjective observation that nothing is wrong.
- Mechanisms of action:
  - **Decrease aqueous inflow** (aqueous production in ciliary body)→ CAIs, β-Blockers, α2-adrenergic agonists, osmotic agents
  - **Neuroprotection** → β-Blockers, α2-adrenergic agonists, NMDA receptor agonists, Calcium antagonists
  - **Increase conventional aqueous outflow** (trabecular meshwork/canal of Schlemm) → Epinephrine, miotics, anti-metabolites, osmotic agents
  - **Increase unconventional aqueous outflow** (uveoscleral) → prostaglandin analogs
- Comparative IOP lowering abilities of current drug options from most potent to least potent:
  - Oral CAIs > Miotics and Prostaglandins > Nonselective β-Blockers >α2 Agonists > Topical CAIs and Betaxolol >Epinephrine

2. Miotics (Parasympathomimetics)

- Miotics are cholinergic agonists that reduce IOP by increasing aqueous outflow.
- **MOA:** Increases acetylcholine which directly/indirectly opens the trabecular meshwork by causing ciliary body and iris sphincter contraction.
- **Examples:**
  - **Pilocarpine** (Ocusert)
    - Used for Acute Angle-Closure Glaucoma patients waiting for surgery. But contraindicated in cases with very high IOP because iris ischemia leads to blood vessel compression making the drug ineffective
    - Most widely used of the miotics, most selective, taken QID.
    - Maximum IOP effect is in 1-2 hours, lasts for 4-6 hrs.
  - **Carbachol** (Miostat)
    - More potent and longer lasting than pilocarpine, but worse corneal penetration
    - Also effects nicotinic receptors (indirect and direct actions) – increases acetylcholine and inhibits acetylcholinesterase makes it more potent and increases the risk of ocular side effects.
    - Taken TID. Typically used as a miotic for surgery.
  - **Ecothiophate Iodide (Phospholine Iodide)**
    - Indirectly acts by inhibiting cholinesterase irreversibly enhancing the effects of acetylcholine in the nerve junction.
    - Low lipid solubility limits its penetration across the blood-brain barrier, allowing for lower effects on the CNS.
    - Miosis onset occurs at 10-45 minutes, and action onsets in 4-8 hours, with maximum effect at 24 hours and duration of 1-2 weeks. BID dosage, necessitates punctual occlusion
    - Should discontinue use prior to ocular surgery to avoid excessive bleeding from conjunctival and episcleral vessels.
  - **Isoflurophate (DFP, Diisopropylfluorophosphate)**
    - An irreversible cholinesterase inhibitor that enhances the effect of acetylcholine in the nerve junction.
    - Drug is highly lipid soluble, and most potent and unstable in solution. It readily penetrates the blood-brain barrier thus causing its effects upon the CN.S
    - Action onsets in 5-10 minutes with its maximum effect at 24 hours, with a duration of 1 week. It can decrease IOP by 10-15%.
    - It has increased CNS effects (anxiety, tremors, convulsions, coma, respiratory distress).
- **Clinical indications**:
  - Primary open-angle glaucoma
  - Acute angle-closure glaucoma
  - Non-inflammatory secondary glaucomas
  - Post-operative conditions: Iris fixed-IOL, prevention of PC IOL pupillary capture
  - Pre-operative conditions: Laser peripheral iridectomy, Corneal transplant in phakic patients
  - Minimal concentrations of pilocarpine used for Adie's tonic pupil diagnosis
  - Differential diagnosis of dilated, fixed pupil (CN III vs. pharmacological dilation with 1% pilocarpine)
- **Contraindications:**
  - Prolonged use in chronic angle-closure glaucoma/narrow angles
  - Malignant glaucoma
  - Younger patients prone to ciliary spasm
  - Cautionary use in patients with retinal disease
  - Asthma (parasympatholytics)
  - Parkinson's
  - Myasthenia gravis drugs
  - Alzheimer's drugs

Miotic	Ocular Side Effects	Systemic Side Effects
Pilocarpine	Ciliary spasm/Accommodative myopia Miosis Vascular congestion and hyperemia Decreased night vision Brow ache, eye pain Lid Myokymia Visual field constriction Shallowing of anterior chamber 8-12% Band keratopathy Retinal detachment	Bradycardia with rebound tachycardia Hypotension (vasodilation) with rebound hypertension Pulmonary edema Bronchospasm GI distress Diarrhea Vomiting, nausea Bladder incontinence
Ecothiophate	Iris cysts Pigment dispersion Cataracts Reactivates uveitis	CNS excitation

3. Epinephrine (Sympathomimetic)

- Epinephrine is a sympathetic agonist that non-selectively agonizes adrenergic α and β receptors.
- **MOA:** There is a slight increase in aqueous production early on due to β2 stimulation on the ciliary epithelium, but then has a β-mediated increase in conventional outflow.
- **Examples:**
  - **Dipivefrin** – dipivalyl epinephrine, a prodrug that is lipophilic, allowing for increased intraocular penetration of the cornea, 17x greater than epinephrine. Taken BID. IOP reduction onset peaks in 2-4 hours, decreases IOP by 15-26% and takes 3 months to achieve full therapeutic efficacy. Can be used concomitantly with topical beta-blockers.
- **Ocular side effects:**
  - Irritation, stinging, allergic reactions
  - Macular edema in aphakes
  - Decreased optic nerve head perfusion
  - Acute-angle closure glaucoma

4. α2-Agonists (Sympathomimetic)

- **MOA:** Stimulation of α2 receptors on the ciliary epithelium leads to G-protein mediated decrease in cAMP, leading to a decrease in aqueous humor production.
- **Examples:**
  - **Apraclonidine (Iopidine)** – somewhat selective
    - Indicated for the treatment and prophylaxis of IOP spikes following anterior segment laser procedures, uveitis, and AACG.
    - Dosed TID, with onset of IOP reduction at 1 hour, and peak of action from 3-4 hrs.
  - **Brimonidine (Alphagen)** – More selective for α2>α1
    - More lipid soluble, able to penetrate blood-brain barrier
    - Significant melanin binding
    - Late increase in uveoscleraloutflow, neuroprotective, Pregnancy Category B
    - Dosage BID
    - FDA approved as initial treatment for glaucoma
  - **Combigan (Timolol + Brimonidine)** – has a decreased allergic reaction
- **Indications:**
  - Treatment of primary and secondary open angle glaucoma.
  - Consider in patients who may not tolerate miosis or brow ache. Not the primary choice of drug since it has less IOP reduction than other hypotensive medications.
  - Not additive with β-Blockers.
- **Contraindications:**

- Very young and very elderly patients (CNS effects)
- Cardiac arrhythmia, hypertension
- Aphakia (ICCE) – increased likelihood of CME
- Hyperthyroidism
- Ischemic heart disease
- Cautionary use in patients with renal impairments
- Soft contact lens wearer
- Narrow angles without a patent iridectomy
- Plateau iris syndrome
- Secondary glaucomas with pigment component

- **Drug interactions:**
  - Discontinue use prior to general anesthesia
  - Concurrent therapy with Tricyclic Antidepressants and/or MAO inhibitors – risk of hypertensive crisis
- **Ocular side effects:**
  - Mydriasis (Aproclonidine), Miosis (Brimonidine)
  - Ocular irritation (stinging, burning)
  - Soft contact lens discoloration
  - Follicular conjunctivitis, allergic blepharitis (Aproclonidine)
  - Conjunctival blanching, eyelid retraction (Aproclonidine)
  - Cystoids Macular Edema (20-30% in aphakes)
  - Vasoconstriction with rebound conjunctival hyperemia
  - Adenochrome deposits in the conjunctiva
  - Corneal epithelial edema
- **Systemic Side Effects:**
  - Headaches
  - Extreme tachyphylaxis (aproclonidine)→intolerable effects in 20-50% of cases
  - α1 effects lead to vasoconstriction, decreased bleeding and blood flow as well as increased ocular side effects

5. <u>β-Blockers (Sympatholytic)</u>

- **MOA**: Decreases chloride ion transport into the posterior chamber by blocking the β2 receptor on the ciliary epithelium, thus decreasing the osmotic gradient, decreasing aqueous production, and IOP.
- β-blockers reduce IOP 20-30%, and can manifest in a 10-15% decrease in the contralateral eye, allowing for monocular treatment.
- The response to some of the β-blockers decreases over time (escapes), especially early in the treatment phase. There is no cross sensitivity to β-Blockers, so one can switch to another if the desired effect is no long reached.
- There is smaller decrease in IOP in those of African descent due to genetic polymorphism and melanin binding.
- β-Blockers are only effective during the daytime due to decreased sympathetic tone at night.
- **Examples:**
  - **Timolol Maleate (Timoptic, Timoptic-XE, Betimol)** – nonselective
    - Onset is in 30 mins with a peak effect in 1-2 hrs, and duration of 12-24 hrs
    - Standardly dosed BID in solution, QD for gel-based Timoptic
    - Standard preservative is BAK with a preservative-free form available
    - Has MSA (membrane stabilizing activity)
  - **Levobunolol (Betagan)** – nonselective
    - Onset is in 1 hour, with a peak effect in 2 hrs, and duration of 12-24 hrs
    - The metabolite of levobunolol has a longer half-life in the plasma than Timolol, and an increased efficacy with chronic therapy
    - Typical dosage is QD or BID
  - **Metipranolol (Optipranolol)** – nonselective
    - Onset is in 30 mins with a peak effect in 2 hrs, and duration of 12-24 hrs
    - Has a long duration

- **Carteolol (Ocupress)** – nonselective
  - Onset is in 30 mins with a peak effect in 1-2 hrs, and duration of 12-24 hrs
  - Has MSA and ISA (intrinsic sympathomimetic activity) which leads to fewer systemic side effects
  - Has a better lipid profile, so it does not cross the blood-brain barrier as easily as other non-selective β-Blockers, so may protect against depression
- **Betaxolol (Betoptic-S)** – β1 cardioselective
  - Onset is in 20 mins with a peak effect in 1hr, and duration of 12-24 hrs
  - Is the β-Blocker of choice for individuals with compromised respiratory systems (COPD, asthma). The selectivity is relative, and is only less likely to induce respiratory complications
  - Comes in a suspension – decreases the stinging upon instillation
  - Has a neuroprotective mechanism as a calcium channel blocker. Additionally the decreased vasoconstricive effect leads to increased perfusion at the optic nerve head compared to other β-Blockers
  - Not as efficacious in its hypotensive effects as Timolol or Levobunolol but does preserve visual field. It combines effectively with Dipivefrin and Epinephrine

- **Indications:**
  - Treatment in open-angle glaucoma, narrow-angle glaucoma, congenital glaucoma, and secondary glaucoma (including neovascular and uveitic)
- **Contraindications (for non-selective β-Blockers):**
  - Bronchial asthma/history of asthma
  - Chronic obstructive pulmonary disease, emphysema
  - Congestive heart failure, 2nd or 3rd degree atrioventricular block, 1st degree heart block with a PR-segment interval >0.24 sec
  - History of myocardial infarct, decreased myocardial contractility
  - Diabetes
  - Thyroid disease – patients prone to develop thyrotoxicosis
  - Hypotension (,100/60), bradycardia (pulse<55beats/min)
- **Drug interactions:**
  - Systemic β-Blockers – wont get added effect with topical due to crossover effect
  - Calcium Channel Blockers – decrease neuroprotective vasodilation effect
  - Heart medications (β-Blockers decrease blood pressure)
  - B-Agonists
  - NSAIDs – p450
- **Ocular side effects:**
  - Stinging
  - Punctate keratitis, dry eye (MSA, BAK)
  - Decreased corneal sensitivity (MSA)
  - Allergic conjunctivitis
  - Hyperemia, lacrimation
  - Orbital pain
  - Pupillary dilation
  - Persistent hypotony
  - Ocular myasthenia gravis – ptosis, diplopia, weakness
- **Systemic side effects:**
  - Respiratory distress, exacerbated asthma, increased airway resistance, bronchospasm, dyspnea, edena
  - Hypotension, bradycardia, decreased cardiac output, arrhythmia, palpitations
  - Masked hypoglycemia in diabetics, prevents usual rebound of plasma glucose concentration
  - CNS effects – depression, sleep disturbances, lethargy, confusion, hallucinations, memory loss
  - Skin rashes, urticaria, alopecia
  - Nausea, emesis, diarrhea
  - Joint pain
  - May mask signs of hyperthyroidism
  - Decreased exercise tolerance

- Decreased libido, impotence
- Syncope
- Sudden death
- Decreased HDL cholesterol, increased LDL

6. Oral Carbonic Anhydrase Inhibitors (CAIs)

- **MOA**: CAIs target carbonic anhydrase 2 and 4 in the ciliary epithelium. By blocking carbonic anhydrase, the production of bicarbonate ions is reduced, decreasing the osmotic gradient that drives aqueous humor formation, decreasing IOP
  - Carbonic anhydrase catalyzes the first step in the following reaction: $CO_2 + H_2O \rightarrow H_2CO_3 \rightarrow H + HCO_3$
  - By altering intracellular pH, metabolic acidosis also helps reduce IOP
- CAIs do not produce a significant or prolonged reduction in IOP due to poor corneal penetration
- Some have shown that systemic administration of these agents produces 45-55% inhibition of aqueous formation
- **Examples:**
  - **Acetazolamide (Diamox)**
    - Maximum IOP reduction occurs after 30 mints to 12 hours
  - **Methazolamide (Neptazane)**
    - More potent, increased duration, decreased protein binding, decreased alkalinization of urine makes it better tolerated
    - 25-50mg tablets
  - **Dichlorphenamide (Datahide)**
    - Faster effect reducing IOP than acetazolamide because it is largely non-ionized at plasma pH. 50mg tablets
- **Indications:**
  - Angle Closure Glaucoma
  - Primary open-angle Glaucoma
  - Altitude sickness
  - Anticonvulsant
  - Diuretic
- **Contraindications:**
  - Liver disease
  - COPD
  - Renal disease
  - Pregnancy
  - Sulfa drug allergies
- **Ocular side effects:**
  - Induced myopia
  - Stevens Johnson Syndrome
- **Systemic side effects:**
  - Alkalinizes urine
  - Metallic taste
  - High intolerance (30-80%) due to carbonic anhydrase presence throughout the body
  - Individual variation – hypotensive effect
  - Blood dyscriasis: thrombocytopenia, agranulocytosis, and aplastic anemia
  - Symptomatic complex: malaise, depression, fatigue, weight loss, decreased libido, GI upset, renal calculi, metabolic acidosis

7. Topical Carbonic Anhydrase Inhibitors (CAIs)

- **MOA**: same as oral CAIs
- **Examples:**
  - **Dorzolamide (Trusopt)**
  - **Cosopt** – combination drop with 2% dorzolamide and 0.5% timolol

- **Brinzolamide (Azopt)** – suspension, decreases instillation irritation
- **Indications:**
    - Primary open angle glaucoma
- **Contraindications:** same as oral CAIs
- **Ocular side effects:**
    - Stinging, burning, tearing (pH)
    - SPK, dry eye, foreign body sensation
    - Blurred vision
    - Blepharitis, hyperemia
    - Ocular discharge
    - Ocular pain
    - Hyperemia
- **Systemic side effects:**
    - Rhinitis
    - Headache
    - Bitter taste
    - Metabolic acidosis

8. Prostaglandin Analogs (PGAs)

- **MOA**: binding of PGAs to PGF2 receptors in uveoscleral pathway leads to increased metalloproteinases which leads to extracellular matrix remodeling that leads to increased scleral flow
    - Prostamide receptors on the trabecular meshwork endothelial cells decrease outflow resistance
    - Reduces IOP by up to 35% but takes 2 weeks to obtain maximum effect
- 90-95% of patients respond well, dosage is qd, and PGAs have 24 hour control
- Is able to be additive to any β-blocker, α2-agonist, or CAI
- **Examples:**
    - **Travaprost (Travatan, Travatan Z)**
        - Travatan Z has borate has a preservative to reduce punctate staining of the cornea. It is the first drug of choice due to relatively mild side effects compared to others in its class. It has the highest potency and highest efficiency.
    - **Latanoprost (Xalatan)**
    - **Bimatoprost (Lumigan)**
        - Amide, has effects on conventional and unconventional outflow pathways
    - **Unoprostone**
        - Partial agonist, has decreased efficacy, milder side effects and a neuroprotective effect
- **Indications:**
    - Effective for treatment of open-angle glaucoma for patients that might be intolerant or not responding sufficiently to other glaucoma meds.
    - Currently used as the first line of treatment
- **Contraindications:**
    - None, other than allergy to preservative
- **Ocular side effects:**
    - Irritation/SPK → all have BAK
    - Conjunctiva hyperemia
    - Irreversible iris color change (darkening)
    - Hypertrichosis – thicker and longer eyelashes
    - Mild burning sensation upon ocular instillation
    - Darkening of periorbital dermis
    - Choroidal detachment –rare
    - Reactivation of CME and uveitis
- **Systemic side effects:**
    - Rare – but bradycardia, chest pain, headache, nasal congestion, flu symptoms, nausea, and vomiting have been documented

8. Topical Hyperosmotic Agents

- **MOA**: Topical Ocular Agents reduce IOP by creating an osmotic gradient between the aqueous fluid and the cornea
- **Examples:**
  - **Glycerin (Osmoglyn, Ophthalgan)**
    - Onset in 10-30 minutes, peak onset at 60-90 minutes
- **Clinical uses:**
  - Acute angle closure glaucoma
  - Reduction of corneal edema
- **Contraindications:**
  - Dehydration
  - Pulmonary edema
  - Diabetes
  - Severe cardiac decompensation
- **Systemic effects:**
  - Arrhythmia
  - Headache
  - Dizziness
  - Dehydration
  - Diarrhea

9. Systemic Hyperosmotic Agents

- **MOA**: Reduce IOP by creating an osmotic gradient between the aqueous fluid and the plasma
- **Examples:**
  - **Isosorbide**
  - **Mannitol (IV)**
- **Indications**: acute angle closure glaucoma
- **Contraindications:**
  - Congestive heart failure
  - Kidney disease
  - Pulmonary edema
  - Dehydration
  - Allergy to organic nitrates
  - Concurrent use of sildenafil
  - Severe hypotension
- **Systemic effects**:
  - Nausea
  - Increased urination
  - Vomiting, nausea
  - Pulmonary congestion
  - Metabolic acidosis
  - Rhinitis
  - Chest pain
  - Hypotension
  - Headache, fatigue
  - Rash

Drug Class	Generic Name	Trade Name	Contraindications	Ocular Side-Effects	Special Notes
Prostaglandins and analogues: enhances uveoscleral outflow	Latanoprost	Xalatan	None	Darkening of irises, Lengthening of eyelashes Ocular hyperemia, macular edema	
	Travoprost	Travatan			Least side effects
	*Bimatoprost	Lumigan			
Beta-Blockers: decreases aqueous production	*Timolol	Timoptic	COPD, asthma, CHF, Hypotension (< 100/60), diabetes, Thyroid - pts prone to develop thyrotoxicosis	Allergic conjunctivitis, Burning and irritation, Dry eye, Corneal hypesthesia, Lacrimation, Ocular myasthenia gravis - ptosis, diplopia, weakness, Superficial punctate keratitis, Orbital pain, Hyperemia, Pupillary dilation	
	Levobunolol	Betagan			
	Betaxolol	Betoptic			Cardioselective
	Carteolol	Cartrol, Ocupress			intrinsic sympathomimetic activity (ISA).
Parasympathetic Agonists: increase TM aqueous outflow	Pilocarpine	"Pilo-"	Neovascular GLC, prolonged use in chronic ACG, Younger patients prone to ciliary spasm, pts w/ predisposition to retinal tears/ detachments, peptic ulcers, urinary tract obstructions, asthma, acute cardiac failure, Parkinson's disease and cardiovascular disease.	Miosis, Accommodative spasm, Decreased night vision, brow ache, eye pain, Myokymia, VF constriction, hyperemia, Shallowing of Ant. chamber of 8-12%, Follicular conjunctivitis, Band keratopathy, Retinal detachment	
	Carbachol	Isopto Carbachol			
	Echothiphate	Phospholine			
	Neostigmine	Prostigmin			
	Physostigmine	Antilirium			
Sympathetic Agonists: increases TM aqueous outflow and decreases aqueous production	Epinephrine	Glaucon	Narrow angles, Cardiac arrhythmia, HTN, aphakia (increased likelihood of CME), Plateau iris, Hyperthyroidism, Ischemic heart disease, TCAs or MAOIs therapy (Risk of hypertensive crisis), D/C prior to general anesthesia	Cystoid macular edema, vasoconstriction with rebound conjunctival hyperemia, Punctal stenosis, Adrenochrome deposits in the conjunctiva, Follicular conjunctivitis, Corneal epithelial edema, Mydriasis	Vasoconstriction during ocular surgery; DDx of episcleritis vs. conjunctivitis
	Dipivefrin	Propine			
	Apraclonidine	Iopidine			alpha-2 adrenergic agonist
	*Brimonidine	Alphagan			
Carbonic Anhydrase Inhibitors: Decrease aqueous production	Acetazolamide	Diamox	Liver disease, COPD, Renal disease, Pregnancy, Allergies to sulfa drugs	Blurred Vision, Blepharitis, FBS, Dry eyes, Photophobia, Nausea, Headache	Oral
	*Dorzolamide	Trusopt			combined with Timolol to produce Cosopt
	Brinzolamide	Azopt			

* most commonly used drugs in practice today

Chapter 19 – Ocular Emergencies & Trauma

OCULAR ADNEXA

1. Blow-Out Fracture

- **Etiology:** Blunt trauma causes a wave of pressure. The orbital floor susceptible to fracture along with blowout into ethmoidal or maxillary sinuses
- **Symptoms**: Anesthesia, diplopia, pain
- **Signs:** Tear drop sign (portion of orbital tissue trapped in maxillary sinus), EOM restriction, Orbital swelling, *Ecchymosis* (bruising), *Enophthalmos* (eye sunken in).
- **Observation, inspection, techniques:**
    - Skull x-ray and orbital CT scan
    - Old photographs
    - EOM, pupils, color vision
    - IOP, palpating eyelid for trapped air
- **Complications associated with blunt trauma:**
    - Hyphema
    - Traumatic iritis
    - Choroidal rupture
    - Retinal detachment
    - Commotio retinae
    - Angle recession glaucoma
    - Optic atrophy

2. Horner's Syndrome

- **Etiology:** Internal carotid dissection, Trauma, Cluster headaches, Herpes zoster infection, Pancoast tumor, Stroke
- **Classic Triad of Signs:** 1) Ptosis 2) Miosis (Anisocoria) 3) Facial Anhydrosis
- **Observation, inspection, techniques**: Catheter angiography, CT angiography, MRI, Magnetic resonance angiography (MRA)

3. Orbital Cellulitis

- **Symptoms:** Red eye, Pain, Blurry vision, Diplopia, Headache, Fever
- **Signs:** Lid swelling (Warm and tender to touch), Proptosis, Restricted EOM
- **Observation, inspection, techniques:** Pupils, EOM, Color vision, IOP, Orbital CT scan
- **Differential diagnosis:** Thyroid disease, Preseptal cellulitis, Orbital blow out fracture, Tumors

4. Malignant Lid Lesions

- **Types:**
    - Squamous cell carcinoma
    - Basal cell carcinoma – Most common type
    - Malignant melanoma
    - Actinic keratosis – Due to long term UV exposure
- **Observation, inspection, techniques**: Biopsy

CRANIAL NERVE PALSY

- **Epidemiology**:
    - Most common palsy (in order of most to least common):
        - CN VI
        - CN III
        - CN IV
    - Most common causes for recent onset nerve palsy:
        - Vascular
        - Diabetes (Should resolve in 3 months)
    - Other causes: tumor, aneurysm, trauma, idiopathic
- **Observation, inspection, techniques:**
    - Case history: Onset, Other neurological signs, Medical history (i.e. vascular risk factors)
    - EOM→Degree of restriction, Direction of increased restriction, Check if palsy is isolated or multiple involvement, Cover test, Warning signs
    - Pupils→ Blown pupil (If not resolved within 3 months, need neuroimaging)
    - Multiple cranial nerve involvement due to lesion at brain stem, cavernous sinus, or orbital apex
- **Third nerve palsy:**
    - Most common etiology (also see above)
        - Intracranial aneurysm: A **true emergency** → send to ER immediately, potentially fatal
        - Diabetes
    - **Ocular Symptoms:** Diplopia, Unilateral blurry vision, sharp eye pain
    - **Associated symptoms:** headache, facial or extremity weakness, fever, change in speech, gait, and coordination
    - **Signs:** pupil dilation**, ptosis, eye down and out
        - Pupil evaluation**
            - Blown pupil = non reactive or sluggish reaction to light
            - Pupil involvement = aneurysm 95-97% of the time
            - Pupil spared = usually diabetes
            - Pathophysiology
                - Pupil fibers of CN III are superficial and more easily compressed with vascular event
            - **Do NOT dilate eyes** →must be able to follow up to see if changes to pupil involvement
    - **Additional tests**: head CT scan, MRA, MRI, Lumbar puncture, Catheter angiogram
    - First symptoms improved with resolution of CN III palsy: Ptosis, Inferior rectus palsy
    - Differential diagnosis
        - Pupil dilation
            - Mydriatics
            - Trauma to ciliary ganglion
            - Adie's pupil
            - Glaucoma
        - Ptosis
            - Myasthenia gravis
            - Botulism
            - Orbital infections
            - Orbital trauma
            - Migraine
        - Chronic progressive external ophthalmoplegia
            - Ptosis
            - Decreased convergence
            - Difficulty with up gaze

LACRIMAL SYSTEM INFECTIONS

- **Acute dacryoadenitis:**
  - Lacrimal gland inflammation
  - Etiology: usually injury complicated by acute bacterial infection
  - **Symptoms**: pain, redness in lacrimal gland region, heat, swelling
  - **Signs:** epiphora, enlarged preauricular lymph nodes, viral milder than bacterial, no pus in viral
  - **Complications:** loss of gland function
  - **Observation, inspection, techniques**: palpation, lid eversion
- **Acute dacryocystitis:**
  - Lacrimal sac inflammation
  - Epidemiology: more often in females
  - **Symptoms:** painful to touch, redness in lacrimal sac region, heat, swelling, sometimes headache
  - **Signs:** epiphora, unilateral, Pus or mucus can be expressed from the sac, no pus in viral (milder than bacterial)
  - **Complications**: Obstruction of the naso lacrimal duct
  - **Observation, inspection, techniques**: palpation, Jones dye test
- **Canaliculitis:**
  - Narrow or inflamed canaliculus
  - Symptoms: similar to dacryocystisis
  - **Signs:** Sulfur granules indicate the presence of actinomyces infection

CONJUNCTIVITIS

- **Observation, inspection, techniques:**
  - Slit lamp exam with lid eversion
  - Preauricular and submandibular lymph nodes in viral infections
- **Bacterial conjunctivitis:**
  - Most common cause is Staphylococcus aureus
  - **Symptoms:** Foreign body sensation, lashes stuck shut upon wakening, redness, no changes in VA
  - **Signs:** Often has lid involvement, mucopurulent discharge, hyperemia greater towards fornices, chemosis, papillae without preauricular adenopathy
- **Viral conjunctivitis:**
  - Most common cause of acute conjunctivitis
  - Common causes: Adenovirus, HSV, HZ (varicella), molluscum contagiosum
  - **Symptoms:** Acute onset; clear, watery discharge; mild VA fluctuations; foreign body sensation; redness
  - **Signs:** Usually unilateral, Usually associated with upper respiratory tract infection, Follicles in palpebral conjunctiva
- **Allergic conjunctivitis:**
  - Types:
    - Atopic/seasonal
    - Vernal
    - Giant papillary (Large papillae in upper tarsal plate, Usually seen in soft contact lens wearers)
    - Phlyctenular:
      - Whitish nodules with excavated center surround by dilated vessels near limbus
      - Secondary reaction to staphylococcus eye lid infections
      - Previously associated with tuberculosis
  - **Symptoms:** Bilateral, itchy eye; burning; tearing, ropey, stringy discharge; redness; foreign body sensation; chemosis

- **Chlamydial Conjunctivitis:**
  - TRIC agent = Trachoma, Inclusion, Conjunctivitis
  - **Symptoms**: Redness, tearing, photophobia, irritation
  - **Signs**: Mild mucous discharge, unilateral, preauricular node, follicles, micropannus, Herbert's pits, iritis
  - **Trachoma;**
    - Most common cause of preventable blindness in the world
    - Pathophysiology of blindness → Chronic conjunctival inflammation induces trichiasis, Corneal scarring
    - Vector: fly
- Pharyngoconjunctival fever (PCF), aka Beal's folllicular :
  - Children <18
  - Preceded by mild fever
  - Recent swimming pool exposure

CONJUNCTIVITIS - RULES OF THUMB	
Age	**Likely organism responsible**
Newborns - 5 days old	Neisseria
5 day old - 5 weeks old	Chlamydia – Infant
5 weeks old - 5 years old	Haemophilus
5 years old - 55 years old	Staphylococcus

EPISCLERITIS/SCLERITIS

- **Episcleritis:**
  - Superficial episcleral plexus inflamed
  - **Epidemiology:** Much more common than scleritis (3/4 cases), In Females > male (2:1) Associated with rheumatoid arthritis, Peak age 40
  - **Symptoms:** Hot gritty feeling, tender, no discharge, tearing. photophobia
  - **Signs:** Wedge shaped region or diffuse vascular engorgement, episcleral edema, dilated vessels. Vessels straight (not lacy), pink colored vessels
  - **Types** (of increasing severity):
    - Simple
    - Nodular:
      - Nodules composed of fluid and inflammatory cells
      - Single nodules not adherent to sclera
    - Periodosis Fugax
      - Spreads over entire globe
- **Scleritis:**
  - More severe, destructive and painful than episcleritis
  - **Epidemiology:** Female > Male; age 40 to 60 years; associated with rheumatoid arthritis, gout, herpes zoster
  - **Symptoms:** Deep boring ache, photophobia, tearing
  - **Signs:** Deep purple colored vessels, possible corneal guttering, possible scleral thinning
  - Types (of increasing severity):
    - Diffuse
    - Nodular
    - Necrotizing

CORNEA

- **Abrasion:**
  - Common causes: Trauma, foreign body, contact lens, trichiasis
  - Symptoms:
    - **Superficial** abrasion: Sandy, gritty feeling; foreign body sensation
    - **Deep abrasion:** Sharp pain, conjunctival injection, decreased VA due to edema, photophobia, nausea
  - **Signs:** Fluorescein staining, epithelial defect
  - **Observation, inspection, techniques**: Slit lamp evaluation (location, Depth – check with optic section, edge quality – look for any epithelial flaps
- **Foreign body:**
  - **Symptoms:** Acute onset of pain:
  - **Observation, inspection, techniques**
    - Slit lamp with lid eversion -Look for foreign body on corneal surface, cul de sac, palpebral conjunctiva
    - Fluorescein
    - Seidel's sign – Rule out penetration or perforation, Look for any aqueous leakage or negative staining with fluorescein
- **Microbial keratitis:**
  - Common causes:
    - Pseudomonas associated with contact lens wear
    - Streptococcus – Very purulent
    - Staphylococcus – Focal stromal infiltrate
    - Acanthamoeba
    - Fusarium
    - Herpes simplex – Dendritic ulcer
  - **Symptoms:** Pain, red eye, mucopurulent discharge
  - **Signs**: Epithelial defect, inflammatory infiltrate, AC reaction
  - **Observation, inspection, techniques:** Fluorescein, culture
- **Chemical burn:**
  - True ocular emergency:
    - Minutes of delay in treatment can result in permanent damage
    - Flush for at least 30 minutes immediately
  - **Symptoms**: Lid swelling, severe pain
  - **Signs:** Conjunctival hyperemia (circumlimbal flush), chemosis, hazy cornea
  - Complications:
    - Corneal perforation
    - Secondary glaucoma due to scarring of episcleral aqueous outflow
    - Corneal meltdown due to closing off of limbal vessels
    - Symblepharon due to penetration of palpebral conjunctiva
  - Acid burn:
    - Damage localized
    - Common types of acid chemicals: battery acid, photo chemicals, bleach
  - Alkali burn:
    - Much more severe than acid
    - Pathophysiology:
      - Rapid penetration
      - Saponification of lipids in cornea
      - Bind mucoproteins and collagen
      - Coagulates blood vessels
      - Eyes will be red for a while then turn white→Necrosis, Blood vessel death
      - Continued effect
    - Common types of alkali chemicals: ammonia, lye, firecrackers, chlorine, cement

UVEITIS

Lab tests - to rule out
ESR - systemic inflammation
ANA - JRA
VDRL - active syphilis
FTA/ABS - previous syphilis
Chest X ray - sarcoids & TB
ACE - active sarcoids
PPD - TB
HLA B27

- **Epidemiology:**
  - Younger patients:
    - Congenital toxoplasmosis
    - Toxocariasis
    - HLA B27
    - Juvenile rheumatoid arthritis
    - Bechet's disease
  - Elderly patients:
    - Toxoplasmosis
    - Herpes zoster
    - Aphakic uveitis
- **Observation, inspection, techniques:**
  - Slit lamp optic section with max intensity – look for KP
  - Anterior chamber conical beam – look for cells/flare
  - Gonioscopy - look for PAS
  - Macula - look for cystoid macular edema
  - Dilated exam - look for posterior synechiae or vitritis
- Most common cause: Idiopathic
- **Non-granulomatous (NG):**
  - HLA B27 – **Ankylosing spondylitis**
    - Unilateral (all HLA B27), lower back pain, more common in males
  - HLA B27 – **Reiter's syndrome**
    - Keratitis & conjunctivitis, urogenital lesions, knee & ankle arthritis
    - "Can't see, can't pee, can't bend the knee"
  - HLA B27 – **Psoriatic arthritis**
  - HLA B27 – **Inflammatory bowel disease** (Crohn's Disease, Ulcerative Colitis)
  - **Juvenile rheumatoid arthritis (JRA)** – Bilateral, more common in white females
  - **Bechet's** – Bilateral, more common in Mediterranean & Japanese males, oral and genital ulcers
  - **Fuch's heterochromic iridocyclitis:**
    - Bilateral, Heterochromia – affected eye changes color, posterior subcapsular cataract
- **Granulomatous (G):**
  - (G) less symptoms than (NG)
  - **Sarcoidosis:**
    - African American, Scandinavian, more common in females
    - Pulmonary involvement
    - Unilateral or bilateral
    - Anterior uveitis
    - Posterior uveitis → candle wax drippings, choroidal granuloma, disc swelling, snowballs
  - **Tuberculosis**
  - **Syphilis:**
    - The great mimicker of ocular infections
    - Argyll Robertson pupils; skin rash of trunk, palm, or soles; fever; malaise
  - **Vogt-Koyanagi-Harada Syndrome (VKH):**
    - Japanese and heavily pigmented individuals
    - Vitiligo, poliosis, alopecia, hearing problems
    - Bilateral, chronic
- **Symptoms:**
  - Deep pain
  - Redness
  - Photophobia – When light on both ipsilateral and contralateral eye
  - Tearing
  - Acute (NG)

- **Signs:**
    - Circumlimbal injection - Bulbar > palpebral
    - Miosis:
        - Sphincter muscle spasm caused by release of prostaglandins in response to iris irritation
        - Differential →Conjunctivitis = normal pupil; acute angle closure = mid-dilated pupil
    - Keratic precipitates:
        - Inferior half of cornea, Arlt's triangle, White blood cells
        - Fine KP (NG), Mutton fat KP (G)
        - Diffuse stellate - Fuch's heterochromic iridocyclitis
    - Cells and flare
    - Hypopyon
    - Iris nodules→ pupillary Koeppe (NG), anterior iris Busacca (G)
- **Complications:**
    - Posterior synechiae
    - Peripheral anterior synechiae (Secondary glaucoma)
    - Band keratopathy
    - Cataracts
    - Corneal edema
    - Macular edema
    - Retinal detachment
- **Glaucomatocyclitic crisis (Posner –Schlossman)**
    - Symptoms: Blurred vision, lasts for few hours to 2 weeks
    - Signs: Unilateral, recurrent, dilated pupil, small KP, heterochromia
- **Posterior Uveitis**
    - Symptoms: No perilimbal injection, little or no pain
    - Signs:
        - Choroidal lesions – Focal, patchy yellow white areas of infiltrate
        - Vitritis
        - Retinitis
        - After resolution, chorioretinal scar
        - Visual field scotoma
- **Panuveitis:**
    - Entire uveal tract
    - Common causes:
        - Bechet's disease
        - VKH
        - Tuberculosis
        - Sarcoidosis
    - **Signs:** Mutton fat KP, Small pupils, possibly with posterior synechiae, Cell and flare, Iris nodules, Vitreal haze

Other Uveal Tract:

- Iris neovascularization (Rubeosis iridis)
    - Causes:
        - Diabetic retinopathy
        - CRVO
        - Chronic uveitis
        - Chronic retinal detachment
        - Tumors
        - Carotid occlusive disease
        - Sickle cell retinopathy
    - Observation, inspection, techniques:
        - IOP

- Careful iris examination with slit lamp
- Gonioscopy

OPTIC NERVE

- **Papilledema**
  - **Definition:** Bilateral optic nerve swelling associated with elevated intracranial pressure (cerebral spinal fluid) Normal CSF <200 mmH_2O
  - **Causes** (many other rare causes not listed):
    - Intracranial space occupying lesion → brain tumors, hemorrhage
    - Cardiovascular disorders → hypertension, CHF, emphysema
    - Infection & Inflammation → encephalitis, Meningitis
    - Toxicity → too much Vitamin A, tetracycline
    - Metabolic/Endocrine disorder → diabetic ketoacidosis, Addison's
    - Trauma
    - Pseudotumor cerebri → idiopathic elevated CSF, common in young, overweight females
  - **Mechanism:** Compression of optic nerve fibers by elevation in CSF leads to thickening of ganglion cell axons → disc swelling due to blockage of axoplasmic transport
  - **Symptoms:**
    - If nausea and vomiting, send to ER immediately = **EMERGENCY!**
    - Early stages → VA, pupils, color vision, and VF NOT affected
    - Late stage → impaired color vision, diplopia due to CNVI palsy, decreased VA, enlarged blindspot on visual field testing
  - **Signs:**
    - Bilateral
    - Asymmetric
    - Disc swelling → obscuration of margins, elevation
    - Disc hemorrhage (Flame shaped)
    - Disc hyperemia → dilated capillaries
    - CWS
    - Loss of spontaneous venous pulsation (SVP)
    - **Paton's lines** → circumferential wrinkles adjacent to disc
  - **Additional tests:** Blood pressure (Rule out systemic HTN), neurologic evaluation (MRI, CT), lumbar puncture
  - Benign differentials:
    - Persistent hyaloids tissue (Bergmeister's papilla)
    - Hyperopia
    - Optic nerve head drusen
    - Myelinated nerve fibers
  - **Complications** if untreated: Optic atrophy → blindness
- **Optic Neuritis:**
  - **Causes:**
    - Inflammation
    - Vascular disorder
    - Demyelination (MS)
  - **Multiple sclerosis:**
    - Epidemiology: Females, age 20-50
    - Systemic symptoms: Loss of balance, paraesthesia, tingling, numbness, weakness
  - **Symptoms:** Acute loss of vision, unilateral, periorbital or ocular pain, altered color vision, diplopia
  - **Signs:**
    - Disc swelling, disc hemes
    - Visual field defect (Variable)
    - APD in affected eye
    - **Uhthoff's sign** – worsening of symptoms with exercise or heat

        - CNS abnormalities: Numbness, paresthesia, weakness
    - Self-limiting → should resolve within a few months, emergency to rule out AION

- **Anterior Ischemic Optic Neuropathy (AION)**
    - **Mechanism:** Poor blood supply or occlusion of posterior ciliary arteries, which supply the optic nerve
    - **Epidemiology:**
        - Non-arteritic:
            - Age <70, more common in Caucasians
            - Incidence: 2 to 10 out of 100,000 age >50
            - Female to male ratio 1.2:1
            - Risk factors: Hypertension, diabetes, heart attacks, smoking, small crowded ONH
        - Arteritic:
            - Age >70, Males
            - Incidence: 20 out of 100,000 age >50
            - Risk factors: Giant cell arteritis, polymyalgia rheumatica
    - **Giant cell arteritis (GCA):**
        - Ocular involvement up to 70% of cases
        - Systemic signs and symptoms:
            - Neck stiffness (highest correlation to GCA)
            - Jaw claudication, scalp tenderness, temporal pain, temporal artery swelling
        - Observation, inspection, techniques: Always dilate
        - Additional tests, ESR lab test, CSR lab test, Temporal artery biopsy
    - **Symptoms:**
        - Acute painless loss of vision, unilateral
        - Amaurosis fugax
        - Dyschromatopsia
        - Much more severe vision loss in arteritic type
    - **Signs:**
        - Disc swelling, disc hemorrhage, CWS
        - APD
        - Visual field defect → Arteritic – dense central scotoma; Non-arteritic – altitudinal
        - Late stage – Disc pallor and cupping
    - **Complications** if untreated
        - Arteritic → progression to blindness within 1-2 days, 70% involvement of contralateral eye within 1 week
        - Non-arteritic → better prognosis,15% involvement of contralateral eye within 5 years

---

RETINA

- **Retinal Detachment**
    - **Symptoms:** Acute onset of flashes or floaters, Dark curtain across field of view
    - Differential diagnosis:
        - Acquired retinoschisis. Rule out because retinoschisis is/has:
            - Usually bilateral, usually inferotemporal
            - No vitreal pigment, no vitreal hemorrhage
            - Snowflakes on inner retinal layers
        - Choroidal detachment. Rule out because:
            - Color
            - Solid appearance
            - Hypotony (↓ IOP)
- **Central retinal artery occlusion**
    - **Causes:** Emboli, GCA, vascular diseases

- **Symptoms:** Acute painless loss of vision, unilateral, amaurosis fugax
- **Signs:** White retinal edema, cherry-red spot in macula, arteriole attenuation

OTHER

- **Endophthalmitis:**
  - Infection of the entire eye
  - **Causes**: Surgery, trauma, secondary infection
  - Common organisms: *Staphylococcus epidermidis, Staphylococcus aureus, Streptococcus*
  - **Symptoms:** Rapidly decreased vision, pain
  - **Signs:** Hypopyon, vitritis
- **Vasovagal Syncope**
  - Patient faints during exam
  - May be unconscious for minutes to hours
  - Epidemiology: Usually late teens to 20s, patients with low blood pressure
  - Usually occurs during Instillation of drops, tonometry, smell of cleaning alcohol
  - Management:
    - Do not leave patient alone in room
    - Cold compress on back of neck
    - Head down, not back
    - Cold water

DIFFERENTIAL DIAGNOSIS FOR ER SYMPTOMS

- **Transient dimming of vision:**
  - Amaurosis Fugax →transient ischemic attack, lasts for few minutes to hours, unilateral
  - Migraine → Lasts 10-60 minutes
  - Optic nerve:
    - Papilledema → few seconds, bilateral
    - Optic nerve drusen
    - Anterior ischemic optic neuropathy
  - Cardiovascular
    - Vertebrobasilar artery insufficiency → bilateral
    - Arrhythmias
    - Cardiac valvular disease
    - Carotid occlusive disease vasospasm
    - Sudden change in blood pressure
  - CNS lesion
  - Orbital mass
- **Sudden, painless loss of vision:**
  - Retinal artery occlusion
  - Retinal vein occlusion
  - Anterior ischemic optic neuropathy
  - Vitreal hemorrhage
  - Retinal detachment
  - Stroke
  - Methanol poisoning
- **Burning sensation:**
  - Dry eye syndrome
  - Conjunctivitis
  - Blepharitis
  - Meibomitis
  - Inflamed pterygium/pinguecula
- **Sudden painful loss of vision:**
  - Acute angle closure glaucoma
  - Optic neuritis
  - Uveitis
  - Endophthalmitis

- Episcleritis
- Superior limbic keratoconjunctivitis

- **Diplopia:**
  - **Monocular:**
    - Refractive error
    - Corneal or lens opacity
    - Dislocated lens
    - Macular disease
    - Retinal detachment
    - CNS lesions
  - **Binocular:**
    - Myasthenia gravis (intermittent)
    - Cranial nerve palsy
    - Thyroid eye disease
    - Tumor
    - CNS lesion
    - Trauma
    - Internuclear ophthalmoplegia
- **Acute ocular pain:**
  - Dry eye syndrome
  - Corneal abrasion
  - Foreign body
  - Corneal erosion
  - Corneal ulcer
  - Anterior uveitis
  - Scleritis
  - Endophthalmitis
  - Acute angle-closure glaucoma
- **Periorbital/orbital pain:**
  - Preseptal or orbital cellulitis
  - Sinusitis
  - Dacryocystitis
  - Dermatitis → HSV or Zoster dermatitis, contact
  - Tumor
  - Optic neuritis
  - Diabetic cranial nerve palsy
  - Migraine
  - Referred pain → dental, sinus
- **Acute red eye**
  - Conjunctivitis
  - Keratitis
  - Recurrent corneal erosion
  - Foreign body
  - Endophthalmitis
  - Anterior uveitis
  - Episcleritis & scleritis
  - Angle closure glaucoma
  - Superior limbic keratoconjunctivitis

Chapter Questions

CHAPTER 1: OPTICS (GEOMETRICAL)

1. Your cycloplegic refraction reveals a 1.00D increase in myopia for a patient who already wears -2.00DS lenses in both eyes. What is the patient's far point?
   A. 1 m
   B. 50 cm
   C. 33 cm
   D. 25 cm
   E. 10 cm

2. You design a -5.00D achromatic doublet using ophthalmic crown glass (Abbe value=58.6) and polycarbonate (Abbe value=30). What is the power of the ophthalmic crown glass?
   A. -10.25 D
   B. +10.25 D
   C. -5.25 D
   D. +5.25 D
   E. -5.00D

3. A sphero-cylindrical lens has +3.00D and +2.00D along the two principal meridians. Where is the circle of least confusion located after the lens?
   A. 1 m
   B. 50 cm
   C. 40 cm
   D. 41.5 cm
   E. 33 cm

4. Your patient has a spectacle prescription of -3.50-1.50x180. You wish to fit her into a toric soft contact lens. If her vertex distance is 10 mm, what is her CL Rx?
   A. -3.75-1.00x180
   B. -3.75-1.00x090
   C. -3.50-0.75x180
   D. -3.50-1.25x180
   E. -3.50-1.00x180

5. Find the focal length of a positive thin lens if the distance of the real object and real image are 90 cm and 45 cm.
   A. 3.33 m
   B. 3.0 m
   C. 0.30 m
   D. 0.03 m
   E. 0.003 m

6. You induce marginal (oblique) astigmatism when you:
   A. decenter a spherical lens
   B. tilt a spherical lens
   C. rotate a spherical lens around optical axis
   D. move a spherical lens closer to the eye
   E. move a spherical lens farther from the eye

7. Your patient's polycarbonate lens has a sag of 0.2mm. What is the dioptric reading on a standard Geneva lens clock (separation between the two stationary pins is 20.8mm)
   A. 5.86D
   B. 2.17D
   C. 3.69D
   D. 1.93D
   E. 1.87D

8. A thick lens (n=1.5) with a center thickness of 2cm has a +6.00D front surface and a -4.00D back surface. If an object is at optical infinity, where is the image located? Assume the lens and object are in air?
   A. 39.7 cm in front of the back surface
   B. 39.7 cm behind the back surface
   C. 64.3 cm in front of the back surface
   D. 64.3 cm behind the back surface
   E. 25cm in front of the surface

9. To neutralize a patient's phoria, you placed a 4 base 060 in front of the OD and a 2 base 150 in front of the OS. What single prism placed in front of the OD eye would also neutralize this phoria?
   A. 4.47 base 33.2 deg OD
   B. 4.47 base 33.2 deg OS
   C. 3.35 base 87.1 deg OD
   D. 3.35 base 87.1 deg OS
   E. 3.25 base 33.2 deg OD

10. Your patient has a right hyperphoria. Using the Maddox rod red lens, you found 4 BD OD. You've decided to split the prism in half for each eye (2 pD per eye). The patient selects a frame that has an A dimension of 47 mm, DBL of 17mm, and B dimension of 38 mm. The prescription is: -2.75-1.25x180 OD and -3.25-1.75x180 OS. Where is the optical center with respect to the prism reference point (PRP) for the OD?

A. 4.0 mm above PRP
B. 4.0 mm below PRP
C. 5.0 mm above PRP
D. 5.0 mm below PRP
E. 4.5 mm below PRP

11. Your patient's phoria can be neutralized with a prism of 4 pD at base 060 over her left eye. If you were to neutralize the phoria during a cover test with loose prisms over her left eye, what combination would you use?

A. 2 pD BI, 3.5 pD BD
B. 2 pD BO, 3.5 pD BU
C. 3.5 pD BO, 2 pD BU
D. 3.5 pD BI, 2 pD BD
E. 2 pd BI, 3 pD BU

12. An object is placed at optical infinity in front of a lens with the power +2.00-1.00x180. Where is the circle of least confusion relative to the lens?

A. 33.3 cm
B. 50 cm
C. 66.7 cm
D. 75 cm
E. 100 cm

13. Last year, your patient was happy with her +8.00 D glasses. Your patient complains that her vision is not as sharp as it could be. However, she says her vision is impeccable if she tilts her glasses to produce a 020 deg pantoscopic tilt. What is MOST likely her new prescription?

A. +8.31-1.10x180
B. +8.31-1.10x090
C. +9.41-1.10x180
D. +9.41-1.10x090
E. +8.31+1.10x090

14. Your -4.00 D myopic patient has a pair of glasses where her optical center is 1.0 cm out and 0.75 cm up relative to the PRP. Cover test over her glasses reveals an orthophoria. If she took her glasses off, what prisms would you use to neutralize her phoria?

A. 4 BI, 3 BD
B. 4 BO, 3 BD
C. 4 BI, 3 BU
D. 4 BO, 3 BU
E. 3 BO, 3 BU

15. You prescribe 2 BO for your 8 year old patient. His mother selected a lens material of 1.60 with an Abbe value of 36. How much lateral chromatic aberration is present at the prism reference point?

A. 0.0556
B. 1.25
C. 0.0335
D. 0.1081
E. 0.1236

16. The human pupil limits the amount of light entering the eye. When we look at someone's pupil, we are actually seeing an image of the pupil. This image is the:

A. exit pupil
B. entrance pupil
C. aperture stop
D. field stop
E. ramsden circle

17. You want to design a +10.00 D achromatic doublet using ophthalmic crown glass (Abbe= 58.6) and dense flint glass (Abbe= 36.6). What power lenses would you choose for the crown glass?

A. +26.64 D
B. -16.64 D
C. -26.64 D
D. +16.64 D

18. A +5.00 D thin lens separates air from a media with n=1.5. An object is placed 50 cm in front of the lens. Which of the following is true about the image?

A. real, inverted
B. real, right-side up
C. virtual, inverted
D. virtual, right-side up
E. none of the above

19. Which of the following instruments uses a telescopic system?

A. indirect ophthalmoscope
B. direct ophthalmoscope
C. lensometer
D. slit lamp
E. retinoscope

20. A +7.00 D lens has a real object located 20 cm from the lens. The conjugate image is:

A. real and located 50 cm from the lens
B. virtual and located 50 cm from the lens
C. real and located 8.30 cm from the lens
D. virtual and located 8.30 cm from the lens
E. real and located 14.30 cm from the lens

CHAPTER 2: OPTICS (PHYSICAL)

1. An anti-reflective coating of an unknown material is used on a spectacle lens. If the thickness of the coating is 100 nm, what is the index of refraction (assume that 555 nm light is hitting the lens)?

A. 1.38
B. 1.66
C. 1.33
D. 1.45
E. 1.56

2. A hyperope looks through his +5.00DS thin lens with a diameter of 3 mm. He can barely resolve two distant point objects illuminated by 600 nm light. How many wavelengths apart are these two points?

A. 4
B. 3
C. 80
D. 12
E. 8

3. 600 nm light in a vacuum enters medium wherein the light reduces to 500 nm. What is the velocity of light in the medium?

A. 5.0×10^8 m/s
B. 1.2×10^8 m/s
C. 3.0×10^8 m/s
D. 1.0×10^8 m/s
E. 2.5×10^8 m/s

4. A ray of light incident on a surface (that is in air) has an angle of 30 degrees. A ray emerges at an angle 45 degrees from the normal. What is the index of refraction of the surface?

A. 1.41
B. 1.00
C. 1.52
D. 0.707

5. A +5.00D surface (n=1.45) is adjacent to water. If an object is placed in the water 15cm in front of the surface, where is the image located?

A. 37.5 cm in front of the surface
B. 37.5 cm in back of the surface
C. 86.9 cm in front of the surface
D. 86.9 cm in back of the surface
E. 63.1 cm in back of the surface

6. Waves can be added together by their amplitudes. If the 2 waves are in phase, what occurs?

A. Diffraction
B. constructive interference
C. destructive interference
D. reflection
E. refraction

7. A screen is held 2 m from an aperture with a 0.1 mm slit. What is the separation between the maxima for a wavelength of 500 nm?

A. 0.1 cm
B. 1 cm
C. 1.5 cm
D. 2 cm
E. 2.3 cm

8. Which of the following in theory perfectly absorbs all radiant energy?

A. Maxwell's spot
B. Phosphene
C. black body radiator
D. gray body radiator
E. Purkinje tree

9. What is the radiant energy emitted per unit time (units in watts)?

A. radiant intensity
B. radiant flux
C. irradiance
D. radiance
E. diffraction

10. A lens is made of glass with a refractive index of 1.65. What would be the refractive index for the ideal anti-reflection coating?

A. 1.28
B. 1.34
C. 1.41
D. 1.49
E. 1.65

11. A lens is made of glass with a refractive index of 1.65. What would be the refractive index for the ideal anti-reflection coating?

A. 1.28
B. 1.34
C. 1.41
D. 1.49
E. 1.65

12. The portion of the spectrum called blue-green by normals is MOST readily confused with the white portion for which of the following types of observers?

A. Trichromats
B. Deuteranopes
C. Tritanopes

13. Young's Double Slit Experiment:
What is the separation between maxima for an aperture with a 0.1mm slit spacing and light of a wavelength of 500nm when the screen is held at a distance of 2 meters?

A. 0.01cm
B. 0.1cm
C. 1cm
D. 10cm
E. 100cm

14. Thin Film Interference
Two flat microscope slides, 10cm long are touching on one side and are separated by 3 microns on the other. How many dark interference bands will appear on the slide if you look at the reflection for 450nm light?

A. 11 bands
B. 12 bands
C. 13 bands
D. 14 bands
E. 15 bands

15. An eye under the influence of an extremely strong miotic agent has a pupil diameter of 1 mm. The resolution of this eye is considered to be limited by:

A. radial astigmatism
B. coma
C. diffraction
D. spherical aberration
E. depth of focus

16. Limits of Resolution
A diffraction-limited eye with a 6mm pupil is looking at an approaching car whose headlights have a wavelength of 550nm and are separated by 1.5m. What is the minimum angular resolution of the eye?

A. 0.00011183 minutes of arc
B. 0.00011183 degrees
C. 0.0064 minutes of arc
D. 0.0064 degrees
E. 0.384 minutes of arc

17. At what distance can you no longer resolve two distinct headlights?

A. at the patient's near point
B. 5.7 miles
C. 8.4 miles
D. 13.412 miles
E. at infinity

18. A slit of width 0.5mm is illuminated with 633nm light. At what angular location is the first minimum observed in the single slit diffraction pattern on a distant screen?

A. 1.27x10-6 radians
B. 1.27x10-5 radians
C. 1.27x10-4 radians
D. 1.27x10-3 radians
E. 1.27x10-2 radians

19. Where is the location of the minimum if the screen is 10m away from the slit?

A. 0.0127cm
B. 0.127cm
C. 1.27cm
D. 12.7cm
E. 127cm

20. A 71-year-old monocular low vision patient has a distance correction of +3.00 DS. Through a single +5.50 DS lens in the trial frame, he can barely read 2M print at 40 cm. What is the SMALLEST print you should expect him to barely read at a distance of 20 cm, through a total lens power of +8.00 DS in the trial frame?

A. 0.6M
B. 0.8M
C. 1.0M
D. 2.0M
E. 4.0M

CHAPTER 3: OPTICS (PHYSIOLOGICAL)

1. Which of the following aberrations cause image mislocation?
    A. spherical aberration
    B. coma
    C. astigmatism
    D. curvature of field
    E. diffraction

2. You are conducting a slit lamp evaluation of your patient who is here for a dilated eye exam. Which of the following structures that you see is not a refractive surface for the Gullstrand 1 exact eye model?
    A. anterior cornea
    B. anterior cortical lens
    C. anterior nuclear lens
    D. anterior surface of the vitreous
    E. posterior cornea

3. An eye under the influence of an extremely strong miotic agent has a pupil diameter of 1 mm. The resolution of this eye is considered to be limited by:
    A. radial astigmatism
    B. coma
    C. diffraction
    D. spherical aberration
    E. depth of focus

4. The Jackson crossed cylinder subjective test is begun with a -1.00 DS -1.75 DC x 090 lens in front of a patient's eye. If the correcting cylinder power is changed to -0.75DC x 090, then the spherical power should now be:
    A. -2.00 DS
    B. -1.50 DS
    C. -1.00 DS
    D. -0.50 DS
    E. +0.50 DS

5. A 21-year-old patient has a history of previously uncorrected simple hyperopic astigmatism of 3.00 D in each eye. Which of the following is MOST likely to be associated with the patient's refractive error?
    A. Eccentric fixation in one or both eyes
    B. Meridional amblyopia in both eyes
    C. Monocular central suppression
    D. Anomalous retinal correspondence
    E. Strabismus secondary to the uncorrected refractive error

CHAPTER 4: OPHTHALMIC OPTICS

1. Examination of a 15-year-old patient reveals the following:
Prescription:
OD: – 2.50DS -0.75DC x 090
OS: +3.25DS -0.50DC x 180
Keratometry:
OD 43.50D @ 180, 43.00D @ 090
OS 39.00DS

Which of the following spectacle lens designs should be the MOST effective in reducing aniseikonia for this patient?

	BC OD	CT OD	BC OS	CT OS
A	+3.75D	2.0mm	+7.50D	3.6mm
B	+3.75D	2.0mm	+3.75D	6.0mm
C	+5.25D	2.5mm	+7.50D	3.5mm
D	+6.25	3.4mm	+6.25D	3.4mm

2. A 22-mm round bifocal lens has a power of +2.00DS, Add +2.50D. What is the "jump" with this bifocal in prism diopters?
   A. 1.50
   B. 2.20
   C. 2.75
   D. 3.75
   E. 4.50

3. An executive bifocal has a base curve of +6.00D and a segment surface of +8.00 D. The ocular surface measures -5.00 D when a lens gauge is placed on it vertically, and -3.00 D when placed horizontally. The Rx is:
   A. +3.00 DS -2.00 DC x 090, Add +2.00 D
   B. +3.00 DS -2.00 DC x 090, Add +3.00 D
   C. +3.00 DS -2.00 DC x 180, Add +2.00 D
   D. +3.00 DS -2.00 DC x 180, Add +3.00 D
   E. +5.00 DS -4.00 DC x 180, Add +2.00 D

4. A convex mirror has a radius of curvature of 100cm. What is the secondary focal length of the mirror?
   A. 100cm in front of the mirror
   B. 100cm behind the mirror
   C. 50cm in front of the mirror
   D. 50cm behind the mirror
   E. At the center of curvature of the mirror

5. A +8.00D lens has a new 020 degree pantoscopic tilt. What's the new power, assuming the lens is made of ophthalmic crown glass?
   A. +7.28D
   B. +8.31D
   C. +8.89D
   D. +9.31D
   E. +9.89D

6. If the standard lens is +25.00D, how much and in which direction must the target be moved from the zero position, when measuring a -5.00D lens?
   A. 2mm toward the observer
   B. 2mm away from the observer
   C. 8mm toward the observer
   D. 8mm away from the observer
   E. Should not need to move target from the zero position

7. A 54mm round CR-39 lens has a c.t. of 2.0mm and Rx of -4.00DS. What is the edge thickness?
   A. 2.108mm
   B. 3.19mm
   C. 4.00mm
   D. 4.93mm
   E. 5.62mm

8. Which of the following would NOT be an option to correct for vertical prism effects?
   A. Slab off
   B. Dissimilar segments
   C. Increasing pantoscopic tilt
   D. Fresnel prisms
   E. Wearing contact lenses instead

9. If incident light is 100%, what is the transmission of a 3.0mm thick lens with a transmittance factor of 0.75/mm. The lens is CR-39, and it is in air.
   A. 36.7%37.8%
   B. 38.9%
   C. 40.1%
   D. 41.2%

10. Which of the following factors would NOT result in a darker photochromic glass lens?
   A. Cooler temperature
   B. Warmer temperature

C. Thicker lens
D. Heat tempered lens

11. Your patient's OS prescription is -6.75-1.50x135. She selects a frame with a 51 mm eye size. The lens is 51 mm round with an index of 1.60. The optical center is 24 mm from the nasal edge of the lens and the edge thickness is 5.3 mm. How thick is the temporal edge of the lens? Use the spherical equivalent.
A. 5.30 mm
B. 5.76 mm
C. 6.25 mm
D. 6.51 mm
E. 7.01 mm

12. You are using a lens clock calibrated for index of 1.70. You have a lens with the prescription +4.75-1.25x075. It is made with a material of index 1.70. What power would you measure along the plus axis?
A. +5.38 D
B. +4.75 D
C. +4.12 D
D. +3.96 D
E. +3.50 D

13. Your patient accidentally sat on her glasses, giving them a 25° pantoscopic tilt. Her prescription is -5.50DS and her glasses are made of index 1.60 mounted in a frame with a 10° pantoscopic tilt. How much additional cylinder is induced?
A. -1.09 DC
B. -1.26 DC
C. -1.34 DC
D. -0.95 DC
E. -0.17 DC

14. The lab makes the following lens prescription in minus cylinder form: -4.50-1.75x030. The lens is made of a material index 1.701. You measure a base curve of +4.00DS. What is the true surface power along the power meridian?
A. -5.95 D
B. -13.56 D
C. -10.25 D
D. -11.24 D
E. -8.50 D

15. The lab sends you a lens with an unknown back vertex power. The only parameters you have are: index of 1.60, front surface power of +8.00D, back surface power of -3.25D, and center thickness 3.5 mm. What is the back vertex power?
A. +4.75 D
B. +4.28 D
C. +4.89 D
D. +3.89 D
E. +3.56 D

16. A 60 year old presbyopic patient who has worn progressive lenses for many years is having difficulty reading through the lenses. You suggest the patient try FT28 bifocals. The prescription is:
OD:-6.25-1.75x180
OS:-5.75-1.25x180 Add:+2.25D
The lens segment top is 3 mm below the distance optical center (DOC) and the reading level is 10 mm below the DOC. Assume there is no segment decentration. What is the displacement at the reading level for the OD lens?
A. +1.125 BD
B. +0.45 BU
C. +0.43 BU
D. +0.43 BD
E. +0.53 BD

17. A patient needs to fill out the following prescription:
OD: +2.25+1.75x090, 2 BO
OS: +2.75+1.25x090, 2 BO Add: +2.75
He selects a frame 49□17. His PD is 63/59. He only wants the distance prescription in the frame. The lens material is 1.60 with an Abbe value of 36. The lens center thickness is 4.75 mm. Taking into account for the decentration of the lens to yield the prism, what is the IPD you would write on the lab order form?
A. 65 mm
B. 60 mm
C. 57 mm
D. 73 mm
E. 81 mm

18. What is the separation of the two outer pins of the generic brand lens clock if the center pin moves 0.075 mm per 1D on the lens clock reading?
A. 17.83 mm
B. 16.28 mm
C. 15.34 mm
D. 16.53 mm
E. 20.30 mm

19. A lensometer measures the power of a lens to be +1.50DS. A lens clock calibrated for CR-39 measures +4.50DS on the front surface and -3.50 on the back surface. What is the refractive index of the lens material?

A. 1.498
B. 1.523
C. 1.58
D. 1.75
E. 1.70

20. A polycarbonate lens has a spherical back surface. The sag of the concave back surface is 2.8mm with a chord length of 50.0mm. What is the power of the back surface?

A. -5.00D
B. -5.25D
C. -5.50D
D. -5.81D
E. -6.12D

21. A -5.00D myope selects a frame with a 52mm eye size. The lab provides you with a CR-39 lens with a 2.0mm center thickness. Assuming the patient's pupils are centered at the frame geometric center, what do you expect the edge thickness of the finished lens to be?

A. 4.35mm
B. 4.67mm
C. 4.91mm
D. 5.23mm
E. 5.39mm

22. If a frame is selected with the following boxed dimensions: A=54mm, B=48mm, DBL=16mm, distance PD=60 mm, and the optical center is at the prism reference point, what is the minimum blank size?

A. 59mm
B. 64mm
C. 67mm
D. 70mm
E. 72mm

23. For the following prescription: -4.50-1.50x090, if the lens diameter is 52 mm round, center thickness=1.8mm, n=1.60, and optical center is at geometric center, what is the temporal edge thickness?

A. 5.18mm
B. 5.23mm
C. 5.34mm
D. 5.67mm
E. 6.45mm

24. An OD lens 55 mm round is made with 2 BI prism. If the temporal edge of this CR-39 lens is 0.5mm thick, what is the nasal edge thickness?

A. 2.709mm
B. 2.813mm
C. 2.645mm
D. 2.13mm
E. 2.209mm

25. Which of the following are not examples of temple styles?

A. riding bow
B. library
C. comfort cable
D. keyhole
E. skull

26. You decide to prescribe today's refraction: -4.50-1.50x090. Your patient chooses a frame with a 52 mm round eye size. The parameters for the lens are: center thickness=1.8mm, n=1.60, and optical center is at geometric center, what is the edge thickness 30 deg from the power meridian?

A. 4.97mm
B. 4.86mm
C. 5.45mm
D. 5.03mm
E. 5.89mm

27. A 34 year-old male engineer presents with a complaint of very slight distance blur with his glasses. You neutralize his glasses and find +2.50D OU. He said that he managed to obtain clear vision by moving his glasses 5mm closer to his eyes. However, he prefers the glasses to sit at their original spot on his nose. What do you predict is his new prescription?

A. 2.47 D
B. 2.53 D
C. 2.58 D
D. 2.62 D
E. 2.76 D

28. What is the focal power of a convex mirror (n=1.80) in air with a radius of curvature of 30 cm?

A. -12D
B. +12D
C. -6D
D. +6D
E. +3D

29. The patient selects a frame with a 52 mm round eye size. You tell the lab that you want a lens with center thickness=1.8mm, n=1.60, and optical center is at geometric center. Your patient's prescription is -4.50-1.50x090. What is the superior edge thickness?

A. 5.18mm
B. 4.34mm
C. 4.23mm
D. 5.67mm
E. 4.89mm

30. Which of the following lens material will have the least amount of lateral chromatic aberration for a given power?

A. ophthalmic crown glass
B. CR-39
C. Polycarbonate
D. highlite glass
E. Hi-index plastic (Abbe=37)

Questions from NBEO

31. A 22-mm round bifocal lens has a power of +2.00 DS, Add +2.50 D. What is the "jump" with this bifocal in prism diopters?

A. 1.50
B. 2.20
C. 2.75
D. 3.75
E. 4.50

32. An Executive bifocal has a base curve of +6.00 D and a segment surface of +8.00 D. The ocular surface measures -5.00 DS when a lens gauge is placed on it vertically, and -3.00 D when placed horizontally. The Rx is:

A. +3.00 DS -2.00 DC x 090, Add +2.00 D
B. +3.00 DS -2.00 DC x 090, Add +3.00 D
C. +3.00 DS -2.00 DC x 180, Add +2.00 D
D. +3.00 DS -2.00 DC x 180, Add +3.00 D
E. +5.00 DS -4.00 DC x 180, Add +2.00 D

33. A 53-year-old male complains of occasional blur at distance and near. His visual acuities are 20/30 in each eye at distance and near with his present lens correction of OU +1.00 DS, Add +1.75 D. Your distance refraction for 20/20+ acuity is OU +1.50 DS. The BEST tentative Add for the new prescription will have a power of:

A. +1.25 D
B. +1.75 D
C. +2.25 D
D. +2.50 D

34. Examination of a 15-year-old patient reveals the following:

Prescription: OD -2.50 DS -0.75 DC x 090
OS +3.25 DS -0.50 DC x 180
Keratometry: OD 43.50D @ 180, 43.00D @ 090
OS 39.00 DS
Which of the following spectacle lens designs should be the MOST effective in reducing aniseikonia for this patient?
Base Curve OD Center Thickness OD
Base Curve OS Center Thickness OS

A. +3.75 D, 2.0 mm, +7.50 D, 3.6 mm
B. +3.75 D, 2.0 mm, +3.75 D, 6.0 mm
C. +5.25 D, 2.5 mm, +7.50 D, 3.5 mm
D. +6.25 D, 3.4 mm, +6.25 D, 3.4 mm

CHAPTER 5: CONTACT LENSES

1. Upon refraction, you found out that your patient has -5.00 DC of with-the-rule astigmatism, Keratometry, however, only found -0.50 DC of with-the-rule astigmatism. Your instructor told you to put a spherical RGP with base curve close to the flat meridian on patient's eye. What kind of fluorescein pattern do you expect to see?
   A. Vertical band of green pooling
   B. Horizontal band of green pooling
   C. Minimal apical clearance (MAC)
   D. Excessive apical touch

2. During proficiency testing, you were told to determine the parameters of an unknown RGP lens. What equipment would you use?
   A. Lensometer, contact lens loupe, radiuscope.
   B. Lensometry, topography
   C. Topography, lensometer, radiuscope
   D. Autorefractor

3. Your contact lenses patient came to see you with a red eye. She stated that she has been using home-made contact lenses solution that is preservative free! You should be expecting to see the following finding:
   A. follicular reaction on the palpebral conjunctiva, watery eyes, conjunctival injection
   B. cells and flare in anterior chamber, vitritis
   C. green discharge, cornea edema, guttata
   D. macular edema, cornea edema, lid chemosis

4. You have an emergency walk in. Patient has severe eye pain immediately after he inserted his contact lenses into his eyes after rinsing with the new solution he bought. He just started using a hydrogen peroxide cleaning solution last night after he got the solution on sale in Target. What seemed to be the problem?
   A. Patient had a hypersensitivity to the solution
   B. Patient had an episode of recurrent corneal erosion
   C. Patient didn't properly neutralize the solution prior to insertion
   D. The solution was on sale. It had poor quality control.

5. You see a ring infiltrate on your patient's cornea. Your patient expressed that he is in extreme pain. He wears soft contact lenses. Although unlikely to occur with proper contact lenses cleaning regimen, what kind of solution is the patient most likely been using?
   A. Chlorobutanol
   B. Thimerosal
   C. Hydrogen peroxide
   D. Polyquad

6. Your patient has a huge corneal abrasion OD. You wanted to fit him with a bandage contact lenses, but what kind of lens materials should you go with?
   A. HDS
   B. Boston XO
   C. PMMA
   D. Hydrogel

7. During contact lenses evaluation, you observed that your patient's contact lenses had changed color and your patient reported that she has been taking antibiotics for an upper respiratory infection. Which medicine has she been taking?
   A. Tetracycline
   B. Prednisone
   C. Augmentin
   D. Brolene

8. For patients who are allergic to preservatives such as thimerosal and chlorhexidine, what are some of the corneal findings that you are expecting to see?
   A. Horner-Trantas dots
   B. Anterior chamber reaction
   C. Bleaching of the limbal blood vessels
   D. Diffuse keratitis

9. Mr. Lee started using a homeopathy eye drop for cataract treatment, which was preserved in Benzalkonium chloride (BAC). He felt that his hydrogel contact lenses had become significantly uncomfortable after he started using the eye drops. What is most likely the cause?

A. Dry eyes
B. Cataracts are getting worse
C. Hydrogel
D. BAC was absorbed into the hydrogel lenses

10. After you started to use lens lubricant while wearing contact lenses, you feel the world is so much sharper and cleaner. What property of the lubricant can be used to explain for this?

A. Your dry eyes have been treated with lubricant
B. Lens lubricants has polyquad cleaning agent
C. It was mental; placebo effect.
D. Lens lubricant contains a low concentration of nonionic surfactant

11. A patient is wearing a -2.00 DS RGP trial lens. The overrefraction is -0.50 DS and you decide to steepen the base curve by 0.75 diopters. What power contact lens should you order?

A. -1.75 DS
B. -3.25 DS
C. -2.25 DS
D. -0.75 DS

12. Consider this patient. Spectacle Rx: -3.00-3.00x 090. Keratometry: 46.50 @ 180, 45.50 @ 090. An RGP has P= -5.00 and Base Curve 45.00. What is the expected overrefraction?

A. +1.75-0.25 x 090
B. +1.50-1.00 x 090
C. -0.50-0.50 x 180
D. +3.50-3.50 x 180

13. Which of the following solutions is most appropriate for a hydrogel contact lens?

A. Polyquad
B. Benzalkonium chloride
C. Chlorobutanol
D. Hydrogen Peroxide

14. A patient is wearing a +5.00 RGP. The Over-refraction is -1.25 DS, and you decide to flatten the base curve by 1.00 D. What power contact lens should you order?

A. +7.25 DS
B. +4.75 DS
C. +2.75 DS
D. +5.25 DS

15. A patient's spectacle prescription is +4.00-2.75 x165, and the trial lens you place on the patient's right eye is rotated 15 degrees nasally. What power contact lens should you prescribe?

A. +3.50-2.75 x 180
B. +4.25-2.75 x 180
C. +4.50-2.50 x 150
D. +4.25-3.00 x 150

16. A patient's spectacle prescription is -2.00-1.50 x035, and the trial lens you place on the patient's left eye has the prescription -2.00-1.50 x 030, and it is rotated 5 degrees nasal. What power contact lens should you prescribe?

A. -2.00-1.50 x 045
B. -2.00-1.50 x 025
C. -2.00-1.50 x 035
D. -2.00-1.50 x 040

17. Consider this patient. Spectacle Rx: +7.00-3.50x 180. Keratometry: 41.50 @180, 44.00 @090. An RGP has P=+2.00 and Base Curve 42.00. What is the expected over-refraction?

A. +5.00-1.00 x 180
B. +4.50-3.00 x 180
C. +5.00-1.50 x 180
D. +5.50-1.87 x 180

18. A patient's contact lens prescription is -4.00-2.00x 175. The over-refraction is -1.00 DS, what should be the patient's spectacle prescription?

A. -4.75-1.75 x 175
B. -5.00-2.00 x 175
C. -3.00-2.00 x 175
D. -5.25-2.25 x 175

19. A patient is wearing an RGP with P=-5.75. Your over-refraction is +0.75, and you decide to flatten the base curve by 0.50 Diopters. What power contact lens should you order?

A. -5.50 DS
B. -7.00 DS
C. -4.50 DS
D. -6.00 DS

20. An RGP wearer has keratometry readings of 46.25 @180, 47.00 @090. He is wearing an

RGP with P=-5.00 DS and base curve 45.00. What would be the most appropriate soft contact lens prescription for this patient?

A. -6.25-0.75 x 180
B. -5.75-0.75 x 180
C. -3.00-0.75 x 090
D. -5.75-0.75 x 090

21. A patient is wearing an RGP with P=+3.00 DS. The over-refraction is -4.25 DS and you steepen the base curve by 0.75 DS. What RGP lens should you prescribe?

A. -1.25 DS
B. -2.00 DS
C. -0.50 DS
D. +6.50 DS

22. A patient's contact lens prescription is +3.50-0.75 x 010. The over-refraction is +0.75 DS. What is the patient's spectacle prescription?

A. +4.00-0.50 x 010
B. +4.25-0.75 x 010
C. +4.50-1.00 x 010
D. +4.50-0.75 x 010

23. A patient's spectacle prescription is -1.00-4.00x 085. The over-refraction is -0.75 DS, and the contact lens is rotated 5 degrees temporally on the right eye. What contact lens should you prescribe?

A. -1.00-3.75 x 090
B. -1.75-3.75 x 090
C. -1.75-3.75 x 080

24. A patient's spectacle prescription is +1.00-2.25x 090 and his keratometry readings are: 43.50@180, 46.00 @ 090. The RGP he is wearing has P=-3.00 and base curve 43.00. What is the expected over-refraction?

A. +7.00-4.75 x 090
B. +1.25-0.25 x 180
C. +5.25-4.75 x 090
D. +3.50-2.00 x 180

25. A patient's contact lens prescription is -6.75-2.25 x 045. The over-refraction is -0.25 DS. What should the patient's spectacle prescription be?

A. -7.50-2.00 x 045
B. -7.50-2.25 x 045
C. -7.00-2.25 x 045
D. -7.50-2.50 x 045

26. Which type of aberration is most likely to be induced by contact lenses?

A. spherical aberration
B. coma
C. chromatic
D. tilt

27. Which has the highest index of refraction (n)?

A. an RGP
B. the cornea
C. the tear film
D. the calibration of the keratometer

28. A patient's RGP prescription is +3.50 DS with a base curve of 42.50 D. Her keratometry readings are: 41.75 @180, 44.00 @090. The over-refraction is +0.75. What is the patient's spectacle prescription?

A. +5.75-2.25 x 180
B. +5.50-2.00 x 180
C. +4.75-2.00 x 180
D. +6.50-2.25 x 090

29. A patient's RGP prescription is -2.25 DS with a base curve of 46.00. His keratometry readings are: 44.75 @180, 47.75 @ 090. The over-refraction is+0.75. What is the patient's spectacle prescription?

A. -0.25-3.00 x 180
B. -1.75-3.00 x 090
C. +0.25-3.00 x 180
D. -1.50-1.50 x 090

30. Which drug is most contraindicated while wearing hydrogel contact lenses?

A. pilocarpine
B. latanoprost
C. epinephrine
D. betaxolol

CHAPTER 6: LOW VISION

1. A stenopaic slit is used to test the eye of a patient with astigmatism. When the slit is held vertically, the patient needs +1.00D to see clearly. When the slit is held horizontally, the

patient needs +2.00D to see clearly. What is the Rx normally needed to correct this patient's vision in minus cyl form?

A. +2.00 -1.00x180
B. +1.00 +1.00x090
C. +2.00 -1.00x090
D. +1.00 -1.00x180
E. +2.00 +1.00x180

2. Your patient brings in a telescope but has no idea what type it is but would like you to prescribe another identical one for his brother. What characteristics would allow you to identify if it is a Galilean or Keplarian?

A. Keplarians are short, light, and have a brighter erect image than Galilean TS
B. Keplarians are long, heavy, and have a dimmer inverted image than Galilean TS.
C. Keplarians are short, heavy, and have a dimmer erect image than Galilean TS.
D. Keplarians are short, light, and have a brighter inverted image than Galilean TS.
E. Keplarians are short, heavy, and have a dimmer inverted image than Galilean TS.

3. Your patient comes in complaining about having trouble using her "Design for Vision" microscopic lens. She says that the images she is seeing are blurry and makes it difficult to use daily. What is your first suggestion to reduce this problem?

A. Microscopic lenses are high minus lenses so aberrations can be reduced using a higher index material.
B. Microscopic lenses are high minus lenses so aberrations can be reduced using an aspheric surface.
C. Microscopic lenses are high plus lenses so aberrations can be reduced using a higher index material.
D. Microscopic lenses are high plus lenses so aberrations can be reduced using an aspheric surface.

4. Your low vision patient wants you to determine a reading Rx for him. His distance VA is 20/100, his near VA is 0.4/2M, preferred working distance is 21cm and he wants to read the equivalent of a 20/30 letter up close. Which would be the best way to determine the necessary add?

A. Kestenbaum: 20/100 = 5.00 add = 5.00D
B. Kestenbaum: 20/100 = 0.4/2M, wants 0.4/0.6M = ~3x mag desired = 12.00D add
C. Kestenbaum: 20/100 = 5x improvement, current working distance 21cm → bring material to 4cm
D. Bailey: 0.6M print at 21cm, currently reads 2M (~3x increase) --> new distance 7cm --> F = 1/0.07m
E. Bailey: 1M print at 21cm, currently reads 2M (~2x increase) → new distance ~10cm → P = 1/0.1m

5. Your suspect your patient has congenital achromatopsia. Which of these statements is most likely true if your suspicion is right?

A. Black letters on a white background will vary exponentially with log luminance up to 10mL
B. Black letters on a white background will vary linearly with log luminance up to 10mL
C. Black letters on a white background will reach max VA at a low luminance and with further increase in retinal illumination, the VA will continue to fall.
D. Black letters on a white background will reach max VA at a high luminance and with further increase in retinal illumination, the VA will continue to rise.
E. Black letters on a white background will reach max VA at a low luminance and with further increase in retinal contrast, the VA will continue to rise.

6. In the magnification equations (**M = I'/I = h'/h = L/L'**), which of these variables is not listed correctly?

A. H' = object height
B. I = object distance
C. L' = emerging vergence
D. L = incident vergence
E. I' = image distance

7. Which is NOT true about the definition of low vision?

A. About 0.2% of the population is legally blind but 85% of this population have some useful vision left.
B. 87% of the legally blind are over 60yo.

C. Almost a third of people over age 80 are legally blind.
D. Generally after age 50, the majority of low vision patients are female.
E. Reduced peripheral acuity to less than 20/100 can be classified as legally blind.

8. Which of the following statements is NOT true about the Bailey-Lovie chart?
A. Each row is of equal difficulty.
B. Letter spacing is not proportional, making it less desirable than a Snellen chart.
C. There are always the same # of letters on each line.
D. There is a log regression of letter size for easy conversion.

9. Which notation is preferred by ophthalmology compared to optometry but runs the risk of non-standardization?
A. Jaeger
B. M notation
C. N notation
D. Snellen
E. Point units

10. The best test to identify a macular defect would be...
A. Red cap test
B. FDT
C. Amsler grid
D. Tangent screen
E. Photostress test

11. Today is Jose's first low vision exam. He is one of the 109,000 Americans who are visually impaired. His mother is wondering what the chances are of Jose being legally blind based on population percentiles and how many other Americans are like Jose.
A. 0.1%, 10,900
B. 0.5%, 54,500
C. 0.2%, 21,800
D. 0.1%, 10,750
E. 0.2%, 24,750

12. A 71-year-old monocular low vision patient has a distance correction of +3.00DS. Through a single +5.50DS lens in the trial frame, he can barely read 2M print at 40 cm. What is the SMALLEST print you should expect him to barely read at a distance of 20cm, through a total lens power of +8.00 DS in the trial frame?
A. 0.6M
B. 0.8M
C. 1.0M
D. 2.0M
E. 4.0M

13. Lauren's mom is a low vision patient due to some very dense cataracts. Lauren is worried that she might also be a low vision patient someday because of her close genetic connection with her mother. Your advice to Lauren would be:
A. That she is at much greater risk and should always wear sunglasses when outside to significantly lower her chances of getting cataracts.
B. That she is at much greater risk and wearing sunglasses won't really decrease her chances of getting cataracts.
C. That there isn't a strong genetic component for cataracts but she should always wear sunglasses when outside to significantly lower her chances of getting cataracts.
D. That there isn't a strong genetics component for cataracts and wearing sunglasses won't really decrease her chances of getting cataracts.

14. Raquel is a low vision patient that comes into your office wanting to be able to read her Bible print. You don't have a Bible at the office but you do have a standard newspaper. She is confident that her Bible print is half the size of standard newspaper print. Raquel can read 1M print at 20 cm with a 2X magnifier. What strength of magnifier will she need to read the Bible print at 20 cm?
A. 10x
B. 6 x
C. 4 x
D. 2 x

15. What is the size of print in M units if it subtends a 15' of arc at 6 meters?
A. 6M

B. 12M
C. 18M
D. 3M
E. 2M

16. A visual acuity of 20/600 is a MAR of what?
A. 35
B. 30
C. 25
D. 20
E. 15

17. If a patient can read 12.5M print at 25 cm, how close does this patient have hold 8M print to be able to read it?
A. 15 cm
B. 16 cm
C. 12.5 cm
D. 18 cm
E. 10 cm

18. Your patient has a constant, long standing superior field defect in her right eye. What treatment option would you offer her?
A. Patch OS and force OD to practice for neural development
B. Use a Fresnel prism over the entire left eye, base down.
C. Use a Fresnel prism over the bottom part of the left eye, base down.
D. Use a Fresnel prism over the entire right eye, base up.
E. Use a Fresnel prism over the top part of the right eye, base up.

19. One of your patients is using a collimating lens. He says the power is sufficient but feels like he is "looking through a straw" instead having a nice wide field of vision. You observe him using the lens about 10 cm away from his eye. You don't want to change the focal length of the telescope. What is one thing you could change to allow him a wider field of view?
A. Power of the objective lens
B. Power of the ocular lens
C. Larger lens diameter
D. Greater telescope EVP

20. A CCTV video-magnifier gives an image that is enlarged by 8x. If the patient is viewing a screen 125 cm what is the Equivalent Viewing Distance?
A. 16.43
B. 1000
C. 1.5625
D. 15.625
E. 1.643

21. A patient with a +2.50 D add, reads 4M print at 32 cm. The pt would like to be able to read a telephone book (0.8M print). A low vision aid would have to provide what EVD in order for the patient to read the telephone book clearly?
A. 6.4 cm
B. 3.7 cm
C. 10 cm
D. 25 cm

22. Which of the following characteristics is similar in both a Galilean and a Keplerian (Astronomical) telescopes?
A. Length
B. Cost
C. Weight
D. Image brightness
E. Image Orientation (erect/ inverted)
F. coincidence of the secondary and primary focal points

23. Your patient has advanced glaucoma and now needs a magnifier. Would it be better to suggest a Keplerian (astronomical) or a Galilean telescope and why?
A. Galilean because it offers the wider field of view
B. Galilean because it offers the smaller field of view
C. Keplerian (astronomical) because it offers the wider field of view
D. Keplerian (astronomical) because it offers the smaller field of view

24. Which of the following is not an example of a distance vision chart?
A. AMA
B. Sloan
C. Feinbloom
D. Bailey-Lovie
E. Greenwich

25. Which of the following is not an advantage of the Bailey-Lovie visual acuity chart?
A. Spacing is the same on each line
B. Follows a log progression down the chart
C. Chosen letters prohibit successful guessing
D. Contains British standard letters
E. Each row is of equal difficulty

26. What visual acuity qualifies a patient as low vision?
A. 20/200
B. 20/40
C. 20/60
D. 20/100

27. What is the length of a 10 x 50 Galilean telescope if the objective is +2D?
A. 0.62
B. 0.45
C. 0.34
D. 0.58

28. When using trial lenses to refract a low vision pt which procedure would be best?
A. Start from nothing and bracket with large dioptric values so as not to miss the endpoint and so that the patient can definitively make a lens selection
B. Start from retinoscopy or an old Rx and bracket with small dioptric values so as not to over prescribe.
C. Start from nothing and bracket with small dioptric values so as not to over prescribe.
D. Start from retinoscopy or an old Rx and bracket with large dioptric values so that the patient can definitively make a lens selection

29. A Galilean telescope with $P_{objective}$ = +5 and P_{ocular} = -20 is being used for distance vision. What is the distance from the objective to the ocular?
A. 0.12 m
B. 0.17 m
C. 0.15 m
D. 0.10 m
E. 0.40 m

30. Amar can just barely read 3.0M print at a distance of 30 cm. What is Amar's acuity?
A. 20/150
B. 20/100
C. 20/200

CHAPTER 7: ACCOMMODATION, VERGENCE AND OCULOMOTOR ANOMALIES

1. Choose the best answer to explain accommodation:
A. It is the natural tendency of the lens to flatten due to the elasticity of the capsule to allow for lens accommodation.
B. Accommodation occurs when the ciliary muscle relaxes, causing zonule relaxation allowing the lens to round up.
C. Accommodation is a passive process when the lens decreases its radius of curvature as the zonule relaxes. This tendency is held in check by normal tension on the zonules.
D. During accommodation, relative power of the eye decreases because lens radius of curvature decreases as the lens bulges forward.

2. If your patient came in with a partially dilated unilateral pupil and said he had "spilled some kind of eye drops in his left eye", which of the following would be your first logical conclusion for what kind of drop it was?
A. A sympathomimetic drug that acts on the iris dilator muscle in a localized fashion to partially dilate the pupil because the dilator muscle is arranged in spoke-like muscles.
B. A sympatholytic drug that acts on the iris sphincter muscle in a localized fashion to partially dilate the pupil because the sphincter is an all-or-nothing muscle.
C. A parasympathomimetic drug that acts on the iris sphincter muscle in a localized fashion to partially dilate the pupil because the sphincter is an all-or-nothing muscle.
D. A sympathomimetic drug that acts on the iris dilator muscle in a localized fashion to partially dilate the pupil because the dilator is arranged in individual spoke-like muscles.

3. If your patient exhibits a severe -4 underaction of their right lateral rectus (RLR) muscle as they turn both eyes to the right, what will you see and what normal law is this a violation of?

A. The right eye will continue to point towards the left since the RLR is normally responsible for abduction. This is a violation of Hering's Law which would indicate that the RLR should be equally yoked to the left medial rectus muscle to correctly compensate for rightward gaze.
B. The right eye will continue to point towards the right since the RLR is normally responsible for adduction. This is a violation of Sherrington's law of reciprocal innervation where the RLR and the RMR should be equally innervated and inhibited, respectively.
C. The right eye will continue to point towards the left since the RLR is normally responsible for adduction. This is a violation of Sherrington's law of reciprocal innervation where the RLR and the RMR should be equally innervated and inhibited, respectively.
D. The right eye will continue to point towards the left since the RLR is normally responsible for adduction. This is a violation of Fick's system because the eyes are moving along an x-axis without any movement in the y- or z-axes.

4. Your 5 year old patient exhibits some unusual eye movements that you suspect could be congenital nystagmus. Which of the following situations would most likely lead you to this conclusion?

A. The movements are pendular, fatiguing, and the patient does not appear to have a null point where the nystagmus is relieved. The patient appears to have normal visual acuity and be developmentally normal, as are most children with congenital nystagmus.
B. The movements are pendular and horizontal in primary gaze. Your patient appears to have a head turn about 15deg to the right and a slight head-bobbing movement which are both very common in congenital nystagmus.
C. The movements are fine, pendular, and rapid, and are often associated with strabismus. Your patient also has a head-bobbing movement that resembles spasmus nutans that is common in patients with congenital nystagmus.
D. The movements are rapid, reflexive, and repetitive in an attempt to foveate any previous head movement inaccuracy. Your patient also seems to be developmentally normal.

5. You suspect that your patient is an accommodative esotrope. Which of the following cases would most lead you to believe?

A. Your patient is a 3 year old male with an intermittent esotropia, high AC/A, and +5.50D refractive error.
B. Your patient is a 3 year old male with an intermittent large esotropia of 40pD and a +2.00 refractive error.
C. Your patient is a 3 year old male with a constant esotropia with varying severity in different fields of gazes and a +2.00 refractive error.
D. Your patient is a 3 year old male with a 6pD intermittent esotrope with reduced stereo and a small central scotoma.

6. Which is a true statement about accommodation?

A. During accommodation, the relative power of the eye increases because the radius of curvature of the anterior lens increases.
B. Accommodation usually occurs in response to a target with decreasing distance from the corneal surface.
C. The main stimulus for accommodation is foveal blur, leading to innervation of the ciliary muscle through short ciliary nerves.
D. Sympathetic innervation of the ciliary muscle via the short ciliary nerves causes contraction of the ciliary body, which can lead to accommodation.

E. The near reflex links accommodation to vergence only, indicating that vergence is the stimulus for accommodation.

7. If your patient has bilateral unequal eccentric fixation, which of the following is true?

A. They will not accommodate when asked to focus on a near target when one eye is covered.
B. Your patient also has anomalous retinal correspondence (ARC) since all patients with eccentric fixation have ARC.
C. You can use an attachment on your indirect ophthalmoscope to measure the degrees of eccentric fixation.
D. Their monocular acuity will be the same in both eyes since all points off the foveola result in the same acuity.
E. Your patient will always see double with both eyes open.

8. Which of the following is NOT a purpose for eye movements?

A. Yoking coordination of both eyes to fuse images.
B. Saccades to maintain eye position as the patient moves their head to the side.
C. Vergence system to align both visual axes and maintain binocular fixation.
D. Pursuit of objects to maintain the retinal image near or on the fovea.

9. Which of the following descriptions of eye movements is NOT correct?

A. The inferior oblique performs elevation, abduction, and extorsion.
B. **The lateral rectus performs abduction and elevation.**
C. The superior rectus performs elevation, adduction, and intorsion.
D. The inferior rectus performs depression, adduction, and extorsion.

10. Which of the following is NOT true about microsaccades?

A. They are small movements of 1-25 arc seconds.
B. They have relatively long durations up to 25msec.
C. They are moderately slow movements that move between 30-40deg/sec.
D. They are a type of fine fixational movements intended to keep the image foveated.

11. How much of their nominal length can EOMs expand and contract?

A. +/- 10%
B. +/- 20%
C. +/- 30%
D. +/- 40%

12. The full actions of the IO are:

A. Elevation, Abduction Intorsion
B. Elevation, Abduction, Extorsion
C. Elevation, Adduction, Intorsion
D. Elevation, Adduction, Extorsion

13. Which type of vergence eye movement is caused by the awareness of the nearness of a given object?

A. Tonic
B. Accommodative
C. Proximal
D. Fusional

14. The latency of vergence eye movements is:

A. less than VOR but greater than saccades
B. less than saccades and VOR
C. less than saccades but greater than smooth pursuits
D. greater than smooth pursuits and saccades

15. What are the three types of fine fixational movements?

A. Microtremors, Microdrifts, Microstrabismus
B. Microstrabismus, Microdrifts, Microsaccades
C. Microdrifts, Microstrabismus, Microsaccades
D. Microtremors, Microdrifts, Microsaccades

16. You diagnose your 2 year old patient with accommodative esotropia. Your optical treatment plan is:

A. Single vision reading glasses that correct the refractive error only
B. Single vision reading glasses that correct the refractive error and also include BO prism
C. Bifocals
D. Bifocals with BO prism for near

17. When examining the extraocular motility of a patient, you notice his left eye has reduced abduction and mildly restricted adduction movements as well. Additionally, his left eye tends to narrow upon medial gaze. The most likely diagnosis is:
A. LR palsy
B. Duane's Retraction Syndrome
C. Mobius Syndrome
D. Brown's Syndrome

18. You suspect your patient has Brown's Syndrome. Their eye movements would thus have:
A. elevation restriction in adduction
B. elevation restriction in abduction
C. equal elevation restrictions in abduction and adduction
D. diplopia

19. The following are true about nystagmus EXCEPT:
A. latent nystagmus occurs only when one eye is covered
B. nystagmus generally decreases with convergence
C. the null point refers to the refractive error that dulls the nystagmus
D. it is generally horizontal and pendular.

20. A patient with reduced NRA will most likely also have:
A. reduced convergence ranges
B. poor accommodation
C. reduced PRA
D. low AC/A

21. A patient is 1XP at distance and 5EP at 40cm. His PD is 57/54. What is his heterophoria at 33cm?
A. 8 eso
B. 6 eso
C. 5 eso
D. none of the above

22. Place in order the key points of the pathway that neurosignals take during constriction of the pupil after leaving the optic nerve:
I. Ciliary ganglion
II. Pretectal nucleus
III. Short ciliary nerve
IV. Edinger-Westphal nucleus
A. i, ii, iii, iv
B. iv, ii, i, iii
C. ii, iv, i, iii
D. iv, iii, i, ii

23. The eye movement with the slowest velocity is:
A. vergence
B. smooth pursuit
C. saccade

24. Your patient has been told by his wife that when he slowly closes his eyes to sleep, his eyes move upward and outwards. He is exhibiting:
A. Bruckner's Reflex
B. Bell's Phenomenon
C. Doll's Head Phenomenon
D. None of the above

25. The following are all characteristics of Spasmus Nutans EXCEPT:
A. jerk nystagmus
B. presents early in life
C. spontaneously resolves
D. can be associated with strabismus

26. Your patient tells you he has a brain tumor, but can't recall the location of the tumor. His OKN response is abnormal, which indicates a tumor in what brain region?
A. Frontal
B. Parietal
C. Temporal
D. Occipital

27. In which experimental method does the subject manipulate the stimulus?
A. Method of Limits
B. Method of Adjustments
C. Method of Constant Stimuli
D. Staircase Method

28. The following data was collected:

	Stimulus detected	Stimulus not detected
Stimulus present	7	3
No Stimulus	2	5

What is the hit rate?
A. 35%

B. 45%
C. 70%
D. 78%

Questions from NBEO

29. In performing the alternating cover test, a patient with normal correspondence reports that the target moves to the right and down as the right eye is uncovered and the left eye is covered. Which of the following deviations is MOST likely present?

A. Double hyper
B. Eso, right hyper
C. Eso, right hypo
D. Exo, right hyper
E. Exo, right hypo

30. The near point of accommodation (NPA) of a patient wearing a +1.25D add over his BEST distance correction is 19cm. If the Add is removed, the NPA would then be approximately:

A. 15cm
B. 20cm
C. 25cm
D. 30cm

31. A 65 year old patient had a cerebrovascular accident and now manifests strabismus. In testing the patient for correspondence, the MOST likely result would be:

A. unharmonious anomalous correspondence
B. harmonious anomalous correspondence
C. normal correspondence

CHAPTER 8: AMBLYOPIA/STRABISMUS

1. Which of these statements are true?

A. The Abney effect is associated with a change in photometric saturation that changes the psychological perception of hue.
B. The Abney effect is associated with a change in photometric hue that changes the psychological perception of saturation.
C. The Abney effect is associated with a change in psychological saturation that changes the psychological perception of purity.
D. The Abney effect is associated with a change in photometric saturation that changes the psychological perception of purity.

2. You suspect your patient is a protanope and you want to present them with two different wavelengths of light to identify if they have a color deficiency. Which statement is most true?

A. 520nm and 580nm since protanopes discriminate hue best above 520nm.
B. 494nm and 500nm since the protanopic neutral point is around 494nm.
C. None because protanopes do not have a color neutral point
D. 499nm and 505nm because protanopes have a neutral point around 499nm.

3. Which of these statements is false?

A. Complementary R + B + G = white
B. When primary colors red and green are mixed, you get yellow, which is sometimes considered a “psychological primary”
C. Complementary R + B = G
D. Complementary G + R = Y

4. Your patient comes in with some difficulties with monocular fixation for 10sec. You are concerned by the slight spring-like horizontal oscillations because... (pick the best answer):

A. opsoclonus is a less severe form of ocular flutter that can be associated with cerebellar disease.
B. ocular flutter can often occur randomly and is often associated with cerebellar disease.
C. square wave jerks are often mistaken with nystagmus and include unwanted saccades that are followed with a corrective saccade.
D. spasmus nutans is often present at birth and can disappear in the 4th -12th month of life.

5. Your patient has noticed a difference in the way he perceives the color of his favorite red sweatshirt. If you suspect red/green changes, what would be a practical next assumption?

A. He has experienced a retinal change since Kollner's rule states that acquired R/G changes are usually caused by retinal or lenticular changes.
B. Ishihara would be an inappropriate test to choose to confirm the severity of the change since Ishihara is only used for B/Y changes.
C. The desaturated D-15 test would be a good choice to use since it picks up even very subtle R/G changes.
D. His family history of glaucoma makes you concerned because glaucoma is often associated with R/G color changes.

6. The Bezold-Brucke effect states that:
A. Stimuli below 500nm (blue-green) appear more green as intensity increases.
B. The change in hue associated with a change in luminance.
C. Stimuli below 500nm appear more yellow when intensity increases.
D. The change in saturation with a change in luminance.

7. Which of the following is NOT true about hue?
A. Hue is a color sensation usually correlated with wavelength or a combination of wavelengths.
B. Hue discrimination is wavelength discrimination– the ability to distinguish a color from a neighboring color.
C. Hue discrimination is best at blue-green (490nm) and yellow-red (590).
D. Hue can be described as the photometric purity of a color.

8. Which is NOT true about the CIE color diagram?
A. The values for the visible spectrum range from 300-760nm.
B. Tristimulus values are the amounts of primary colors necessary to get your desired color.
C. If you take any two colors on the chromaticity diagram, the mixture of these will always be a point on a line between the two colors.
D. Two spectral wavelengths that can be mixed to match white are called complementary wavelengths.

9. Which of these statements about photoreceptors is FALSE?
A. S cones (short wavelength) - B cone 420 to 430nm.
B. M cones (middle wavelength) - G cones 535nm.
C. L cones (long wavelength) - R cones 565nm.
D. Cones have greatest sensitivity at green-yellow (555nm).
E. Rods have greatest sensitivity at green (505nm).

10. Sensory fusion requires a number of different factors. Which of these statements is not true?
A. Sensory fusion can be either color or form, but color fusion is understood to be less important.
B. If there is simultaneous perception or diplopia, no fusion occurs.
C. There can be flat fusion of two similar objects, resulting in true sensory fusion without stereopsis.
D. There can be stereopsis (second-degree fusion) occurs when there is a disparity between images that results in the perception of a three-dimensional object in visual space.

11. A male patient with an inherited color vision defect will most likely need what amount of luminance of a yellow stimulus in order to match the brightness of either a pure red or pure green stimulus:
A. A greater amount
B. An equivalent amount
C. A lesser amount
D. Cannot determine

12. You have correctly diagnosed a patient as an anomalous trichromat. This patient's neutral point is closest to which wavelength:
A. 494 nm
B. 499 nm
C. 570 nm
D. The patient has no neutral point

13. You find that as you add intensity to a stimulus of 580 nm, the stimulus appears more

yellow to a normal individual. This phenomenon illustrates the following principle:

A. Abney Effect
B. Bezold-Brucke Effect
C. Kollner Effect
D. Purdy Effect

14. Which of the following conditions violates Kollner's Rule?

A. Nuclear sclerosis
B. ARMD
C. Leber's optic atrophy
D. Primary Open Angle Glaucoma

15. A 75 year old color normal individual with no history of ocular trauma or surgery and with normal fundi would most likely have which pattern of defects on a Farnsworth D-15 test:

A. Deutan
B. Protan
C. Tritan
D. No pattern

16. Which of the following is most affected by nuclear sclerosis:

A. Simultaneous color contrast
B. Successive color contrast
C. Color contingent aftereffects
D. Color constancy

17. For which are the following patients would a color vision test be least indicated:

A. A 5-year old Caucasian male who has no problems his preschool class
B. A 65-year old African American female with complaints of bumping into fire hydrants
C. A 25-year old native American female with unequal VA's and a history of crossed eyes.
D. A 20-year old Caucasian male with an acute, painless loss of vision in his right eye.

18. You suspect your patient may have ARMD. What color vision test decide to administer:

A. Ishihara
B. Dvorine
C. Nagel anomaloscope
D. Farnsworth D-15

19. Which of the following conditions would be most detrimental to a patient trying to become certified as electrician:

A. Early cataracts
B. A genetic defect that prevents his body from producing erythrolabe
C. A genetic defect that causes the body to produce a mutated form of erythrolabe
D. Untreated strabismus

20. The Munsell Color System uses all the following attributes to describe the color, except:

A. Hue
B. Value
C. Wavelength
D. Chroma

21. A patient fixates eccentrically by five prism diopters, you expect her VA's to be:

A. 20/40
B. 20/80
C. 20/120
D. 20/160

22. You measure your patient's esotropia with an anomaloscope at H=+20. The subjective angle S=+15, and the anomalous angle A=+5. What is the best treatment method for this patient:

A. Base-out prisms
B. Plus lenses
C. Minus lenses
D. Leave well enough alone

23. When improving foveal resolution an amblyopic patient using a red lens coloring book:

A. The dominant eye should receive the red lens, so that the non-dominant eye can see the print
B. The non-dominant eye should receive the red lens, so that the dominant eye can see the print
C. The striations should be oriented on the dominant eye, vertically
D. The striations should be oriented on the non-dominant eye, vertically

24. Which of the following characteristics is not used to describe suppression:

A. Depth
B. Laterality
C. Size
D. Comitance

25. A rod monochromat being treated for esotropia will have trouble with which of the following vision therapy techniques:

A. Brock String
B. Tranaglyph
C. Aperture rule trainer
D. Vectograms

26. When measuring Hirschbergs, you find a 1.5 mm asymmetry. This corresponds to a deviation of:

A. 10 prism diopters
B. 15 prism diopters
C. 25 prism diopters
D. 30 prism diopters

27. Which of the following conditions has the poorest prognosis for amblyopia treatment:

A. Amblyopia due to anisometropia with age of onset at 12 months
B. Visual acuity of the deviating eye is 20/80, with eccentric fixation at three prism diopters
C. Eccentric fixation is steady and vertical
D. Suppression is present

28. Bifoveal stimulation would not be indicated in a patient with ARC when:

A. Visual acuity is greater than 20/40
B. The deviation is constant and comitant
C. HARC is present in free space
D. Angle H is less than 20 prism diopters

29. Your two year-old patient's mother reports that she noticed her daughter's eyes have been crossed since three months of age. The retinoscopy reveals a refractive error of +7.00 DS (OD) and +5.00 DS (OS). You might expect all of the following symptoms and signs except

A. Enlarged blind spot
B. Poor depth perception
C. Eye strain and headache
D. Photophobia

30. Your 15-year-old patient reports seeing one red light and one green light, simultaneously, when you administer a standard worth four-dot test, green lens over the right eye and red lens over the left eye. Your patient is probably:

A. Suppressing one eye
B. Demonstrating ARC
C. Demonstrating UARC
D. Malingering

CHAPTER 9: PERCEPTUAL FUNCTION/COLOR VISION

1. In a left superior oblique palsy, what would happen when using the Parks 3-Step method?

A. Left eye is deviated upward, deviation is greater in right gaze, and deviation is greater on left head tilt.
B. Right eye is deviated upward, deviation is greater in left gaze, and deviation is greater on left head tilt.
C. Left eye is deviated upward, deviation is greater in left gaze, and deviation is greater on right head tilt.
D. Right eye is deviated upward, deviation is greater in right gaze, and deviation is greater on right head tilt.

2. Which of the following is NOT a pictorial monocular depth cue?

A. Retinal image size
B. Elevation horizon
C. Linear perspective
D. Looming

3. Which form of myopia might contaminate the blur in the binocular refractive balance test?

A. Night myopia
B. Space myopia
C. Dark focus
D. Instrument myopia

4. Point A is directly in front of you. There is another point B that lies closer than A and is on a line between A and the right eye. You are asked to fixate A and then to fixate B. What happens to the right eye?

A. It does not move.
B. It first moves left and then right.
C. It first moves right and then left.
D. None of the above.

5. Your patient has normal binocular vision and is looking at a frontoparallel plane. You present a lens in front of the left eye that magnifies the

image in that eye vertically. How would the patient's perception of the plane change?

A. It would appear to be slanted left side near and right side far.
B. It would appear to be slanted right side near and left side far.
C. It would appear to be slanted top edge near and bottom edge far.
D. It would appear to be slanted top edge far and bottom edge near.

6. Which wavelength is most effective at bleaching rhodopsin?

A. 420 nm
B. 507 nm
C. 555 nm
D. 610 nm

7. The cones are exposed to a bright light source that bleaches much of their photopigment. After 3 minutes in the dark, what percentage of the bleached cone photopigment has recovered?

A. 25%
B. 50%
C. 75%
D. 100%

8. Which of the following acuities is most related to increment threshold?

A. Resolution
B. Recognition
C. Minimum detectable
D. Vernier

9. When foveally fixated, a small target (0.5 deg) of which of the following wavelengths will be least visible?

A. 430 nm
B. 535 nm
C. 565 nm
D. 610 nm

10. Which of the following cues to depth is much more useful at near distances than at farther distances?

A. Interposition
B. Retinal disparity
C. Linear perspective
D. Motion parallax

11. Your 12-year old patient is in a bicycle accident and isn't wearing his helmet. He now complains of running his shoulders into poles while walking down the street. Looking at his fundus, you note pallor on the nasal half of each nerve. What sort of visual field defect do you expect on a threshold field, and where is the most likely site of injury?

A. Bitemporal hemianopsia with injury at the chiasm
B. Bitemporal hemianopsia with injury at the visual cortex
C. Binasal hemianopsia with injury at the chiasm
D. Binasal hemianopsia with injury at the visual cortex

12. Your patient complains of sudden onset constant diplopia. During EOM testing, the patient exhibits what appears to be a bilateral limitation of adduction, however her convergence is normal. You note a gaze nystagmus as each eye abducts. What is your diagnosis?

A. supranuclear disorder secondary to injury to the medial longitudinal fasciculus
B. supranuclear disorder secondary to multiple sclerosis
C. internuclear opthalmoplegia secondary to injury to the medial longitudinal fasciculus
D. internuclear opthalmoplegia secondary to multiple sclerosis

13. The patient in your chair complains of diplopia. You find vertical and a large cyclo component to her deviation. The deviations are worse during downgaze, with the right eye seemingly affected. What are the most likely diagnosis and treatment option after running imaging tests to confirm it?

A. Unilateral trochlear palsy; bifocals and immediate surgery
B. Unilateral trochlear palsy; patch and wait 6 months to see if it resolves, then surgery
C. Unilateral third nerve palsy; bifocals and immediate surgery
D. Unilateral third nerve palsy; patch and wait 6 months to see if it resolves, then surgery

14. All the following are considered kinetic depth cues except:

A. Looming
B. Convergence
C. Motion parallax
D. Observer motion

15. Your patient's right lateral rectus is paretic. When you present a monocular target to his right eye's temporal field, and ask him to point out it, he will point:
A. To the left of the object
B. Directly at the object
C. To the right of the object
D. Cannot determine

16. Binocular suppression would be expected to develop in a 7-year old patient with which of the following uncorrected refractive errors:
A. OD: +3.00, OS: +2.00
B. OD: +5.00, OS: +2.00
C. OD: -2.00, OS: -3.00
D. OD: -2.00, OS: -5.00

17. When measuring visual acuities, your nine year old, deaf patient performs better when you test her with single letter Lea optotypes, then she does with Snellen tumbling E's. What condition do you suspect:
A. Amblyopia
B. Usher syndrome
C. Functional visual loss
D. Alport syndrome

18. With respect to the contrast sensitivity function of your 68 year old patient, a generalized depression would be expected with which condition:
A. Glaucoma
B. ARMD
C. Charles Bonnet syndrome
D. Cataracts

19. Emmert's Law can be explained by:
A. Lightness constancy
B. Size constancy
C. Color constancy
D. Shape constancy

20. The brighter the background stimulus, the bigger the change in brightness of target stimulus is necessary for the detection of an absolute difference. This describes:
A. Weber's Law
B. Devries-Rose Law
C. Bloch's Law
D. Ricco's Law

21. When performing an EOG, how many minutes of dark adaptation would be minimally necessary to measure the dark trough:
A. 2 minutes
B. 4 minutes
C. 6 minutes
D. 8 minutes

22. A patient with which of the following conditions might be expected to see a single flash if they are presented with the stimulus flash twice with the threshold number of quanta and a 70-second gap in between:
A. Cone monochromacy
B. Rod monochromacy
C. Dichromacy
D. Anomalous trichromacy

23. Your astute patient complains that, while wearing his new sunglasses, objects moving in a pendular path appear to be traveling elliptically – appearing closer as they move to the right and farther as they move to the left. You suspect that:
A. The right lens is tinted darker than the left lens
B. The left lens is tainted darker than the right lens
C. Your patient has a monocular cataract in his left eye
D. Your patient has a hemifield defect

24. A patient with a lesion in the striate cortex affecting direction-specific movement detectors, is the least likely to appreciate which affect:
A. Autokinetic effect
B. Stroboscopic motion
C. Plateau spiral
D. Brucke-Bartley Effect

25. At how many degrees per second of motion does dynamic visual acuity begin to drop?
A. 10
B. 30
C. 50
D. 70

26. All of the following are determinants of critical fusion frequency except:
A. Test stimulus size
B. Retinal location
C. Age
D. Refractive error

27. A stimulus of constant intensity is presented intermittently at just below 10 cps. This stimulus will appear to be:

A. Less bright than a continuously illuminated target of equal intensity
B. As bright than a continuously illuminated target of equal intensity
C. More bright than a steady target of the same intensity
D. Cannot determine from the information given

28. The masking stimulus has the effect of:

A. Raising the threshold for the test stimulus
B. Lowering the threshold for the test stimulus
C. Dampening the perceived contrast of the test stimulus
D. Amplifying the perceived contrast of the test stimulus

29. What is the high frequency cut off of the temporal CSF?

A. 60 Hz
B. 50 Hz
C. 40 Hz
D. 30Hz

30. A patient reports that the world swims as he looks from one object to another. This patient's condition violates:

A. The Pulfrich Effect
B. Saccadic Suppression
C. The Troxler Effect
D. Sub-fusional flicker phenomenon

CHAPTER 10: VISUAL AND HUMAN DEVELOPMENT

1. Which of the following is the same in adults and infants?

A. Inability to see short wavelengths of visible light
B. Sensitivity to slow moving objects
C. Ability to see high frequency contrast sensitivity gratings
D. Accurate accommodation

2. A condition caused by pattern deprivation can also be caused by all of the following EXCEPT?

A. Ptosis
B. Cataracts
C. corneal scarring
D. age related macular degeneration

3. Normal threshold for a test with a rapidly blinking light is reached by what age?

A. 2 Years
B. 5 years
C. 2-4 months
D. 6-8 weeks

4. Which of the following age-related changes is not a result of changes in the ocular media?

A. glare recovery
B. light sensitivity
C. visual fields
D. dark adaptation

5. A child that has difficulty finding a particular object on a cluttered desk might do poorly on which of the following tests?

A. Beery-Butenica
B. Gardener test of visual perceptual skills (TVPS)
C. Rosner test of Visual Analysis Skills (TAS)

6. A baby born 3 months premature is expected to have what refractive error?

A. -6.00DS
B. -0.50DS
C. Plano
D. +3.00 DS

7. A baby born full-term is expected to have what refractive error?

A. -6.00DS
B. -0.50DS
C. +2.00DS
D. +4.00DS

8. When is accommodation fully developed?

A. at birth
B. 3-4 months

C. 1-2 years
D. 3-4 years

9. You have a 75 year old patient who you've seen for the past 25 years. When reviewing her past charts, you notice her convergence ability has:
A. Increased with age
B. Decreased with age
C. Remained stable over time

10. The limiting factor in the onset of stereopsis is:
A. Accommodative ability
B. Cortical development
C. Cone spacing
D. Convergence

11. Failure to treat amblyopia can cause:
A. Loss of depth perception
B. Cosmetic defects
C. Educational and occupational restrictions
D. All of the above

12. The main reason why newborns are unable to see high frequency targets is because:
A. their pupils are too large
B. they have poor accommodative ability
C. foveal cones are spaced too far apart
D. not enough retinal cells are present at birth

13. A hallmark sign of Retinopathy of Prematurity (ROP) is a:
A. dragged macula
B. retinal detachment
C. optic nerve drusen
D. nystagmus

14. All of the following may cause morbidity in newborns if the mother is exposed during the first trimester EXCEPT:
A. Toxoplasmosis
B. Rubella
C. Syphillis
D. Hepatitis

15. The ability to dark adapt decreases with age primarily because:
A. the ability to quickly regenerate rhodopsin deteriorates over time
B. yellowing of the lens decreases the quality of light reaching the retina
C. pupil miosis decreased the amount of light reaching the retina
D. rod sensitivity decreases over time

16. You are asked to examine a 3 month old newborn. What can you reasonably expect in terms of the baby's behavior?
A. The baby will preferentially look at a patterned page over a blank page.
B. The baby's eyes will follow moving objects.
C. The baby will reach for your retinoscope.
D. The baby will point at what he's looking at.

17. Which of the following decreases the lease with age?
A. Visual acuity
B. Temporal vision
C. Visual field
D. Glare sensitivity

18. Bruckner's Reflex is used primarily to determine:
A. Presence of amblyogenic risk factors
B. Eccentric Fixation
C. Optic nerve size
D. Response time of an infant

19. The critical period for humans is usually between:
A. 2-3 months
B. 4-5 months
C. 6-8 months
D. 10-12 months

20. Which develops first?
A. Monocular OKN
B. Binocular OKN
C. Monocular and binocular OKN develop concurrently.

21. The most common cause of amblyopia is?
A. Strabismus
B. Congenital cataracts
C. Refractive Error
D. Anisometropia

22. The corneal diameter reaches adult size at:
A. Birth
B. 6 months
C. 12 months
D. 24 months

23. Which infant would you expect to have the steepest cornea?
A. A premie
B. A full-term newborm
C. A 6-month old
D. A teenager

24. You examine a newborn and notice an optic nerve coloboma. What other systemic abnormalities would you expect?
A. Heart problems
B. Genital abnormalities
C. Ear deformation
D. All of the above

25. In terms of visual deprivation:
A. monocular deprivation is more severe than binocular deprivation
B. binocular deprivation is more severe than monocular deprivation
C. monocular and binocular deprivation are equally damaging

Questions from NBEO

26. Which of the following tests would be LEAST appropriate for assessing visual information processing skills
A. Gardner Reversal Frequency Test
B. Visual Motor Integration Test
C. Test of Visual Perceptual Skills
D. The Grooved Pegboard Test

27. When an elderly person is driving toward a sunset, his vision is disturbed MOST by the normal aging changes in:
A. tear film
B. pupil size
C. dark adaptation
D. the crystalline lens

CHAPTER 11: LIDS/LASHES/LACRIMAL SYSTEM/OCULAR ADNEXA/ORBIT ANATOMY

1. The following pass through the cavernous sinus
A. CN II, CN III, CN IV, V_1 branch of CN V, internal and external carotid
B. CN III, CN IV, V_1 and V_2 branch of CN V, CN VI, internal carotid
C. CN III, CN IV, V_1, V_2, V_3 branches of CN V, CN VI, internal carotid
D. CN III, CN IV, V_1, V_2, V_3 branches of CN V, CN VI, internal and external carotid

2. Damage to the abducens nucleus would most likely involve what other cranial nerve?
A. Oculomotor
B. Trochlear
C. Trigeminal
D. facial

3. Which of the following is true?
A. Meibomian glands are sebaceous glands and are associated with hair follicles
B. Zeiss glands are sebaceous glands that are associated with hair follicles
C. Moll glands are sweat glands located in the tarsal plate
D. Infection of Meibomian glands can result in an external hordeolum

4. Which of the following pairs of arteries DO NOT form an anastomosis?
A. Dorsal nasal and angular
B. orbital branch of middle meningeal and recurrent meningeal
C. supraorbital and supratrochlear
D. inferior lacrimal and zygomatic

5. Which of the following does not apply to the veins of the orbit?
A. They are bidirectional and do not have valves as in the rest of the body
B. Infection can spread more easily through the veins in the orbit than the rest of the body
C. Draining of different compartments is easy in the orbit
D. Do not form anastomoses like arteries

6. Which of the following nerves stimulate tear production and through which foramina do they pass?
A. Oculomotor and Facial – oculomotor and stylomastoid foramen
B. Oculomotor and Autonomic - Oculomotor and superior orbital fissure
C. Facial and Autonomic -stylomastoid foramen and inferior orbital fissure

D. Trigeminal and Facial superior orbital fissure and stylomastoid foramen

7. CN IV shares the following characteristic with CN III, CN V_1, CN VI
   A. It innervates the orbital side of an EOM
   B. It exits the dorsal side of the brainstem
   C. It crosses the midline to innervate the opposite eye
   D. It enters the orbit through the same opening

8. Which of the following antibiotics is matched correctly with its site of action and targeted organisms?
   A. Cephalosporin, cell membrane, Gram + and Gram –
   B. Polymyxin B, cell membrane, only Gram –
   C. Neomycin, cell wall, Gram + and Gram –
   D. Tetracycline, protein synthesis, only Gram +

9. You suspect that your patient may be infected with Pseudomonas Aeruginosa. What do you prescribe, including dosing frequency?
   A. Tobramycin, every one to two hours initially, tapering for 7-10 days.
   B. Erythromycin lubricant at night
   C. Natamycin, every two hours initially, tapering for 7-10 days
   D. Vancomycin, 4 times a day for 1 week

10. Select the correct order of in utero developmental events
   A. tendons of recti muscles fuse with sclera, sutures of the orbit close, motor nerves are well developed
   B. motor nerves are well developed, sutures of the orbit close, tendons of the recti muscles fuse with the sclera
   C. motor nerves are well developed, tendons of recti muscles fuse with sclera, sutures of the orbit close
   D. sutures of the orbit close, motor nerves are well developed, tendons of recti muscles fuse with sclera

11. Which of the following is correct regarding a patient who walks into your office with vesicles at the tip of the nose:
   A. it is referred to as positive Hutchinson's sign when there is an absence of painful vesicular eruptions at the tip of the nose
   B. is related to the fact that the anterior ethmoidal nerve is a branch of the nasociliary nerve
   C. can be of prognostic value in patients with suspected herpes zoster ophthalmic infection
   D. both b and c are correct

12. A patient walks into your clinic complaining of dry eye symptoms, and behind the slit lamp, you measured a tear break-up time (TBUT) of 4 seconds OU. Which eye structure most likely causes the lowered TBUT?
   A. Meibomian glands
   B. lacrimal glands
   C. goblet cells
   D. accessory glands of Krause and Wolfring

13. In a patient with hemianopsia in which the pupil constricts when light is directed to the normal side of the retina, but fails to constrict when light is directed to the retina's blind side
   A. the visual field of the two eyes often exhibit a heteronymous defect
   B. this is referred to as the Wernicke's sign.
   C. the lesion is usually in the central portion of the sensory visual pathway, after the entrance of the optic tract into thalamus

14. Which of the following is least likely to be observed in a patient who recently suffered a stroke that damaged the right midbrain?
   A. reduced ability to depress the left eye when adducted
   B. loss of accommodation, mydriasis and reduced direct, consensual and near pupillary response of the right eye
   C. drooping of the right upper lid
   D. reduced function of the left superior rectus
   E. dry eye on the ipsilateral side

15. In the reflex pathway for papillary dilation:
   A. the preganglionic neurons are in the cilio-spinal center of Budge-Waller, which is located in the lateral horn of the

spinal cord, usually at the level of C8-T3.

B. the postganglionic fibers usually travel in the external carotid nerve
C. the central neurons lie in the thalamus and their axons usually undergo a partial decussation in the lateral columns of the spinal cord
D. all of the above are correct
E. none of the above are correct

16. Which of the following would likely be a primary effect of damage to the 7th Nerve?

A. jaw clenching
B. ptosis of ipsilateral upper eyelid
C. numbness of ipsilateral external auditory meatus
D. dry eye" on the contralateral side

17. Which is incorrect regarding oculomotor developments in infants?

A. Methods for evaluating eye movements include direct observation, monitoring the location of the corneal reflex, infrared limbal trackers and electrooculography (EOGs)
B. The OKN response has a subcortical and cortical pathway
C. Horizontal smooth pursuit develops before vertical pursuit
D. Adults who were blinded at an early age show normal VOR responses.

18. Which is correct regarding saccadic eye movements in newborns?

A. saccades are functional at birth
B. infant saccades show a shorter latency to initiate compared to adults
C. infants do not use multiple saccades to reach the visual target
D. the effective visual field for eliciting saccades decreases after birth

19. A 37-year old Caucasian man presents in your office and reports taking a fall while skiing yesterday, and upon awakening this morning noted a change in his appearance. He reports a headache and recalls having multiple episodes of right side head pain over the last two weeks. Your patient's right pupil does not respond to direct or consensual testing. Your ocular findings were: Ptosis of the right superior eyelid, Anisocoria, OD larger than OS 2° to a parasympathetic defect, and Exotropia, O.D. What is your tentative diagnosis?

A. involutional ptosis
B. mechanical ptosis
C. neurogenic ptosis

20. Which of the following is least likely to cause lacrimation if the fibers were activated?

A. nasociliary nerve
B. anastomosis between zygomatic nerve and the inferior division of lacrimal nerve
C. greater superficial petrosal nerve
D. nerve of pterygoid canal
E. medial branch of internal carotid nerve

21. When you ask a patient to shrug his shoulders, which cranial nerve are you evaluating?

A. Vagus
B. Glossopharyngeal
C. Spinal accessory
D. Hypoglossal
E. Trigeminal

22. What are the borders of Tenon's capsule?

A. the sphenoid and ethmoid bones
B. the nerve of Kobelt and the annulus of Zinn
C. the edge of the optic nerve and the corneal margin
D. the pial artery and the supraorbital artery

23. What is the narrowest muscle?

A. superior rectus
B. inferior oblique
C. medial rectus
D. superior oblique
E. inferior rectus

24. In patients with Argyll-Robertson (A-R) pupil:

A. the condition is usually bilateral, the pupils are usually miotic in longstanding cases and the direct and consensual responses are usually quite poor.
B. the near response is usually normal
C. the lesion is in the sympathetic pathway to the pupil and may be secondary to diabetes, alcoholism, or syphilis.
D. both a and b are correct.
E. all of the above are correct.

25. With regards to anti-infective agents, ones that affect the cell membrane is/are:

A. Penicillins
B. Bacitracin
C. Tobramycin
D. Sulfonamides
E. Polymyxin B

26. Which of the following antiviral drugs do not block RNA and DNA synthesis?

A. Nystatin
B. Cytarabine
C. Interferons
D. methisazone

27. Which of the following structures is/are usually found in the pterygopalatine fossa?

A. Vidian nerve
B. infraorbital nerve
C. maxillary division of the trigeminal nerve
D. both a and c are correct answers
E. all of the above are correct answers

28. Anterior ischemic optic neuropathy (AION):

A. refers to a pathology that typically involves both the laminar and retrolaminar portions of the optic disc
B. is thought to arise from a reduction in the blood that is supplied to the retrolaminar portion of the optic disc by the pial plexus
C. is thought to arise from a reduction in the blood that is supplied to the prelaminar or laminar portion of the optic disc
D. may have an acute onset
E. both c and d are correct

29. With respect to the geometry of the bony orbit

A. with the eye in primary position, the angle btw the visual axis and the orbital axis approximates 22.5 degrees
B. the angle btw the medial wall and the lateral wall is approximately 45 degrees
C. the angle between the orbital axis of the right orbit and the orbital axis of the left orbit is about 90 degrees
D. both a and b are correct
E. all of the above are correct

30. In cases of relative afferent pupillary defect (RAPD):

A. lesion is typically in the optic nerve or the retina
B. visual acuity can be assessed, usually lowered in the affected eye
C. during swinging flashlight test, both pupils usually constrict when the normal eye is illuminated and dilate when the affected eye is illuminate
D. all of the above

Questions from NBEO

31. What is the final position of the eye after being abducted 10 degrees and elevated 20 degrees from the straight-ahead position?

A. Primary
B. Secondary
C. Tertiary

CHAPTER 12: CONJUNCTIVA/CORNEA/ REFRACTIVE SURGERY

1. Your 20-year-old patient wanted to get fitted with contact lenses so you performed keratometry and found egg-shaped mires with distortion. What type of refractive error shift do you expect in this patient who had -3.00DS OU prescription from 3 years ago?

A. Hyperopia, astigmatism
B. Hyperopia
C. Myopia
D. Myopia, astigmatism

2. During slit lamp examination, you found out that your patient's TBUT was 1 sec OU, which gland is not functioning?

A. Accessory gland
B. Krause gland
C. Wolfring gland
D. Goblet cells

3. You had the opportunity to put a piece of fresh donor cornea under microscope. You noticed that the cornea is infected with bacteria. What are some of the cells of the stromal layer that would help the cornea to fight against infection?

A. Lymphocyte
B. Macrophage
C. Lymphocyte and macrophage
D. Wandering cells

4. Urgent care patient came to your clinic with extreme pain OD. History revealed that a piece of moderately high speed velocity metal flew into his eye. You successfully took the metallic foreign body out and treated with topical antibiotics. You saw the patient back in 1 year and you saw a corneal scar where the foreign body was. Which layer of the cornea had the metal penetrate through?

A. Descemet's membrane
B. Epithelium
C. Endothelium
D. Bowman's

5. After your patient woke up and opened her eyes, she had a sharp pain sensation that gave her red eye epiphora for about 2 hours, then the pain went away. What kind of corneal condition did the patient most likely have?

A. Fuch's endothelial dystrophy
B. Arcus
C. Kruckenburg spindle
D. Recurrent corneal erosion

6. You see multiple sharp refractile linear lesions on the cornea. With optic section beam through the cornea, you saw that the lesion is at the stroma layer. Patient also complained of occasional sharp eye pain in the morning. Which corneal condition do you think the patient has?

A. Lattice dystrophy
B. EBMD
C. Arcus
D. Fuch's endothelial dystrophy

7. What of the following surgical technique reduce astigmatism by creating deep straight incisions parallel to the limbus?

A. LASEK
B. Astigmatic Keratotomy (AK)
C. Clear Lens Extraction
D. LASIK

8. You see a pair of funny looking plastic claw on your patient's iris. Your patient told you that he had a really complicated cataract surgery and the surgeon put these claws on his iris inside the anterior chamber. Which of the following should you definitely NOT do?

A. Check pupillary response
B. Dilate the patient
C. EOM
D. Check IOP

9. How are LASEK different/similar to LASIK?

A. Flaps are created for both procedures
B. One corrects for astigmatism while the other for myopia
C. LASIK requires a much longer healing time post-op
D. Pupil size is important for determining the surgical success of LASIK, but not LASEK.

10. You patient was swimming with his 3 months old focus dailies contact lenses. He came to you clinic today complaining of severe eye pain. Slit lamp examination revealed an 3 mm opaque base corneal epithelium defect, 3+ anterior chamber reaction, 3+ bulbar conjunctiva 360 OS. What does the patient have?

A. Infectious corneal ulcer
B. Sterile corneal ulcer
C. Marginal keratitis
D. Anterior uveitis

11. Your patient complains of severe eye pain, but only moderate epithelial staining with fluorescein on the cornea is observed What is the most likely explanation (assuming everything else was unremarkable)?

A. Patient is a malinger
B. Patient is HIV + so he is more sensitive to pain
C. Cornea has very rich nerve innervations so exposed nerve endings can lead to pain
D. Epithelial staining is pathognomonic for corneal ulcer

12. Your patient complains of blurry vision after he wakes up so you think he has Fuchs endothelial dystrophy. What corneal findings would you see in this patient to confirm your diagnosis?

A. Corneal guttata
B. Increased endothelial cell density
C. Decreased pleomorphism
D. Decreased polymegethism

13 You see a metallic foreign body stuck on your patient's right cornea, which doesn't stain with fluorescein. Patient is asymptomatic. Which layer is the foreign body most likely to be located in?

A. Epithelium
B. Stroma
C. Endothelium
D. Descemet's membrane

14. Your patient just recently had a baby and she brought her 6-month-old son for a pediatric eye exam, what do you think his refractive error is and why?

A. Hyperopia – infant's corneal is flatter than adult's
B. Hyperopia – infant's corneal is steeper than adult's
C. Myopia – infant's corneal is flatter than adult's
D. Myopia – infant's corneal is steeper than adult's

15. Your 35-year-old -5.00 D myopic patient has corneal thickness of 535 microns. Is he a good candidate for LASIK? Answer yes/no following a true statement assuming your patient has unremarkable ocular health.

A. Yes; flap is only 250 micron
B. Yes; stromal bed is only 250 micron
C. No; flap is only 150 micron
D. No, stroma is only 150 micron

16. Your patient is 89-year-old. You are expecting to see the following findings, EXCEPT?

A. Vogt limbal girdle
B. Decreased corneal sensitivity
C. Arcus
D. Conjunctival Injection

17. You want to fit your patient with RGP contact lenses, but accidentally rinse the contact lenses with ice-cold water from the faucet (you live in Tahoe and it's winter and snowing right now), your patient jumps out of her chair. You try again after you rinse her contacts with warm water, she feels some mild discomfort, but it's not as bad as the 1st time, why is this?

A. Cornea has adapted to RGP during the 2nd try
B. Cornea is more sensitive to cold than hot
C. Patient is over-reacting the 1st time you insert the RGP into her eyes
D. There are some protein deposits on the contact lenses

18. Your patient is a 35-year-old white female. She has erythematous skin on her cheeks with telangiectatic vessels. Her chief complaint is dry and gritty eyes. What condition does she have and what would be an appropriate treatment?

A. Uveitis – steroid
B. Hypertensive retinopathy – laser
C. Ocular rosacea – artificial tears
D. Iritis – pilocarpine

19. Which forms the conjunctival and corneal epithelium (development)?

A. Ectoderm
B. Mesenchyme/Mesoderm
C. Ectoderm and Mesenchyme
D. Endoderm

20. Your patient has Sjogren's syndrome, what would be the best eye drop to prescribe to help with his mild eye irritation?

A. Artificial tears
B. Pilocarpine
C. Antihistamine
D. Eye drops will not help

21 What is the difference between Rose Bengal and fluorescein staining?

A. No difference
B. Only different in the colors of the dye
C. Fluorescein takes longer to stain than Rose-bengal.
D. Rose-bengal stain does not stain stroma

22. What anesthetic is found in Fluress?

A. Benoxinate
B. Proparacaine
C. Sorbic acid
D. Benzalkonium chloride

23. What are the two mechanisms of anesthetics?

A. Calcium channel blocking and sodium channel blocking
B. Calcium channel blocking and Potassium channel blocking
C. Calcium channel blocking and water channel blocking

D. Potassium channel blocking and sodium channel blocking

24. The sensation of corneal pain is primarily transmitted through which of the following nerves?
A. Oculomotor
B. Infraorbital
C. Nasociliary

25. Which of the following preservative is MOST likely to disrupt the corneal epithelium?
A. Benzalkonium chloride
B. Chlorobutanol
C. Sorbic acid
D. Chlorhexidine

26. The MOST frequent etiology of a unilateral or bilateral proptosis in an adult is?
A. Orbital pseudotumor
B. Cavernous hemangioma
C. Painful ophthalmoplegia
D. Graves' disease

27. What is the thickness of the epithelium of the cornea?
A. 50 micron
B. 500 micron
C. 5 micron
D. 130 micron

28. What is the anterior limiting membrane of the cornea?
A. Bowman's layer
B. Epithelium
C. Endothelium
D. Stroma

29. How does the size of the cornea change from birth to full grown adult?
A. 10 mm for newborns and 12 mm for adults
B. The same
C. 5 mm for newborns and 13 mm for adults
D. 10 mm for newborns and 8mm for adults

30. What are Hassall Henle bodies?
A. Tumor cells
B. Localized thickening of Descemet's membrane seen with aging
C. Sub-conjunctival hemorrhages
D. Iris nodules

CHAPTER 13: LENS/CATARACT/IOL/PRE AND POST OPERATIVE CARE

1. Going from most internal to most external of a lens:
A. Embryonic→fetal→adult→cortex
B. Cortex→embryonic→fetal→adult
C. Fetal →embryonic→adult→cortex
D. Embryonic→fetal→cortex→adult

2. During slit lamp examination, you found this suture-like opacity on the anterior part of the crystalline lens. Your attending doctor said it was normal and asked you draw the opacity on the chart. What should you draw on the lens?
A. An erected Y suture
B. An X shaped suture
C. You don't remember
D. An inverted Y suture

3. The HOYA representative told you that their spectacle lens can block UVC. Which eye structure would benefit the most from this lens characteristic?
A. Cornea
B. Lens
C. Iris
D. Conjunctiva

4. You are having a lot of trouble at night due to glare. Your optometrist told you that you have cataracts. Why do cataracts increase your sensitivity to glare?
A. Cataracts change the color if the crystal lens
B. Cataracts make the already disorganized crystalline protein even more disrupted, which became noticeable to human eyes.
C. Cataracts are not the cause of your sensitivity to glare at night.
D. Clear crystalline lens gives you minimal light scatter due to the regular arrangement of the crystalline protein within the fiber cells, but cataracts disrupt this highly organized pattern.

5. Which of the following is not a risk factor for developing cataract?

A. Age
B. UV exposure
C. Nutritional and metabolic deficiencies
D. Male > female

6. Your 30-years-old Hispanic patient complained of blurry vision. She confessed to you that she has really poor control of her diabetes. Last blood sugar measurement was 400mg/dL. Which of the following conditions is most likely a cause of your patient's reduction in vision?

A. Neovascularization of the optic nerve head
B. Age-related macular degeneration
C. Cataract
D. Corneal opacity

7. Your 46 years old patient, who was a truck driver, told you that he bought a pair of glasses with yellow lenses, which helped him with his vision when he is driving. How can the yellow lens improve your patient's vision?

A. Yellow lens enhances the amount of yellow light entering the eyes.
B. Yellow lens block blue light from entering the eyes.
C. Yellow lens enhances the amount of blue light entering the eyes.
D. Yellow lens block yellow light from entering the eyes.

8. Which of the following tests is the LEAST pertinent in determining the effect of a cataract on a patient's vision?

A. Color
B. Visual acuities
C. Pupils
D. Contrast sensitivity

9. Cuboidal shaped cells in the lens elongate to form new fibers. Which of the following MOST closely describes the location on the lens of these mitotic cells?

A. Nucleus
B. Cortex
C. Thinnest part of capsule
D. Thickest part of capsule

10. Which type of cataract has the most profound effect on vision PRIMARILY due to its location?

A. Anterior subcapsular
B. Posterior subcapsular
C. Cortical
D. Nuclear

11. An absolute presbyope reports that her near vision has recently improved. Which slit lamp beam is BEST for assessing changes in the lens?

A. Retroillumination
B. Oblique beam
C. Conical beam
D. Parallel piped

12. In one classic type of cataract, the lens undergoes a biochemical change as a result of decreased soluble protein content. What would be the MOST likely complaint from patients?

A. Near blur
B. Color changes
C. Reduced contrast sensitivity
D. Glare due to light scatter

13. Which of the developmental nuclei are NOT composed of secondary fibers?

A. Fetal
B. Infantile
C. Embryonic
D. Adult
E. Epinucleus

14. The loss of which mature lens fiber component is responsible for lens transparency?

A. Cytoskeleton
B. Crystallins
C. Organelles
D. Actin
E. Cholesterol

15. What type of lens suture would you expect to find in the lens cortex?

A. Erect Y
B. Inverted Y
C. Simple star
D. Star
E. Complex star

16. Which of the following is NOT part of the mechanism by which the mature lens receives its nutrients?

A. Aqueous humor

B. Vitreous
C. Tunica vasculosa lentis
D. Epithelial tight junctions
E. Na/K ATPase

17. Which of the following is NOT one of the major UV absorbers in the lens?
A. Aromatic amino acids
B. Glutathione
C. Fluorophores
D. Yellow pigments

18. Which type of crystallin protein is the MOST responsible for the lens' refractive properties?
A. Alpha
B. Beta
C. Gamma

19. From which of the following tissues does the lens originate?
A. Endoderm
B. Neuroectoderm
C. Cranial neural crest cells
D. Surface ectoderm
E. Mesoderm

20. Which of the following structures did the lens zonules differentiate from?
A. Lens capsule
B. Ciliary body
C. Ciliary muscle
D. Vitreous
E. Trabecular meshwork

21. What type of cataract is caused by disorganized differentiation of epithelial cells into fibers?
A. Anterior subcapsular
B. Posterior subcapsular
C. Nuclear sclerosis
D. Cortical
E. Morganian

22. Which of the following cataracts has decreased soluble proteins?
A. Nucleus sclerosis
B. Cortical
C. Spokes
D. Lamellar

23. Which of the following risk factors is LEAST likely to cause cataracts?
A. Glaucoma surgery
B. Renal failure
C. Diabetes
D. Hypertension
E. Corticosteroids

24. Which of the following is fixed for linearly polarized light?
A. Magnitude
B. Direction
C. Amplitude
D. Intensity

25. What factor generates circular polarization for two harmonic polarized harmonic plane waves?
A. Magnitude
B. Direction
C. Amplitude
D. Intensity
E. Phase

26. Which of the following COULD be Brewster's angle for light entering the eye at the lens surface?
A. 43 degrees
B. 45 degrees
C. 46 degrees

27. A patient has concussive trauma. Where on the lens is the first place to look for changes if the capsule is not ruptured?
A. Capsule
B. Subcapsular region
C. Cortex
D. Nucleus

28. What transmission axis for polarized glasses BEST reduces glare while driving?
A. 45 degrees
B. 90 degrees
C. 135 degrees
D. 180 degrees

29. Which of the following BEST describes the orientation of secondary lens fibers?
A. Radial
B. anterior to posterior
C. circumferential
D. web-like

30. Which of the following BEST describes the stage of development of the lens before its opening closes off into a vesicle?

A. lens placode
B. lens pit
C. lens vesicle
D. lens plate

31. Which of the following MOST accurately describes the distance at which accommodation allows the emmetropic eye to focus objects?

A. All distances
B. Less than 6m
C. Less than 100cm
D. Less than 40cm

32. When light is split as it passes through the lens, what color is normally focused on the retina?

A. White (all wavelengths)
B. Red (600-700nm)
C. Yellow (570-600nm)
D. Blue (440-500nm)

33. A 72 year old female manifests lenticular changes and an increase in myopia. Which type of cataracts is MOST likely responsible for this clinical signs?

A. Anterior cortical
B. Nuclear
C. Cerulean
D. Posterior pole

Short answer style questions:

34. How does index of refraction change with age?
35. Where is the capsule thickest?
36. What is the lens placode?
37. Where are the primitive lens fibers in an adult lens?
38. Where are the majority of insoluble lens proteins located?

Questions from NBEO

CHAPTER 14: EPISCLERA/ SCLERA/ ANTERIOR UVEA

1. Which of the following mydriatics is used systemically in the treatment of motion sickness?

A. Atropine
B. Hydroxyamphetamine
C. Scopolamine
D. Homatropine

2. Which of the following is the best choice for treating moderate to severe recurrent anterior uveitis?

A. Loteprednol etabonate
B. Prednisolone acetate
C. Mydrysone alcohol
D. Dexamethasone acetate

3. The minor circle of the iris is located in the

A. Stroma of the ciliary body
B. Iris anterior border layer
C. At the iris root
D. Iris stroma

4. The pars plicata of the ciliary body

A. Contains 70 to 80 ciliary processes
B. Extends into the anterior chamber
C. Terminates at the ora serrata
D. Is the location of the transition between retinal and ciliary epithelium

5. Which of the following is not significant in the diagnosis of chronic uveitis?

A. Bilaterality
B. Presence of KPs
C. Decreased vision
D. Presence of posterior synechiae

6. Ocular side effects of corticosteroids therapy do NOT include:

A. Cataracts
B. Glaucoma
C. Ocular infection
D. Cushing's syndrome

7. A patient presents with a red, painful photophobic right eye. Slit lamp exam reveals a miotic pupil with 2+ cells and flare in the anterior chamber, IOP is 28 mmHg OD and 20 mmHg OS. The potential treatments of this condition include all of the following EXCEPT:

A. Cyclopentolate 1%
B. Homatropine 5%

C. Pilocarpine 4%
D. Prednisolone acetate 1%

8. The least indicated treatment of episcleritis is:
A. Fluorometholone 0.1%
B. Topical decongestants
C. Tobramycin
D. Prednisolone 1%

9. The least indicated treatment for mild anterior uveitis is:
A. Atropine 1%
B. Fluorometholone 0.1%
C. Homatropine 5%
D. Prednisolone acetate 1%

10. A young Caucasian female presenting with recurrent nongranulomatous anterior uveitis and low back pain should suspect
A. Sarcoid
B. Syphilis
C. Ankylosing spondylitis
D. Inflammatory bowel syndrome

11. When administering pilocarpine, which muscles of the ciliary body become a concern for inducing a retinal detachment?
A. Longitudinal
B. Radial
C. Sphincter
D. Circular
E. Dilator

12. A miotic pupil, unable to dilate in low light conditions, may be the result of a lesion in all of the following EXCEPT:
A. Superior Cervical Ganglion
B. Nasociliary branch of V1
C. Carotid Sympathetic Plexus
D. Superior Branch of III cranial nerve
E. Sympathetic portion of the ciliary ganglion

13. The role of IOP in development of the anterior chamber and angle includes:
A. Induction of the ingrowth of corneal endothelium
B. Produces an outflow path from the Canal of Schlemm to scleral veins
C. Condenses anterior scleral tissue
D. Causes the absorption of mesodermal tissue in the periphery of the anterior chamber
E. Produces a stasis pressure which dilates distal veins causing anastomoses and formation of the Canal of Schlemm

14. Which of the following muscles originates from the cytoplasm of epithelial cells?
A. Ciliary Body
B. Iris Sphincter
C. Recti muscles
D. Iris Dilator
E. Muller's Muscle

15. A patient with suspected Adie's tonic pupil should be administered which of the following ophthalmic solution to help in the diagnosis?
A. Direct Acting cholinergic agonist
B. Cholinergic antagonists
C. Non-selective α/β Adrenergic agonist
D. $\beta1/\beta2$ non-selective antagonist
E. $\alpha1$ antagonist

16. A 27 year old female presents with a history of Juvenile Rheumatoid Arthritis and pain in the right eye. Following SLE a diagnosis of iridocyclitis is made. What clinical signs would you LEAST expect?
A. Photophobia
B. Limited ocular motility.
C. Cells in the anterior chamber
D. Flare in the anterior chamber
E. Fixed, mid-dilated pupil

17. The sympathomimetic action of phenylephrine can result in which of the following side effects?
A. Posterior synechia
B. Conjunctival injection
C. Widening of the palpebral fissure
D. Miotic cysts when used concomitantly with echothiopate
E. Ciliary spasm

18. All of the following characteristics of Hydroxyamphetamine are true EXCEPT:`
A. Has little to no effect on accommodation
B. Results in mydriasis in patients with preganglionic sympathetic denervation
C. Induces vasoconstriction
D. Results in mydriasis in patients with post-ganglionic sympathetic denervation

E. Increases release of norepinephrine from adrenergic nerve terminals.

19. The characteristics of Timolol as a glaucoma treatment include all of the following EXCEPT:
   A. Decreased aqueous humor production
   B. Increased aqueous outflow
   C. 5-10 times more potent than propanolol
   D. Superior control of IOP over other nonselective β-blockers
   E. Ability to treat open-angle, aphakic, and secondary glaucomas.

20. A patient arrives at the clinic with a detachment of the lateral rectus at its insertion. Which layer of the globe is likely to be compromised?
   A. Sclera
   B. Episclera
   C. Bulbar conjunctiva
   D. Tenon's capsule
   E. Suprachoroidal space

21. When administering a cholinergic agonist to a 25 year old, all of the following can be expected EXCEPT:
   A. Decrease in anterior chamber depth
   B. Anterior shift of peripheral retina
   C. Accommodative spasm
   D. Increase in trabecular space
   E. Decrease in the "spaces of Fontana"

22. Which of the following signs/symptoms can help differentiate scleritis and episcleritis?
   A. Photophobia
   B. Lacrimation
   C. Engorged blood vessels
   D. Degree of pain
   E. Gender

23. An 8-year old patient arrives at the clinic with anterior uveitis. Which of the following is LEAST likely to be the etiology?
   A. HLA-B27 disease
   B. Congenital toxoplasmosis
   C. Toxocariasis
   D. Herpes Zoster
   E. Peripheral uveitis

24. While performing a slit lamp examination of a patient with a suspected uveitis, all of the following are critical areas of observations to make EXCEPT:
   A. Debris on lids/lashes
   B. Perilimbal injection
   C. Cells and flare in anterior chamber and retrolental space
   D. Pupillary light response
   E. Iris hyperemia

25. Which of the following is an observable IOP shift and its associated etiology in a patient with uveitis?
   A. Increase in IOP due to increase in aqueous production
   B. Increase in IOP due to decreased uveoscleral outflow
   C. Decrease in IOP due to decrease in aqueous production
   D. Decrease in IOP due to increased uveoscleral outflow
   E. There is typically no observable change in IOP

26. All of the following are true of the iris EXCEPT:
   A. It is the most anterior extension of the uveal tract
   B. It is thickest at the collarette
   C. It contains several types of pigment
   D. It is under the control of both sympathetic and parasympathetic innervations
   E. Is made up of a pupillary portion and ciliary portion

27 All of the following are commonly found with posterior uveitis EXCEPT:
   A. Perilimbal flush
   B. Choroidal lesions
   C. Retinitis
   D. Minimal photophobia
   E. Granulomatous presentation

28. Which of the following ciliary body tissues and their origin are INCORRECTLY paired?
   A. Ciliary muscle- Mesoderm
   B. Ciliary vessels- Mesoderm
   C. Inner epithelial layer- Neural ectoderm
   D. Ciliary processes- Mesodermal core
   E. Outer epithelial layer- Mesoderm

29. Which structure is found between the uveal and corneoscleral meshwork?
   A. Ciliary body
   B. Schwalbe's line

C. Iris
D. Scleral spur
E. Choroid

CHAPTER 15: VITREOUS/RETINA/CHOROID

1. Which of the following is the strongest area of vitreal attachment?
   A. optic nerve head
   B. macula
   C. ora serrata
   D. retinal blood vessels
   E. posterior lens surface

2. What two layers of the retina are split apart in an acquired retinoschisis?
   A. outer and inner segments of photoreceptors
   B. inner and outer nuclear layers
   C. photoreceptors and RPE
   D. photoreceptors and bipolar cells
   E. inner nuclear and outer plexiform layer

3. What part of the retina has the thickest nerve fiber layer?
   A. near the ora serrata
   B. at the fovea
   C. papillomacular bundle
   D. at the equator
   E. nasal retina

4. Which of the following is NOT a risk factor for retinal detachment?
   A. posterior vitreous detachment
   B. lattice
   C. cystic retinal tufts
   D. hyperopia
   E. trauma

5. What is the earliest sign of diabetic retinopathy?
   A. cotton wool spots
   B. intraretinal microvascular abnormalities
   C. pre-retinal hemorrhage
   D. microaneuryms
   E. venous beading

6. Which of the following is not a classical sign of histoplasmosis?
   A. spots of chorioretinal atrophy
   B. vitreal cells
   C. peripapillary atrophy
   D. maculopathy

7. Your patient has recently had an ischemic central retinal venous occlusion. Which of the following gonioscopy findings would you MOST likely see as a result of the CRVO?
   A. angle recession
   B. peripheral anterior synechiae
   C. neovascularization
   D. iris processes
   E. hyphema

8. Which of the following layers is NOT present at the foveola?
   A. RPE
   B. outer plexiform layer
   C. nerve fiber layer
   D. photoreceptors
   E. external limiting membrane

9. Which of the following is the type of retinal glial cell that has a phagocytic role?
   A. hyaluronic acid
   B. astrocytes
   C. Muller cells
   D. microglia
   E. amacrine cells

10. Which of the following is the MOST likely concern with age-related macular degeneration?
   A. choroidal neovascularization
   B. rhegmatogenous retinal detachment
   C. nerve fiber layer loss
   D. macular branch venous occlusion
   E. angioid streaks

11. Which of the following is LEAST associated with macular holes?
   A. positive Watzke Allen sign
   B. surrounding fluid cuff
   C. red lesion at macula
   D. visual acuity better than 20/40
   E. central scotoma

12. From which of the following tissues does the RPE develop?
   A. Endoderm
   B. Neuroectoderm
   C. Cranial neural crest cells
   D. Surface ectoderm
   E. Mesoderm

13. The formation of retinal layers begins with the establishment of which layer?

A. Photoreceptors
B. Bipolar cells\
C. Inner plexiform layer
D. Ganglion cells
E. RPE

14. Which of the following MOST accurately describes the type of photoreceptors in the macula?

A. Rods and cones
B. Short thick cones
C. Tall thin cones

15. Which vitreous is described as a dense avascular packing of very fine fibers?

A. Primary
B. Secondary
C. Tertiary

16. Which of the following MOST closely describes the diameter of the foveola?

A. 150um
B. 350um
C. 1.5mm
D. 3mm
E. 5.5mm

17. Which of the following dictates the direction of retinal layers?

A. Amacrine cells
B. Bipolar cells
C. Horizontal cells
D. Ganglion cells
E. Muller's fibers

18. Which of the following do NOT have cell nuclei in the inner nuclear layer?

A. Amacrine cells
B. Bipolar cells
C. Horizontal cells
D. Ganglion cells
E. Muller's fibers

19. What type of junctions connect the RPE cells?

A. Adherens
B. Gap
C. Tight
D. Desmosome

20. Which of the following MOST accurately describes the apical face of the RPE?

A. Microvilli
B. Smooth
C. Convoluted infolds
D. Ciliated

21. Which of the following is the blood supply for the outer retinal layers?

A. Retinal blood vessels
B. Central retinal artery
C. Posterior ciliary arteries
D. Diffusion from the choriocapillaris

22. What is the major component of the blood retinal barrier in the retinal capillaries?

A. Epithelium
B. Endothelium
C. Pericytes
D. Fenestrations

23. Which of the following arteries feeds into the choroid to make up the Circle of Haller-Zinn?

A. Central retinal
B. Long posterior ciliary
C. Short posterior ciliary
D. Anterior ciliary
E. Muscular

24 Which is NOT a vein that blood from the retina and choroid passes through when leaving the eye?

A. Superior ophthalmic
B. Inferior ophthalmic
C. Anterior ciliary
D. Orbital
E. Vortex

25. The venous perfusion pressure of intraocular veins depends on the IOP. Where does the greatest resistance to the retinal venous outflow occur?

A. Vortex veins
B. Optic nerve rim
C. Lamina cribosa
D. Posterior pole

26. Rhodopsin is regenerated in the RPE MOST directly from what structure?

A. Retinol

B. 11-cis-retinal
C. All-trans retinal
D. Retinyl esters

27. Which of the following results in photoreceptor transduction?
A. Sodium influx
B. Potassium influx
C. Blocked sodium influx
D. Blocked potassium influx

28 Which vascular structure of the choroid completes its development first?
A. Posterior ciliary artery
B. Stroma
C. Choriocapillaris
D. Vortex veins
E. Bruch's membrane

29. Which vitreal component is responsible for the viscosity of the vitreous?
A. Water
B. Hyaluronic acid
C. Collagen type I
D. Collagen type II

30. Which of the following cells gives feedback to adjust the sensitivity of the bipolar-ganglion synapse?
A. Amacrine
B. Bipolar
C. Ganglion
D. Photoreceptor
E. Horizontal

31 Which of the following do NOT synapse with bipolar cells?
A. Amacrine
B. Muller
C. Ganglion
D. Photoreceptor
E. Horizontal

32. Which is the excitatory neurotransmitter in the photoreceptor-bipolar synapse?
A. Acetylcholine
B. GABA
C. Glutamate
D. Glycine

33. Which of the following ophthalmoscope and lens systems gives the highest magnification?
A. Direct ophthalmoscope
B. Binocular indirect with a 20D lens
C. Binocular indirect with a 60D lens
D. Noncontact fundoscopy with a 90D lens

Questions from NBEO

34. Occlusion of the short posterior ciliary arterioles will MOST likely cause necrosis of which of the following retinal layers?
A. Inner nuclear
B. Ganglion cell
C. Nerve fiber
D. Outer nuclear

Short answer style questions

35. What are the 4 layers of the choroid?
36. What are the 2 types of blood vessels in the choroidal stroma?
37. What is the major blood supply for the posterior choroid?
38. Which veins drain the anterior ½ of the choroid?
39. What are the 7 layers of Bruch's (choroidal) membrane?
40. What are the 4 locations of vitreous attachment? Which is the strongest?
41. What is Cloquet's canal?
42. What is the area of Martegiani?
43. What are the 10 retinal layers (outer to inner)?
44. What is the blood supply to the photoreceptors? What supplies most of the retina?
45. What is the layer of Henle?
46. When is the choriocapillaris complete?
47. Which tissues gives rise to the primary and secondary vitreous?
48. Where is the secondary vitreous located relative to the primary vitreous?
49. Which are the first retinal receptors to develop?
50. When is macular development complete?
51. Which part of the ophthalmic artery degenerates during development?
52. What does the CRA develop from?
53. What % of the vitreous is H2O?
54. When do syneresis and liquefaction of the vitreous occur?
55. What is dark current?
56. What is the pedicle?

CHAPTER 16: OPTIC NERVE/NEURO-OPHTHALMIC PATHWAYS

1. Your patient was at the dentist yesterday. He mentions experiencing some ocular pain while his dentist was performing dental procedure for an abscessed tooth . This phenomenon also known as "referred pain" is caused by an overload of sensation carried by which of the following nerves?
   A. Facial nerve
   B. Lacrimal nerve
   C. Infraorbital nerve
   D. Ophthalmic nerve

2. Your patient has damaged his trochlear nucleus during an automobile accident. You predict that the affected muscle is:
   A. Ipsilateral superior oblique muscle
   B. Contralateral superior oblique muscle
   C. Both superior oblique muscles
   D. No EOM would be affected

3. While performing EOM on your patient, you noticed the left eye is elevated in primary gaze and unable to move down in the adducted position. Which muscle/nerve would you suspect to be injured?
   A. Right trochlear nerve
   B. Left trochlear nerve
   C. Right inferior oblique muscle
   D. Left inferior oblique muscle

4. Your third patient of the day is a 29 year old healthy Caucasian male here for his first eye exam. While evaluating the patient's optic nerve head, you noticed a white lesion with distinct borders that appears to be raised and is located in the middle of the optic nerve head. What is the most likely diagnosis for this lesion?
   A. Cotton wool spot
   B. Bergmeister's papilla
   C. Mittendorf's dot
   D. Myelinated nerve fiber layer

5. Your 45 year old Asian male patient complains of constant headache and feels like he is not seeing as well as he used to. This is his 30-2 visual field result. After analyzing it, you suspect a specific area had been interrupted. Where would that area be:

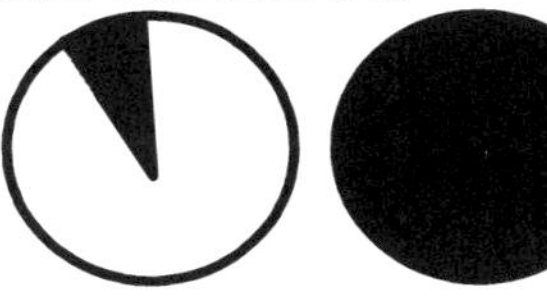

   A. midline of the chiasm
   B. area in the left optic radiation involving Meyer's loop
   C. at the chiasm, slightly toward the right optic nerve tract with right anterior knees of Willebrand involvement
   D. interruption in the right posterior striate cortex

6. While performing pupil testing, you notice your patient pupils are not equal in size. The anisocoria is much more noticeable in the dark. Your patient is an alcoholic and a poorly controlled Type 2 diabetic for the past 17 years. With the light directly in front of OD, you see poor direct response OD and normal consensual response OS. With the light directly in front of OS, you see normal direct response OS and poor consensual response OD. Which is the more severely affected eye? Which condition would cause this? And what test you should do next?
   A. Right eye, Diabetic neuropathy, near response test.
   B. Left eye, neurosyphilis, near response test.
   C. Left eye, alcoholic neuropathy, swinging light test
   D. Right eye, alcoholic neuropathy, instill 0.125% pilocarpine into the larger pupil and wait for the pupil to constrict.
   E. None, benign anisocoria, start refraction.

7. A 30-2 visual field of the left eye shows a homonymous hemianopic VF defect with a 5 degree zone of preserved vision around fixation. What is the MOST likely location for a corresponding cortical lesion?
   A. Temporal at Meyer loop
   B. Occipital lesion
   C. Frontal lesion
   D. Parietal lesion

8. A 54 year old female complains of occasional double vision, especially at the end of the day, and dry eyes. Your patient tells you that she just moved into a new house and the temperature in that house never feels right. She said it is either always too hot or too cold. She also has not slept very well lately and is quite concerned that it might affect her vision. What do you suspect the patient has?

A. Severe dry eye syndrome
B. Grave disease
C. An ocular tumor
D. Paget's disease

9. A 35 year old Caucasian woman complains of visual fluctuation, muscle weakness, ataxia, urinary disturbances, parasthesia with onset of one week. She also reports history of acute vision loss in the left eye two years ago, but her vision has since recovered. Her BCVA OD 20/20, OS 20/30. Red Cap test reveals some red color deficiency in the left eye. During NCF, you note pink and healthy discs OD and pallor OS. What type of condition do you think your patient is suffering from?

A. Grave disease
B. Myasthenia Gravis
C. Multiple Sclerosis
D. Ischemic Optic Neuropathy

10. You are having a hard time determining the C/D in a patient's right eye because you are unable to identify the disc margin. Your patient also reports sudden onset of decreased in vision in the right eye, starting 2 days ago. Vision slowly improved over the past 2 days. HVF 30-2 OD show superior temporal defect that respects the vertical midline. What do you think the patient has?

A. Optic neuritis
B. Ischemic Optic Neuropathy
C. Marcus Gunn Pupil
D. Optic pit
E. Melanocytoma

11. A lesion to the left temporal loop of the optic radiations results in this type of visual field defect:

A. Bilateral left inferior quadranopsia
B. Bilateral right superior quadranopsia
C. Bilateral left superior quadranopsia
D. Bilateral right inferior quadranopsia

12. A bilateral inferior quadranopsia visual field defects results from damage to this structure:

A. Optic chiasm
B. Temporal optic radiations
C. Parietal optic radiations
D. Upper calcarine fissure

13. The density of blue cones peaks here:

A. The fovea
B. 1 degree from the fovea
C. 5 degrees from the fovea
D. 10 degrees from the fovea

14. If a probe is inserted into the visual cortex at a right angle to the surface, which is true about the cells stimulated?

A. The cells have the same orientation preference
B. There is a systematic change in the orientation preference.
C. The cells have difference ocular dominance.
D. The cells have no orientation preference

15. A neuron in the visual cortex that is stimulated by both eyes but responds more to the ipsilateral eye is classified into which ocular dominance group or groups?

A. Group 2 and 3
B. Group 4
C. Group 5 and 6
D. Group 7

16. The first synapse of the parasympathetic pathway from the eye to the iris is in this nucleus:

A. Red nucleus
B. Edinger-Westphal nucleus
C. Ciliary ganglion
D. Pretectal Nucleus

17. What is the name of the phenomenon in which a constantly applied stimulus is no longer perceived by the brain?

A. Adaptation
B. Habituation
C. Negative Feedback
D. Imprinting

18. Where do the sensory neurons of reflex motion synapse with the motor neurons?

A. The cerebellum
B. The white matter of the spinal cord

C. The grey matter of the spinal cord
D. The brain stem

19. If you are listening to music, which cranial nerve is being stimulated?
A. Glossopharyngeal
B. Vagus
C. Facial
D. Vestibulocochlear

20. Where does the myelination of the optic nerve end in most humans?
A. The lamina cribosa
B. 12-13mm behind the eye
C. The meniscus of Kuhn
D. The optic chiasm

21. Which type of systemic cancer is most commonly associated with pupillodilator dysfunction?
A. Breast
B. Lung
C. Liver
D. Pancreatic

22. What is the most common cause of cranial nerve palsies?
A. Head trauma
B. Idiopathic
C. Neoplasm
D. Aneurysm

23. If your patient is having difficulty speaking, which cranial nerve is MOST likely to be the cause?
A. Glossopharyngeal
B. Vagus
C. Hypoglossal
D. Facial

24. A 50 year old male presents with sudden decrease in VA in the right eye. During your exam you find that in the right eye there is red desaturation, +RAPD, swollen and hyperemic optic nerve head, and pain with eye movements. What is the most likely cause?
A. Papilledema
B. Optic nerve head drusen
C. Anterior ischemic optic neuropathy
D. Papillitis

25. An 80 year old patient presents with temporal headaches, fatigue, neck pain, and transient blur. Which of the following tests will be most helpful in determining the cause?
A. Ultrasound
B. Goldman Visual Fields
C. Sedimentation rate
D. Confrontation Visual Fields

26. A patient presents with a face turn to the left and you notice that the left eye has severely limited abduction and that the left palpebral fissure gets smaller with adduction. Which is mostly likely to be the cause?
A. 6th cranial nerve palsy
B. Partial 3rd cranial nerve palsy
C. Duane's Retraction Syndrome
D. 4th cranial nerve palsy

27. Which test will not help you to test the Vestibular Ocular reflex?
A. Rotating Drum
B. Caloric nystagmus (COWS)
C. Doll's head maneuver
D. Post rotatory nystagmus

28. A lesion in which of the following brain areas is most likely to result in difficulty coordinating motion, abnormal gait, and poor muscle tone?
A. Motor cortex
B. Brain stem
C. Cerebellum
D. Frontal Lobe

29. A 40 year old female presents with ptosis and diplopia, which of the following is not on the differential diagnosis?
A. Multiple sclerosis
B. Perinaud's Syndrome
C. 3rd cranial nerve palsy
D. Myasthenia gravis

30. A 55 year old male presents with sudden loss of vision in the left eye, a left RAPD, as well as pallor and swelling of a temporal sector of the optic nerve head, which of the following is the most likely diagnosis?
A. Anterior ischemic optic neuropathy
B. Optic Neuritis
C. Papilledema
D. Temporal arteritis

CHAPTER 17: PHARMACOLOGY

Questions are dispersed throughout the chapter regarding ocular anatomy specific pharmacology

CHAPTER 18: GLAUCOMA

1. During gonioscopy of the inferior angle, the most posterior structure in the view is posterior aspect of Descemet's membrane. What structures are present?
   A. ciliary body, scleral spur, and posterior trabecular meshwork
   B. scleral spur, posterior and anterior trabecular meshwork
   C. trabecular meshwork and Schwalbe's Line
   D. Schwalbe's Line

2. Which part of the ciliary body is responsible of producing aqueous humor?
   A. Pars plicata
   B. Pars plana
   C. Supraciliaris
   D. Pigmented epithelium

3. Which of the following is NOT considered a glaucoma visual field defect?
   A. Nasal step
   B. Superior or Inferior Arcuate
   C. Ring scotoma
   D. Nasal paracentral scotoma
   E. Central tubular fields

4. What type of glaucoma is a patient who recently had a central retinal vein occlusion at MOST risk for?
   A. Neovascular Glaucoma
   B. Normal Tension Glaucoma
   C. Primary Open Angle Glaucoma
   D. Pigmentary Glaucoma
   E. Exfoliative Glaucoma

5. Common signs of glaucoma include all of the following EXCEPT:
   A. Notching of rim tissue
   B. Drance hemorrhage
   C. Nerve fiber layer defect
   D. Vitreous hemorrhage
   E. Enlarged C/D ratio

6. If a patient presents with frontal headaches, blurred vision, photophobia, nausea, and pain, they MOST likely have:
   A. Acute angle-closure glaucoma
   B. Ocular hypertension
   C. Chronic angle-closure glaucoma
   D. Angle-recession glaucoma
   E. Glaucomatocyclitic Crisis

7. Which of the following glaucoma agents is NOT correctly paired with the correct class of drugs?
   A. Apraclonidine: selective, alpha adrenergic agonist
   B. Carbachol: sympatholytic agent
   C. Brinzolamide: Carbonic Anhydrase inhibitor
   D. Levobunolol: beta-adrenergic receptor blocking agent
   E. Pilocarpine: cholinergic parasympthomimetic agent

8. Which of the following drugs would be contraindicated for management of secondary angle closure glaucoma caused by Uveitis or Chronic inflammation?
   A. Prednisolone acetate 1% ophthalmic solution
   B. Homatropine 5% ophthalmic solution
   C. Timolol 0.5% ophthalmic solution
   D. Travaprost 0.004% ophthalmic solution
   E. Brimonidine 0.2% ophthalmic solution

9. All of the following are conditions associated with neovascular glaucoma EXCEPT:
   A. central retinal vein occlusion
   B. Diabetic retinopathy
   C. Chronic uveitis

D. Central retinal artery occlusion
E. Posterior Vitreous Detachment

10. Which of the following medications would be most appropriate to use if your patient has pulmonary disease?
A. Timolol
B. Carteolol
C. Betaxolol
D. Levobunolol
E. Metipranolol

11. Which of these structures is derived from myoepithelial cells?
A. ciliary body
B. iris dilator muscle
C. iris sphincter muscle
D. zonules

12. Phacodonesis is observed in a patient with pseudoexfoliation. Which structure is MOST likely to be compromised?
A. lens capsule
B. iris pigmented epithelium
C. zonule
D. ciliary body process
E. pars plicata

13. A patient presents with a complaint of severe eye pain and central retinal vein occlusion with a duration of four days. Gonioscopy reveals a closed angle. Which of the following is the most likely cause?
A. Neovascularization of the disc
B. Retinal Neovascularization
C. Neovascularization of the angle
D. Swollen ciliary body

14. When measuring intraocular pressure by Goldmann applanation tonometry, which patient would theoretically have a true intraocular pressure lower than what you measure? Central corneal thickness measurements are provided below.
Patient A: 480 microns
Patient B: 500 microns
Patient C: 550 microns
A. Patient A
B. Patient B
C. Patient C

15. For a patient with kidney stones and asthma, which glaucoma medication is the MOST suitable as initial treatment?
A. Timolol
B. Trusopt
C. Cosopt
D. Alphagan

16. For a patient with pulmonary sarcoidosis and uveitic cystoid macular edema, which glaucoma medication is the MOST suitable treatment option?
A. Xalatan
B. Betagan
C. Trusopt
D. Combigan

17. When performing gonioscopy you observed that the angle is open to the trabecular meshwork. Which of the following structures is NOT visible to you?
A. Scleral Spur
B. Descemet's membrane
C. Iris processes
D. Schwalbe's Line

18. Angle recession involves a tear between which of the following two structures?
A. Longitudinal and circular muscles of the ciliary body
B. Sphincter and dilator muscles
C. Pars plana and pars plicata
D. Trabecular meshwork and scleral spur

19. You placed a patient on pilocarpine for chronic angle closure glaucoma. The patient returns 30 minutes after the first instillation with eye pain and an increase in intraocular pressure from 19 to 48. What is the MOST likely pathophysiology of his symptoms?
A. Anaphylactic reaction to pilocarpine
B. Choroidal detachment
C. Malignant glaucoma
D. Anterior rotation of the ciliary body

20. A patient has a myopic refractive error shift. Which of the following is not likely to cause this shift?
A. Acetazolamide
B. Nuclear sclerosis cataract
C. Pilocarpine
D. Idiopathic central serous chorioretinopathy

21. A diabetic patient presents with severe eye pain, nausea, a cloudy cornea, and an

intraocular pressure of 69. Which of the following medications is contraindicated?

A. Iopidine
B. Diamox
C. Glycerin
D. Timolol

22. Laser peripheral iridotomy prevents acute angle closure by opening communication between which two cavities?

A. The anterior chamber and the vitreous
B. The posterior chamber and the vitreous
C. The anterior chamber and the posterior chamber
D. The anterior chamber and Schlemm's Canal

23. A patient is placed on a medication for glaucoma and begins experiencing headaches, lack of energy, and shallow breathing. The patient cannot remember the name of the medication. Which of the following is MOST likely to cause these symptoms?

A. Acetazolamide
B. Alphagan
C. Lumigan
D. Travatan

24. For a patient who has a history of myocardial infarction, chronic obstructive pulmonary disease, and sulfa drug allergy, which of the following medications is LEAST contraindicated?

A. Betaxolol
B. Levobutanol
C. Timolol
D. Methazolamide

25. Which drug has a mechanism of action that is MOST different from the others?

A. Epinephrine
B. Iopidine
C. Timolol
D. Dorzolamide

26. A patient presents with a patent laser peripheral iridotomy and has a shallow central and peripheral anterior chamber, a cloudy cornea, and an intraocular pressure of 46. Which of the following could NOT be the cause of her symptoms?

A. Relative pupillary block
B. Aqueous misdirection
C. Plateau iris
D. Choroidal detachment

27. After examining a patient you note an iris insertion anterior to the scleral spur, broad peripheral anterior synechiae, and correctopia. Which of the following could NOT be the cause?

A. Anterior Chamber Syndrome
B. Iridocorneal Endothelial Syndrome
C. Plateau Iris
D. Posterior Polymorphous Dystrophy

28. A patient with pseudoexfoliation is undergoing cataract extraction. Which of the following complications is MOST likely in a patient with this condition?

A. Retinal detachment
B. Corneal edema
C. Vitreous loss
D. Endophthalmitis

29. In a patient with a blind and painful eye, to which eye structure can one apply laser to inhibit aqueous production?

A. Pigmented epithelium of the iris
B. Trabecular meshwork
C. Pars plana
D. Pars plicata

30. Which of the following is NOT an effect of pilocarpine?

A. Miosis
B. Anterior displacement of the ciliary body
C. Zonular laxity
D. Flattening of the anterior aspect of the lens

CHAPTER 19: OCULAR EMERGENCIES AND TRAUMA

1. Which the following emergencies must be treated the MOST immediately?

A. Blow out fracture
B. Central retinal venous occlusion

C. Vitreal detachment
D. Alkali burn
E. Bacterial conjunctivitis

2. Which of the following is the MOST appropriate test during a work up for a patient with a foreign body?
A. Seidel test
B. Jones Dye Test
C. Schirmer's test
D. Pachymetry
E. pH testing

3. Which of the following is a malignant lid lesion?
A. Phlyctenule
B. Squamous cell papilloma
C. Dermoid
D. Squamous cell carcinoma
E. Pemphigoid

4. Your patient presents with mutton fat keratic precipitates, cells in the anterior chamber, and a hazy view of the fundus. What is the most likely diagnosis?
A. Traumatic cataract
B. Panuveitis
C. Foreign body
D. Retinal detachment
E. Anterior ischemic optic neuropathy

5. Which of the following would be an appropriate test to order for 16.4?
A. Chest X-ray
B. B-scan
C. OCT
D. MRI
E. Fluorescein angiography

6. Which of the following is NOT a sign or symptom of acute angle closure glaucoma?
A. Eye pain
B. Corneal edema
C. Nausea and vomiting
D. IOP spike
E. Darkening of vision Amaurosis Fugax

7. Which of the following is NOT on the list of differential diagnosis for acute eye pain?
A. Dry eye syndrome
B. Uveitis
C. Orbital cellulitis
D. Corneal abrasion
E. Retinal detachment

8. In which of the following conditions would you be LEAST likely to see an afferent pupil defect?
A. Advanced glaucoma
B. Optic neuritis
C. Ischemic optic neuropathy
D. Macular degeneration
E. Central retinal vein occlusion

9. Your new patient has a blown pupil. Which of the following tests is the LEAST appropriate to perform?
A. Dilated fundus exam
B. Extraocular muscles
C. Pupil testing
D. Blood pressure
E. Visual fields

10. Which of the following is LEAST likely to be seen in your patient with severe bacterial conjunctivitis?
A. Mucous discharge
B. Hypopyon
C. Lid edema
D. Papillae
E. Chemosis

11. Your walk-in patient complains of reduction in vision and severe eye pain from a racquetball accident. He also has restricted ocular motility. How would you manage this patient?
A. Refer to ophthalmologist immediately
B. Give patient Tylenol #3 and follow-up in 1 week
C. Refer to ophthalmologist, next available appointment
D. Perform a dilated fundus exam and follow-up in office next day

12. Your patient brings in her 8- year-old son and tells you that he got hit by a basketball. Her son does not experience any pain or reduced vision, but he has a dark bruise below his eye near the orbital floor. How would you manage this young patient?
A. Refer to ophthalmologist immediately
B. Refer to ophthalmologist in 24-48 hours
C. Refer to your colleague down the street who specialized in binocular vision and vision therapy
D. Send him to emergency room

13. All the following are signs of orbital compartment syndrome, EXCEPT?
A. Limited ocular motility
B. (-) RAPD
C. Out of proportion reduction in vision
D. Unable to open eyelids

14. Which type of sub-conjunctiva hemorrhage is considered most alarming for your patient who gets hit by a golf ball?
   A. Flat
   B. Bullous
   C. Petechial
   D. Dot-blot

15. Seidel test is not an appropriate test to perform under which circumstances?
   A. Patient has a corneal transplant 1 week ago
   B. Patient has cataract extraction 1 week ago
   C. Patient has a fast traveling metallic foreign body stuck on his cornea
   D. Patient with mild trichiasis

16. Your patient has bleach splashed into her right eye when she was doing laundry. How would you not manage this patient?
   A. Sweeping the fornix
   B. Copious irrigation
   C. Frequent pH testing
   D. Refer to emergency room immediately without irrigation if cornea is involved.

17. Which of the following chemical causes more severe and serious ocular burn?
   A. Battery acid
   B. Bleach
   C. Vinegar
   D. Wet cement

18. What posterior segment findings would you not see in your patient with a recent ocular trauma?
   A. Commotio retinae
   B. Lattice degeneration
   C. Macular hole
   D. Retinal breaks

19. Which of the following is not true about retained metallic foreign body?
   A. Zinc causes severe inflammation
   B. Aluminum causes minimal inflammation and may be encapsulated
   C. Pure copper causes acute endophthalmitis and rapid vision loss
   D. Copper alloys may causes sunflower cataract

20. Signs and symptoms of retained iron in the eye may include all the following, EXCEPT?
   A. Nyctalopia and decreased vision
   B. Concentrically restricted visual field
   C. Optic atrophy and peripheral retinal degeneration
   D. Retinal detachment

21. Your patient brings his adopted child for an infant-toddler exam. His baby looks irritable and tired. During the eye exam, you found some retinal hemorrhages and cotton wool spots at the back of the baby's eyes. Now, you are suspecting that the baby has:
   A. Shaking baby syndrome
   B. Retinopathy of prematurity (ROP)
   C. Branch retinal vein occlusion
   D. Branch retinal artery occlusion

22. Your patient has acute painless vision loss, all of the following are included in your differential diagnoses, EXCEPT?
   A. Central retinal artery occlusion
   B. Retinal detachment
   C. Vitreous hemorrhage
   D. Map-dot dystrophy

23. Which of the following is more likely to causes hyphema?
   A. Iritis
   B. Primary open angle glaucoma
   C. Cataract
   D. Corneal transplant

24. You think your patient has acute angle closure glaucoma (AACG), which of the below signs helps you to conclude the diagnosis?
   A. Very elevated IOP with eye pain
   B. No visual complaint
   C. Patient had his first episode of eye pain before he went to bed last night
   D. IOP = 15 mm Hg in the right eye and 13 mm Hg in the left eye

25. During slit lamp, you see track-like fluorescein staining on your 49 year old patient's cornea, injection, mild AC reaction and your patient thinks that he might gotten something into his eye when he was gardening, what is the first item on your differential?
   A. Corneal abrasion
   B. Conjunctival abrasion
   C. Dry eyes syndrome
   D. Ocular allergy

26. You have been treating your patient with antibiotic for acute red eyes, but the condition is worsened so you decide to run some lab tests.

Which of the following media is incorrectly matched with the bacteria that grow it?

A. Chocolate agar – Haemophilus, Neisseria
B. Blood agar – Most bacteria
C. Sabouraud dextrose – Fungus
D. Lowenstein-Jensen – Virus

27. Your patient complains of acute eye pain right after he wakes up that occurs two times per week and the last episode is 3 days ago. With slit lamp, you don't see any epithelial defects or abrasion, but there are some negative fluorescein staining, what is the first item on your differential diagnoses?

A. Iritis
B. Dry eyes syndrome
C. Recurrent corneal erosion
D. Malingerer

28. The etiologies of vitreous hemorrhage include all of the following, EXCEPT?

A. ARMD
B. Retinal detachment
C. Diabetes
D. Pigmentary dispersion syndrome

29 How would you manage your patient with moderate anterior uveitis, who also complains of photophobia and eye irritation?

A. Steroid with cycloplegia
B. Observe with no treatment
C. Glaucoma eye drops to lower IOP
D. Refer to emergency room

30. Which are not signs of orbital cellulitis?

A. Painful red eye
B. Headache
C. Blurry and or double vision
D. Impaired vision

Answers to Chapter Questions

CHAPTER 1: OPTICS (GEOMETRICAL)

1. Answer: C. The patient requires -3.00D correction and is thus a 3.00D myope. The far point for a myope is in front of the eye. The far point here is 1/-3.00D = -0.33 m = 33 cm in front of the refracting surface. Therefore, with accommodation relaxed, the patient can only see 33 cm in front of his eye.

2. Answer: A. *We desire the total power of the system to be -5.00D. The power of the doublet consists of the powers of the individual materials.*
$P_{total}=P_1+P_2= -5.00D$

A doublet is designed to eliminate chromatic aberration, therefore the total desired amount of CA (sum of the individual CA of each material) should add up to zero.
CA_{total}=total chromatic aberration of the system=$CA_1+CA_2=0$
CA=P/v
$CA_{total}=P_1/v_1 = P_2/v_2=P_1/58.6 + P_2/30 = 0$

Now combine the above two formulas and compute the individual powers of the materials:
$P_1/58.6 = -P_2/30$
$P_1= P_{total} - P_2 = -5 - P_2$
$(-5 - P_2)/58.6 = - P_2/30$
$-5 - P_2 = -1.953P_2$
$5 = 0.953P_2$
$P_2 = 5.25$ D
$P_1 = P_{total} - P_2 = -5 - 5.25 =$ -10.25 D

3. Answer: C. The average power of the two meridians is (2+3)/2 = 2.5. The circle of least confusion is the reciprocal of the average power which is 1/2.5=0.40m or 40cm.

4. Answer: D. Determine how much spectacle power is correcting each meridian.
-3.50D @ 180
-5.00D @ 090
Determine the amount of power reaching the plane of the eye along the 180 meridian by taking into account vertex distance. Assume that parallel light enters the lens.
U=0
P=-3.50D
V=-3.50D
v=1/-3.50=-0.2857m
-0.2857+(-0.010)=-0.2957 m
1/-0.2957=-3.38D reaching the eye at 180

Determine the amount of power reaching the plane of the eye along the 090 meridian by taking into account vertex distance. Assume that parallel light enters the lens.
U=0
P=-5.00D
V=-5.00D
v=1/-5.00=-0.20m
-0.20+(-0.010)=-0.210 m
1/-0.210=-4.76D reaching the eye at 090

Determine the cylindrical power.
-3.38-1.38x180
Based on the above numbers, the closest CL Rx is -3.50-1.25x180

5. Answer: C. A real object produces diverging light. It is located in front of a lens. Therefore, u=location of object= -0.90 m. The distance is negative because the object is located in front (to the left) of the lens.

A real image is formed by converging light. It is located in back of a lens. Therefore, v=location of image= +0.45 m. The distance is positive because the image is located in back (to the right) of the lens.

Use the lens maker formula to calculate the power.
U=1/u=1/-0.90=-1.11D
V=1/v=1/+0.45=+2.22D
P=V-U=+3.33D
Focal length for a thin lens is calculated by the formula f=1/P=1/+3.33D=0.30m

6. Answer: B. Oblique astigmatism occurs when a bundle of rays meet a lens surface obliquely (e.g., from below), and the beam forms an ellipse with a shorter tangential axis and a longer sagittal axis. Hitting a lens obliquely is like tilting the lens.

7. Answer: D. Use equation $r=(h^2/2s)+(s/2)$ where s=0.2mm, h=20.8/2=10.4mm and Δn=0.523 (on Geneva lens clock) so that r=0.2705 and using $P=\Delta n/r$, P=1.93D

8. Answer: B. Treat each surface as a thin lens, but the media separating the two surfaces has n=1.5
$U_1=0 \rightarrow V_1=P_1=+6 \rightarrow v_1=1.5/6=0.25$m
u_2=0.25-0.02-0.23
U_2=1.5/0.23=6.5217D
$V_2=P_2+U_2$= -4 +6.5215 = 2.5217D
v_2=1/2.5217=0.397m

9. Answer: A. Each prism can be thought of as a vector with a magnitude and direction. Separate each one into its corresponding horizontal and vertical components
OD: Z_H=Zcos060=4cos060=2 BI
Z_V=Zsin060=4sin060 = 3.46BU
OS: Z_H=Zcos030=2cos030=1.732 BI
Z_V=Zsin030=2sin030=1 BU
Combine the results with respect to OD
OD: Z_H=2BI +1.732 BI = 3.732 BI
Z_V= 3.36BI + 1BU = 2.46 BU
Determine resultant vector using data calculated above
$Z_r=\sqrt{(Z_H^2+Z_V^2)}$ = 4.468
Angle=$\tan^{-1}(Z_V/Z_H)$ = 33.2 deg

10. Answer: C. Given: Z=-2 BD, P=-4.00 D
The prism reference point (PRP) is the point on the lens where prism is measured. It is where the eye is located along the meridian of the lens to achieve the prismatic effect. Use $Z=h_{cm}P$ to find h_{cm}. The value of h_{cm} is the distance from the lens pole in cm. If the optical center (OC) is up or out from the PRP, h_{cm} is positive. It the OC is down or in from the PRP, h_{cm} is negative.
h=+0.50 cm=OC is 5 mm above PRP

11. Answer: B. Separate 4 base 060 into its horizontal and vertical components.
Z_H=4cos060=2 BO
Z_V=4sin060=3.5 BU

12. Answer: C. Determine power along the horizontal and vertical meridians.
P_{hor}= +2 D, P_{vert}= +1 D
Determine outgoing vergences (V).
U=0 because object at infinity
$V_{hor}=P_{hor}$ + 0= +2 D
$V_{vert}=P_{vert}$ + 0= +1 D
C.O.C.= $(V_{hor}+V_{vert})/2$=1.50 D
1/1.5 D = 0.667 m

13. Answer: D. The patient is looking through a different power when she tilts the lens. To calculate the power, use:
$P_{ns}=P_o[1+\sin^2\langle/2n]$
= 8(1+[($\sin^2$020)/2(1.523)]) = +8.31D
$P_c=P_{ns}\tan^2\langle$= 8.31$\tan^2$020=+1.10D
New lens power=+8.31+1.10x180 because pantoscopic tilt changes power along 090 and not 180. The Rx is transposed to +9.41-1.10x090

14. Answer: A
Use Prentice's eq: $Z=h_{cm}P$
P=-4, h (vert)=+0.75, h(hor)=+1
Z_{hor}=(-4)(1)= -4= 4 BI
Z_{vert}=(-4)(0.75)= -3= 3 BD

15. Answer: A. LCA= Z/Abbe=2/36= 0.0556

16. Answer: B. What we see when we look at someone's eye is the image of the human pupil. The pupil acts as an aperture stop. Thus, we are looking at the entrance pupil, which is the image of the aperture stop.

17. Answer: A
$P_{total}=P_1+P_2$= +10 D
$CA_{total}=CA_1+CA_2$=0
CA=P/Abbe value
CA=0= P_1/58.6 +P_2/36.6
P_1= -58.6P_2/36.6
P_2 + (-58.6P_2/36.6)=10
P_2[(-58.6/36.6)+1]=10
P_2= -16.64 D
P_1=26.64 D

18. Answer: A
u= -0.5m
U=1/-0.5= -2 D
V= 5-2= +3 D
v= 1.5/3= 0.5 m behind the surface, thus image is real.
M=U/V= -2/3, if M<0 then image is inverted

19. Answer: C The lensometer uses a telescopic system to focus the target. None of the other choices use a telescopic system. The BIO images the object through the condensing lens to produce an upside down and inverted image. The DO directly views an object and magnifies it using a mirror built into the head, The slit lamp uses a microscope to produce the images. The retinoscope emits light that hits the patient's retina and is reflected back as a reflex.

20. Answer: A

CHAPTER 2: OPTICS (PHYSICAL)

1. Answer: A. For an anti-reflective coating to work, it must meet the path and amplitude conditions.
Path condition (to achieve destructive interference): $t = \lambda/(4n_c)$
Amplitude condition: $n_c = \sqrt{(n_1\, n_2)}$
Where t = thickness,
n_c = index of ARC,
n_g = index of the material
$n_c = \lambda/4t$ = (555 nm)/ 4(100 nm)= 1.38

2. Answer: E. First determine the angle made by the two point sources at the eye using the Rayleigh criterion.
$\theta_{min}=1.22\ \lambda/d$
d=diameter of aperture = 3 mm = 3×10^{-3} m
λ = 600 nm = 600×10^{-9} m
$\theta_{min} = 1.22\ (600 \times 10^{-9}\ m)/\ (3 \times 10^{-2}\ m) = 2.44 \times 10^{-4}$ radians
Now determine the distance between the two points. $\tan \theta_{min} = x/y$, where x = separation between the two point objects, y = distance the eye is from the point objects
In this example, y = the secondary focal length of the lens = 1/ (+5.00D) = 0.20 m.
We can use the small angle approximation here where $\tan \theta_{min} = \theta_{min}$.
Thus, $x = \theta_{min}\ y = (2.44 \times 10^{-5})(0.20) = 4.88 \times 10^{-5}$ m.

Since we have the separation of the two point objects in meters, we can calculate the distance in wavelength equivalence.
$(4.88 \times 10^{-5}\ m)/(600 \times 10^{-9}\ m)$ = 8.1 wavelengths

3. Answer: E. c=speed of light=3.00×10^{8} m/s= λf
f=frequency=$c/\lambda=(3.00\times10^{8})/600\times10^{-9} = 5 \times 10^{14}\ s^{-1} = 5 \times 10^{14}$ Hz
When light enters a medium, the frequency does not change. Thus, f=5×10^{14} Hz
$v_{medium}=\lambda f$ = (500 nm)(5×10^{14} Hz) = 2.5×10^{8} m/s

4. Answer: D. Use Snell's Law: $n_1\sin\theta_1 = n_2\sin\theta_2$
n_1=1.00 because the material is in air
θ_1=30
θ_2=45
1.00 sin (30) = n_2 sin (45)
n_2= 0.707

5. Answer: A
u=-0.15m → U =1.33/u
V=P+U=-3.867D
v=n/V=1.45/-3.867=-0.375m

6. Answer: B. When two waves are in phase, constructive interference occurs where the amplitudes are additive.

7. Answer: B
$y=m\lambda s/a=0$ for m=0
for m=1, $y=[1(500\times10^{-9})(2)]/0.0001 = 0.01$ m

8. Answer: C. A black body radiator is the thermal source of energy. The surface absorbs all radiant energy incident on it. Therefore, it appears black.

9. Answer: B. Radiant flux is the radiant energy emitted per unit time (units in watts).

10. Answer: A
11. Answer: A $n_c = \sqrt{n_g} = \sqrt{1.65} \approx 1.28$
12. Answer: B. Refer to the CIE diagram.

13. Answer: C
For m=0, $y=(m\lambda s)/a=0$ for m=0
For m=1, $y=(1\times500\times10^{-9}\times2)/(0.1\times10^{-3})$ =0.01m = 1cm

14. Answer: D
$$t_{destr} = \frac{m\ \lambda}{2\ n_{air}}$$
For m = 0, t = 0
For m = 1, t = 0.225
For m = 2, t = 0.450
For m = 3, t = …

A dark band occurs whenever the thickness changes by 0.225 microns.

(3/0.225) = 13.33 so the last band occurs when m = 13 Therefore, there are 14 dark bands (there is one for m = 0).

15. Answer: C
Two point resolution is limited by diffraction (the phenomena which occurs when a wave encounters an obstacle).

16. Answer: E
$\theta min = (1.22\lambda)/a = (1.22 \cdot 550x10^{-9}/6x10^{-3})$
= 0.00011183radians
=0.0064degrees
=0.384minutes of arc

17. Answer: C
$y_{min} = 1.5m = 1.22x550x10^{-9}s/6x10^{-3}$
s = 13,412.8m = 13.412km = 8.4miles

18. Answer: D
$Sin\ \theta = m\lambda/a = [(1)(633x10^{-9}) / 0.5x10^{-3}]$
$= 1.27x10^{-3}$ radians
Using the small angle approximation,
$\Theta = 1.27x10^{-3}$ radians

19. Answer: C
$\Theta = 1.27x10^{-3}$ radians
$Y = 10tan\Theta \approx 10 \cdot \Theta = 1.27cm$

20. Answer: C

CHAPTER 3: OPTICS (PHYSIOLOGICAL)

---

1. Answer: D. The first three choices cause image blur, not image mislocation. Curvature of field does not cause deviation from a spherical converging wavefront, but the wavefront is moved from the ideal position. This causes a crisp image to be formed in the wrong location.
2. Answer: D
The 6 Gullstrand 1 surfaces are
-ant/post cornea
-ant/post cortical lens
-ant/post nuclear lens
3. Answer: C
4. Answer: B
5. Answer: B

CHAPTER 4: OPHTHALMIC OPTICS

1. Answer: D
Axial ametropia: try to equalize the shape factor.

$Ms = 1/ (1\text{-}t/nP1)$

Therefore, choose the same P1 (BC) and same thickness.

2. Answer: C. For image jump, use the equation, $Z=P_{add}h_{cm}$ For a round 22mm seg, the r value is 11mm, so for this problem, we calculate Z=(+2.50)(1.1)=+2.75.

3. Answer: C. Since there is a difference in the BC reading, you know that this is a one-piece bifocal (add is due to change in curvature). Taking the difference between +8 to +6, you know the add must be +2.00. Sometimes, you will get help from the equation:

$$P_{true} = P_{clock} \frac{(n_{true}-1)}{(n_{clock}-1)}$$

4. Answer: D
The convex mirror is a diverging mirror.
r= -100cm
f2 = (r/2) = -50cm
For incoming plane waves, a virtual image would be formed 50cm behind the mirror. An observer looking at the mirror would see the virtual image.

5. Answer: B
For OCG, n=1.523.
$Pns=Po[1+\sin^2\alpha/2n]$
$= +8.00[1+(\sin^2 020/2(1.523))$
= + 8.31D

6. Answer: D
$x=P_{unk}/(P_{std}P'_{std})^2$
$x= (-5.00)/(+25.00)^2$
x= -0.008m; target moved 8mm away from the observer (for a minus lens, you move the target away)

7. Answer: D
For CR-39, n=1.498.
$\Delta s = Ph^2/2\Delta n$
$\Delta s = (-4.00)(0.027)^2/2(1.498-1.000)$
Δs = -2.93mm
Δs = ct-et so et = ct-Δs
Et = 2.0-(-2.93) = 4.93mm

8. Answer: C
Vertical prism effects can be compensated by all other choices.

9. Answer: C
Steps:

1) For CR-39, n = 1.498.
2) Find Rf.
   $Rf = [(1.498-1)/(1.498+1)]^2 = 0.0397$
3) Find transmittance.
   $T=(If-Rf)(1-Rb)q^x$
   $T=(1-0.0397)^2(0.75)^3$ (assume Rb=0)
   T=0.3890 = 38.9% transmission

10. Answer: B
Photochromic lenses are darker in:

- cooler temperatures
- thicker lenses (more photochromic materials contained in lens)
- heat tempered photochromics are darker than chemically tempered photochromics
- brighter environmental conditions cause the lens to darken more due to more UV

11. Answer: C
Use Δs= ct – et = $Ph^2/(2\Delta n)$ to find ct.
Given: P= -7.50 D, et= 5.3 mm, h= 24 mm, n=1.60
$Ct=[(-7.5)(0.024)^2/(2(1.60-1))] + 0.0053 = 0.0017$ m
$Et= ct - Ph^2/(2\Delta n) = 0.0017 – [(-7.5)(0.027)^2/(2(1.60-1))]= 0.00625$ m

12. Answer: E
Plus axis is along the 165 meridian
$P_T=P_C[(n_T-1)/(n_C-1)]$ = (3.5) [(1.7-1)/(1.7-1)] =+3.50 D

13. Answer: A
$P_{ns}=P_o[1+(\sin^2\theta/2n)]$
$P_C=P_{ns}\tan^2\theta$
n=1.60
P_o=-5.50D
Pantoscopic tilt is on 180 meridian
Calculate the actual Rx with a 10 deg tilt: -5.55-0.17x180
Calculate the actual Rx with a 25 deg tilt: -5.81-1.26x180
Determine the additional cyl
-1.26-(-0.17)= -1.09

14. Answer: B. Minus cylinder lens form has +4.00DS on the front (base curve) and -8.50-1.75x030 on the back. The power along the "power meridian" is -10.25 DS.
$P_T=P_C[(n_T-1)/(n_C-1)]$
n_T=1.701
n_C=1.53
P_C=-10.25D
Thus, P_T=-13.56 D

15. Answer: C
n=1.60
P_1=+8.00D
P_2=-3.25D

T=3.5 mm

$P_v=P_2+[P_1/(1-(t/n)P_1)]=+4.89D$

16. Answer: B. The lens segment top is 3 mm below the distance optical center (DOC). The vertical distance from the segment top to the segment optical center (SOC) is 5 mm in a flat top 28 bifocal segment. Thus, the total distance from the DOC to the SOC is 3+5=8 mm. We know that the reading level (RL) is 10 mm below the DOC. Now we need to calculate the distance from the reading level to the SOC. The SOC is 10-8=2 mm above the RL, therefore h=+0.2 cm. The vertical displacement at the reading level only depends on the add power, and is independent of the distance power. Therefore, we use P=+2.25D. We plug these numbers into Prentice's equation:

Z=hP=(+0.2)(+2.25)=+0.45 BU

17. Answer: D

Use Prentice's eq: Z=hP

OD: +2 BO=h(+4)

h=0.5 cm=5 mm out wrt PRP

OS: +2 BO=h(+4)

h=0.5 cm

(FPD-pt's PD)/2=(49+17-63)/2=1.5 mm=PRP is

1.5 mm in wrt GC

5-1.5=3.5=OC is 3.5 mm out wrt GC

IPD=distance between optical centers

DOC's=FPD+2(3.5)=66+7=73 mm

18. Answer: A

s=(+4D)(0.075mm/1D)=0.0003m

$s= Ph^2/(2\Delta n)$

$h^2=(s \times 2\Delta n)/P= (0.0003m)(2)(1.53-1)/4 = 0.0000795$

h=0.00892 m. Separation between outer pins=2h=17.83 mm

19. Answer: D

Given: $P_T=+1.50D$, $n_c=1.498$, $P_{1,c}=+4.50D$, $P_{2,c}=- 3.50D$

Determine the true front and back surface powers using $P_T=P_C[(n_T-1)/(n_C-1)]$

$P_{T,1}=P_{C,1}[(n_T-1)/(n_C-1)]=(4.50/1.498-1)(n_T-1)=9.036(n_T-1)$

$P_{T,2}=-7.028(n_T-1)$

Back vertex power=$P_V=P_T=+1.50D= P_{T,1}+ P_{T,2}=9.036(n_T-1)+ -7.028(n_T-1)=2.008(n_T-1)$

$n_T=1.75$

20. Answer: B

Since back surface is concave, sag value is negative. Given: s=-2.8mm, h=1/2(50.0mm)=25.0mm, n=1.586

Use $s= Ph^2/(2\Delta n)$

$P=(s)(2\Delta n)/h^2=2(0.586)(-0.0028)/(0.025)^2= -5.25D$

21. Answer: E

Given: P=-5.00D, h=26.0mm, n=1.498, ct=2.0mm.

Use $\Delta s= ct - et = Ph^2/(2\otimes n)$ to find et.

$\Delta s= 2.0 - et = (-5)(0.026)^2/[2(1.498-1)] \times 1000= -3.39$ mm

et=2.0-(-3.39)=5.39 mm

22. Answer: B

Decentration=(FPD-IPD)/2=[(54+16)-60]/2=5.0mm in

MBS=ED+(2x dec/lens)=54+2(5)=64mm

23. Answer: A

Given: P=-6.00D, h=26.0mm, n=1.60, ct=1.8mm.

Use $\Delta s= ct - et = Ph^2/(2\otimes n)$ to find et.

$\Delta s= 1.8 - et = (-6)(0.026)^2/[2(1.60-1)] \times 1000= -3.38$ mm

et=1.8-(-3.38)=5.18mm

24. Answer: A

Use $\Delta t=Zh/100(n-1)$ =2(55)/100(0.498)=2.209mm

Nasal edge=2.209+0.5=2.709mm

25. Answer: D

Keyhole is a type of frame bridge.

26. Answer: A

30° from power meridian: $\langle$=060

$P_{\langle}=P_s+P_c\sin^2\langle=-4.50+-1.50\sin^2 060=-5.625D$

Use $\Delta s= ct - et = Ph^2/(2\otimes n)$ to find et.

$\Delta s= 1.8 - et = (-5.625)(0.026)^2/[2(1.60-1)] \times 1000= -3.17$ mm

et=1.8-(-3.17)=4.97mm

27. Answer: B

Since the new position of the lens solves the patient's problems, they are looking through the effective power instead of the intended power of +2.50D.

$P_{eff}=P_o/(1-dP_o)$

P_o=power at old vertex distance=+2.50D

D=vertex distance change=5mm=0.005m

$P_{eff}=2.5/[1-(.005)(2.5)]=2.53D$

28. Answer: A

Use P= -2n/r for a mirror in air.

The value r is positive for convex mirrors.

Thus, P=-2(1.8)/0.3=-12D

29. Answer: B

Given: P=-4.50D, h=26.0mm, n=1.60, ct=1.8mm.

Use $\Delta s= ct - et = Ph^2/(2\otimes n)$ to find et.

$\Delta s= 1.8 - et = (-4.5)(0.026)^2/[2(1.60-1)] \times 1000= -2.535$ mm

et=1.8-(-2.535)=4.34mm

30. Answer: A
The material with the least amount of lateral chromatic aberration will have the largest Abbe value. This is based on the equation LCA=P/abbe value. The Abbe values are: glass=59, CR-39=58, polycarbonate=30, highlite glass=31, and given Hi-index plastic=37. Glass has the highest Abbe value and, therefore, has the least amount of lateral chromatic aberration.

NBEO Questions
31. Answer: C
32. Answer: C
33. Answer: B
34. Answer: D

CHAPTER 5: CONTACT LENSES

1. Answer: A. With-the-rule cornea is the steepest vertical. Spherical RGP will reveal a vertical band of pooling, where the RGP is not closely matched to the curvature of the cornea.
2 Answer: A. Power can be verified with the use of a lensometer. Diameter: can be verified with a contact lens loupe. Base curve: can be verified with a radiuscope.
3. Answer: A. Preservative in the contact lenses solution is added to prevent and kill the growth of bacterial and viral pathogens. Viral infection would include a follicular response with watery/red eyes. Bacterial infection would include heavy discharge, significant red eye and anterior chamber reaction.
4. Answer: C. ClearCare is an example of a hydrogen peroxide contact lenses cleaning system, where the solution needs to be neutralized with a platinum catalyst, enzyme catalase, sodium pyruvate or sodium sulfite for at least 6 hours prior to insertion. Patient had chemically burned his cornea by coming in contact with hydrogen peroxide.
5. Answer: C. Hydrogen peroxide is a very effective antibacterial and antiviral and helps maintain clean lenses but is not effective against the protozoan Acanthamoeba. Keratitis secondary to Acanthamoeba develops ring infiltrates later and patient has pain out of proportion to ocular signs.
6. Answer: D. Hydrogel lenses absorb topical medication well and are an effective lens choice for bandage contact lenses.
7. Answer: A. Systemic medications, such as tetracycline, phenazopyridine, phenolphthalein, and nitrofurantoin can also lead to contact lenses discoloration.
8. Answer: D. Corneal toxicity induced by incompatible contact lenses solution can lead to diffuse superficial punctuate keratitis.
9. Answer: D. Hydrogel lenses are not cleaned or compatible with BAC because BAC is absorbed into the lens and later released, which is toxic to the cornea.
10. Answer D.
Lens lubricants contain a low concentration of nonionic surfactant to help keep lenses clean, a polymer to lubricate the lens, and buffering agents.

11. Answer B
12. Answer D
13. Answer A
14. Answer B
15. Answer D
16. Answer D
17. Answer A
18. Answer D
19. Answer C
20. Answer A
21. Answer B
22. Answer A
23. Answer B
24. Answer A
25. Answer D
26. Answer A
27. Answer A
28. Answer C
29. Answer A
30. Answer C

CHAPTER 6: LOW VISION

1. Answer: A
2. Answer: B
3. Answer: D
4. Answer: D
5. Answer: C
6. Answer: A
7. Answer: E
8. Answer: B
9. Answer: A
10. Answer: C
11. Answer: C
12. Answer: C
13. Answer: C. That there isn't a strong genetic component for cataracts but she should always wear sunglasses when outside to significantly lower her chances of getting cataracts.
14. Answer: C
15. Answer: E
16. Answer B
17. Answer B
18. Answer E. Use a Fresnel prism over the top part of the right eye, base up.
19. Answer: C. Larger lens diameter
20. Answer D
21. Answer A
22. Answer F
23. Answer A. Galilean because it offers the wider field of view
24. Answer E
25. Answer C. Chosen letters prohibit successful guessing
26. Answer C
27. Answer B
28. Answer D. Start from retinoscopy or an old Rx and bracket with large dioptric values so that the patient can definitively make a lens selection
29. Answer C
30. Answer D

CHAPTER 7: ACCOMMODATION, VERGENCE AND OCULOMOTOR ANOMALIES

1. Answer: C
2. Answer: D
3. Answer: A
4. Answer: B
5. Answer: A
6. Answer: C
7. Answer: A
8. Answer: B
9. Answer: B
10. Answer: C
11. Answer B.
12. Answer. B
13. Answer C. Proximal is caused by nearness of an object.
14. Answer D. Compared to all eye movements, vergence eye movements have the greatest latency (takes the longest to become stimulated into action.)
15. Answer: D. Microstrabismus is not a fine motor eye movement.
16. Answer: C. The generally preferred therapy is bifocals along with either patching or using cycloplegics regularly on the good eye. The bifocals should correct the refractive error and relax accommodation, without the use of prism.
17. Answer: B. Duane's. Duane's can sometimes look like a LR palsy because of the restricted abduction, but the key is to look for retraction of the eye and narrowing of the palpebral fissure upon medial gaze.
18. Answer B. Brown's Syndrome is sometimes mistaken for a SO palsy because of the restriction in elevation during abduction. It is usually congenital, so diplopia is not commonly a symptom.
19. Answer C. Null point is the position of both eyes where these is no nystagmus. Patients tend to develop a head turn in order to keep their eyes at the null point.
20. Answer: A. With NRA, plus lenses are used to relax accommodation and cause eyes to diverge, but stimulates compensatory convergence in order to maintain binocular single vision. A low NRA thus would mean the patient has excess accommodation and poor convergence.
21. Answer B. His calculated AC/A is 8.1/1. Set at 33cm, his new heterophoria is ~6 eso.
22. Answer: C. Signal travels from optic nerve to pretectal nucleus, then onto EW nucleus. The signal then travels down CNIII to the ciliary ganglion before entering the

orbit via the short ciliary nerves to innervate the sphincter muscles.
23. Answer: A. Pursuits are the slowest (21 deg arc/sec) compared to saccades (1000 deg arc/sec) and smooth pursuits (40 deg arc/sec).
24. Answer: B. Bell's Phenomemon is when eyes move upwards and outwards upon bilateral closure of the eyelids.
25. Answer A. All are correct except A, since Spasmus Nutans is associated with fine, pendular nystagmus.
26. Answer B. A brain lesion affecting the visual radiations in the parietal lobe will cause an abnormal OKN response.
27. Answer B. Method of Adjustments is when the subject manipulates the stimulus and after a
set number of trials, the average reading is recorded.
28. Answer C. Hit rate is Hits/(Hits+Misses), or 7/10.

NBEO Questions
29. Answer B
30. Answer C
31. Answer C

CHAPTER 8: AMBLYOPIA/STRABISMUS

1. Answer: A
2. Answer: B
3. Answer: C
4. Answer: B
5. Answer: C
6. Answer: B
7. Answer: D
8. Answer: A
9. Answer: E
10. Answer: D
11. Answer: B
12. Answer: D
13. Answer: B
14. Answer: D
15. Answer: C Tritan – this is a result of increased brunescence of the natural lens over time.
16. Answer: D
17. Answer: C. A 25-year old Native American female with unequal VA's and a history of crossed eyes.
Not (a) bc a baseline should be established, especially for young males to avoid potential problems in school.
Not (b) bc peripheral field loss could indicate glaucoma; you would expect to find a B-Y defect in early glaucoma.
Not (d) acute optic neuropathy may present with color vision loss.
18. Answer: D. Farnsworth D-15 – the D-15 is the most appropriate test of those listed because it reveals tritan as well as deutan and protan defects.
19. Answer: B. A genetic defect that prevents his body from producing erythrolabe – an electrician is required to differentiate different colored wires in order to perform his job properly.
20. Answer: C
21. Answer C. 20/120 – MAR = EF + 1
22. Answer: D. Leave well enough alone – this patient has unharmonious ARC; treating the patient endangers him of intractable diplopia.
23. Answer: A. The dominant eye should receive the red lens, so that the non-dominant eye can see the print.
24. Answer D. Comitance
25. Answer B. Tranaglyph – this is the only technique that requires color discrimination.
26. Answer D. 30 prism diopters
27. Answer C. Eccentric fixation is steady and vertical .
28. Answer D. Angle H is less than 20 prism diopters.
29. Answer A. Enlarged blind spot – the signs and symptoms above describe an amblyope; amblyopia does not cause an enlarged blind spot.
30. Answer: D. Malingering – it is impossible for the patient to see the scenario described.

CHAPTER 9: PERCEPTUAL FUNCTION/COLOR VISION

1. Answer: A In a left SO palsy, left eye is hyper, worse on right gaze, worse on left head tilt.
2. Answer: D Looming is a kinetic monocular depth cue, not a pictorial one.
3. Answer: B Space myopia may contaminate the binocular balance
4. Answer: C Hering's Law of Equal Innervation dictates that both eyes make a version to the right, but the right eye must make a vergence back to the left to focus on the point.
5. Answer: A When magnifying the left eye's image vertically, it appears that the left side is closer because it is larger, and the right side is farther because it is smaller, so the plane appears to be slanted.
6. Answer: B The scotopic visual system is most sensitive to 507 nm because this wavelength is most effective at bleaching rhodopsin.
7. Answer: C After 1.5 min, 50% of the photopigment has regenerated and 50% remains bleached. Over the next 1.5 minutes, 50 percent of the remaining photopigment recovers. Consequently, the total amount of cone photopigment that recovers after 3 minutes is 50% + 25% = 75%.
8. Answer: C
9. Answer: A
10. Answer: B
11. Answer: A
12. Answer: D. internuclear opthalmoplegia secondary to multiple sclerosis.
13. Answer: B. Unilateral trochlear palsy; patch and wait 6 months to see if it resolves, then surgery.
14. Answer: B
15. Answer: C. To the right of the object - though the patient's eye cannot make the vergence movement necessary for the target, the feedback mechanism makes him believe he is pointing in the correct direction; consequently, he will point too far in the direction of the paretic muscle.
16. Answer: B. OD: +5.00, OS: +2.00 – the difference in the hyperopia is likely to result in amblyopia if left uncorrected.
17. Answer: A
18. Answer: D
19. Answer: B
20. Answer: A
21. Answer: D
22. Answer: B
23. Answer: A. The right lens is tinted darker than the left lens – this patient is experiencing the Pulfrich Effect.
24. Answer: C
25. Answer: C
26. Answer: D
27. Answer: C.
28. Answer A.
29. Answer: A
30. Answer B

CHAPTER 10: VISUAL AND HUMAN DEVELOPMENT

1. Answer: B. Infants have one log unit less sensitivity than adults for wavelengths below 450nm. By 2 months, infants can use smooth pursuits for low velocities. High frequency contrast sensitivity gratings and accurate accommodation are achieved later
2. Answer: D. Pattern deprivation can cause amblyopia. Ptosis, cataracts and corneal scarring can all inhibit visual information from reaching the brain. If this happens at an early age, amblyopia can occur. AMD does not cause amblyopia
3. Answer C. The test with a rapidly blinking light is CFF (critical flicker frequency) and normal threshold is reached by 2-4 months of age
4. Answer: D. Dark adaptation decreases because of inadequate regeneration of rhodopsin and decreased ability to metabolize vitamin. Increased glare can be caused by light scattering due to cataracts. Light sensitivity decreases because retinal illuminance decreases because less light reaches the retina due to opacification of ocular media. Visual fields decrease in part because of nuclear lens sclerosis (also because of senile miosis and decreases retinal illumination). This is why you have to enter an age when you do visual fields. A normal 80-year-old's VFs will be very different from a 13-year old's.

5. Answer: B. The Gardener test of visual perceptual skills (TVPS) has a visual figure ground section. For this section the patient must find a particular shape amidst a distracting background.
6. Answer: B. The average refractive error of premature babies is -0.50DS.
7. Answer: C. The average refractive error for fullterm babies is +2.00DS.
8. Answer: B. Accommodation develops fully by 3-4 months.
9. Answer: C. Convergence ability generally stay the same over time because of the unlimited use of accommodative convergence.
10. Answer: B. The limiting factor is cortical development. If ocular dominance columns do not emerge after birth, then stereopsis is not possible.
11. Answer: D. All of the above, as well as irreversible visual field defects and loss of binocularity.
12. Answer: C. At birth, all retinal cells are present (mitosis has ended) but cones are spaced more apart. Therefore, visual signals must be stronger at birth in order to stimulate more cones.
13. Answer: A. A dragged macula caused by temporal blood vessels pulling on the macula.
14. Answer: D. A quick pneumonic to remember for causes of fetal morbidity is TORCH – Toxoplasmosis, Other (syphilis, AIDS), Rubella, Cytomegalovirus, Herpes Simplex.
15. Answer: A. While all are correct, the first answer is the most accurate in terms of dark adaptation.
16. Answer: D. Pointing at objects isn't expected until close to 1 year of age.
17. Answer: A. Visual acuity.
18. Answer: A. Bruckner's reflex (difference in color or brightness of retinal reflex between the two eyes) is used to look for amblyogenic factors such as anisometropia, strabismus, or media opacity.
19. Answer: C. 6-8 months.
20. Answer: B. Binocular OKN is present at birth, monocular OKN develops by 6-8 months.
21. Answer: A Strabismus.
22. Answer: D. Corneal diameter reaches adult size (~11-12mm) by 2 years of age.
23. Answer: A. Premies will have the steepest corneas (~54D). By age 1, the average is 44D.
24. Answer: D. Colobomas are associated with CHARGE disorders: Coloboma, Heart problems, Atresia, Retardation, Genital abnormalities, Ear deformation and abnormalities.
25. Answer: A. Monocular deprivation is worse since it drives visual pathways in the cortex visual to develop for one side but not the other. In binocular deprivation, acuity will be decreased symmetrically in both eyes.

NBEO Questions
26. Answer: D.
27. Answer: D.

CHAPTER 11: LIDS/LASHES/LACRIMAL SYSTEM/OCULAR ADNEXA/ORBIT ANATOMY

1. Answer: B
2. Answer: D
3. Answer: B. Zeiss glands are sebaceous glands that are associated with hair follicles
4. Answer: C.
5. Answer: D.
6. Answer: C.
7. Answer: D.
8. Answer: B.
9. Answer: A. Tobramycin, every one to two hours initially, tapering for 7-10 days.
10. Answer C. motor nerves are well developed, tendons of recti muscles fuse with sclera, sutures of the orbit close.
11. Answer D. Because the nasociliary branch of cranial nerve V (trigeminal) innervates the globe, the most serious ocular involvement develops if this branch is affected. Classically, involvement of the tip of the nose (Hutchinson's sign) has been thought to be a clinical predictor of ocular involvement. Herpes simplex infections do not manifest on the nose.
12. Answer: A. The stability of the tear film is dependent upon the integrity of the meibomian glands which secrete oil to keep the tears from evaporating.
13. Answer: B. Wernicke's sign is associated with lesion in the peripheral portion of the sensory visual pathway, prior to the entrance of the optic tract into the thalamus. The visual field of the two eyes

exhibit a homonymous defect. The near reflex is frequently normal.
14. Answer: E. The likely result from a brain lesion that was confined to the superior salivatory nucleus in the pons is reduced lacrimation on the ipsilateral side.
15. Answer: A. The postganglionic fibers travel in the internal carotid nerve. The central neurons lie in the hypothalamus.
16. Answer: C. The sensory root (nervus intermedius) supplies the tongue, the external auditory meatus (earhole), and part of the soft palate and pharynx.
17. Answer: D. Adults blinded at an early age show abnormal VOR responses.
18. Answer: A. Infant saccades show a longer latency to initiate compared to adults. They use multiple saccades to reach a visual target. Also, the effective VF for eliciting saccades increases after birth.
19. Answer C. Neurogenic ptosis is ptosis secondary to 3rd nerve.
20. Answer: E. Nasociliary nerve, anastomosis between zygomatic nerve and the inferior division of lacrimal nerve, the greater superficial petrosal nerve and the nerve of pterygoid canal all innervates lacrimation in some way.
21. Answer: C. The spinal accessory nerve provides motor innervation from the central nervous system to two muscles of the neck: the sternocleidomastoid muscle and the upper part of the trapezius muscle. The ternocleidomastoid muscle tilts and rotates the head, while the trapezius muscle has several actions on the scapula, including shoulder elevation. Range of motion and strength testing of the neck and shoulders can be measured during a neurological examination to assess function of the spinal accessory nerve. Limited range of motion or poor muscle strength is suggestive of damage to the spinal accessory nerve, which can result from a variety of causes.
22. Answer: C. The edge of the optic nerve and the corneal margin surround Tenon's capsule.
23. Answer: D. Superior oblique is the longest and thinnest EOM.
24. Answer: D. This affects the parasympathetic system. Pupils fail to dilate in dim light, and usually related to tertiary syphilis.
25. Answer: E. Penicillin and bacitracin inhibits peptidoglycan cross-link formation of the cell wall. Tobramycin affects the protein synthesis by blocking the 30S and 50S ribosomes. Sulfonamides act as competitive inhibitors of the the enzyme dihydropteroate synthetase (DHPS).
26: Answer: D. Nystatin is a polyene antifungal drug to which many molds and yeast infections are sensitive, including *Candida* spp. Methiazone blocks protein synthesis.
27. Answer: D. The Vidian nerve and the infraorbital nerve are usually found in the pterygopalatine fossa.
28. Answer: E. AION affects the pre-laminar or laminar portion of the optic nerve.
29. Answer: D. The angle between the orbital axis of the right orbit and the orbital axis of the left orbit is about 45 degrees, not 90 degrees.
30. Answer: D In RAPD, there is decreased visual acuity due to retinal pathology or opacity in the lens (ie. Cataract scattering light), there is pronounced sensory loss in one eye. Patient's pupil dilates instead of constricts when light swings from the unaffected "good" eye to the affected "bad" eye.

NBEO Questions
31. Answer: C

CHAPTER 12: CONJUNCTIVA/CORNEA/ REFRACTIVE SURGERY

1. Answer: A. Patients with keratoconus often have a hyperopic astigmatic shift in refractive error due to inferior steepening of the cornea.
2. Answer: D. Goblet cells secret mucus (the bottom layer of the tear), which helps to stabilize the adhesion of tear film to cornea.
3. Answer: C. Macrophage and lymphocyte cells can be found inside the stroma. Their main purpose is to fight infection
4. Answer: D. Foreign body that passes through the Bowman's membrane will leave a scar on the cornea.
5. Answer: D. Recurrent corneal erosion can lead to sharp eye pain after the patient

woke up and opened eyes. Epithelium is loosely attached the cornea in the morning for patient with RCE and this corneal layer can be easily removed with lid opening leading to sharp eye pain.

6. Answer: A. Macular, granular and lattice dystrophies belong to the stromal layer.

7. Answer: B. Astigmatic keratotomy (AK) is a refractive surgical procedure that can correct or reduce astigmatism. This procedure can be performed in additional to other refractive surgeries if the surgeon feels that a further reduction in post-op astigmatism is needed.

8. Answer: B. Your patient had an iris-claw lens in his eyes s/p cataract surgery. The lens is fixed onto the iris inside the anterior chamber so you should not dilate this patient. A referral is needed if the patient needs to be dilated.

9. Answer: A. LASIK uses a keratome to cut open a partial thickness corneal flap and laser is applied to the underlying stroma to reshape the cornea for refractive correction. LASEK also has a flap, but it is only composed of a thin layer of epithelium. LASIK and LASEK both reduce the healing time and post-op pain compared to PRK.

10. Answer: A. Infectious corneal ulcer can be secondary to gram + or – microbial organism. Most common cause of all bacterial ulcers is Pseudomonas. Seen more in warmer climates. CL wearers are at greater risk. Subjectively, patients usually complain of irritation, progressing to increased lacrimation, photophobia, reduced VA due to edema and infiltrates, and finally deep seated pain. Objectively, ulcer usually locates centrally with edema, larger epithelial defect and more anterior chamber reaction compared to sterile corneal ulcer.

11. Answer: C. Cornea has the richest sensory innervation in the body, but exposed nerve ending secondary to dry eyes can cause a lot of eye discomfort, especially if the epithelial staining is central.

12. Answer: A. Signs of Fuchs endothelial dystrophy include corneal guttata, decreased endothelial cell density, increased pleomorphism, increased polymegathism, early stromal edema, late epithelial edema, bullae, and fibrosis.

13. Answer: B. The five layers of cornea in order are: epithelium, Bowman's layer, stroma, Descemet's membrane and endothelium. The appearance of superficial lesions (epithelial defects) can be accentuated with fluorescein. Foreign bodies that penetrated past Bowman usually cannot be stained if epithelium has re-epithelized/regenerated. Lesions that travel past Bowman's layer lead to stromal scarring.

14. Answer: A. Infants/Children often have hyperopia. At birth, the corneal curvature is flatter than the adult's. On average, at age 4, children have about +1.00 D hyperopia and emmetropization is completed when they are around age 10.

15. Answer: B. Average cornea is about 535 microns, epithelium is about 50 microns, stromal bed is about 250 microns and LASIK flap is about 150 microns. So 535- (150 +250) = 135 microns is what the surgeon has left to work with. Assuming removing 10 microns corrects 1D myopia, 5 x 10 =50 microns needed to be removed to correct for -5.00D of myopia, which is plenty since the surgeon has 135 microns to work with.

16. Answer: D. Other aging changes of the cornea also include increase in light scatter, stippling of Bowman's membrane, thickening of Descemet's membrane, Hassall-Henle bodies and endothelial cell loss.

17. Answer: B. Cornea is highly sensitive to both touch and pain, with pain threshold about ten times higher than the touch threshold. Moreover, cornea contains many cold sensing spots, but the sense of heat is almost entirely absent. This explains why it is usually more comfortable for a hard contact lens wearer to rinse his lenses in warm water, whereas cold water produces discomfort when the lens is placed upon the eye.

18. Answer: C. Ocular rosacea is more common in white females in their 30 to 50's. It is a chronic inflammatory disease that affects the eyes. Acne rosacea is often associated with ocular rosacea and some objective signs can include: erythematous skin, telangiectatic vessels, follicular pustules and raised papules, thickened skin on the nose and sebaceous gland hypertrophy.

19. Answer: A. Ectoderm specializes forming conjunctival and corneal epithelium as well as glands.

20. Answer: A. Sjogren's syndrome is an autoimmune condition which affects the exocrine glands that produce tears and saliva. Patient has dry eyes and mouth.

These patients are often treated with artificial tears, and sometimes steroid and non-steroid anti-inflammatory agents.
21. Answer: D. Fluorescein is a water-soluble compound and easily dissolves in tear. It is repelled by intact corneal and conjunctival epithelium and attracted to corneal stroma. Rose-bengal stains devitalized epithelial cells a bright purples color. It will not stain stroma or healthy cells and is slower to stain than fluorescein.
22. Answer: A. Proparacaine is commonly used anesthetic, but since benoxinate inhibits the fluorescence of fluorescein less, it's the anesthetic that is used in Fluress.
23. Answer: A. Anesthetics compete for receptor sites of calcium channels and directly inhibit the permeability of the nerve to sodium. Most anesthetics last for about 10-30 minutes.
24. Answer: C. Corneal innervation is derived from ophthalmic division of cranial nerve V primarily by long nasociliary nerves; some innervation is by short ciliary nerves, which are branched from ciliary ganglion.
25. Answer: A. BAK or Benzalkonium chloride is a common preservative used in ophthalmic products.
26. Answer: D. Graves' disease is autoimmune disease that causes over-activity of the thyroid gland, causing hyperthyroidism. Some ocular signs include proptosis, exophthalmos, and diplopia.
27. Answer: A. Corneal epithelium is 50 micron.
28. Answer: A. Bowman's layer is also called anterior limiting membrane and anterior elastic lamina. It's 8-14 microns thick and indistinguishable from stroma.
29. Answer: A. 10 mm for newborn and 12 mm for adults
30. Answer: B. Localized thickenings in the peripheral cornea are called Hassall Henle bodies, which increase with age and appear as dark spots or holes in endothelium

CHAPTER 13: LENS/CATARACT/IOL/PRE AND POST OPERATIVE CARE

1. Answer: A
2. Answer: A. Y-sutures are the insertions of the lens fiber. Erect Y shape is on the anterior surface and an inverted Y is on the posterior surface
3. Answer: A Cornea absorbs UVC while lens absorbs UVA and UVB.
4. Answer: D
5. Answer: D In additional to choice A, B and C, trauma and genetics also may play a role in cataract development
6. Answer: C Diabetes can lead to rapid cataract development. Diabetic patients have an elevated glucose level in the aqueous and the glucose goes through sorbitol pathway leading to an increase in sorbitol concentration within the lens fiber and draw water into the fiber. This causes lens to swell and disrupts the lens fiber. Lens thus, loses its transparency.
7. Answer: B. Yellow filter does not improve contrast, but does cut down the amount of blue light entering into the eyes. Blue light has short wavelength and is most easily scattered causes vision impairment Therefore, some patients may experience an improvement in vision with yellow glasses
8. Answer: A. The effect on color is negligible and patients are usually unaware of the difference until after cataract surgery. Pupil testing includes checking for an APD to evaluate the extent that light is being obscured.
9. Answer: D. The thinnest part of the capsule is the posterior pole and the thickest is the equator.
10. Answer: B. PSC is located on the posterior pole, which is the nodal point of the eye.
11. Answer: B. Second sight is when a presbyope reports being able to read again and occurs with a myopic shift in the lens, usually with diabetes or nuclear sclerosis. An oblique beam is the best way to assess for nuclear sclerosis. Both retroillumination and oblique beam are useful methods to assess a PSC.
12. Answer: D. This describes cortical spoking cataracts. Near blur is a complaint due to reduced accommodation reported by patients with PSC. Color change is rarely a complaint, but it would most likely occur with NS due to yellowing of the lens.
13. Answer: C. The embryonic nucleus contains the original lens fiber cells formed

in the lens vesicle. The epinucleus is not defined as a developmental nucleus. It describes the area between the hardened embryonic/fetal core and the softer infantile/adult nucleus.

14. Answer: C. Actin is in all lens fibers. Cholesterol is the major sterol in the lens. Along with a major saturated fatty acid and phospholipid, cholesterol is responsible for a highly ordered membrane.

15. Answer: E. The erect Y suture is in the anterior fetal nucleus and the inverted is in the posterior fetal nucleus. The cortex, comprised of the newest lens fibers, will have the most complicated suture.

16. Answer: C. The tunica vasculosa lentis is present before the lens has matured. The Na/K ATPase is necessary for ion transport through the lens capsule.

17. Answer: B. Aromatic amino acids that absorb UV include tyrosine, phenylalanine, and tryptophan. Glutathione is a tripeptide antioxidant that has several functions. It maintains lens transparency by preventing crystalline aggregation, aids amino acid transport, and protects cells against oxidative damage from free radicals. Glutathione is found in high concentrations in the epithelial layer.

18. Answer: A Alpha crystallins has a more significant effect as it is found in all lens cells (both the epithelial cells and fibers). Beta and gamma are only in elongated cell fibers.

19. Answer: D. Neuroectoderm: neural retina, RPE, iris muscle and pigment epithelium, vitreous. optic nerve. **Cranial neural crest cells**: cornea, sclera, trabecular meshwork, ciliary muscles, orbital bones. **Surface ectoderm**: conjunctival epithelium, lacrimal glands, lens, vitreous **Mesoderm**: extraocular muscles, endothelial lining of blood vessels, vitreous, temporal sclera.

20. Answer: D. The zonules are formed from the tertiary vitreous.

21. Answer: B. Anterior subcapsular cataracts are usually caused by trauma or UV. It is a metaplastic change between the epithelium and the capsule. New epithelial cells are pushed around the equator to the posterior side of the lens. Posterior cells get pushed more posterior and then elongate.

22. Answer: A. The total amount of protein is the same in nucleus sclerosis, but only the amount of soluble protein decreases. In cortical cataracts, there is an overall decrease in lens proteins. In spoking cataracts, a group of fibers are affected. In lamellar cataracts, fibers of a particular shell are affected.

23. Answer: D. Although hypertension can be a risk factor for cataracts, the rest have higher risk for cataracts with renal failure and glaucoma being the highest.

24. Answer: B.

25. Answer: E

26. Answer: C. This can be solved without a calculator. You need to know:

1) Brewster's law
2) The path of light (anatomy)
3) The relative indices of refraction (not exact)
4) Basic trigonometry

Brewster's angle = $\tan^{-1}(n_2/n_1)$

The index of refraction of the aqueous humor is 1.336. The index of refraction of the lens is a gradient and can range from 1.386 at the outer edges to 1.406 at the center. For all parts of the lens, the index of refraction (n_2) is greater than the index of refraction of the aqueous humor (n_1).

n_2/n_1 will always be greater than 1.

$\text{Tan}^{-1}(1) = 45$ degrees or $\pi/4$

$\text{Tan}_{-1}(>1) = >45$ degrees

$\text{Tan}_{-1}(<1) = < 45$ degrees

27. Answer: B

28. Answer: B The surface that creates the glare is the road, which is horizontal. A vertical transmission axis would block out the most light.

29. Answer: C

30. Answer: B

31. Answer: B Accommodation is not required to focus objects beyond 6m.

32. Answer: C Longer wavelengths (red light) are transmitted faster and are focused behind the retina. Shorter wavelengths (blue light) are transmitted slower and are focused in front of the retina.

NBEO Question

33. Answer: B

Short answer

34. Increases

35. The equator, where the zonules insert

36. The portion of the surface ectoderm that is in direct contact with the neural ectoderm at the optic outgrowth

37. At the center of the lens

38. In the nucleus

CHAPTER 14: EPISCLERA/ SCLERA/ ANTERIOR UVEA

1. Answer: C
2. Answer: B. PredForte (prednisolone acetate) for moderate to severe anterior uveitis
3. Answer: D. The major circle of the iris is located in the stroma of the ciliary body
4. Answer: A. Pars plicata extends into the posterior chamber
5. Answer: C. Usually asymptomatic
6. Answer: D. Cushing's syndrome is caused by long term systemic CORT use
7. Answer: C. Pilocarpine will cause ciliary spasm, not appropriate for anterior uveitis.
8. Answer: C Not an infection
9. Answer: A
10. Answer: C
11. Answer: A
12. Answer: D
13. Answer: E. Produces a stasis pressure which dilates distal veins causing anastomoses and formation of the Canal of Schlemm
14. Answer: D
15. Answer: A
16. Answer: B
17. Answer: C
18. Answer: D. Results in mydriasis in patients with post-ganglionic sympathetic denervation
19. Answer: B. Increased aqueous outflow
20. Answer: A
21. Answer: E. Decrease in the "spaces of Fontana"
22. Answer: D
23. Answer: D
24. Answer: A
25. Answer: C. Decrease in IOP due to decrease in aqueous production
26. Answer: C.
27. Answer: A
28. Answer: E.
29. Answer: D.

CHAPTER 15: VITREOUS/RETINA/CHOROID

1. Answer: C Strongest adhesion is at the vitreal base. The second strongest attachment is at the ONH.
2. Answer: E. These are the layers, not cell types
3. Answer: C. The NFL thins towards the ora serrata.
4. Answer: D. Myopia is a higher risk factor.
5. Answer: D. Microaneurysms are the earliest signs of non-proliferative diabetic retinopathy. Neovascularization and pre-retinal hemorrhage are seen in proliferative diabetic retinopathy, which is a severe form of diabetic retinopathy.
6. Answer: B Presumed ocular histoplasmosis syndrome (POHS) is characterized by the triad of:
1. Midperipheral yellow-white lesions
2. Macular neovascularization
3. Peripapillary atrophy

7. Answer: C. Central Retinal Vein Occlusion (CRVO) is caused by a blood clot in the CRV, which slows or stops blood from leaving the retina. As a result, blood and fluid are backed up which causes retinal injury and loss of vision. Over time as the retina becomes "ischemic" (which means starved for oxygen-containing blood).
8. Answer: C. Henle's Fiber Layer is OPC
9. Answer: D Microglia are a type of glial cell that are the resident macrophages of the brain, and thus act as the first and main form of active immune defense in the central nervous system (CNS). Microglia must be able to recognize foreign bodies, swallow them, and act as antigen-presenting cells activating T-cells.
10. Answer: A. Photodynamic therapy with verteporfin is aimed at treating patients with subfoveal choroidal neovascularization (CNV) caused by age-related macular degeneration (ARMD).
11. Answer: D VA usually worse than 20/200
12. Answer: B. Neuroectoderm: neural retina, RPE, iris muscle and pigment epithelium, vitreous, optic nerve **Cranial neural crest cells**: cornea, sclera, trabecular meshwork, ciliary muscles, orbital Bones. **Surface ectoderm**: conjunctival epithelium, lacrimal glands, lens, vitreous

Mesoderm: extraocular muscles, endothelial lining of blood vessels, vitreous, temporal sclera
13. Answer: D
14. Answer: C. In the macula, the cones are the same volume but elongated to accommodate for the extremely dense crowding.
15. Answer: B. The primary vitreous is a mass of fibers vascularized by the hyaloid artery. The secondary vitreous is avascular.
16. Answer: B. 150um is the diameter of the umbo (the very center of the fovea) 1.5mm is the diameter of the fovea 3mm is the diameter of the macula lutea 5.5 mm is the diameter of area centralis, which includes all of the above and corresponds with the posterior pole.
17. Answer: E. Muller's fibers extend from the inner limiting membrane (as its basement membrane) to the external limiting membrane and communicate with the RPE.
18. Answer: D. Ganglion cell nuclei are in their own cell layer. The outer nuclear layer contains rod and cone nuclei. The inner nuclear layer contains the cell bodies of the horizontal, Muller, bipolar, and amacrine cells.
19. Answer: C
20. Answer: A. The apical membrane of the RPE is the side facing the photoreceptors. This membrane needs to have long projections to envelope the photoreceptors to phagocytose the discs shed by the photoreceptor outer segments. Melanin granules are also present in the apical projections to absorb excess light that would otherwise cause scatter. Convoluted infolds are found on the basal membrane.
21. Answer: C. The retinal arteries branch from the central retinal artery and supply the inner retinal layers. The RPE acts as a blood-retina barrier, so blood cannot passively diffuse from the choroid.
22. Answer: B. The 2 layers of the retinal capillaries are the endothelium and the surrounding layer of pericytes. One function of endothelium is to be a blood-retina barrier. The function of the pericytes is local control of retinal blood flow. Fenestrations are pores in blood vessels that are permeable to macromolecules and are found in the choriocapillaris.
23. Answer: C. The central retinal, anterior ciliary, and muscular arteries are all branches of the ophthalmic artery. The long posterior ciliary supplies the anterior half of the choroid and makes up the Major arterial supply. The short posterior ciliary supplies the posterior half of the eye.
24. Answer: D
25. Answer: C
26. Answer: B
27. Answer: C. Transduction is the conversion of light input into electrical signals. In the dark, Na is normally flowing in while K is flowing out to produce a "dark current." Depolarization of Na stops when light hits the retina and photoisomerizes the photoreceptor disc membranes.
28. Answer: C. The choriocapillaris is complete by 6 weeks. Bruch's membrane (as randomly oriented fibers) begins to form around this time. The larger vessels form after small vessels.
29. Answer: B. Water makes up 99% of the vitreous. Collagen type II is the most common protein in the vitreous.
30. Answer: A
31. Answer: B
32. Answer: C. Ach is excitatory for amacrine cells. GABA is inhibitory for horizontal and amacrine cells. Glutamate is excitatory for photoreceptor, bipolar and horizontal cell synapses. Glycine is inhibitory for amacrine cells.
33. Answer: A. As the power of the lens increases, the magnification decreases and the field of view increases. The magnification with direct ophthalmoscope is 15x. The BIO with 20D condensing lens gives 3x magnification and with the 60D 1x.

<u>NBEO Question</u>
34. Answer: D

<u>Short Answers</u>
35. Bruch's membrane, choriocapillaris, stroma, suprachoroidia
36. Haller's (large), Sattler's (small)
37. Short posterior ciliary arteries (Circle of Haller-Zinn)
38. Anterior ciliary veins via the limbal plexus
39. RPE basement membrane, inner collagenous, elastic, outer collagenous, basement membrane of the choriocapillaris, intercapillary, terminal
40. Ciliary body, peripapillary, macula, posterior lens (hyaloideocapsillary ligament)
41. Empty channel through the vitreous that is a remnant of the hyaloid vessel

42. Area of flaring out of Cloquet's canal near the ONH
43. RPE, photoreceptors, external limiting membrane, outer nuclear layer, outer plexiform layer, inner nuclear layer, inner plexiform layer, ganglion cell layer, nerve fiber layer, inner limiting membrane
44. Choroid, central retinal artery
45. Thick outer plexiform layer of the parafovea
46. At the end of 6 weeks of gestation
47. Primary – neural exctoderm, surface ectoderm and mesoderm & secondary – only neural ectoderm
48. Secondary surrounds primary
49. Ganglion cells
50. 3-4 months after birth
51. Ventral degenerates, dorsal remains
52. Hyaloid artery
53. 19. 99%
54. Occurs during adolescence but becomes clinically significant by age 40
55. Resting conduction of Na+ and K+ ions in the photoreceptors
56. Cone terminal in the outer plexiform layer

CHAPTER 16: OPTIC NERVE/NEURO-OPHTHALMIC PATHWAYS

1. Answer: C
2. Answer: B, the contralateral superior oblique muscle should be affected.
3. Answer: B
4. Answer: B
5. Answer: C
6. Answer: A
7. Answer: B. the only place there is a clear separation of optic radiation is in the macula. Therefore a VF that has macula sparing must be in occipital lobe.
8. Answer: B. Please read section on Grave disease. Answer c can also be an acceptable answer if pt also complaint of severe HA and transient visual blur.
9. Answer: C. Please read section on MS.
10. Answer: A
11. Answer: B. This is also known as "pie in the sky". First, it's on the left side because a lesion posterior to the chiasm will affect the visual field on the opposite side, having separated after the chiasm. Also, in the temporal and parietal lobes, the superior and inferior fibers are centimeters apart, and the most common temporal loop lesions tend to affect the superior visual field.
12. Answer: C. This lesion is the "pie on the floor". Parietal lobe lesions usually involve the inferior visual field, and the lesion is after the chiasm, so the left and right side fibers have already separated.
13. Answer: B. Blue (S) cones are not concentrated in the fovea, instead they peak 1 degree away. S Cones also make up <10% of all cones.
14. Answer: A. The visual cortex is organized into columns that go down through the cortex layers. Each column is sensitive to information from the same eye and also to a specific orientation, so sticking a probe 90 degrees to the surface will hit cells that are within one column, but a probe placed at another angle will hit multiple columns and so there is a systematic change in orientation sensitivities.
15. Answer: C. This question references how the ocular dominance of a particular cell in an ocular dominance column is classified. Cells in Group 1 are only stimulated by the contralateral eye. Groups 2 and 3 are co dominant to both eyes, but respond more to the contralateral eye. Group 2 responds more the contralateral eye than Group 3. Group 4 responds equally to both eyes. Groups 5 and 6 respond to both eyes, but more to the ipsilateral eye. Group 6 responds more to the ipsilateral eye than Group 5. Group 7 responds only to the ipsilateral eye.
16. Answer: D. Parasympathetic fibers run from the eye through the LGN and synapse in the pretectal nucleus first, then to the Edinger-Westphal nucleus and though the 3rd CN to the iris. The fibers never actually touch the red nucleus and do not move into the cortex.
17. Answer: A. Adaptation to a sensory stimulus occurs by mechanisms at the receptor site and in the brain. It's the reason we can wear contacts and clothes. Habituation on the other hand is a decrease in a behavioral response to a repeated stimulus which occurs at the level of the synapse usually, reducing the nerve's ability to respond over time. Negative feedback describes a self-limiting biological process

where the end products accumulate and inhibit the cells or proteins at the initial step. Imprinting is learning that occurs at a particular age or a particular life stage that is rapid and apparently independent of the consequences of behavior

18. Answer: C. These are the spinal cord reflexes and these are not processed by the brain. The sensory and motor neurons synapse in the grey matter of the spine which houses the cell bodies of these nerves. These signals are modified by input from the brain, though the nerves do not physically travel there.

19. Answer: D. If you are listening to music then the nerve for hearing is stimulated and this is Cranial Nerve 8, the Vestibulocochlear nerve, a purely sensory cranial nerve.

20. Answer: A. In most humans, optic nerve myelination ends at the lamina cribosa. The entire length of the optic nerve is myelinated up to this point. The central retinal artery inserts into the optic nerve 12-13mm behind the eye. The meniscus of Kuhn is where the inner limiting membrane of Elschnig fills in the optic cup.

21. Answer: B. Pupillodilator Dysfunction is another name for Horner's Pupil. The preganglionic fibers exit the spinal cord at the T1 and T2 segments wrapping around the tip of the lungs before traveling along the internal carotid and into the eye. However, Horner's pupil is seen in less than 5% of lung cancer patients.

22. Answer: B. Nerve palsies are most commonly idiopathic. The second most common is from vascular problems like diabetes, HTN, and atherosclerosis. The third most common is heat trauma.

23. Answer: B. The motor fibers of the Vagus nerve innervated the larynx and allow for phonation. The Hypoglossal nerve innervates the tongue muscles for motility, which does assist in shaping words but not the generation of sound. The Facial and Glossopharngeal nerves are responsible for the sense of taste.

24. Answer: D. Papilledema refers specifically to optic nerve head swelling related to raised intracranial pressure. This is usually bilateral and vision is only transiently lost and there is no pain with eye motion. AION usually is unilateral with a transient loss of vision and papillary defect, but the optic nerve tends to be pale and there is no pain. Optic nerve head drusen typically do not involve hyperemia and the vision loss would not be sudden. Papillitis or Optic Neuritis is unilateral, with a swollen, hyperemic disc and pain with eye motion and a RAPD.

25. Answer: C. First, this patient is presenting with common symptoms for temporal arteritis. Symptoms also can involve jaw pain, scalp sensitivity, fever, and tongue pain. Second, the SED rate is generally very high in these patients, but it can be normal in about 20% of patients, so even if the SED rate is normal, a temporal biopsy should be done as well. In this case, visual fields and ultrasound do not historically rule out this condition.

26. Answer: C. In a 6th nerve palsy, there is a head turn to the affected side, but there is usually no lid involvement. In a 4th nerve palsy, the head is directed away from the affected side not towards it and there are no fissure changes. In a partial third nerve palsy, there may be limited ADduction, but not ABduction. Duane's syndrome patients usually are esotropic and amblyopic in the affected eye.

27. Answer: A. Rotating Drum is the only test that doesn't help you to test the Vestibular Ocular Reflex, instead this is used to test Optokinetic nystagmus, where the clinician is looking for asymmetry in the movements between the two eyes or in the direction of movement.

28. Answer: C. The cerebellum is involved in coordination of motion, controlling posture, and controlling limb movement. It receives input from the motor and parietal cortices to initiate planned movement and compares sensory feedback to output to fine tune motion. The brain stem typically involves vegetative functions like heart rate and breathing.

29. Answer: B. Parinoud's syndrome generally involves eyelid retraction, though this associated with 20-30 year women who have multiple sclerosis. Diplopia and ptosis are symptoms in 75% of Myasthenia gravis patients, the 3rd nerve innervates the lids and most of the eye muscles and multiple sclerosis patients report diplopia as one of the earliest symptoms and is mainly associated with women 15-55.

30. Answer: A. This is a case of AION. It's unilateral, +RAPD, with pallor and sectoral swelling of the ONH. In Optic neuritis, generally the nerves are hyperemic and swollen with pain upon eye movement. Papilledema is typically bilateral due to raised intracranial pressures and this patient is a little young for temporal arteritis and there are no other symptoms to contribute to this diagnosis given.

CHAPTER 17: PHARMACOLOGY

Answers to questions are dispersed throughout the chapter questions regarding ocular anatomy specific pharmacology

CHAPTER 18: GLAUCOMA

1. Answer: D. "I Can See The Line" is the mnemonic for the structures, posterior to anterior, in the anterior chamber angle (Iris, Ciliary body, Scleral Spur, Trabecular Meshwork, Schwalbe's Line). Schwalbe's line is the name given to the posterior part of Descemet's membrane.
2. Answer: A. Pars plicata is responsible for producing aqueous humor. Pars plana produces mucopolysaccharides for vitreous humor.
3. Answer: E. Tubular fields that manifest centrally, without any retinal findings, are known as non-organic visual field defects. Some end-stage glaucoma patients may have a temporal island of vision remaining. A ring scotoma is formed when a superior and inferior arcuate defect manifest in the same eye. Nasal steps, nasal paracentral scotoma, and arcuates are common nerve fiber bundle defects seen in glaucoma.
4. Answer: A. A patient who has recently suffered from a CRVO experiences ischemia. This causes new blood vessels to grow at the area where non-perfusion meets perfusion, and this happens to be at the angle.
5. Answer: D. A vitreous heme is more commonly seen in proliferative diabetic retinopathy. A drance heme is a nerve fiber layer heme that crosses the disc margin.
6. Answer: A. A. AACG patients present with all those symptoms. Patients with the diagnosis of Ocular hypertension, Chronic ACG, and Angle recession glaucoma are usually asymptomatic. Glaucomatocyclitic Crisis patients (aka Posner-Schlossman Syndrome) usually experience mild pain and decreased vision without nausea.
7. Answer: B. Carbachol is cholinergic parasympathomimetic, therefore causing miosis and falls into the same category as pilocarpine. It is not a sympathetic antagonist or beta blocker.
8. Answer: D. Since the Uveitis or Chronic inflammation is causing the ACG, you would want to treat the uveitis as well. This is done with an Anti-inflammatory agent (Prednisolone) and Mydriatic-cycloplegic agent (Homatropine 5%). They you would also treat the elevated pressured. Travaprost, a prostaglandin, is contraindicated because it is known to increased inflammation which could make the situation worse. To reduce pressure, aqueous suppressants would be the drugs of choice: a beta-blocker (Timolol), alpha-agonist (brimonidine), and a carbonic anhydrase inhibitor.
9. Answer: D. All of the above conditions can cause neovascularization of the angle except a PVD.
10. Answer: C. Out of all the beta blockers, Betaxolol is Beta 1 selective and is the best drug of choice for someone who has pulmonary problems. Carteolol has intrinsic sympathomimetic activity and demonstrates less risk for cardiac patients along with less CNS side effects
11. Answer: B. The sphincter and ciliary body are both derived from mesenchymal cells, but the dilator is derived from myoepithelial cells.
12. Answer: C. Phacodonesis is tremulous of the lens due to a defect in the zonules.
13. Answer: D. CRVOs typically result in neovascularization of the iris or the angle as opposed to BRVOs that can result in retinal neovascularization. However, neovascularization almost never occurs in 4 days, so a swollen ciliary body is the best choice.
14. Answer: C. Goldmann applanation tonometry assumes a corneal thickness of

500 (even though avg corneal thickness is about 530). Therefore, if the corneal thickness is higher than 500, the measured IOP is lower than the actual IOP.
15. Answer: D. Beta blockers are always contraindicated in patients with asthma, and carbonic anhydrase inhibitors are contraindicated in patients with renal disease.
16. Answer: C. Again, beta blockers are contraindicated in patients with lung disease, and Xalatan has been associated with the development of CME.
17. Answer: A. Iris processes extend into the trabecular meshwork, and Descemet's membrane is on the cornea which is clearly visible with gonioscopy, but the scleral spur is more posterior than the trabecular meshwork.
18. Answer: A. As is evident with gonioscopy, the tear that results in angle recession involves the ciliary body. The connections between the longitudinal and the circular muscles are the most susceptible to damage in the ciliary body.
19. Answer: D. Anaphylaxis to pilocarpine causes many other systemic signs, but a sudden large increase in IOP is not typically associated with pilocarpine. Choroidal detachments can occur after a decrease in IOP, but they take much longer to occur than 30 minutes. To be classified as malignant glaucoma, a patent LPI must be present. Anterior rotation of the CB is fairly common with pilocarpine and it can close the angle.
20. Answer: D. ICSC is a type of CME, and any swelling in the retina leads to a hyperopic shift, the other choices typically lead to myopic shifts.
21. Answer: C. Although glycerin is only a relative contraindication in patients with diabetes, it should be avoided if necessary because it can lead to a spike in the patient's blood sugar.
22. Answer: C. Angle closure attacks are caused by the iris being pushed against the trabecular meshwork blocking drainage. Pressure builds up in the posterior chamber causing the iris to remain pushed against the TM. LPIs equalize the pressure between the anterior and posterior chamber preventing the iris from being permanently pushed forward.
23. Answer: A. CAIs can lead to metabolic acidosis, causing the symptoms in this question.
24. Answer: A. CAIs contain sulfur, so methazolamide is contraindicated in this patient. Betaxolol is the only B-blocker that appears to be safe for patients with COPD.
25. Amswer: A. Iopidine, timolol, and dorzolamide all decrease inflow, but epinephrine affects outflow.
26. Answer: A. A patent LPI would prevent an angle closure attack caused by relative pupillary block, but it would not prevent an increase in IOP from the other 3 choices.
27. Answer: C. Plateau iris does not cause corectopia or PAS.
28. Answer: C. Although RD, corneal edema, vitreous loss, and endophthalmitis are all possible complications of cataract surgery, vitreous loss is more likely to occur in a patient with PXF due to the fact that many of the ocular structures are compromised in patients with PXF.
29. Answer: D. The pars plicata is the part of the CB that produces aqueous, so applying laser will inhibit aqueous production.
30. Answer: D. Pilocarpine can cause an accommodative spasm, which results in the anterior aspect of the lens becoming more rounded.

CHAPTER 19: OCULAR EMERGENCIES AND TRAUMA

1. Answer: D. Alkali burns must be flushed immediately with water for at least 30 minutes to minimize corneal damage.
2. Answer: A. Look for penetration of the cornea (contents leak from anterior chamber)
3. Answer: D
4. Answer: B. Panuveitis causes inflammation in the anterior and posterior segment. The hazy view is caused by inflammation in the vitreous, retina, and/or choroid.
5. Answer: A. Common causes of pan-uveitis are Bechet's, VKH, tuberculosis, sarcoidosis, syphilis. Rule out tuberculosis, sarcoidosis with Chest X-ray. The rest of the tests are not useful in diagnosing panuveitis.
6. Answer: E. Dimming of vision is associated with amaurosis fugax (monocular, transient vision loss).
7. Answer: E. No pain is associated with retinal detachment
8. Answer: D. RAPD suggest optic nerve disease or very asymmetric loss of sensory information to one eye. Macular degeneration is not a disease of the optic nerve and affects only a small portion of the retina.
9. Answer: A. Blown pupil is an informal medical term used by medical providers to refer to sudden pupillary dilation and loss of ability to constrict in response to light. You should never dilate a blown pupil because it will become impossible to assess for changes in pupil status.
10. Answer: B. Hypopyon is associated with severe bacterial keratitis.
11. Answer: A. For patient with a history orbital fracture/trauma, refer immediately if your patient has grossly limited ocular motility, reduced vision and orbital pain.
12. Answer: B. Refer within 24-48 hours for asymptomatic pediatric orbital fractures.
13. Answer: B. Orbital compartment syndrome include +RAPD, tense orbit (increased resistance to retropulsion), increased IOP, proptosis, reduction in vision out of proportion to optics, limited ocular motility and inability to open eyelids due to optic.
14. Answer: B. Bullous sub-conjunctiva hemorrhage is suggestive of a ruptured globe.
15. Answer: D. trichiasis is a condition where eyelashes are turning/growing inward toward the eyeball, but it usually doesn't perforate the globe. Seidel test is performed to rule out globe perforation.
16. Answer: D. Always irrigate first for patient with an ocular acid or alkali burn. Obtain ophthalmology consultation if necessary.
17. Answer: D. Alkali burn is more severe and serious than acid burn because alkali causes saponification. Alkali include wet cements, lye, refrigerants, fertilizers, sparklers and wet plaster, Acid include industrial cleaner, bleach, battery acid, HCl and vinegar.
18. Answer: B. Posterior segment complications may include choroidal rupture, chorioretinal ruptures, commotio retinae, macular hole, retinal breaks, traumatic maculopathy and traumatic retinopathy (bone spiculing). Lattice degenerations are more commonly seen in patients with myopia.
19. Answer: A. Retained zinc and aluminum cause minimal inflammation and may be encapsulated in the eye with time. Copper alloys may also cause Kayser-Fleischer ring, greenish discoloration of the iris and aqueous particles, and metallic flecks in the retinal vessels and macula.
20. Answer: D. Other signs of retained iron foreign body may include iris heterochromia, pupillary mydriasis, arterial attenuation and cataract.
21. Answer: A. Babies with shaking baby syndrome often have retinal hemorrhages, cotton wool spots, retinal folds, schisis cavities along with other systemic findings.
22. Answer: D. Central retinal vein occlusion and stroke can also cause painless vision loss.
23. Answer: A. Iritis is also known as anterior uveitis
24. Answer: A. Patient with AACG often has the following signs/symptoms: elevated eye pressure, eye pain in the morning, blurry vision, seeing color halos around lights, frontal headache, nausea, and vomiting.

25. Answer: A. Patient with corneal abrasion often complained of sharp eye pain, photophobia, foreign body sensation, epiphora and had a history of abrasion.
26. Answer: D. Lowenstein-Jensen is the media for Mycobacteria and Nocardia, esp. post LASIK. Non-nutrient with Escherichia coli overlay is the media for acanthamoeba while thioglycolate broth is the media for aerobic and anaerobic bacteria.
27. Answer: C. Recurrent corneal erosion (RCE) often occurs in the morning. Patient has recurrent attacks of ocular pain, photophobia, epiphora and foreign body sensation. Patient might also has history of anterior/epithelial basement membrane dystrophy.
28. Answer: D. Retinal break, retinal vein occlusion, PVD, sickle cell disease, trauma, intraocular tumor, Eales disease and subarachnoid or subdural hemorrhages can also cause vitreous hemorrhages.
29. Answer: A. PredForte 1% every 1 hour with atropine 1% twice or four times a day is a common dose regimen for treating anterior uveitis
30. Answer: D. color vision is usually not impaired unless optic nerve is damaged or involved.